# Assessment of the Lower Limb

*For Churchill Livingstone*

*Editorial Director:* Mary Law
*Project Editor:* Dinah Thom
*Project Manager:* Valerie Burgess
*Project Controller:* Nicola Haig/Pat Miller
*Copy Editor:* Sukie Hunter
*Design Direction:* Judith Wright
*Sales Promotion Executive:* Hilary Brown

# Assessment of the Lower Limb

Edited by

**Linda M. Merriman** MPhil DPodM MChS CertEd
Head of School, Northampton School of Podiatry, Nene College, Northampton, UK

**David R. Tollafield** DPodM BSc(Hons) FPodA
Associate Specialist in Podiatric Surgery, Walsall and Dudley,
Senior Lecturer (part time), Nene College, Northampton, UK

CHURCHILL LIVINGSTONE
EDINBURGH  HONG KONG  LONDON  MADRID  MELBOURNE  NEW YORK  AND  TOKYO  1995

CHURCHILL LIVINGSTONE
Medical Division of Pearson Professional Limited

Distributed in the United States of America by Churchill
Livingstone Inc., 650 Avenue of the Americas, New York,
N.Y. 10011, and by associated companies, branches and
representatives throughout the world.

© Pearson Professional Limited 1995

First published 1995

## ISBN 0-443-05030-9

**British Library Cataloguing in Publication Data**
A catalogue record for this book is available from the British Library.

**Library of Congress Cataloging in Publication Data**
Assessment of the lower limb/edited by Linda M. Merriman, David R.
  Tollafield.
    p.  cm.
    Includes index.
    ISBN 0–443–05030–9
    1. Leg—Examination. 2. Foot—Examination. I. Merriman, Linda
M. II. Tollafield, David R.
    [DNLM: 1. Leg—physiopathology. 2. Leg Injuries—diagnosis.
3. Foot Diseases—diagnosis.   WE 850 A8464 1995]
RD779. A86  1995
617.5'8075—dc20
DNLM/DLC
for Library of Congress
                                                94–44955
                                                CIP

The
publisher's
policy is to use
**paper manufactured
from sustainable forests**

Produced by Longman Singapore Publishers (Pte) Ltd.
Printed in Singapore

# Contents

# Contributors

**S. J. Avil** DPodM BSc (Hons) CertEd
Lecturer, Northampton School of Podiatry,
Nene College, Northampton, UK

**John Cairns** FIBS
Laboratory Manager, Haematology Department,
Heartlands Hospital, Birmingham, UK

**Christopher J. Griffith** BSc(Hons)
Principal Lecturer, Wessex School of Podiatry,
Southampton, UK

**Janet Hughes** BA MPhil MCSP
Formerly Research Officer, Division of
Molecular Rheumatology, Northwick Park
Hospital and Clinical Research Centre, Harrow,
Middlesex. Honorary University Research
Assistant, Department of Orthopaedic and
Accident Surgery, Royal Liverpool Hospital,
Liverpool, UK

**Timothy E. Kilmartin** FPodA
Specialist in Podiatric Surgery, Ilkeston
Hospital, Chesterfield and North Derbyshire
Royal Hospital NHS Trust, Doncaster
Community Trust, UK

**Patrick Laing** FRCS
Consultant Orthopaedic Surgeon, Wrexham
Maelor Hospital and Robert Jones and Agnes
Hunt Orthopaedic Hospital, UK

**David Lodwick** BSc PhD
Lecturer in Molecular Biology, University of
Leicester, Leicester, UK

**Jacqueline McLeod-Roberts** BSc(Hons) MSc DPodM
Senior Lecturer, Northampton School of
Podiatry, Nene College, Northampton. External
Examiner, Access to Medicine Course, Norfolk
College, Kings Lynn, Norfolk, UK

**Linda Merriman** MPhil DPodM MChS CertEd
Head of School, Northampton School of
Podiatry, Nene College, Northampton, UK

**Jean Mooney** BSc(Hons) MA DPodM FChS FSFCP SRCh
Senior Teacher, The London Foot Hospital and
School of Podiatric Medicine, London, UK

**Patricia S. Nesbitt** DPodM MChS PGD(BioEng)
Senior Lecturer, Northampton School of
Podiatry, Nene College, Northampton, UK

**Kate Springett** PhD FChS SRCh DPodM
Clinical Research Unit, Department of Podiatry,
University of Brighton. Private Practitioner,
Hove and Eastbourne, UK

**David R. Tollafield** DPodM BSc(Hons) FPodA
Associate Specialist in Podiatric Surgery, Walsall
and Dudley. Senior Lecturer (part-time),
Northampton School of Podiatry, Nene College,
Northampton, UK

**Ian F. Turbutt** BSc(Hons) FPodA FChS
Specialist in Podiatric Surgery, South
Bedfordshire Community Health Care Trust and
Luton and Dunstable Hospital. Visiting Lecturer
in Podiatric Radiology at Department of Podiatry,
University of Brighton and at Wessex School of
Podiatry, University of Southampton, UK

**Warren Turner** BSc(Hons) DPodM
Lecturer, Northampton School of Podiatry,
Nene College, Northampton, UK

**Steven West** BSc(Hons) FChS MBES
Dean of the School of Human and Health
Sciences and Head of Department of Podiatry,
University of Huddersfield, UK

# Preface

Many textbooks make reference to the assessment of the lower limb but very few are dedicated entirely to this purpose. Those that are tend to focus on only one of the components of the process, e.g. locomotor, vascular. The purpose of this book is to produce a textbook which encompasses all aspects of lower limb assessment. Problems affecting the lower limb can lead to discomfort, pain, reduction or loss of mobility and loss of time from work. Effective and efficient management of these problems can only be based on a thorough assessment.

Throughout the book the term 'practitioner' is used in its broadest sense to denote any person who has an interest in the management of lower limb problems. Although the podiatrist has a natural claim to specialising in caring for the foot, the range of practitioners with an interest in the lower limb includes bioengineers, diabetologists, general medical practitioners, nurses, occupational therapists, orthopaedic surgeons, orthotists, physiotherapists and rheumatologists.

The book is divided into four parts: Approaching the Patient, Systems Examination, Laboratory and Hospital Tests, Specific Client Groups. Approaching the Patient provides an introduction to the assessment process and covers in detail the assessment interview, the presenting problem and the reliability and validity of clinical measurements.

Systems Examination covers the separate components of lower limb assessment: medical history, vascular, neurological, locomotor, skin and nails and footwear. Details relating to anatomy and physiology have been discussed where relevant.

Laboratory and Hospital Tests focuses on those tests which may be performed to confirm, support or clarify the clinical examination: blood analysis, urine analysis, microbial identification, histopathology, radiographic imaging and methods of quantifying gait and foot ground interface systems. Reliance on tests without the appropriate clinical examination is unwise, creates elevated costs, may worry the patient unnecessarily and overworks support departments. It is intended that this part of the book demonstrates when and how these tests can be used to aid the assessment process.

The last part of the book, Specific Groups, looks at the main areas of foot disease: the 'at risk' foot, the child's foot, sport injuries and the painful foot. Although Systems Examination covers the range of assessments and can be applied to all age groups, the assessment of children and sports people is worthy of independent discussion. Pain in the foot can arise due to a multitude of factors, affects all age groups and has a highly morbid effect on our lives; for this reason it has been given a separate chapter. The early diagnosis of the 'at risk' foot is recognised as a means of reducing morbidity, mortality and minimising the cost of in-hospital care for these patients.

Some of the chapters, particularly those in Systems Examination and Specific Groups, are supported by case histories and comments. These have been used to illustrate certain points and reflect real life experiences. Where appropriate, black and white photographs, figures and tables have also been used to support and further illustrate points raised in the text. A section of colour plates have been specifically used to support Chapters 6, 9 and 17. Each chapter has been referenced and some indicate further reading.

The design of this book has left little opportunity for discussion of pathological changes. The editors consider that other books exist to fill this gap, such as *The Foot*, edited by B. Helal and D. Wilson (1988) and published by Churchill Livingstone.

It is obvious that there is more than one approach to undertaking an assessment. Assessment of the Lower Limb has been written to support good practice in a wide range of outlets for all professionals with an interest in the foot. Whatever approach the practitioner adopts, it is hoped that this text will be a valuable asset.

Northampton, 1995                              L.M.M.
                                               D. R. T.

# Acknowledgements

We are indebted to those who have given their help and encouragement throughout the development and production of this textbook. In particular our partners, Robert Merriman and Jill Tollafield—only they know how much the word 'tolerance' really meant.

Special thanks are due to the radiographers and radiologists of the Diagnostic Imaging Department in the Luton and Dunstable NHS Trust Hospital, Bedfordshire, in particular, Lorraine Nuttall, Superintendent Radiographer, who willingly assisted Ian Turbutt in the production of chapter 11.

Many experts in the field gave willingly of their time to review chapters of the book: Anne Marie Carr, Charles Fox, Ralph Graham, Damian Holdcroft, Tim Kilmartin, Jackie McLeod-Roberts, Catherine Pioli, Gregory Quinn, Alan Sutton, Paul Stepanczuk. We would like to thank Sarah Burgon who acted as a model for some of the Chapter 8 illustrations.

Finally we would also like to thank the staff at Churchill Livingstone, especially Dinah Thom and Mary Emmerson Law, for their encouragement, advice and continued support.

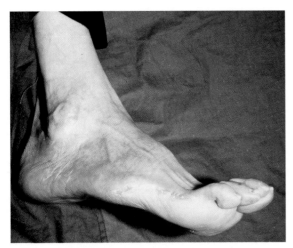

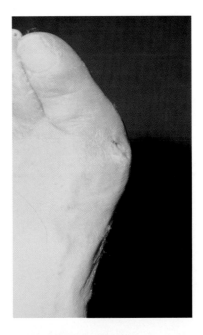

**Plate 1** An ischaemic foot. The superficial tissues are atrophied. The fifth ray has been excised.

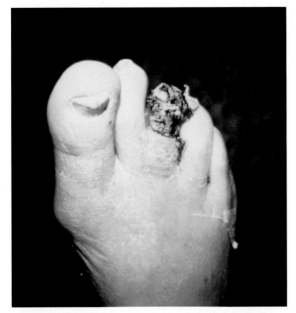

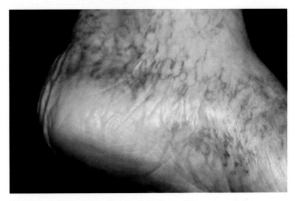

**Plate 4** Telangiectasias: distortion of the superficial venules secondary to varicosity

**Plate 3** 'Dry' gangrene, involving two toes. The necrotic area is surrounded by a narrow band of inflammation. The toes have become mummified, due to loss of the local blood supply.

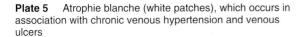

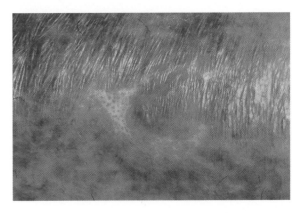

**Plate 5** Atrophie blanche (white patches), which occurs in association with chronic venous hypertension and venous ulcers

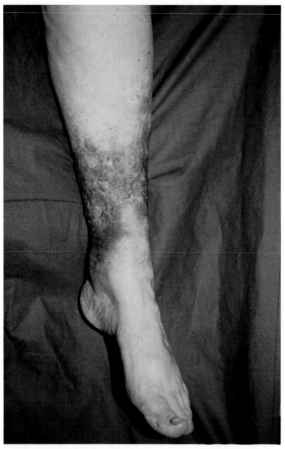

**Plate 6** Gravitational (varicose, stasis) eczema and haemosiderosis

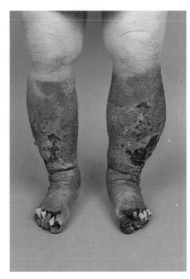

**Plate 7** Venous ulceration in association with gross oedema and haemosiderosis (from Wilkinson J, Shaw S, Fenton D 1993 Colour guide to dermatology. Churchill Livingstone, Edinburgh, Figure 179)

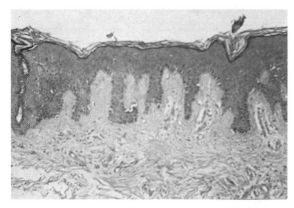

**Plate 8** Histology section of normal hairy skin stained with haematoxylin and eosin. Light microscopy × 60

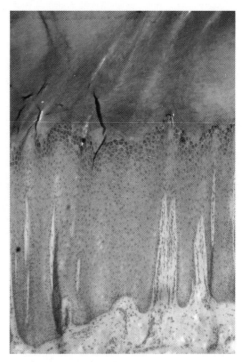

**Plate 9** Histology section of normal plantar skin stained with haematoxylin and eosin dye. Light microscopy × 60

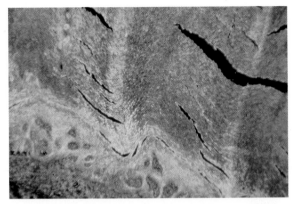

**Plate 10**  Darkfield illumination of plantar skin stained with haematoxylin and eosin, × 40, showing marked refraction of light at the stratum compactum, at the base of the stratum corneum and superficial to the stratum granulosum

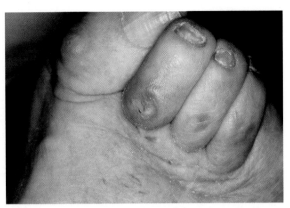

**Plate 11**  Chronic inflammation of a dorsal lesion shows colour changes of atrophie blanche and cyanosis

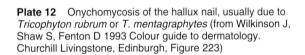

**Plate 12**  Onychomycosis of the hallux nail, usually due to *Tricophyton rubrum* or *T. mentagraphytes* (from Wilkinson J, Shaw S, Fenton D 1993 Colour guide to dermatology. Churchill Livingstone, Edinburgh, Figure 223)

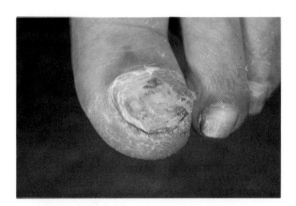

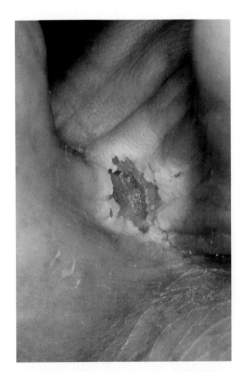

**Plate 13**
Dry fissures develop when the skin is too brittle to conform to external and internal mechanical stresses (tension and shear particularly) They are a frequent complication of anhidrosis and atrophy.

**Plate 14**  Hyperhidrosis, particularly interdigitally, leads to over-moist skin (macerated) which tears easily when mechanically stressed, sometimes exposing the dermis as seen here. Complications of hyperhidrosis include dermatophyte, yeast and bacterial infections.

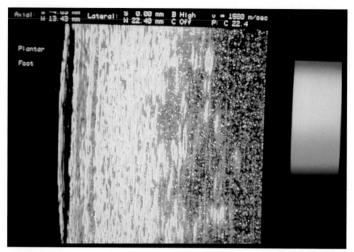

**Plate 15** B-scan ultrasound image of normal plantar skin. The stratum corneum entry echoes are on the left and deep tissue echoes on the right. The more echogenic tissues, like the stratum corneum and collagen, are shown in yellow and orange.

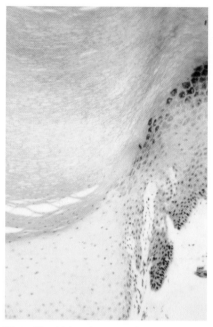

**Plate 16** Light micrograph (× 100) of a corn where the granular layer is absent and parakeratosis (nuclear remnants are still visible within the keratinocytes) is evident within the stratum corneum

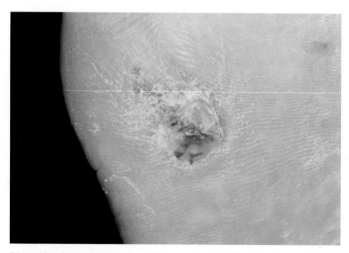

**Plate 17** A corn with extravasation, suggesting that the site is subject to marked mechanical stress.

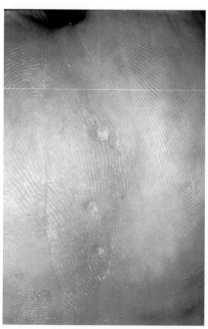

**Plate 18** Seed corns (heloma milliare)

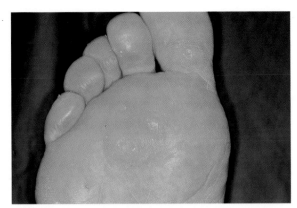

**Plate 19** Hard corns, which appear as darker, more dense areas within a layer of callus tissue (differential diagnosis includes foreign body, early plantar wart)

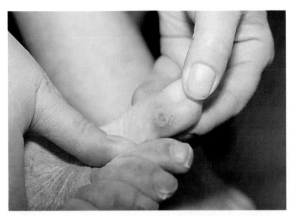

**Plate 20** Soft corn (heloma molle). These corns usually develop interdigitally where the interphalangeal joints are compressed together or against a metatarsal head and transepidermal water loss is therefore restricted.

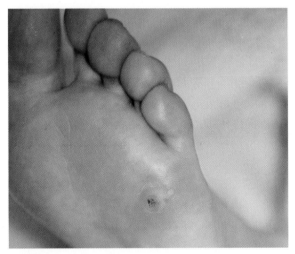

**Plate 21** Appearance of a previously treated satellite verruca

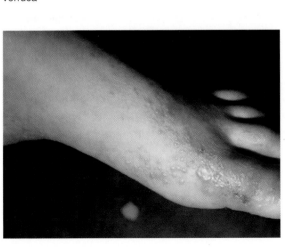

**Plate 23** Juvenile chronic dermatosis

**Plate 22** Contact dermatitis: an allergic response to rubber-based adhesive strapping.

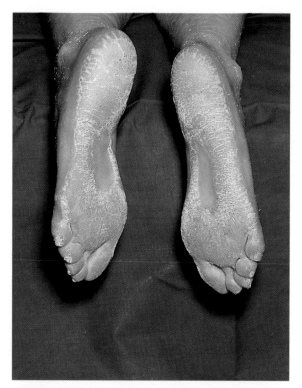

**Plate 24** Ichthyosis tylosis (reproduced by kind permission of the Dermatology Department, Oxford)

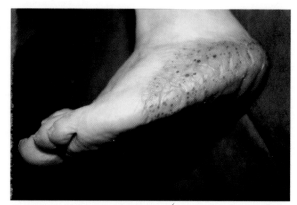

**Plate 25** Pustular psoriasis

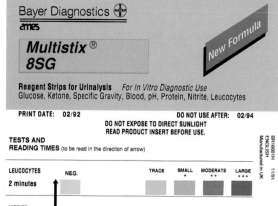

| TEST | | | | | | | |
|---|---|---|---|---|---|---|---|
| LEUCOCYTES 2 minutes | NEG. | | | TRACE | SMALL + | MODERATE ++ | LARGE +++ |
| NITRITE 60 seconds | NEG. | | | | POSITIVE (any degree of uniform pink colour) | | |
| PROTEIN 60 seconds | NEG. | g/L | TRACE | 0.30 + | 1 ++ | 3 +++ | ≥ 20 ++++ |
| pH 60 seconds | | 5.0 | 6.0 | 6.5 | 7.0 | 7.5 | 8.0 | 8.5 |
| BLOOD 60 seconds | NEG. | NON-HAEMOLYZED TRACE | HAEMOLYZED TRACE | | SMALL + | MODERATE ++ | LARGE +++ |
| SPECIFIC GRAVITY 45 seconds | 1.000 | 1.005 | 1.010 | 1.015 | 1.020 | 1.025 | 1.030 |
| KETONE 40 seconds | NEG. | mmol/L | TRACE 0.5 | SMALL 1.5 | MODERATE 4 | LARGE 8 | 16 |
| GLUCOSE 30 seconds | NEG. | mmol/L | 5.5 TRACE | 14 + | 28 ++ | 55 +++ | ≥111 ++++ |

HANDLE END

**Plate 27** Multistix 8SG: the range of biochemical tests available from one urine sample (reproduced by kind permission of Bayer Diagnostics UK Ltd)

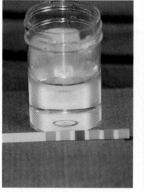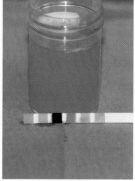

**Plate 26** The sample of urine on the left is normal; the sample on the right is cloudy and tinged with blood, indicating infection

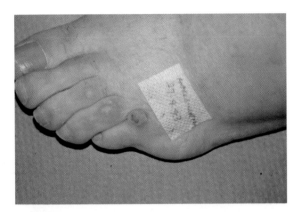

**Plate 28**  Pyogenic granuloma

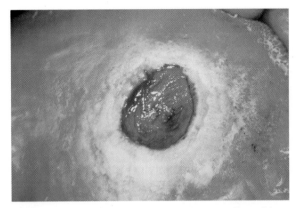

**Plate 29**  A neuropathic ulcer on the plantar surface of the foot

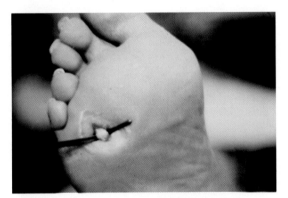

**Plate 30**  Deep neuropathic ulcer which penetrates to the plantar tendons; there is no cellulitis or abscess formation. The patient was a non-insulin-dependent diabetic.

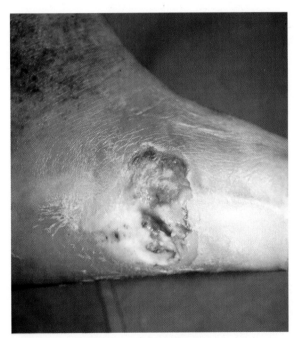

**Plate 31**  Typical neuro-ischaemic ulceration over the lateral aspect of the midfoot in a non-insulin-dependent diabetic, showing deep erosion of soft tissues, sloughy base, heavy peripheral callosity and maceration of superficial tissues

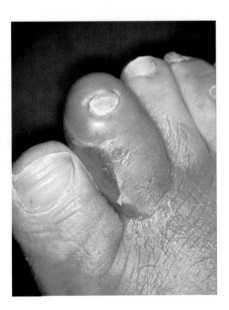

**Plate 32**  Cellulitis affecting the soft tissues of the second toe and spreading to involve the dorsum of the foot of a patient with diabetes mellitus, showing the typical characteristics of redness and swelling. It was very painful as the patient did not have a sensory neuropathy.

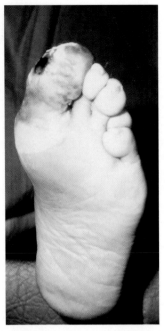

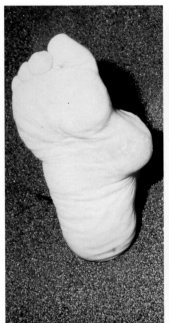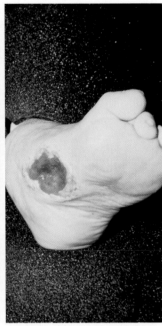

**Plate 33**   Wet and infected gangrene in a diabetic patient, involving the medial forefoot. The tissues of the great toe have become necrotic, with a wide area of proximal cellulitis.

**Plate 34**   Bilateral arthropathy of the midtarsal joint, with ulceration of normally non-weightbearing soft tissues, in an insulin-dependent diabetic with peripheral neuropathy

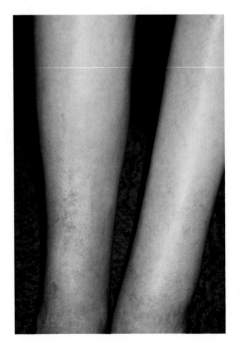

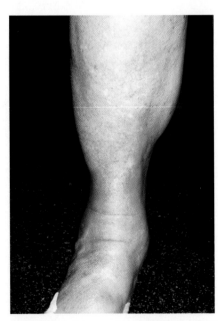

**Plate 35**   The lower limbs of a 84-year-old female with a stenosis at the bifurcation of the right popliteal artery. The right foot and lower part of the right leg are cold and red/cyanotic. The patient was in very great pain and unable to sleep in bed; hence both legs are somewhat oedematous

**Plate 36**   A champagne leg due to the chronic effects of deep venous thrombosis, with woody oedema, fibrosis and haemosiderosis

# Approaching the patient

# 1

# Assessment

*L. Merriman*
*D. R. Tollafield*

## INTRODUCTION

Patients present with a range of signs and symptoms for which they are seeking relief and if possible a cure. However, before this can be achieved, it is essential to undertake a primary patient assessment. Ineffective and inappropriate treatment may result if the practitioner has not taken into account information obtained from the assessment. This chapter discusses the assessment process.

## Why undertake a primary patient assessment?

Information from the assessment helps the practitioner to:

- arrive at a differential diagnosis or definitive diagnosis
- identify the likely cause of the problem (aetiology), e.g. trauma, pathogenic microorganism
- identify any factors which may influence the choice of treatment, e.g. poor blood supply, current drug regime
- assess the extent of pathological changes so that a prognosis can be made
- establish a baseline in order to identify whether the condition is deteriorating or improving
- assess whether a second opinion is necessary.

All the above information is essential if the practitioner is to provide effective treatment and care for his/her patients.

## THE ASSESSMENT PROCESS

Figure 1.1 outlines the assessment process; each aspect will be considered in turn.

## Presenting complaint

It is essential to establish the presenting problem or concern. On account of the demands on his/her time it is often necessary for the practitioner to differentiate those patients who need immediate attention from those who do not. Table 1.1 lists the presenting problems which should be given high priority.

## Assessment

The components of an assessment are outlined in Table 1.2. Each of these components is considered in turn in the remainder of this book.

A good assessment requires the practitioner to demonstrate listening and observational skills and to know when and which questions to ask. Research has shown that most diagnoses are based on observation and information volunteered by the patient (Sandler 1979).

Clinical, laboratory and hospital based tests provide additional data. Clinical tests involve physical examination of the patient (e.g. assessing ranges of motion at joints, taking a pulse) as well as near-patient tests such as assessing blood

**Table 1.1** Presenting problems which should be given high priority

| Problem | Features |
|---|---|
| Pain | Constant, weightbearing and non-weightbearing Affects patient's normal daily activities |
| Infection | Raised temperature (pyrexia) Signs of acute inflammation Signs of spreading cellulitis Lymphangitis, lymphadenitis |
| Ulceration | Loss of skin May or may not be painful May expose underlying tissues |
| Acute swelling | Unrelieved pain Very noticeable swelling May have associated signs of inflammation |
| Abnormal skin changes | Distinct colour change Discharge may be malodorous Itching Bleeding |

**Table 1.2** Components of an assessment

| Component | |
|---|---|
| Assessment interview | Presenting problem Personal details Medical history Family history Social history Current health status |
| Observation and clinical examination | Vascular Neurological Locomotor Skin and nails Footwear |
| Laboratory and hospital tests | Urinalysis Microbiology Blood tests Histology Gait analysis X-ray Other imaging techniques ECG Nerve conduction |

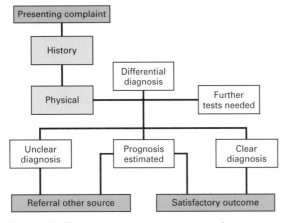

**Figure 1.1** The assessment process—presenting complaint to outcome.

glucose levels with a glucometer. Most clinical tests are relatively quick and inexpensive to carry out and in most instances give fairly reliable and valid results. Laboratory- and hospital-based tests are more expensive and can be time-consuming. Such a test should only be used when it is necessary to confirm a suspected diagnosis; in cases of differential diagnosis or when the outcome of the test will have a positive influence on treatment.

## Diagnosis and differential diagnosis

Arriving at a diagnosis is a complex activity which is affected by a variety of factors (Table 1.3). The practitioner has to sift and interpret the information gained from the patient, identify the important points and then relate this to his/her knowledge base and previous clinical experience. Laboratory and sophisticated hospital tests can be used to aid this process. From the information gained from the patient, observation and tests the practitioner generates hypotheses as to the likely diagnosis.

There can be enormous differences between practitioners both in their assessment findings and their diagnoses. For example, Comroe & Botelho 1947 described a study in which 22 doctors were asked to examine 20 patients and note whether cyanosis was present. Under controlled conditions these patients were assessed for cyanosis by oximeter. When the results of the clinical assessment were compared with the oximeter results, it was found that only 53% of the doctors diagnosed cyanosis in subjects with extremely low oxygen content. 26% said cyanosis was present in subjects with normal oxygen

**Table 1.3** Factors which influence making a diagnosis

Current level of knowledge and research

Practitioner's knowledge base

Practitioner's professional update

Previous clinical experience

Availability of clinical equipment

Access to laboratory and hospital tests

Interaction between practitioner and patient

Previous clinical experience

Patient's needs

Patient's expectations

Geographical variations

Cultural variations

**Table 1.4** Factors which should be taken into consideration when making a differential diagnosis

| Social history | Age |
| --- | --- |
| | Gender |
| | Race |
| | Social habits |
| | Occupation |
| | Leisure pursuits |
| Medical history | Family history |
| | Medication |
| Symptoms | Onset |
| | Type of pain |
| | Aggravated by/relieved by |
| | Seasonal variation |
| Signs | Site |
| | Appearance |
| | Symmetry |
| Specific tests | Imaging techniques |
| | Urinalysis |
| | Microbiology |
| | Blood analysis |
| | Biopsy |
| | Foot pressure analysis |
| | Electrical conductive studies |

content. Unfortunately, making a diagnosis is not a precise science: errors can and do occur. Practitioners should always keep an open mind when making a diagnosis, reflect on the process they have used, keep up to date with current literature and technology and request a second opinion when unsure.

Sometimes the practitioner may have generated more than one possible diagnosis; in these instances the practitioner has to undertake a differential diagnosis, i.e. decide which is the most likely from a number of possibilities. When arriving at a differential diagnosis the practitioner should take into account the factors listed in Table 1.4. For example, a number of conditions affect specific age groups (e.g. the osteochondroses) while other conditions have specific presenting features (e.g. the sudden, acute, nocturnal pain associated with gout).

When a diagnosis cannot be made or the cause of the problem cannot be isolated, the manner in which the condition evolves over a period of time and/or the effects of treatment may make a definitive diagnosis or identification of the cause possible at a later date.

## Aetiology

Information from the assessment can enable the practitioner to identify the cause of the problem. A variety of aetiological factors can result in disorders of the lower limb. These can be divided into hereditary, congenital (present at birth) or acquired.

**Hereditary conditions** may manifest immediately after birth, e.g. epidermolysis bullosa, or may not appear until some years after, e.g. Huntington's chorea.

**Congenital conditions** include chromosomal abnormalities, e.g. Down's syndrome, developmental defects, e.g. spina bifida, or birth injuries such as cerebral palsy.

**Acquired conditions** are those which arise after birth. Infection by a pathogenic organism resulting in sepsis is a common example of an acquired condition affecting the lower limb.

Many conditions occur as a result of more than one factor, i.e. they are multifactorial. Atherosclerosis is thought to be due to the interplay of a number of factors, including dietary intake, familial high cholesterol level, high blood pressure, sedentary life style and stress. In some cases there have to be predisposing factors present in conjunction with an exciting factor before the condition manifests. An example is a septic toe, where there has to be a portal of entry in order for the bacteria to gain entry into the skin and multiply.

If the cause can be identified (e.g. lack of shock absorption, contamination by a pathogen) then treatment can be aimed at eradicating or reducing its effects. Knowing what has caused a problem can assist in identifying the most appropriate treatment and help to produce an accurate prognosis. For example, if the cause of pain in the foot is chronic ischaemia due to atherosclerosis, the prognosis may be poor unless radical (bypass) surgery is performed. Conversely if the foot pain is due to acute ischaemia that has occurred as a result of hosiery constricting the peripheral circulation, the prognosis is good and advice may be all that is required. Unfortunately, it is not always possible to isolate the cause; in these cases the term *idiopathic* (unknown cause) is used.

## TIME MANAGEMENT

The assessment process is fundamental to a satisfactory outcome for both patient and practitioner. However, practitioners often find themselves working within strict time constraints and may feel they have insufficient time in which to undertake a full primary patient assessment. It is important that the practitioner does not compromise the assessment process in order to save time. Such action, although it may deliver a short-term time saving, may result in unfortunate long-term effects. The practitioner who has not obtained important information or failed to recognise salient clinical findings may reach an incorrect diagnosis and/or implement treatment which puts the patient at considerable risk. In the long term this will lead to avoidable patient suffering and extra time being spent in dealing with the complications arising from treatment.

In order to use time effectively it is important to plan and prioritise activities. The time allotted to a primary assessment may be as little as 5 minutes or may stretch to 30 minutes plus. On average practitioners should be able to undertake a routine assessment in 10 minutes; further time may be required if the problem is complex,

**Table 1.5** The essential components of an assessment. These should be carried out with all patients. Further tests and examination should be used if indicated from the information obtained from the essential assessment

| | |
|---|---|
| Observation | Gait as the patient walks into the room in order to detect abnormal function |
| | Facial features for signs of current health status |
| Interview | Presenting problem |
| | Personal details |
| | Medical history |
| | Family history |
| | Social history |
| | Current health status |
| Observation | Skin and nails to detect trophic changes and abnormal lesions |
| | Position of lower limb to note deformity, malalignment |
| | Footwear |
| Tests | Pulses, capillary filling time |

if a definitive diagnosis cannot be reached or if laboratory or hospital tests are required. Table 1.5 identifies the essential components of any assessment.

## RE-ASSESSMENT

Assessment should not be something that is only undertaken on the patient's first visit. Every time the patient attends the clinic a mini-assessment should be undertaken in order that the following can be noted:

- Changes to the patient's general health status
- Changes to the status of the lower limb
- Patient's perception of previous treatment
- Effects of previous treatment
- Information about treatment from other practitioners.

The process of assessment, diagnosis, treatment should be an uninterrupted loop: at every subsequent consultation the patient should be re-assessed and evaluated (Fig. 1.2).

## RECORDING ASSESSMENT INFORMATION

Information gained from the assessment should be accurately and clearly noted in the patient's record. This record is the storehouse of knowledge concerning the patient and his/her medical history. It should contain a summary of the main points from the assessment and sufficient data to justify the diagnosis.

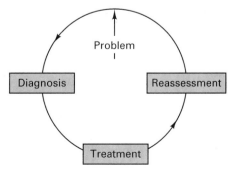

**Figure 1.2** The assessment loop.

Two methods may be used to record the assessment information. The first involves using a blank piece of paper on which the practitioner writes, in a logical sequence, assessment and diagnostic details (see Fig. 5.3). The other involves the use of a pro-forma; this may vary from a form with a few headings to a very detailed format with boxes in which to write specific details. Such pro-formas can be self-designed or purchased from specialised suppliers.

Whatever the method used, it is important that all details are written in such a way that practitioners not involved with the assessment can familiarise themselves with the salient details and any previous treatment. Practitioners need to be able to write succinct notes that are not too time-consuming to complete or read. Pollock & Evans (1993) noted that long, unnecessarily detailed patient records were usually due to one of the following factors: inexperience on behalf of the practitioner, the fact that during training records have to be filled in great detail or a fear of leaving out something important.

Abbreviations should be avoided. All entries should be dated and signed. In particular, details regarding the patient's medication should always be dated as the medication may have been changed by the time the patient attends for his/her next appointment. Records should always be written in such a way as not to be offensive or contain subjective opinions.

Records may be handwritten or typed; typed records are preferable as they are more legible but they do have resource implications. The use of computers is already having an impact: it is likely computers will eventually be the prime means of recording patient data.

The information recorded from the assessment may be used for:

- ensuring contraindicated treatments are not used
- clinical and epidemiological research
- audit
- planning
- legal purposes.

Retrospective and prospective analysis of patient records is commonly used for clinical and epidemiological research, audit and planning. If well documented they can provide a wealth of information. However, one of the problems with patient records is that there is no standardised manner in which information is collected. For example, the use of clinical terms can be ambiguous.

The International Statistical Classification of Diseases, Injuries and Causes of Death was established by the World Health Organization as a universal system for collecting data. The system was originally designed for mortality statistics but has evolved to cover a broad range of diseases. It is updated every 10 years to keep abreast of the constantly changing information base. This system can be used to record diseases for the purpose of clinical and epidemiological research and audit.

In the late 1980s Dr J. Read founded the Read code system. This system aims to standardise the way in which health professionals describe all aspects of their work; it therefore includes treatment as well as diagnostic categories. The Read system has been purchased by the National Health Service for use in the UK. It is still being developed but in the future it will offer a means of collecting standardised information about diagnosis and treatment throughout the UK.

## CONFIDENTIALITY

The information volunteered by the patient and recorded in the patient's notes is the property of the organisation dealing with the patient, e.g. NHS trust, private practice. The information can be made available to all those involved with the care of that patient. However, information should not be divulged to any other party without the consent of the patient. Requests for information about a patient occur in the following instances:

- The patient or the patient's representative is contemplating taking proceedings against the practitioner or the organisation who employs the practitioner

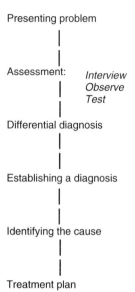

**Figure 1.3**  The stages of assessment summarised.

- The patient is engaged in litigation with a third party which does not involve the practitioner or the organisation who employs the practitioner.

In either instance the patient must give his/her written consent to the release of the information. The only exception to this is when a court issues a subpoena which requires the person responsible for the records to bring them to court on a particular date.

Care must be taken with the storage of patient data, especially where this is committed to computer disk.

## SUMMARY

This chapter has stated the purpose of assessment and outlined the assessment process (Fig. 1.3). If undertaken well it leads to the drawing up of appropriate and effective treatment plans. It is therefore an activity which should be seen as pivotal to good patient–practitioner interaction.

## REFERENCES

Comroe J H, Botelho S 1947 The unreliability of cyanosis in the recognition of arterial anoxemia. American Journal of the Medical Sciences 214: 1–6

Pollock A, Evans M 1993 Surgical audit. Butterworth Heinemann, London, p 101–102

Sandler G 1979 Costs of unnecessary tests. British Medical Journal 1: 1686–1688

# 2

# The interview

*L. Merriman*

## INTRODUCTION

Research has shown the interview, as opposed to any other method of assessment such as clinical tests and examinations, is the most efficient method in reaching an initial diagnosis (Sandler 1979). This chapter examines the purpose of the interview, the skills required, how it should be structured and the pitfalls to avoid. It concludes by examining the features of a good assessment interview.

### Is an interview different from a normal conversation?

An interview is based upon a conversation between two or more people. As individuals we converse with a broad range of people. Conversation serves a multitude of purposes. The conversation in an interview differs from ordinary conversation in a number of ways:

• It is an opportunity for one person to gain information from another
• It has a specific purpose, e.g. to solve a problem
• It has an outcome, e.g. a course of treatment
• The time and place of the assessment interview is set by the interviewer
• It has less flexibility than an ordinary conversation
• The interviewer has a perceived position of authority/power over the interviewee. It is important that this power is not abused. Every effort should be made to put the interviewee (the patient) at his/her ease

- A written record of the interview is usually kept.

Practitioners may be involved with other types of conversation with patients such as counselling, teaching and advising. These are discussed in the accompanying text to this book: *Clinical skills in treating the foot.*

# THE PURPOSE OF THE ASSESSMENT INTERVIEW

This assessment interview is a conversation between the practitioner and the patient. Patients present with problems which may have physical, psychological and social dimensions. Patients have their own ideas and concerns about one or more problems. They also have expectations about the medical care they may or may not receive. Likewise, practitioners approach the interview with perceptions of their role. These will have been influenced by training, past experiences, attitudes and beliefs. The availability of resources and facilities will contribute to the practitioner's response to the patient. It is essential that the practitioner and the patient develop common ground during the interview and that both are aware of each other's perspectives. If this cannot be achieved the interview may be an unsatisfactory experience for both of them.

The prime purpose of the interview is for the cause of the patient's concerns to be identified and appropriate action taken. This is best achieved by the patient and the practitioner working in partnership to reduce or resolve these concerns.

It is essential that the practitioner provides ample opportunity for the patient to convey his/her concerns and worries. In other words the interview should be patient-centred. Research has shown that this is not always the case. A few years after qualification most practitioners are confident that they are good at taking histories and explaining things to patients. Is this confidence justified? A detailed analysis of the recordings of over 2500 doctor/patient interviews showed that 77% of them were doctor-centred, compared to 21% classed as patient-centred (Byrne & Long 1975).

Information gathered collectively from the interview and examination should facilitate the identification of the cause of the patient's anxiety. Where appropriate a diagnosis can be made. As well as aiding the diagnostic process, the interview serves other important purposes:

- The information gained may be of help when drawing up a treatment plan. For example, the interview can provide a picture of the patient's social circumstances which may affect the manner of, or the actual advice given
- It provides an opportunity to gain the patient's trust and confidence in you as a practitioner
- It facilitates the development of a working relationship between you and the patient.

## Communication skills

Good communication skills are essential if you are to achieve an effective assessment interview. What is meant by communication? In its simplest form it can be seen as the transmission of information from one person and the receiving of information by another. Unfortunately, the communication process is not that simple; if it were there would not be communication breakdowns or misunderstanding between people as to what has been communicated.

When people transmit information they first need to assemble their thoughts and identify what they wish to communicate. They then need to put this into words and vocalise the information. In going through this process the message that is finally transmitted may be affected by a variety of factors such as the intelligence of the person, his/her limited vocabulary, lack of clarity, confusion, mumbling or a speech impediment, to name just a few.

During transmission, the message may be distorted by surrounding noise, e.g. a telephone ringing or loud music. The person receiving the information may have poor hearing, may not be listening properly or may not be interested in the information. What information the receiver does pick up must then be interpreted. Receivers of communication will place their own perceptions and meaning, either accidentally or deliberately, on what has been received. At this point the receiver may decide to transmit a message back. With so many opportunities for these forms of interference, it is not surprising the original message may become distorted.

Communication involves a combination of the following:

- Non-verbal communication
- Verbal communication
- Written communication.

**Non-verbal communication**. This involves all forms of communication apart from the purely spoken (verbal) message. It includes body language such as gestures, mannerism, expressions and paralanguage. The term 'paralanguage' denotes the vocalisations associated with verbal messages, e.g. tone, pitch, volume, speed. It is said that we primarily communicate non-verbally. Remember the old adage 'a picture says a thousand words'. Your body language and paralanguage will send an array of messages to your patient prior to you saying anything. Non-verbal communication serves many useful purposes. It can be used to replace or complement speech. It may be used to regulate the flow of and control verbal communication. We also use non-verbal communication as a means of providing feedback to the person who is transmitting the message, e.g. looking interested. Non-verbal communication is the main mode of conveying our emotional state.

**Verbal communication**. This involves the spoken word. In general we tend to have greater control over the verbal messages we send than the non-verbal messages. It is certainly easier to lie verbally than non-verbally. Think of the child who says he has not been naughty when guilt is written all over his face.

**Written communication**. This involves writing, either using conventional paper and pen techniques or via modern technologies. Increasingly computers and telecommunications are being used to convey the written message.

All three forms of communication may be used during the interview. Different forms of communication are interpreted at different rates by the receiver. We speak quicker than we write. Speech varies between 100 and 200 words a minute whereas, on average, we can write 30 words a minute. We hear quicker than we read: on average, we can take in 400 spoken words per minute. Reading averages out at approximately 80 words a minute. By looking at a picture we can take in and analyse the information contained in the picture in seconds. It would take a lot longer if the information was in written form.

Non-verbal communication accounts for 70% of most communication. It is through this medium that we create first impressions of people. Once made, first impressions are often difficult to change, yet research has shown they are not always a reliable means of making judgements about people.

A common question asked is, 'are good communicators born or is it a skill you can learn?' The answer has to be, it's a bit of both. We can all think of people we consider to be good communicators; these people appear to have an inherent skill. For others, communication may not come so easily. With assistance and motivation, good communication skills can be developed. It is important for health practitioners to be aware of and develop effective communication skills. Such skills are essential in order that good rapport and effective care of patients can be achieved.

Research has shown that interview skills, over a period of time, may deteriorate rather than improve. First-year medical students, when interviewing simulated mothers, obtained more personal information on disease than third-year students or residents (Helfer 1970). This is probably explained by the first-year students having less medical knowledge than third-year students. As a result they are much more interested in what the patient says about their concerns, their psychological reactions and the social difficulties they have experienced. Once medical students increase their knowledge about conditions, there is a tendency to make quick provisional diagnoses and confine the patient during the rest of the interview to answering questions the practitioner considers relevant. Such a response is not helpful if you wish to discover the patient's anxieties, nor is it helpful if the practitioner has jumped to an incorrect diagnosis.

A myriad of books are available on the subject of communication skills. However, just reading a book does not automatically mean you become a good communicator. Observing others, noting good and bad points, receiving feedback from others, role-play exercises, video- and audiotaping of interactions, practising in front of a mirror or with friends are all helpful ways in which skills can be developed. Communication is a skill you are constantly learning and updating. Constructive criticism is an essential part of learning but not always an easy method to accept.

## SKILLS REQUIRED TO UNDERTAKE AN EFFECTIVE INTERVIEW

In order to achieve an effective interview, it is essential that the practitioner sends appropriate messages to the patient and receives and understands the messages transmitted by the patient. In other words, the practitioner must be able to:

- Transmit appropriate non-verbal messages to the patient
- Demonstrate effective questioning skills
- Demonstrate active listening skills
- Produce an accurate written record of the interview.

Each of these skills will be considered in turn.

## TRANSMISSION OF NON-VERBAL MESSAGES BETWEEN PRACTITIONER AND PATIENT

From the first moment the patient meets you they will be receiving an array of non-verbal messages from you. It is essential practitioners are aware of the types of non-verbal message they are sending. Ideally positive rather than negative messages should be transmitted. The following methods of non-verbal communication can be used.

## Body language

### Eye contact

Eye-to-eye contact is frequently the first stage in any verbal communication. It is the way we attract the other person's attention. Direct eye-to-eye contact creates trust between two people; hence the innate distrust felt of someone who avoids eye contact. However, we do not keep constant eye-to-eye contact throughout a conversation. The receiver looks at the speaker for approximately 25–50% of the time, whereas the speaker looks at the other person for approximately half as long. Too much eye contact is interpreted as staring and is seen as a hostile gesture. Too little is interpreted as a lack of interest, attention or trustworthiness. Interviewers cannot afford to look inattentive because the patient may interpret this as meaning that he has said enough and as a result may stop talking. Conversely, withdrawing eye contact may be used as a legitimate way of getting the patient to stop talking.

Interestingly, psychiatrists often use a technique where their patient lies on a couch while they sit behind or to the side of the couch. This positioning reduces the opportunity for eye-to-eye contact. It is considered by some psychiatrists to facilitate patients to disclose more about themselves as the normal eye-to-eye contact is suppressed. These psychiatrists believe patients can find eye-to-eye contact embarrassing if they are imparting confidential information.

The practitioner should be aware of the frequency and duration of eye-to-eye contact they give their patients. Certainly eye-to-eye contact is recommended at the beginning of the interview, to gain rapport and trust, and at the end of the interview by way of closing the interview. Its use during the interview should be based on the professional judgement of the practitioner.

## Facial expression

It is via our facial expression we communicate most about our emotional state. Smiling together with judicious eye-to-eye contact signifies a receptive and friendly persona and inspires a feeling of confidence and friendliness. It is important that practitioners are aware of their facial expressions. For example, if upset over a personal matter, the practitioner should, where possible, avoid transmitting this to the patient. At the same time practitioners, when they come into contact with unsightly lesions or marked deformity, should avoid exhibiting a facial expression associated with disgust or shock.

## Posture and gestures

The manner in which we hold ourselves and the way in which we move says a lot about us as individuals. Four types of posture have been identified:

- **Approaching posture**, which conveys interest, curiosity and attention, e.g. sitting upright and slightly forward in a chair facing towards the person you are communicating with
- **Withdrawal posture**, which conveys negation, refusal and disgust, e.g. distance between the receiver and the communicator, shuffling, gestures indicating agitation
- **Expansion**, which conveys a sense of pride, conceit, mastery, self esteem, e.g. expanded chest, hands behind head with shoulders in air, erect head and trunk
- **Contraction**, which conveys depression, dejection, e.g. sitting in a chair with head drooped, arms and legs crossed or head held in hands, avoiding eye contact.

Leaning forward towards the patient has been shown to be associated with higher levels of patient satisfaction.

When we speak we tend to use our arms and hands to reinforce and complement the verbal message. When people are constrained from using their arms and hands, they experience greater difficulty in communicating. Self-directed gestures such as ring-twisting, self-stroking and nail-biting indicate anxiety. Be aware of self-participation in these types of activities as you may convey a non-verbal message of anxiety to your patient while verbally you are trying to convey a confident approach. Also you should look out for the patient using self-directed gestures, as he/she may be conveying a message of anxiety although he/she is not verbally communicating that message.

## Touch

The extent to which touching is permissible or encouraged is related to culture. The British are not known as a nation of 'touchers'. During the assessment it may be necessary to touch the patient in order to examine a part of his/her body. This type of touching, known as *functional touching*, is generally acceptable to most patients. People from certain cultures may find it difficult to accept, even in medical settings. Prior to functional touching of a patient, it is important that you inform the patient what you intend to do.

During the interview you may wish to use *therapeutic touch*. This may be used as a means of reassuring the patient, to show empathy or as a sign of care and concern. A hand lightly placed upon a shoulder or holding a patient's hand are means· of showing concern and giving re-assurance. It is difficult to produce guidelines for when therapeutic touching should or should not be used. Practitioners must feel confident and happy to use this form of touch, and must also take into account a multitude of communication cues from the patient before deciding whether it is appropriate.

## Personal space

All of us have a sense of our own personal territory. When someone invades that territory, depending upon the situation, we can be fearful, disturbed or pleased and happy. As with touch, our sense of personal space is affected by culture. In some cultures individuals have a large personal space whereas in others they have a very small personal space. Encroaching on someone else's personal space can be perceived as intimidation and, in the case of the assessment interview, may put the patient on their guard. As a result they may become reluctant to disclose relevant information. Hall (1959) defined the four zones of personal space. These relate to situations where eye-to-eye contact occurs. They do not include such instances as sitting back to back, as on a train, where no eye contact is possible.

- Intimate zone: 0–0.5 m
- Personal zone: 0.5–1.2 m
- Social/consultative zone: 1.2–3 m
- Public zone 3 metres plus.

The assessment interview usually takes place in the social/consultative and the personal zone. During the interview it may be necessary to enter the intimate zone. Prior to doing this, notify the patient in order to justify any actions requiring closer contact.

## Appearance

We use our clothing and accessories to make statements about ourselves to others. Clothing can be seen as an expression of conformity or self-expression, comfort, economy or status. Uniforms are used as intentional means of communicating a message to others; often the message is to do with status. Uniforms are also used in the health care professions for cover and protection. Whether one wears a uniform (white coat, coloured top and trousers) for the interview is open for debate. Not only should attention be paid to the cleanliness and appearance of the uniform but also to hair, hands, footwear and accessories such as jewellery. They all send messages to the patient. In particular the patient will often pay attention to the footwear worn by the practitioner. Avoid giving conflicting verbal and non-verbal messages, e.g. by wearing high-heeled slip-on shoes while advising patients that they should not wear this type of shoe.

## Smell

Olfactory senses are usually very acute. Odours and smells can often prompt early childhood memories of a range of occasions, e.g. the smell of grandma's house. The clinic will have a distinctive smell, usually affected by the use of antiseptics. Clinical smells associated with auto-claves and antiseptics can have an adverse effect on patients. They may remind the patient of an unpleasant experience at a clinic or a hospital. Conversely, they can be reassuring to the patient by transmitting messages of cleanliness and hygiene and as a result patients feel they are in safe hands.

Personal odour will also send messages to the patient. The spicy food you enjoyed the night before may not be so pleasant for the patient the next day. It is essential that practitioners are aware of their personal hygiene and use breath fresheners and deodorants after regular washing. The judicious use of after shaves and perfume needs to be considered. Odour should not just be masked.

Besides being aware of the messages you are conveying via your own non-verbal behaviour, be aware of those conveyed by the patient. A patient may be verbally communicating one message but non-verbally communicating another. The non-verbal message often comes across a lot clearer than the verbal one.

## Paralanguage

This involves the manner in which we speak. It includes everything from the speed at which we speak to the dialect we use. An individual who speaks fast is often considered by the receiver to be intelligent and quick, whereas a slow drawl may be associated with a lower level of intelligence. When talking to patients we should be careful not to speak too quickly as they will not understand what we say. Conversely, if speech is too slow, the patient may not have confidence in the practitioner.

When we speak we use pitch, intonation and volume to affect the message we transmit. Individuals who speak at a constant volume and do not use intonation and/or alter their pitch often come across as monotonous, dull and boring. Such speech is often difficult to listen to. Intonation and pitch should be used to highlight the important parts of your question. Volume should not be changed too regularly. Shouting at the patient should be avoided. It certainly does not guarantee that the patient will listen more to what you say.

The fluency with which we speak also tends to convey messages about mental and intellectual abilities. Repeated hesitations, repetitions, interjections of 'you know' and false starts do not inspire confidence in the receiver. We all experience occasions when we are not as fluent as at other times. These occasions tend to occur when we are tired or under great stress.

Dialect conveys which part of the country we originate from. It may also cause us to use vocabulary a person from another part of the country is not familiar with. Avoid using colloquial terms. Dialect, on the other hand, is not so easy to alter. The only time it should be considered is when patients cannot understand what the practitioner is saying.

## QUESTIONING SKILLS

The prime purpose of the assessment interview is to gain as much information as possible from the patient in order that a diagnosis and treatment plan can be arrived at. In order to achieve this the practitioner uses a range of questioning skills.

There are four categories of question:

- Closed
- Open
- Leading
- Probing.

### Closed questions

Closed questions limit the responses a patient may give. They usually require a one word response. Closed questions may:

- require a yes/no response, e.g. Do you suffer from rheumatoid arthritis?
- require the patient to select, e.g. Is the pain worse in the morning or the afternoon?
- require the patient to provide factual information, e.g. How long have you been a diabetic?

Closed questions serve useful purposes during the assessment interview. They provide a quick means of gaining and verifying information. Patients often find them easier to answer than the more open type of question. They can be used to focus the assessment interview in a particular direction. On the other hand, if used too much they limit what the patient can say. As a result the patient may not volunteer important information.

### Open questions

Open questions invite the patient to give far more than one-word answers. The patient is in a much better position to construct the response he/she wishes to give. Examples of open questions are:

- What happened when you went into hospital?
- What do you look for when buying a pair of shoes?
- What do you think is causing the problem?

This sort of question can elicit information from the patient you had not expected. Open questions are often preferable to closed questions such as 'When you were in hospital did they test your blood sugar or give you an X-ray?' The patient may legitimately answer 'no' to these direct questions and fail to tell you that they undertook a test you have not mentioned.

### Leading questions

Leading questions should be avoided where possible. In general they give responses that the professional expects to receive. Examples of leading questions are:

- You don't smoke, do you?
- That doesn't hurt, does it?
- You said you get the pain a lot; that must mean you get it every day?

### Probing questions

Probing questions are a very useful adjunct to open and closed questions. In general they aim at finding out more from the patient. In particular, they are useful in gaining in-depth rather than superficial information. Examples include:

- Could you describe the type of pain it is?
- What makes you think it might be linked to your circulation?

## General pointers when questioning patients

The following points should be born in mind when interviewing patients:

- Show empathy. Authier (1989) defined empathy as: '[being] attuned to the way another person is feeling and conveying that understanding in a language he/she understands'.
- Use language that is simple, direct and understandable. Avoid medical and technical terms. The 'fog index' can be used to assess the complexity of a piece of communication (Table 2.1). It is primarily used in written communication but has also been used, although less frequently, to analyse the complexity of the spoken word. It involves a mathematical equation that produces a score. For example, tabloid newspapers have a fog index score between 3 and 6, whereas government policy documents can achieve a score of 20+. Applying the fog index to spoken communication or a foot health education leaflet will give an indication of the complexity of that particular communication. If it receives a high fog index score, the average patient may find it very difficult to understand.
- Avoid presenting the patient with a long list of conditions. This is especially important

**Table 2.1** The fog index

Take a passage of about 100 words, ending in a full stop. Work out the average sentence length. This is achieved by dividing the number of sentences into 100. Then work out the number of words of three or more syllables. Ignore two-syllable words that have become three syllables with plural or endings like -ed or -ing, technical words and proper nouns. Add the average sentence length to the number of difficult words and multiply by 0.4. The result will give you the reading score (fog index)

during medical history taking. It is unlikely that a patient has experienced more than one or two of the problems on a list. They may fall into the habit of replying 'no' to all the items on the list and fail to respond in the affirmative to ones they do suffer from. Strategies that can be used to avoid this situation include a pre-assessment questionnaire (see Ch. 5) or breaking up the list of closed questions with some open questions.

- Don't ask the patient more than one question at a time. For example, if asking a closed-type question do not say, 'Could you tell me when you first noticed the condition, when the pain is worse and what makes it better?' By the end of the question the patient will have forgotten the first part.
- Attempt to get the patient to give you an honest answer using their own words. Avoid putting words into the patient's mouth.
- Clarify inconsistencies in what the patient tells you.
- Get the patient to explain what he/she means by using certain terms, e.g. 'nagging pain'. Your interpretation of this term may differ from the patient's.
- Pauses are an integral part of any communication. They allow time for participants to take in and analyse what has been communicated and provide time for a response to be formulated. Do allow the patient time to think how he/she wishes to answer your question. Avoid appearing as if you are undertaking an interrogation.
- In the early stages of the interview it is often better to use the term 'concern' rather than 'problem'. Asking a patient what concerns them may elicit a very different response from asking them what the problem is. Some patients may feel they do not have a problem as such but are worried about some symptom or sign they have noticed. Asking them what concerns them may get them to reveal this rather than a denial that they have any problems.
- Asking personal and intimate questions can be very difficult. Do not start the interview

with this type of question; wait until further into the interview when hopefully the patient is more at ease with you. Try to avoid showing any embarrassment when asking an intimate question as this may well make the patient feel uncomfortable.

- It is important that the patient understands why you are asking certain questions. Remember that the assessment interview is a two-way process: besides gathering information from the patient it can be used for giving information to him/her.
- Some patients, on account of a range of circumstances such as deafness, speech deficit or language difference, may not be able to communicate with the practitioner. In these instances it is important that the practitioner involves someone known to the patient to communicate on his/her behalf, e.g. relative, friend or carer.
- The patient may have difficulty listening and interpreting what you are saying through fear, anxiety, physical discomfort or mental confusion. Be aware of non-verbal and verbal messages that can give clues to the patient's emotional state.

## ACTIVE LISTENING SKILLS

Listening is an active not a passive skill. Do not limit your attention to that which you want to hear or expect to hear. Listen to all that is being said and watch the patient's non-verbal behaviour. As mentioned previously the average rate of speech is 100–200 words a minute. We can assimilate the spoken word at around 400 words per minute. As a result the listener has 'extra time'. It is important that you don't let your mind wander on to unrelated thoughts such as what you are going to do after the interview. Before you know it you have missed a good chunk of what the patient has been telling you and have most probably missed important and relevant information.

Many people ask questions but do not listen to the response. A common example is the general introductory question 'How are you?' Most responses tend to be in the affirmative:

'Fine', 'OK'. Occasionally someone responds by saying they have not been too well, only to get the response from the supposed listener 'Great; pleased to hear everything is fine'.

In order to be a good listener you need to set aside your own personal problems and worries and give your full attention to the other person. It is inevitable that, at times, one's attention does wander. This may be due to lack of concentration, tiredness or because the patient has been allowed to wander off the point. In the case of the former do not be afraid to say to the patient, 'Sorry, could I ask you to go over that again?' In the latter case, politely interrupt the patient and use your questioning skills to bring him/her back to the subject in hand.

During the interview the techniques of *paraphrasing, reflecting* and *summarising* can be used to aid listening and ensure you understand what the patient is trying to convey.

Paraphrasing is used to clarify what a person has just said to you in order to get him/her to confirm its accuracy or to encourage him/her to enlarge. It involves re-stating, using your own and the patient's words, what the patient has said. Reflecting is used to encourage the patient to continue talking about a particular issue that may involve feelings or concerns. It may be used when the patient appears to be reluctant to continue or is 'drying up'. It involves the practitioner repeating in the patient's own words what he/she has just said.

Summarising is used to identify what you consider to be the main points of what the patient is trying to tell you. It can also be a useful means of controlling the interview when a patient continues to talk at length about an issue. To summarise, the practitioner draws together the salient points from the whole conversation. At the end of the summary the patient may agree with, add to or make corrections to what the practitioner has said. Summarising serves a useful purpose in checking the validity, clarity and understanding of old information, it does not aim to develop new information.

The basic skills of a good listener are highlighted in Table 2.2.

**Table 2.2** Skills of a good listener

- Look at the patient when he/she starts to talk
- Use body language such as nodding, leaning forward to demonstrate to the speaker that you are interested in what is being said
- Do not keep looking at the time
- Adopt a relaxed posture
- Use paraphrasing, reflecting and summarising to show the patient that you are listening to and understanding what he/she is/are saying

## WRITTEN RECORD OF THE INTERVIEW

It is essential either during or at the end of the assessment to make a permanent record of the findings of the interview. This record is essential as an aide memoire for future reference when monitoring and evaluating the treatment plan and as a means of communicating your findings to another practitioner who may collaborate in treating the patient.

Currently most permanent records are on paper. The use of computerised records is on the increase. It may well be in the future that paper records are discarded completely, and replaced by computerised techniques. Whatever the future may hold, the need for clear, accurate recording of information will still be the same. The recording of assessment findings, together with the recording of treatment provided, forms a legal document. Patient records would certainly be used if action was taken by a patient against a practitioner, or if certain agencies required detailed evidence of management and progress in the case of disability awards.

Patient records may take a variety of forms: at the simplest level a plain piece of paper may be used. If using plain paper it is essential to adopt an order to the presentation of your assessment findings, e.g. name, address, doctor, age, sex, weight, height, main complaint, medical history, etc. This is considered further in Chapter 5. A variety of patient record cards exist in the NHS and private practice. Many practitioners and health authorities produce their own tailor-made record card. The Association of Chief Chiropody Officers produced a standard record

in 1986 for charting foot conditions, diagnoses and treatment progress.

Handwritten recording of information requires the following:

- The writing is legible and in permanent ink, not pencil. If another practitioner cannot read your writing the information is of no use.
- The information is set in a clear and logical order. It is essential to use an accepted method.
- Accurate recording of location and size of lesions or deformities. The use of prepared outlines of the feet are very good for indicating anatomical sites and save additional writing.
- Abbreviations are avoided where possible. What is obvious to you may not be so obvious to another practitioner.
- Entries are dated. Recording the medication a patient is taking is useless unless it is dated. Once dated the information can be updated as and when there is a change.
- Each entry should be signed and dated by the practitioner.

## STRUCTURING THE ASSESSMENT INTERVIEW

### Prior to the interview

In order to achieve a good assessment interview it is essential you prepare yourself for the interview. The following should be taken into consideration.

#### Purpose

It is essential that the practitioner is clear as to the purpose of interview. In some instances the assessment interview may be used as a screening mechanism to identify patients for further assessment. It may be used to gain information from patients in order that their needs can be prioritised and those judged to be urgent can be seen first. On the other hand the assessment interview may be aimed at undertaking a full assessment of the patient, with treatment provided at the end of the interview.

## Letter of application

Was the patient referred or self-referred? If the patient was referred by another health care practitioner there should be an accompanying letter of referral. Read this carefully so you are fully informed of the reasons for referral. This information should be used as a starting point for the assessment.

If patients have referred themselves directly (self-referred) they should complete any appropriate documentation prior to the interview. Information on application forms can be used to prioritise patients and ensure they are seen by the most suitable practitioner. If no application form or letter of referral is available the practitioner has very little information prior to the interview, possibly only the patient's name.

You may wish to give the patient a short health questionnaire to complete prior to the assessment (Appendix, pp. 73–74). This questionnaire may be sent to the patient prior to the interview or the patient may be asked to fill it in on arrival. These questionnaires provide the practitioner with important information before the start of the interview. The patient should be allowed time to complete the questionnaire in order that he/she can think about his/her responses. The advantage of such a questionnaire is that the practitioner does not have to ask the patient a series of routine questions during the interview. However, some patients may be reluctant to fill in a form without having met the practitioner or reluctant to disclose information in writing.

Prior to the interview try to read all the information you have about the patient. You can then come across to the patient as well informed and as someone who has taken an interest in them.

## Patient expectations

Does the patient know what to expect from the assessment interview? Some new patients, prior to attending their assessment appointment, are sent an information sheet or booklet explaining

**Table 2.3** Information booklet for patients to read prior to the interview

The booklet should contain the following information:
- The purpose of the assessment interview
- How long the interview should take
- What will happen during the interview
- Specific information the patient may be asked to provide, e.g. list of current medication
- Specific items the patient may be asked to bring, e.g. footwear
- Examples of questions he/she is likely to be asked
- The possible outcomes of the assessment interview, e.g. whether the patient will receive treatment at the end of it.

The booklet may also contain a health questionnaire for the patient to complete and bring to the assessment interview

the purpose of the assessment interview and what will happen during it. Such an initiative is helpful. The cause of a poor interview may be that the patient's expectations of what will happen are very different from what actually happens. For example, a patient who expected immediate treatment and had not envisaged any need for history taking may well say 'Why are you asking me all these questions?' Table 2.3 highlights what should be contained in a patient information booklet.

## Waiting room

Patients can spend a lot of time in the waiting room, especially if they arrive too early or are kept waiting due to unavoidable circumstances. Try sitting in the waiting room in your clinic. Look around you: how welcoming is it? The waiting room sets the scene for the rest of the interview. Where possible ensure that it is in good decorative order, clean, with magazines to read and informative, eye-catching posters or pictures on the wall. Make the most of a captive audience to put over important health education information. TV monitors showing health promotion videos may be used.

The name of the practitioner displayed outside the clinic may be useful. Some clinics, like a number of high street banks, have a display of photographs with the names and titles of those within the department or centre.

*Interview room*

The assessment interview may be carried out in an office or in a clinic. Both have advantages and disadvantages. Using an office prevents the patient being put off by surrounding clinical equipment. It facilitates eye-to-eye contact by sitting in chairs, and provides a non-clinical environment. This is especially useful if treatment is not normally provided at the end of the assessment. On the other hand, using a clinic ensures that clinical equipment is readily to hand and the patient can be moved into different positions if there are controls on the couch.

During the interview you should ensure that you are not disturbed. If there is a phone in the room, redirect calls. Ensure the receptionist does not interrupt. While the patient is in the room you should be giving him/her your undivided attention. Constant disturbances not only makes the assessment interview a protracted occasion but can prompt the patient into feeling that his/her problem is not worthy of your attention.

# The assessment interview

The assessment interview has three stages:

- Introduction
- Data gathering
- Conclusion.

## Introduction

When the patient enters the room, welcome him/her to the clinic, preferably by name. This personalises the occasion for the patient and at the same time ensures that you have the correct patient. If you have difficulty with the patient's name, ask politely how to pronounce it rather than doing so incorrectly. Introduce yourself. As part of the Patient's Charter you should be wearing a name badge but a personal introduction is usually preferable, especially if the patient's eyesight is poor. It is useful to shake the patient by the hand. While this is a personal preference, touch can allow rapid assimilation of information about health. The importance of touch is also related to non-verbal communication as previously mentioned.

At this stage you may find it helpful to make one or two general conversation points about the weather, the time of year or some news item. This enables patients to see you as a fellow human. Remember that during the interview they are going to give a lot of themselves to you. It is important that they feel you are someone they wish to disclose information to. Use the introduction as an opportunity to explain the purpose of the interview and what will happen.

The positioning of patient and practitioner can influence the success of the assessment interview. Ideally you and the patient should be at the same level in order to facilitate eye-to-eye contact (Fig. 2.1). Barriers such as desks are often used in medical interviews. They can be considered as means of making the interview formal. Standing over a patient who is sitting down or lying on a couch may be intimidating.

## Data gathering

It is essential that the practitioner is clear as to what areas should be covered in the interview. A logical and ordered approach should be adopted. However, it is not always possible or desirable to stick to an ordered approach. Patients tend to talk around issues or elect to give information about a question you asked earlier at the end of the interview. You must make allowances for this.

Effective and efficient use of time is paramount. Experienced practitioners combine the interview with the examination. This is achieved by, for example, feeling pulses and skin temperature while simultaneously asking questions about medical history. This technique is a matter of preference; some prefer to complete the interview before commencing the examination.

After each assessment interview reflect upon it. Ask yourself how you could improve your performance and how you could make better use of the time. This will help you to make the best use of the data-gathering stage of the interview. Peer appraisal is another mechanism that you

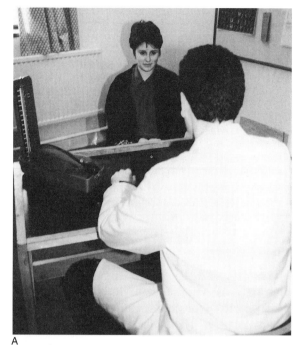

A

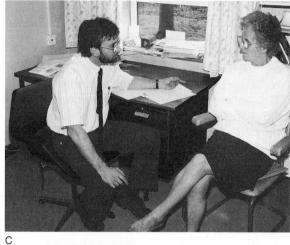

C

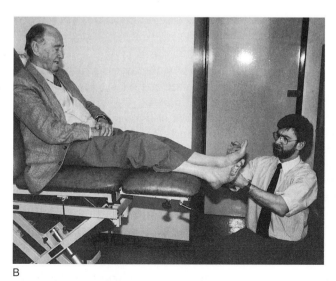

B

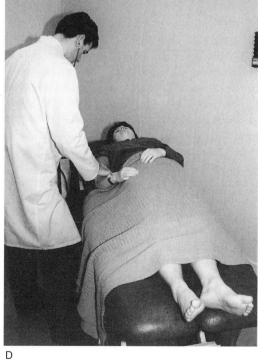

D

**Figure 2.1**    Positioning of patient and practitioner may influence the success of the interview under certain circumstances. The figures show four positions commonly encountered:    **A.**  A desk separates the patient and practitioner    **B.**  The patient is elevated higher than the practitioner    **C.**  The practitioner places the patient alongside the desk removing the barrier effect **D.**  The practitioner stands over the patient.

may find helpful in aiding you to develop good data-gathering skills.

## Closing the interview

Bringing the assessment interview to a close is a difficult task. When do you know you have enough information? This is a difficult question to answer. Some presenting problems, together with information from the patient, can be easily diagnosed. Others are not so easy and may require further questioning and investigations.

General medical practitioners have been shown to give their patients, on average, 6 minutes of their time. Psychotherapists, on the other hand, spend an hour or more on each assessment. Unfortunately the demands on practitioners' time means they are often not in a position to give the patient as much time as they would like.

As a general rule of thumb the interview should be brought to a close when the practitioner feels the patient has been given an opportunity to talk about the problem. Body language can be used to convey the closing of the interview. Standing up from a sitting position, shuffling of papers, withdrawing eye-to-eye contact are all ways in which the end of the interview can be conveyed to the patient, together with a verbal message.

The patient should not leave the interview without fully understanding what is to happen next and without an opportunity to ask questions. A range of outcomes may result from the assessment interview (Table 2.4). Patients should know which outcome applies to them. They should always be given the opportunity to raise any queries or concerns they may have prior to leaving the assessment. This is one of the most important parts of the assessment and should not be hurried. The patient must leave the assessment fully understanding the findings of the assessment interview and what action, if any, is to be taken.

It is helpful to provide written instructions as a follow-up to the interview. For example, if the patient is to be offered a course of treatment what will the treatment involve, when will it be given, who will give it, what problems may the patient experience?

**Table 2.4**   Outcomes from the assessment interview

- Treatment is not required; the patient requires advice and reassurance
- The patient can look after the problem once appropriate self-help advice has been given
- A course of treatment is required; the patient should be informed as to whether treatment will commence straight after the assessment interview or at a later date
- The patient needs to be referred to another practitioner for treatment
- Further examination and investigations are required before a definitive diagnosis can be made
- A second opinion is required
- The urgency for treatment should be prioritised

## Confidentiality

The information the patient divulges during the interview is confidential. It should not be disclosed to other people unless the patient has given consent. The Data Protection Act 1984 requires that all personal data held on computers should be 'secure from loss or unauthorised disclosure'. The General Medical Council (1991) and the National Health Service (1990) have laid down guidelines on confidentiality.

# WHAT IS A GOOD ASSESSMENT INTERVIEW?

The prime purpose of the assessment interview is to draw out information, experiences and opinions from the patient. It is the duty of the interviewer to guide and keep the interview to the subject in hand. At the same time, it is equally important to encourage the patient to talk and to clear up any misunderstandings as you go along. Keeping the balance between these two competing aims is not an easy task. One way of checking on this is to ask yourself who is doing most of the talking. Is it you or the patient? If you are to achieve the aims of the assessment interview it should be the patient.

It is not essential that you like the patient you are interviewing. What is important is that you adopt a professional approach, demonstrate empathy and deal with the patient in a competent and courteous manner. It is essential that you do not make value judgements based on your own biases and prejudices. Respect the patient; avoid stereotyping. Do not jump to conclusions before reaching the end of the interview.

As highlighted earlier, the assessment interview should be patient-centred; its prime purpose is to gain information from the patient. However, one sometimes comes across patients who appear unable to stop talking. What can the practitioner do in these instances?

The first question to ask is why the patient is talking so much. Is it because he/she is lonely and welcomes the opportunity to talk, is he/she very self-centred, is he/she avoiding telling you what the real concern is by talking about minor issues? The reason will influence the action you take. If you feel the patient wants to tell you something but is finding it difficult, try reflecting or summarise what you think has been said. Ask if there is anything else the patient would like to discuss. Encourage patients by telling them that you want to be able to help as much as you can; the more they tell you about their concerns the more you can help them.

On the other hand if you feel you need to control a talkative patient you may find the following techniques helpful:

• Use eye contact and your body language to inform the patient that you are bringing a particular section of the interview to a close
• Politely interrupt the patient, summarise what he/she has said and say what is to happen next
• Ask questions that bring the patient back to the topic under discussion.

The converse of talkative patients are those who are reluctant to disclose information about themselves. This may be because they do not see the purpose of the questions you are asking, they are shy, they cannot articulate their concerns, they are fearful of what the outcomes may be or they are too embarrassed to disclose certain information. Your response will depend on the cause of the reticence.

Explaining why you need to know certain information will be helpful if the patient is hesitant. For example, a patient may wonder why you need to know what medication he/she is taking when all he/she wants is to have a corn treated. If you feel the patient cannot articulate what he/she wants to say, you may find that closed questions can help. This type of questioning limits responses but can be helpful for a patient who has difficulty putting concerns and problems into words. You need to use a range of closed questions and avoid leading questions if you are to ensure you reach an accurate diagnosis.

The shy or embarrassed person may find self-disclosure very difficult. It has been shown that people tend to disclose more about themselves as they get older. In general, females disclose more than males. When privacy is ensured and the interviewer shows empathy, friendliness and acceptance, patients have been shown to disclose more information. Reciprocal disclosure can also be helpful.

### Feedback

In order to develop your interview technique it is important that you obtain feedback on your performance. Mention has already been made of self- and peer assessment of the interview. This is a valuable process which should be ongoing. Patient feedback is another valuable mechanism. Questionnaires (postal or self-administered), structured or unstructured interviews are ways in which patient reactions to the interview can be obtained. Suggestions as to how to improve interviews should be welcomed.

## SUMMARY

The interview is the process of initiating an assessment of the lower limb. The relationship created between the practitioner and the patient during the interview will hopefully lead to an effective diagnosis. A good interview can provide the majority of the information required without having to resort to numerous tests and unnecessary examination. There is no one formula which can be applied to all assessment interviews. Each patient should be treated as an individual with specific needs. Practitioners should develop their interviewing skills in order that the interview achieves a successful outcome for the patient and the practitioner.

REFERENCES

Authier J 1986 Showing warmth and empathy. In: O Hargie (ed) A handbook of communicating skills. Routledge, London

Byrne P, Long E 1976 Doctors talking to patients: A study of verbal behaviour of general practitioners consulting in their surgeries. HMSO, London

Data Protection Act 1984. HMSO, London

General Medical Council 1991 Professional conduct and discipline: Fitness to practice. GMC, London

Hall E 1959 The silent language. Doubleday, New York

Helfer R, Ealy K 1972 Observation of paediatric interviewing skills. American Journal Dis Child 123: 556–560

National Health Service Circular No 1990 (Gen) 22, 7 June 1990 A code of practice on the confidentiality of personal health information. London

Sandler G 1979 Costs of unnecessary tests. British Medical Journal 1: 1686–1688

# 3

# The presenting problem

*L. Merriman*

## INTRODUCTION

Most patients consult a practitioner because they have concerns about or problems with their lower limbs. Problems are usually quite specific and focused. Patients may have problems with painful feet, an ingrowing toe nail or difficulty accommodating a bunion in footwear. Concerns are where the patient is worried or anxious about something. Patients may have concerns related to a problem, e.g. they are worried about an ulcer that is taking a long time to heal. Conversely a patient may have concerns but no specific problems, e.g. a patient may be concerned that an asymptomatic mole on their leg may be a malignant melanoma.

The role of the practitioner is to discover what are the patient's concern(s) and problem(s) in order that an effective management plan can be drawn up and implemented. This may involve anything from giving reassurance, e.g. that the mole is not a melanoma, to implementing a treatment plan aimed at resolving or reducing the effects of a specific problem, e.g. pain in the foot.

During the assessment interview the patient should be given ample opportunity to express their concerns and talk about any problems they may have. The remainder of this chapter concentrates on acquiring information about the patient's presenting problem(s). However, the practitioner should always remember it is also important to identify any concerns the patient may have.

## THE PROBLEM

What one person perceives as a problem another may accept as being normal. A major concern for one person may be a minor issue to another. Defining what is normal and acceptable, and what is abnormal or unacceptable and therefore a problem, is fraught with difficulties.

When patients attend for their appointments they bring with them their own ideas of what is a problem and what is normal. A variety of factors can influence a patient's perception (Table 3.1). For example, if media coverage emphasised a link between verrucae and cancer of the cervix this might result in a number of females who had previously ignored their verrucae seeking treatment. Having a friend who has developed a malignant melanoma may make a person more vigilant for signs associated with this condition and prompt him/her to seek advice when previously he/she may have been oblivious to the situation. People from socioeconomic groups 1 and 2 are more likely to seek medical assistance than those from socioeconomic groups 4 and 5 (Townsend & Davidson 1982).

It is important that the practitioner allows the patient to describe the problem in his/her own words. The practitioner's perception of the problem is not always the same as that of the patient. For example a mother may be concerned that her 3-year-old child has flat feet. The practitioner considers this to be normal for a child of that age. However, during the consultation, the practitioner notices a small verruca on the apex of the right second toe and suggests that it is treated. The mother accepts the treatment but leaves the clinic still concerned about her child's flat feet. The practitioner has failed to identify the mother's main concern. An effective solution would have consisted of advice and reassurance regarding the flat feet as well as treatment of the verruca.

### Encouraging the patient to tell you about concerns and problems

How can you encourage patients to tell you why they have sought your help? A whole range of factors can make it difficult for the patient to articulate the problem in words. Some patients may be frightened or embarrassed, others may be concerned that they are wasting your time and others that you will think they are silly to be concerned about a minor problem. It is essential that patients are made to feel that they are not wasting your time and that you are genuinely interested in their concerns and problems.

Most patients present with discomfort or pain. For example, a patient may present with discomfort from a bunion rubbing on footwear. The patient may also be concerned about the appearance of the bunion and scared that she will develop a deformity similar to her grandmother's. A skilled practitioner will identify all the anxieties the patient is experiencing: the problems with the current discomfort, the difficulty in finding appropriate shoes to wear, the worry about the unsightly appearance of the bunion and the fear that it may get worse.

It is important that you consider how best to start the conversation. Asking the patient 'What are you complaining of?', 'What's the problem?' or 'What is it that's wrong with you?' are probably not the best ways to start. The last question may result in the patient responding 'That's what I've come here for you to find out'. 'How can I help you?' or 'Would you like to tell me about what concerns you?' may be preferable. Open questions should be used. The patient should not feel rushed; avoid interrupting and

**Table 3.1**   Factors that influence a patient's perceptions of what is normal and what is a problem

Age

Gender

Culture

Socioeconomic base

Knowledge base

Previous experiences

Views of family and friends

Media

Socioeconomic background

Life expectations

putting words into the patient's mouth. Record in the patient's own words what he/she is concerned about and what he/she sees as a problem. Avoid medical jargon wherever possible.

Having obtained an idea of the patient's concerns, you may find it helpful to find out if he/she has any thoughts as to the cause. Ask the reason for such conclusions. The answers to these questions may reveal whether patient and practitioner share the same view.

When patients do reveal what is worrying them avoid being judgemental and making comments such as 'Oh, that's nothing!' or 'I don't know why you are so worried!' Remember it is a problem to the patient even if it is relatively innocuous to you. Patients may not reveal their real reason for coming to see you until they are just about to leave. This can be a source of annoyance to the busy practitioner. Do try and give the patient time even if it is at the end of the consultation.

## Patients with special needs

Some patients may experience other difficulties in telling you about their concerns and problems than simply having poor powers of description. The patient may be deaf and dumb, have suffered a stroke, have a speech impediment or have learning or language difficulties. It is important you give these patients extra time. Avoid jumping to too many assumptions. If the patient can write ask him/her to write down the nature of their complaint. Friends or relatives may be able to provide valuable details and information or act as interpreters.

## Why did the patient seek your help?

A variety of factors can influence why a patient has chosen to visit your practice. Table 3.2 gives the usual reasons for a patient choosing a particular practitioner. It is important to find out what made the patient choose you. For example, a patient who has been referred by a friend or relative may find it very easy to disclose his/her concerns to you. The friend/relative may have been very complimentary about your abilities. On the other hand, a patient who is seeking a

**Table 3.2** Reasons for a patient choosing a practitioner

- Applied for treatment at their local health service
- Found your name in the yellow pages
- Saw an advertisement
- Noticed your plate outside the practice
- Were advised by a friend or relative to seek your help
- Were referred by another health practitioner, e.g. GP
- Are seeking a second opinion because they were unhappy with the response of the first practitioner

second opinion may want you to give a different diagnosis from the one given by the previous practitioner. As a result he/she may not disclose all the salient features of the problem. It is important to remember that outstanding legal claims for lower limb injuries may affect the patient's perspective.

## ASSESSMENT OF THE PROBLEM

This involves acquiring information about the history of the problem. The history must be taken logically and systematically. An assessment of the current level of pain and discomfort should also be undertaken.

## History of the problem

History taking involves finding answers to a range of questions (Table 3.3). Many diseases can be identified by the pattern of symptoms they display. Research has shown that history taking can be more effective in diagnosing a problem than clinical tests alone (Sandler 1979).

**Where is the problem?** Locating the problem is very important. Getting the patient to show you by pointing is the best way. If the patient has difficulty reaching the area, you may find it helpful to present an outline of the lower limb and ask him/her to mark the area affected. For example, pain may start in one area but then radiate to other areas. Some problems may have a precise location; others may be far more diffuse or have multiple sites. These variations may yield helpful clues to diagnosis. Isolating a localised area in the case of pain can be very helpful

**Table 3.3**  The history of the problem: questions to ask the patient

- Where is the problem?
- How did it start?
- How long have you had the problem?
- Where is the problem?
- When does it trouble you?
- What makes it worse?
- What makes it better?
- What treatments have you tried?
- Are you treating it at the moment?

in differentiating enthesopathy from the more general discomfort associated with congestion of the heel pad. During the physical examination you may touch the area and attempt to elicit the symptoms in order to make sure you have isolated the area. Do not forget to tell the patient that this is what you are going to do. Palpation should use no more pressure than necessary to elicit symptoms and isolate the particular anatomy affected. It is essential that you record, either on a diagram or in words, the location of the problem and give an indication in the records as to whether it is well localised or diffuse. For example, a patient with plantar digital neuritis (Morton's neuroma) may complain of acute pain at one particular site, but may also describe a paraesthesia which radiates towards the apex of the toes. Diagrams may be preferable to written descriptions. Another practitioner treating the patient on a different occasion can see exactly where the problem lies. This allows the progress to be monitored for improvement or deterioration. It is essential that dimensions of skin lesions are recorded (see Ch. 9).

**How did it start?** It is important to identify how the problem started. The problem may have had a sudden or an insidious onset. For example, rheumatoid arthritis may have an acute sudden onset accompanied by raised temperature and severe joint pains, or more commonly a slow insidious onset with general aches and pains which gradually get worse and more regular. Besides trying to locate the start of the condition, it is also important to record the symptoms the

patient initially experienced. For example, was there anything visible at the start, such as a rash, swelling or erythema? Were there any symptoms, e.g. the throbbing associated with acute inflammation? Initial symptoms may be different from the patient's current symptoms, especially if the condition had an acute onset but is now chronic.

**How long have you had the problem?** It may be necessary to jog the patient's memory, especially if the problem started some time ago. Using family occasions such as weddings or births, national events or the season of the year may help the patient to pinpoint which time of the year it started.

**When does it trouble you?** Some conditions may give rise to constant symptoms. Others may occur especially at night or during the day. For example, one of the distinguishing features of gout is nocturnal pain. Chronic ischaemia is associated with pain in the calf muscle (intermittent claudication) after a period of walking and the maximum distance the patient can walk prior to experiencing pain gives an indication of the severity of the problem.

**What makes it worse and what makes it better?** Some conditions may improve on rest, others can deteriorate. Patients may discover all sorts of ways to alleviate their symptoms, e.g. wearing particular shoes, adopting a different walking pattern. Such information can provide valuable clues. In instances where patients alter their gait because of a problem affecting one part of their foot or leg they may develop secondary problems elsewhere. It is essential that the practitioner identifies the original problem as treatment for the secondary problem will not be successful until the initial problem is identified.

**What treatments have you tried? Are you treating it at the moment?** It is important to find out if the patient has or is presently using any medications. Sometimes treatments can mask or alter the clinical features of a problem and make diagnosis difficult. For example, using 1% hydrocortisone cream on a fungal infection of the skin may mask the inflammatory response and blur the distinctive border between infected and non-infected areas.

It is important that you record the information the patient gives you in response to all these questions. All critical events should be dated.

## Dimensions of pain

Pain is a subjective, multidimensional phenomena that can be affected by social and psychological factors. In the same way as individuals differ over what they perceive as a problem, individuals also differ when it comes to the assessment of their pain. Pain caused by apparently similar conditions affects individuals in very different ways. Practitioners should avoid making assumptions about the severity of pain an individual is experiencing. Patients vary in their abilities to cope with pain. Some are more than willing to complain about mild discomfort whereas others make no complaint despite being in considerable pain.

Tolerance and coping are subjective concepts which are difficult to quantify. A patient's state of mind and personal circumstances may make their pain worse or demand that they ignore it. For example, it is well known that runners may continue to run in a race despite having sustained an injury.

The assessment of pain requires information about its character, distribution, severity, duration, frequency and periodicity. This information, coupled with the history of the problem and details of the patient's concerns, helps the practitioner to arrive at the correct diagnosis and draw up an effective treatment plan.

### Character

Pain can be superficial or deep. Pain arising in the skin often gives rise to a pricking sensation if brief or burning if protracted. Deep pain is more nebulous and is often associated with a dull ache. Patients may use a variety of adjectives to describe their pain (Table 3.4).

### Distribution

Pain may be localised, diffuse or radiating. Initially, a problem may give rise to localised

**Table 3.4** Descriptors used to describe pain

| | |
|---|---|
| Vice-like | Deep |
| Tooth ache | On touching |
| Throbbing | On weightbearing |
| Sharp | Intermittent |
| Stabbing | |
| Shooting | |
| Bursting | |

pain but as it becomes chronic and the disease process spreads it can affect a wider area. Radiating pain can result from the extent of the disease or from pain being referred from one site to another; for example, a trapped spinal nerve can lead to pains in the leg. Usually, referred pain does not get worse when direct pressure is applied to the site affected. However, if the pain has a localised cause it usually worsens when direct pressure is applied.

### Severity

Certain conditions give rise to severe pain, e.g. myocardial infarction. However, a patient's ability to tolerate and cope with pain differs so much that a description of the severity of the pain must be assessed alongside the other features.

### Duration

Pain may be fleeting or may be persistent. Ascertaining the duration of the pain can provide valuable information. For example, pain due to intermittent claudication may last a few minutes to half an hour. The pain associated with a deep vein thrombosis is persistent. These differences can be helpful in differential diagnosis.

### Frequency and periodicity

Some conditions lead to pain occurring in a regular pattern; others result in a less predictable pain pattern. It may be that the pain recurs infrequently or regularly.

## Techniques for assessing pain

A range of techniques can be used to provide more objective information about the dimensions of pain experienced by a patient.

### Pain rating scales

These may involve descriptors or a numerical scoring system. Different dimensions such as severity, frequency and duration can be assessed. For example, a patient may be asked to score the frequency of his/her pain using a 1–5 scale, 1 signifying persistent, present all the time and 5 very infrequent, less than twice a week. Descriptive scales can also be used. Severity can be assessed by the following descriptors: slight, quite a lot, very bad, agonising (Seers 1987).

### Visual analogue scales (VAS)

These can be used to assess the severity of pain. The technique involves asking the patient to indicate how severe their problem is. Figure 3.1 illustrates two different types of visual analogue scale.

### Descriptors

Various descriptors have been used to assess pain. The McGill Pain Questionnaire was devised to elicit the adjectives patients use to describe their pain. Use of this questionnaire indicates that a patient who describes their pain as frightening usually does not understand what is causing it (Melzack 1975).

### Charts

Charts can be used for patients to indicate where the pain occurs and, by using different symbols, the type of pain that occurs (Fig 3.2). Pain charts have been used as an aid to the psychological evaluation of patients with low back pain (Ransford et al 1976). This method should be used with great caution and with the assistance of a suitably qualified psychologist in order to prevent incorrect conclusions being reached.

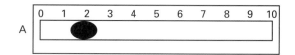

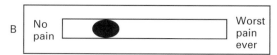

**Figure 3.1** Visual analogue scales  **A.** Numerical **B.** Descriptive.

### Pain diaries

It may be helpful, especially if a patient is rather vague about the duration and frequency of his/her pain, to get the patient to complete a diary of the pain over a specific period of time. Figure 3.3 illustrates a pain chart. The categories used in the chart were devised by the Pain Research Institute, Liverpool. While pain diaries can be helpful, they may lead patients to focus on their problem and could even exacerbate it.

The information gained from a patient presenting with a painful first metatarsophalangeal joint is shown in Table 3.5. The data used for this example suggests a diagnosis of gout. Laboratory tests and further assessments, i.e. medical and social history, may confirm this diagnosis.

## SUMMARY

It is essential that the practitioner acquires a clear and accurate understanding of the patient's concern(s) and problems in order to devise an effective management plan. These terms have been emphasised in different ways in this chapter, although 'problem' and 'concern' may be used synonymously elsewhere.

If the basic history part of the assessment concerning the presenting problem is inadequately dealt with or not undertaken the result of an inaccurate diagnosis occurring is all too clear to see. Some of these issues are emphasised in more detail in Chapter 5, which forms a prerequisite for systems analysis by functional enquiry and physical examination.

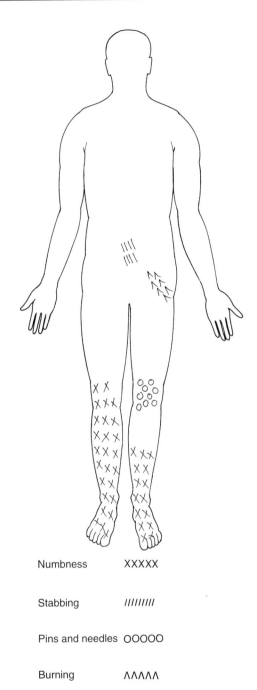

| | Mon | Tues | Wed | Thur | Fri |
|---|---|---|---|---|---|
| 6.00 7.00 8.00 9.00 10.00 11.00 12.00 13.00 14.00 15.00 16.00 17.00 18.00 19.00 20.00 21.00 22.00 | | | | | |

5 Excruciating

4 Very severe

3 Severe

2 Moderate

1 Just noticeable

0 No pain

S Sleeping

**Figure 3.3**   Pain diary.

Numbness            XXXXX

Stabbing            /////////

Pins and needles  OOOOO

Burning             ΛΛΛΛΛ

**Figure 3.2**   Pain chart.

**Table 3.5**   Information gained from assessment of a patient with a painful first metatarsophalangeal joint

| | |
|---|---|
| The problem(s) | 'I've got a very painful big toe. I can't sleep at night for the pain.' |
| The concern(s) | 'Do you think it is something serious?' 'Will I have to have my foot off?' |
| Where is the problem? | The big toe joint on my left foot. |
| How did it start? | The pain started one night. I woke up in a lot of pain. My toe was bright red and throbbing. The next day it was really swollen. |
| How long have you had the problem? | It started about a week ago. |
| When does it trouble you? | It hurts all the time, especially at night. |
| What makes it worse? | If I knock it at all and when I walk on it. |
| What makes it better? | The pain eases a bit when I take a painkiller but when the tablet wears off the pain is just as bad again. |
| What treatments have you tried? | Just painkillers. I have been taking quite strong ones these last few days. |
| Are you treating it at the moment? | See above. |

## REFERENCES

Melzack R 1975 The McGill Pain Questionnaire: major properties and scoring methods. Pain 1(3): 277–299

Ransford A O, Cairns D, Mooney V 1976 The pain drawing as an aid to the psychologic evaluation of patients with low-back pain. Spine 1(2:6): 127–134

Sandler G 1979 Costs of unnecessary tests. British Medical Journal 2: 21–24

Seers K 1987 Perceptions of pain. Nursing Times 83(48): 37–39

Townsend P, Davidson N 1982 Inequalities in health: the Black Report. Penguin, Harmondsworth, p 76–89

# 4

# Clinical measurement

## C. J. Griffith

## INTRODUCTION

Clinical measurement is closely intertwined with assessment and evaluation of the lower limb. The term 'measurement' refers to the discovery of the extent of an observation and to the result obtained. 'Assessment' and 'evaluation' are terms that refer to the process of interpreting the meaning of a measurement. Measurements are used for a number of reasons. They are fundamental to the processes of diagnosis, prognosis, prescription of treatment, case management and assessment of outcomes.

The lower limb consists of a number of inter-related complex body systems. Bones, joints, muscles, nerves, blood vessels and other soft tissues all contribute to the health and function of the lower limb. With so many diverse structures and physiological functions in each of these body systems, it is not surprising that a wide variety of techniques have evolved to measure their performance.

Some clinical observations are amenable to objective scientific measurement and others are not. To gain as much clinically useful information as possible about patients and their responses to treatment, both objective and subjective measurement methods can be employed.

## TYPES OF MEASUREMENT

There are three types of clinical measurement technique:

• Quantitative measurement

- Qualitative measurement
- Semi-quantitative measurement.

All three types of measurement provide valuable but different types of clinical information.

## Quantitative measurement

Quantitative measurements measure quantity in the true scientific sense, being objective and typically consisting of two parts: a numerical value and a unit of measurement. The numerical value denotes the magnitude of an observation, defined against certain norms or standards called *units of measurement*. Units of measurement give a dimension to the numerical value. The language of scientific measurement is the Système International (SI), also known as the metric system. Examples of SI units of measurement appropriate to the clinical setting are kilograms (mass), metres (length), pascals (pressure), newtons (force), hertz (frequency), degrees (angle), and degrees Celsius (temperature). Because quantitative measurements have both magnitude and dimension they can be recorded and communicated exactly and concisely.

All results obtained from quantitative measurements are classed as either interval or ratio levels of data. It is useful to know which category data falls into because it affects its interpretation.

The numeric points or graduations on any quantitative measurement scale have equal intervals between them. This is an important feature because the results can be compared arithmetically. They can also be used in the most powerful inferential statistical tests. A clinical example will make the concept clear. If a plantar ulcer had a diameter of 1.5 cm and a depth of 0.5 cm this would convey the size of the lesion exactly. With treatment it would be hoped that the ulcer would resolve. The progress of the ulcer could be monitored over time. If on a subsequent occasion the ulcer was found to have a diameter of 0.75 cm and a depth of 0.25 cm it would demonstrate that the ulcer was exactly half its previous dimensions.

A wide range of equipment is available to measure clinical observations quantitatively. Instrumentation may be quite basic in its design, such as a rule for measuring a lesion's size or more advanced such as a flexible electrogoniometer system for measuring static and dynamic joint motion.

## Qualitative measurement

Qualitative measurements, as the name suggests, measure quality. They are subjective and essentially descriptive measures dependent upon human perceptions. This type of measurement results in an observation expressed in words. There is some debate as to whether qualitative observations are measurements in the true sense. Qualitative researchers argue a strong case for the legitimacy of these measures. They can provide extremely valuable clinical information where clinical features cannot be quantified. Returning to the ulcer example, qualitative measurement would include descriptions about the appearance of the ulcer. Qualitative descriptions of size could include 'large', 'small', 'deep' and 'shallow'. Comparison of size before and after a period of treatment can be indicated by using phrases such as 'larger than', 'smaller than', 'shallower than' and so on. Qualitative descriptions are clearly less exact in terms of magnitude than are quantitative measures. It would not be possible to say by how much the ulcer had improved or deteriorated over time. Quantitative measurement is clearly superior in the context of magnitude. On the other hand qualitative measures can make a major contribution to the understanding, description and communication of clinical observations. Considerable credence would be given to the colour of the ulcer's base and discharge, the shape of the lesion's edges and walls, and perhaps any odour noticed. Changes in these characteristics are clinically useful indicators of the status of an ulcer and whether it is improving or deteriorating.

## Semi-quantitative measurement

Semi-quantitative measurement techniques involve an association of quantitative and qualitat-

**Table 4.1** Medical Research Council rating scale for muscle strength

| Rating | Characteristic |
|--------|----------------|
| 0 | No movement |
| 1 | Palpable contraction but no visible movement |
| 2 | Movement but only with gravity eliminated |
| 3 | Movement against gravity |
| 4 | Movement against resistance, but weaker than the other side |
| 5 | Normal power |

ive methods to assess quality. They are extremely varied in their design and application and represent attempts to quantify quality where real quantitative methods are not appropriate. This type of measurement allows a common approach to obtaining, recording and communicating information. Results based on objective measurements tend to be modified and supported as more data is acquired (Calnan 1989). The following will exemplify some principles of semi-quantitative measurement.

### Rating (grading) scales

Scores are allocated to each of a logical order of observations, with each score in some way being better or worse than another. The scale may indicate, for instance, the level of function of some system or activity, and range from normal function to absence of function. The Medical Research Council (MRC) grading for muscle strength (Table 4.1) allocates scores from 0–5 to classify function in patients with peripheral nerve damage. This is considered in Chapter 8 as part of essential locomotor assessment.

The six ratings or gradings are placed in rank order of increasing muscle power from 0 (no movement) to 5 (normal power). It is possible to record muscle power on a single occasion, or by taking a series of measurements monitor improvement or deterioration in muscle power over time.

This type of data is classed as ordinal data. It is important to remember that the different scores on an ordinal scale cannot be compared in an arithmetic way because the intervals between the points on the scale are not equal. With reference to Table 4.1 it will be noted that the difference between 1 and 2 is not the same as the difference between 4 and 5. Also a score of 4 is better than, but not twice as good as, a score of 2.

### Indices

Ankle–brachial, footprint and pulsility indices are commonly referred to in the literature. Each index is a ratio calculated from two quantitative values. The ankle–brachial index, for instance, is calculated by dividing the systolic ankle blood pressure by the systolic brachial pressure of the arm, e.g. $110/120 = 0.92$. Indices are often referred to as quantitative measures. Arguably they may best be considered as semi-quantitative measures because they lack two important characteristics of quantitative measures. Indices are dimensionless, as they have no units of measurement, and their numerical values cannot be treated arithmetically. For example, comparison of indices should be treated in a similar way to ordinal data. An ankle–brachial index of 0.4 indicates an ischaemic condition but it cannot be said that the condition is twice as bad as an index of 0.8.

### Nominal categorisation

This is essentially a very simple classification system where an observation is placed into one of two categories. The observation of interest could be either present or absent, and given arbitrary labels, perhaps A (present) and B (absent), or 1 and 2. For instance, a group of patients could be classified as hallux valgus present and hallux valgus absent. Data treated in this manner are described as *nominal*. This is the most basic level of data and gives the least amount of detail about an observation. The hallux valgus is denoted simply as present or absent with no indication as to the severity of the condition. Only the simplest of arithmetic calculations can be carried out, and the data can only be used in the weakest types of statistical test.

## Three types of measuring

In practice, techniques selected from the three types of measurement may be used together to obtain a comprehensive clinical picture. This is illustrated by discussion of the results of measurements obtained for a patient presenting with walking difficulties, shown in Table 4.2. The relevant case history concerns a fall 1 year previously when a fractured pelvis was sustained. Following healing and discharge from hospital the left leg and foot have become progressively weaker.

**Qualitative measurement.** There appears to be a motor deficit in the anterior compartment of the leg. This may be due to impingement of a peripheral nerve related to the pelvic fracture. The lack of ankle dorsiflexion during the swing phase is being compensated proximally, by elevation of the trunk and excessive flexion of the hip and knee, so that the toes can clear the ground.

**Semi-quantitative measurement.** A score of 3 on MRC muscle strength grading scale. This indicates the level of impairment of the anterior muscle group. There is a deficit of motor power. The patient can dorsiflex the foot against gravity but not against resistance of the practitioner's hand.

**Table 4.2** Assessment results

| Type of measurement | Method | Results |
|---|---|---|
| Qualitative | Visual observation of gait | Stance phase: The left foot slaps noisily against the ground at each step Swing phase: The left foot is plantarflexed, the hip and knee are flexed excessively and there is upper body sway to the right |
| Semi-quantitative | MRC muscle strength grading scale | The anterior muscle compartment score of 3 (i.e. movement against gravity) |
| Quantitative | Goniometric measurement | Active ankle dorsiflexion $-10°$ Passive ankle dorsiflexion $-5°$ |

**Quantitative measurement.** Active dorsiflexion can be quantified with a goniometer, e.g. $-10°$ dorsiflexion. The measurement of $-10°$ dorsiflexion indicates that with maximum contraction of the anterior muscle group the foot still remains 10° plantarflexed at the ankle. With assistance from the practitioner the maximum range of dorsiflexion can be obtained ($-5°$). Although an additional 5° of dorsiflexion was obtained with the practitioner's help the foot remained plantarflexed at the ankle. Comparison with the unaffected ankle and known normal values will enable the practitioner to determine the extent of the reduction in ankle dorsiflexion and identify the probable cause. The calf may have shortened if there is a loss of power in the anterior antagonist muscle group. Future measurements can be used to quantify improvement or deterioration of ankle dorsiflexion.

The example above demonstrates the value of each type of measurement. A complete picture of the case can be constructed where evidence from one measurement complements another. Evaluation of the evidence then enables the practitioner to infer the cause of the changes in gait pattern with more than a reasonable degree of confidence. A thorough understanding of the problem gained in this manner enables an appropriate diagnosis and management plan to be decided.

It could be argued that all measurements for the patient could have been quantitative. Gait analysis could have been recorded with video and the movements of the limb segments digitised to allow quantification. Muscle power could have been quantified with a dynamometer. Nevertheless, the example represents the most usual clinical situation where the practitioner would only have access to a goniometer. An important issue for consideration has been raised. If a number of different measurement options are available, how does the practitioner select the most appropriate method?

## SELECTION OF AN APPROPRIATE MEASUREMENT TECHNIQUE

Selection of an appropriate measurement technique can be a dilemma, particularly for students with relatively little experience. Many factors influence the choice of a measurement technique. The main factors are:

- Practitioner
- Patient
- Resources.

## The practitioner

Choice of measurement technique will be influenced significantly by professional education, experience, personal beliefs, skills and knowledge of the patient. Consequently, some tests will be used more frequently than others. Knowledge and skills should be greater for those techniques used more often. Where less frequent or novel situations arise, a relevant and sensible measurement technique for the observation of interest must be selected. The MRC grading for muscle strength described earlier is suitable for patients with peripheral nerve damage causing muscle flaccidity. It is not a valid technique for patients with hypertonicity. To avoid the possibility of selecting an inappropriate technique a sound theoretical knowledge of the measurement techniques under consideration is needed. The situations that might arise when selecting a measurement technique for a particular patient are:

- Seemingly similar observations (as above) may not be amenable to the same measurement technique
- Some observations can be measured by a number of techniques and there may be no particular clinical advantage in any one
- It may be clear that one particular technique is preferred.

## The patient

Each patient is unique. Although there may be similarities between patients, no two cases are identical. An individual patient's characteristics will affect his/her suitability for different measurement techniques. Age, mental state, build and current medical status are characteristics that commonly influence decisions about the choice

of measurement. This may result in a modification to the measurement procedure, selection of an alternative technique, or even a decision not to perform the measurement at all. Techniques that require a patient to adopt a particular position may require modification if the patient has arthritic joints, poor balance, is excessively obese, very old or very young.

## Resources

These have a significant influence on the availability of measurement techniques. Funding, accessibility to equipment, professional skills, time and space will determine which measurements can be conducted. Practitioners will have facilities for routine measurements. Should the need arise, referral to colleagues who specialise in complementary fields can be arranged.

## TERMS USED IN CLINICAL MEASUREMENT

The notion of an ideal measurement is one that is accurate, precise, repeatable, reliable and valid. To gain an awareness of both the value and limitations of contemporary measurement methods, an understanding of the terms associated with measurement is needed.

### Accuracy

This concerns a result which reflects the true value of the observation or phenomenon being measured.

### Precision

This is the degree of refinement in a measurement and relates to the size of the intervals on the measurement scale. A rule with graduations of 1 mm would allow greater precision than one with graduations every 5 mm. The intervals between the graduations on the measurement scale should always be appropriate for the observation of interest. If they are unnecessarily large and the measurement indicator falls between graduations the practitioner is forced to make an estimate of the reading, increasing the potential for error.

## Repeatability

This is determined by measuring the same patient with the same technique on two or more occasions and comparing the results. Inevitably there will be differences. An experimental research design can be used to determine statistically if any differences in repeated measurement results are large enough to be significant. A statistically significant difference between the results would indicate that the measurement technique is not repeatable, and consequently of limited clinical value.

## Reliability

This is the extent to which a measurement procedure produces similar results under constant conditions on all occasions. Repeatability is a measure of reliability. Clinical measures which quantify or semi-quantify the extent of a problem can also be used to detect change. In this context the measurements are used both repeatedly and often by different people. Consequently it is important to know how much any difference is due to real change and how much is caused by error (Wade 1992). In this way real improvements or deterioration in a patient's condition can be determined. Where the repeatability of a technique is known and variation in measurement falls within clinically acceptable limits, the practitioner can interpret the results and make clinical decisions with confidence. Reliability can be reduced by many factors. There are four main sources of uncertainty when comparing two or more results of the same measure:

- Variation in the patient's state
- The instrument may vary with time
- The same observer may differ when measuring (intraobserver reliability)
- Different observers may differ when measuring (interobserver reliability).

**Patient's state.** Differences in the patient's state between measurements may adversely affect the results. There may be changes in physical and mental states, motivation and fatigue levels. Some observations are known to be affected by the time of day that they are taken.

**Instrument variation.** As instruments age their performance tends to deteriorate. They may also be affected by environmental changes. For example, temperature and humidity may affect the performance of pressure transducers.

**Intraobserver reliability.** This concerns the variation between the results of repeated measurements obtained by the same observer. Statistical techniques are used to determine whether the differences in results are significant. Intraobserver variation can be attributed to many human characteristics. Variation in results may be due to differences in fatigue, motivation and stress levels as well as inconsistencies in technique. Intraobserver reliability differs from one individual to another; some demonstrate greater proficiency by obtaining more consistent results.

**Interobserver reliability.** This concerns the variation between results of repeated measurements between two or more observers. The more observers involved the greater the opportunity for differences to occur between them. There is evidence to show that intraobserver reliability is greater than interobserver reliability. For example, one study of repeated goniometric measurements concluded that reliability is increased if only one observer takes the measurements (Boone et al 1978). Simple, well defined measurement techniques have been shown to be more reliable, presumably because observers can follow the procedures more closely. Reliability of measurement improves with training, education and experience (Bovens et al 1990, Diamond et al 1989). Ideally one should be aware of one's own measurement capabilities, and evaluation should be made at periodic intervals. Where the same patient may be measured by different practitioners over time, the interobserver reliability between the individuals in the group should be known. This facilitates interpretation of the differences in results to interobserver error or to real change. The determination of whether a measurement technique is reliable has obvious clinical importance because a reliable technique will enable the practitioner to make useful clinical judgements. However, reliability should not be considered exclusively. It should be considered in context with other measurement characteristics.

## Validity

This is concerned with whether the measurement actually does measure what it is supposed to measure (Bowling 1991). The validity of footprint parameters used as measures of the height of the medial longitudinal arch has been questioned. The arch angle, footprint index and arch index described by various authors were compared with a direct measure of arch height (Hawes et al 1992). It was concluded that these footprint parameters were no more than indices and angles of the plantar surface of the foot itself, and were invalid measures of arch height. Even when the footprint measurements were categorised semi-quantitatively they were poor predictors of high, medium and low arches. All of the footprint parameters had previously been found to be reliable. Presumably this means that the footprint pattern and data measured from it are repeatable, but the indices derived cannot be assumed to be valid indicators of arch height. Sensitivity and specificity can be used to test validity.

**Sensitivity** is the ability of a measurement or test to identify positive cases of the observation of interest.

**Specificity** is the ability of the measurement or test to exclude negative cases of the observation of interest.

A hypothetical example will illustrate the principles of sensitivity and specificity. If we suppose that the traditional approach to screening for hallux valgus was to X-ray each patient's feet it might be thought beneficial to devise a method which did not depend on X-rays. Practitioners could be trained to use a new clinical measurement technique to determine whether patients had hallux valgus or not. If X-rays are assumed to give the true result, the practitioners' results could be compared with the X-rays. Two groups of symptomatic patients, one group with and the other without hallux valgus, would be selected from the X-ray results. If the practitioners' measurements were completely valid then all the patients with a positive X-ray for hallux valgus and those with a negative X-ray would be appropriately identified. This never occurs in practice. There are always some false positives, i.e. those identified as having the condition when they do not, or false negatives, i.e. those identified as not having the condition when they do. Table 4.3 illustrates the main principles.

*Sensitivity* is the percentage of patients correctly identified as having hallux valgus. Calculations from the tabulated data show that the sensitivity is high, at 95%, indicating that most patients with hallux valgus were identified by the practitioners. The *specificity* is the percentage of patients without hallux valgus who were identified as not having hallux valgus. The specificity is low at 45%. This means that 55% of patients without hallux valgus were falsely diagnosed as having hallux valgus. The practitioners identified nearly half as many false positives (61) as true positives (129). With so many false positives identified the new clinical measurement technique would not be considered a useful screening test for hallux valgus.

Acceptable values for sensitivity and specificity depend to some extent on the particular situation. Sensitivity of good tests is likely to be between 80% and 100%. Specificity should be in excess of 95%, particularly for screening tests where most of the population are likely to be negative, otherwise more false positives than true positives may occur.

**Table 4.3** Sensitivity and specificity

| Practitioners' measurements | X-ray results | |
|---|---|---|
| | Hallux valgus present | Hallux valgus not present |
| Hallux valgus present | 129 | 61 |
| Hallux valgus not present | 7 | 49 |
| Total | 136 | 110 |
| Sensitivity | = 129/136 × 100 = 95% | |
| Specificity | = 49/110 × 100 = 45% | |

## ERROR IN MEASUREMENT

A significant problem with taking measurements is error. All results from measurements have two components: the true value of the observation of interest and an error component. The error component can be further divided into two parts.

**Random errors.** These occur by chance and because of their random nature cannot be identified, controlled or eliminated. In research studies an appropriate research design and use of inferential statistical tests take random errors into account. This type of error will not be considered further.

**Systematic errors.** These relate to potential sources of measurement error that can usually be postulated or identified. Once a source of error has been identified, action can be taken to try and reduce its occurrence. In all measurements conducted on patients there are five main potential sources of systematic error:

- Clinical environment
- Procedure
- Equipment
- Practitioner
- Patient.

## The clinical environment

Lighting must enable the practitioner to see clearly so that information can be gathered and recorded with ease. Careful planning of the lighting arrangements is essential. Assessment areas should be well lit so that vital clinical features are not obscured. Special lighting facilities are sometimes necessary. For example, a light box is essential for clear interpretation and measurement from radiographs.

Clinical space is often at a premium. It is essential that there is sufficient space for a selected measurement procedure to be undertaken. Gait analysis requires a walkway of at least 6 m so that a representative walking style can be seen. The ambient clinic temperature should be controlled at $21°C \pm 2°C$. This is not only important for the comfort of the practitioner and patient but essential for vascular and neurological measurements. Significant adverse effects on vascular measurements are caused by factors that change peripheral arterial resistance (Johnson & Kassam 1985).

Background noise, interruptions and distractions during consultations should be kept to minimum levels as they impair concentration, communication and patient relaxation.

## Procedure

Standardisation of measurement techniques reduces the potential for error in measurement. Consequently it can improve repeatability, reliability, accuracy and in most circumstances validity. Standardised techniques have clearly specified procedures which must be followed closely. Unfortunately, standardisation cannot remove error completely. The extent of measurement error that is clinically acceptable is determined by the type of observation, research and statistical methods. Where different techniques measure the same type of observation, the one that produces the least error can be selected. An understanding of the size of the error enables practitioners to understand the limitations of the techniques they use. They can also interpret their clinical measurements realistically and cautiously.

Research reports should be read with care. Special attention should be paid to the quality of the procedure before adopting a new or alternative technique. It is important to balance gains in accuracy, precision, reliability and validity claimed, particularly if they are marginal, with the clinical costs and benefits for patients.

## The equipment

Equipment indirectly involved with measurement can affect results. The examination couch should permit a variety of positions to suit the many types of examination that may be performed. Practitioner fatigue will be reduced if the appropriate height of couch is used or if the height can be adjusted. Instrumentation used directly on the patient should be comfortable to handle and easy to use.

Calibration of instrumentation is an essential and fundamental process of measurement. The purpose of calibration is to minimise the error caused by the equipment. It is a process of setting up the instrument so that its readings are as accurate as possible throughout the range of measurement. The instrumentation is tested against known standards. Calibration curves are plotted so that the accuracy can be determined and the error quantified. An example will make things clear. To calibrate weighing scales they must be placed on a horizontal surface. The measurement indicator is aligned to zero. Known loads are applied at intervals throughout the measurement range. A comparison is made between the output reading on the measurement scale and the known load (kgf). By plotting the two variables a calibration curve can be produced. Ideally the curve would be linear throughout the measurement range. Errors are identified and the measurement tolerances calculated and specified.

Where instruments are precalibrated, errors may be specified as a percentage error within the measurement range. For example, most manufacturers of equipment for measuring foot pressure claim an accuracy within 10%. It is therefore not possible to know whether marginal differences are real or due to error.

Some instruments are designed to measure a series of values during cyclic activities. Pressure transducers measure pressure under discrete areas of the foot. A transducer located under the second metatarsal head would measure the progressive loading and unloading pressures applied during one gait cycle. Static calibration of the transducer is carried out by applying a series of known loads and then progressively removing them. A graph is produced in the form of a loop. This phenomenon is known as *hysteresis*. Figure 4.1 shows that the output readings for known loads differ between the ascending and descending modes. A dashed line drawn from the horizontal axis at 5 kg loading, to intersect with each curve, shows the disparity in output readings during ascending and descending modes at points (a) and (b) respectively on the vertical axis. Hysteresis is defined as the maximum difference in any pair of readings,

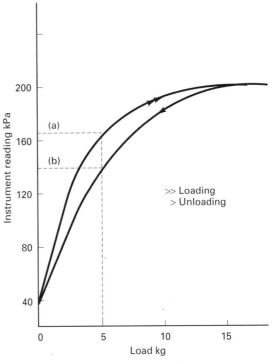

**Figure 4.1** Hysteresis from elastomeric pressure transducer. Pressure is recorded against load applied for static calibration for a VP1 pressure pad. The plot shows loading and unloading as two curves. The hysteresis is represented by gap between the curves (adapted from Tollafield 1990).

one in the ascending mode and one in the descending mode, during one cycle of calibration and is expressed as a percentage of full scale output (Dainty et al 1987).

The performance characteristics, particularly of electronic equipment, must be suitable for the intended purpose. Transducers convert mechanical signals into electrical signals for processing. Characteristics associated with transducers such as hysteresis, sensitivity, threshold, linearity, frequency response, response time, damping and repeatability should be matched with the observation of interest.

Ground reaction forces are measured by force platforms. Different force platforms contain different types of transducer, and some are more suited for one purpose than another. For example, the Kistler multicomponent measuring platform transducers contain quartz elements, which produce a piezoelectric effect. Vertical, anterior and posterior, and lateral shear forces can be measured simultaneously. The Kistler is suitable for obtaining walking and running force data (dynamic performance), but is probably less appropriate for measuring quasi-static motions (seemingly static performance). A force platform using strain gauge technology such as the AMTI six-component biomechanical platform would be more suitable. Other specifications such as the size of the platform and the potential problems related to the patient targeting a small surface area should be considered.

Measurement instrumentation is prone to aging and wear and tear, increasing the potential for error. Obvious changes in mechanical instruments may be noticed where the measurement scale becomes difficult to read, or its components become damaged or loose. Electronic components tend to age less noticeably. Noise is generated by electrical circuitry and it tends to increase as equipment ages. The level of noise must not be so large as to interfere significantly with measurements. Everyday examples of noise include the background hum of audio speakers, or interference with visual information on a display monitor, rather like the lines produced on a television screen as an unsuppressed motor vehicle passes by. It is important to ensure that intrinsic noise produced by the instrumentation and electrical equipment in the vicinity do not cause unacceptable interference.

Careful monitoring and maintenance of equipment will reduce the potential for error caused by loss of calibration, aging and wear and tear.

# The practitioner

Errors made by the practitioner can be reduced if a good practitioner–patient relationship is established. Effective communication and patient compliance is essential. Efficiency and confidence are usually transferred to the patient through verbal and non-verbal communication channels. Instructions given to the patient must be clear, so that they understand exactly what they must do. Children, ethnic minorities, the physically and mentally disabled usually require

more careful and considered approaches. Adequate time must be allowed for the measurements to be completed satisfactorily.

## Qualitative measurements

Qualitative measurements involve an internal appreciation and processing of the observations made. Qualitative techniques are subjective in nature and mainly involve the perceptions of sight, hearing and touch. Some senses are more acute in some individuals than in others. Different life experiences, education, state of health or mind and environmental factors will affect these perceptions. Qualitative measurements are therefore more prone to bias errors in practitioners than are quantitative measures. An awareness of the problems associated with subjectivity is important, because different individuals may perceive the same observation in different ways.

Often, preconceived ideas lead to mistakes, as illustrated in Figure 4.2A. When first seen most people read the legends incorrectly as 'Paris in the spring', 'Once in a lifetime', and 'Bird in the hand'. We have a tendency to see what we expect to see and ignore what we consider unimportant. This may happen in diagnosis, when a feature associated with a particular condition is given greater importance than it should receive and assumptions lead to a rapid, poorly considered diagnosis. It may be that other clinical features indicate a different pathology but these may go unnoticed, be ignored or be regarded as of little significance. By remaining as objective as possible and adopting a systematic problem-solving approach this tendency will be reduced.

The brain may interpret the same observation in different ways, as shown in Figure 4.2B. The same observation may not only differ between individuals but differ in the same individual on different occasions or as they make a closer study.

Some quantitative measurement procedures depend on some subjective decisions by the practitioner. The location of pulses, anatomical landmarks and alignment of instrumentation all rely on subjectivity, thus increasing the potential for bias error. It is important to be aware of the

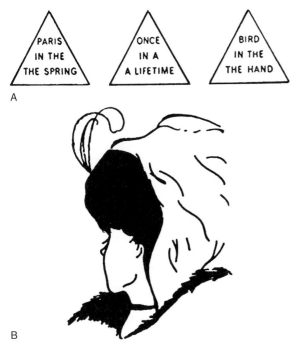

**Figure 4.2   A.** The three triangles. Failure to see the duplicated words is common. We see only what we want to see.   **B.** How old is she? Some observers see a young woman, others an old woman. The chin and neck of the former become the nose and mouth of the latter and vice versa (Munro & Edwards 1990).

subjective qualitative factors which may impair objective measurement so that attempts can be made to control them.

### Vision

Vision plays a major part in quantitative assessments. During clinical training a student practitioner develops a 'trained eye'. Recognition of pathology develops with time and practice into a fine skill, where even subtle signs may alert the practitioner to a problem.

Visual information may be impaired if lighting is inadequate. Apart from the more obvious difficulties caused where lighting levels are low, shadows cast on to a part of the limb may adversely affect subjective aspects during biomechanical examination. *Eyeballing* describes a subjective visual technique that can be used to align joints before measurement, or to identify

midpoints across skin surfaces as goniometric reference points. Passive examination of the subtalar joint range of motion and neutral position is considered to be an important element in understanding abnormal function of the foot. Inappropriate placement of reference lines, particularly on the curved surface of the back of the leg, is more likely to occur if one side of the leg is adequately lit and the other is not. A true vertical bisection of the leg may not be obtained. Consequently, the proportions of inversion and eversion contributing to the total range of motion, and determination of the neutral position, would be incorrect.

**Parallax error** is a potential source of measurement error particularly associated with joint position and movement. Parallax is an apparent difference in position or direction of an object caused by a change or relative change of observation point, as shown in Figure 4.3. Viewing an object or patient at right angles will eliminate parallax error. Measurement error will increase if the measurement instrument is not aligned with the plane of motion. A 90° alignment must also be ensured when reading analogue measurement scales. Parallax error up to 3° was noted in one study (Griffith 1988).

The patient must be advised on the need for appropriate clothing if normal indoor dress inhibits a particular observation. Body parts must be clearly exposed where feasible. Shorts and a T-shirt, for example, allow a relatively uninhibited view of posture and movement.

### Touch

Touch involves many forms of direct and indirect (using instrumentation) physical contact with patients. During orthopaedic examinations various components of the lower limb may be pushed, pulled, pressed, squeezed and twisted. The amount of force used is determined by feedback through the practitioner's proprioceptive pathways, the patient's response, sound and visual information. It is very subjective. The force used to test joint ranges of motion will need adjustment for different patients and different joints. Fluidity of the joints, muscle

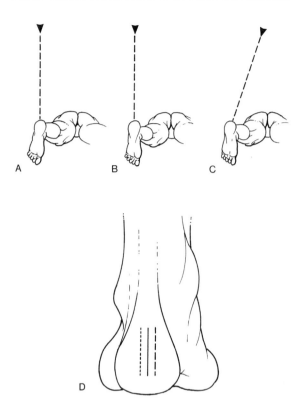

**Figure 4.3** The effect of parallax on observation of the midpoint of the posterior aspect of the leg and heel **A**. Inappropriate positioning of the patient's leg leads to parallax error **B**. With the patient's leg and the practitioner's eyes correctly aligned parallax error is eliminated **C**. Inappropriate positioning of the practitioner's eyes leads to parallax error **D**. The actual and apparent midpoints obtained from the relative eye and leg positions adopted in diagrams **A**, **B** and **C**.

tone and the weight of the limb will all influence the force required to examine a joint effectively.

Instruments used in neurological and vascular assessments must be applied to the appropriate area and with an appropriate amount of force. Using neurotips, tuning forks and cotton wool requires a systematic approach and correct technique. For instance, inadvertently tickling the patient with cotton wool when testing for light touch will be interpreted through pain pathways rather than light touch receptors, invalidating the result.

Measurement of lower limb temperature can be obtained quantitatively with a digital thermo-meter, but most practitioners rely on touch. The practitioner's hand temperature will influence his/her appreciation of the patient's limb temperature. This can be demonstrated with a simple experiment. If both hands are inserted in a bowl of tepid water, having previously had one in cold and the other in hot, a clear difference in appreciation of temperature of the tepid water by each hand is noted. The subjective appreciation of temperature is therefore a relative phenomenon and a patient's limb will feel warmer to a practitioner with cold hands than one who has warm hands.

*Hearing*

Audible signals representing the velocity of blood flow are generated by Doppler ultrasound units. A normal arterial audio spectrum is triphasic, representing forward, reverse and forward blood flow. Differentiation of normal and abnormal sound patterns is a highly skilled process. Considerable experience is necessary to develop the appropriate listening skills so that normal and abnormal sounds can be distinguished. However, abnormal sounds or artifacts can be produced if the application of the probe over the blood vessel is imprecise and an artery and a vein are isonated simultaneously. If the probe angle is incorrect the signal strength is reduced. A probe with an appropriate frequency must be selected, depending on the depth of the vessel of interest, so that an adequate signal strength can be obtained.

## The patient

The patient may be responsible for measurement errors for many reasons. General intelligence, mental disorder, impaired hearing or sight or language difficulties could affect his/her ability to understand what is required. Patients may not follow instructions or respond appropriately or truthfully. They may be non-compliant. If the patient is anxious or annoyed increased adrenaline levels will elevate the basal metabolic rate, e.g. the pulse rate could be increased. Patients who are emotionally distressed may be less able to comply with the requirements of some types of measurement procedure.

It is not unusual for patients to find difficulty in relaxing during passive biomechanical measurements. Joint ranges and fluidity of motion can appear reduced. Forefoot varus or supinatus could be erroneously diagnosed if the patient fails to relax the tibialis anterior muscle, because contraction of this muscle inverts the forefoot relative to the hindfoot.

Neurological sensory tests may require a verbal response from the patient so that the result can be obtained. Assuming that the test is applied correctly, the patient must interpret the sensation felt. This relies greatly on patient subjectivity. Higher vibration thresholds have been associated with sensory loss. It may not be the best indicator of neuropathic change because, in addition to environmental influences, psychological factors may also lead to error (Drysdale 1989). Although the cause is uncertain, there is evidence to show that touch and pressure sensitivity increase during the day and are more acute in women (Mooney 1987). While interpretation of these results should be approached with caution, it is important not to miss the early signs of neurological disorder.

If the patient is embarrassed, poorly motivated, self-conscious or in pain, his/her walking pattern and speed may be altered. If patients are required to step on a specific target such as a force or pressure plate they may adjust walking speed or step length as they activate the transducer mechanism, giving an atypical result. Controlling walking speed is a major factor in foot pressure measurement. Step length, cadence, stance phase gait and peak pressure have all been shown to vary with walking speed (Hughes et al 1991).

Some underlying pathological conditions can influence the measurement results. Doppler ultrasound waves are attenuated when they pass through fat, haematoma or scar tissue, resulting in a weak signal. Calcification of arterial walls prevents collapse of the artery when a blood pressure cuff is applied. The abnormally high reading obtained would invalidate the ankle–brachial index.

## PROBLEMS WITH COMMONLY USED MEASUREMENT TECHNIQUES

Many commonly used measurement techniques have been shown to be prone to substantial error. Two examples of research, one on vascular and the other on goniometric measurement have been selected from the literature. These subject areas are used to raise some general measurement issues and to highlight specific problems in each field. Those interested in improving measurement proficiency, devising or researching a measurement technique must examine the problems associated with measurement carefully. A useful way of approaching this task would be to consider the potential sources of systematic error under the five main headings described earlier. To illustrate this suggestion, findings from each research paper will be followed by consideration of the sources of error and some suggestions for minimising them under the headings Clinical environment, Procedure, Equipment, Practitioner and Patient. It should be appreciated that comments made under clinical environment and procedure are general points and not specifically aimed at the papers under discussion.

### Vascular measurement

Dorsalis pedis and posterior tibial pulses are traditionally palpated to evaluate the blood supply to the foot. An investigation of observer variation in assessment of dorsalis pedis and posterior tibial pulses by palpation and Doppler ultrasound was conducted (Magee et al 1992). The study concluded that palpation of pedal pulses in patients with arterial disease is subject to substantial error.

A consultant, registrar, senior house officer and a nurse measured 33 claudicants and five controls. Following palpation of the claudicants' pulses all observers agreed on the presence of a dorsalis pedis pulse in 67% of limbs, and the presence of the posterior tibial in 53% of limbs. In contrast, with Doppler ultrasound, all observers agreed on the presence of a dorsalis pedis pulse in 58% of limbs, and the presence of a posterior tibial pulse in 78% of limbs. The poor reliability of these measurement procedures has obvious clinical implications and warrant consideration.

**The clinical environment.** Temperature and background noise levels must be controlled to reduce the potential for error. High and low temperatures alter peripheral resistance, affecting the validity of the measurements.

**The procedure.** Standardised procedures for each measurement should be followed. The subject's acclimatisation time before measurements are taken is particularly important. Subjective decisions by observers involved in location of pulses with fingertips and use of the Doppler probe are difficult to standardise.

**The equipment.** Noise and artifacts caused by movement of the Doppler probe could lead to error because of distortion of the audio spectrum. Systems which can provide a permanent visual record of the vascular flow waveform would permit identification of artifacts, thus reducing the potential for error in interpretation. If different Doppler units were used, even of the same make and model, there could be differences in the results they produce.

**The practitioner(s).** More experienced observers may be more skilful and better able to locate weak pulses. There may be differences in sensitivity in the fingertips between observers. Angulation of the Doppler probe over the dorsalis pedis vessel is technically difficult due to the vessel's anatomical site. There is a tendency for the probe to lose contact with the skin and coupling gel as the probe is brought to the appropriate angle. This could cause differences in detection of the pulse between observers. The amplitude of the signal depends on the probe-to-vessel angle. Using probes with preset angles may reduce this source of error.

**The patient.** Anatomical variations, blood vessel abnormalities and oedema could cause variation in results between examiners.

## Goniometric measurement

Goniometric measurement of the subtalar joint has been shown to be unreliable by many re-searchers. Accuracy, repeatability and reliability have been shown to vary with the joint measured and the technique used. A particular difficulty involves alignment of conventional mechanical goniometers to the plane of joint motion and to the joint axis. However, the need for subjective alignment of an instrument is thought to be eliminated with flexible electrogoniometers.

A study using flexible goniometers investigated the effects of patient position, measurement method, active and passive measured motion and symmetry between the left and right foot on subtalar joint measurements (Ball & Johnson 1993). The results showed an *interobserver* variation of up to 7° for the subtalar joint neutral position. The *intraobserver* variation was only 2.5°. The influences of measurement method and patient position produced statistically significant differences between measurements. Reliability of measurement of the range of joint motion improved when measurement started from a resting subtalar joint position rather than from a point determined by palpation of talonavicular congruency.

**The clinical environment.** This should be conducive to the measurements required.

**The procedure.** The study demonstrated that different measurement methods produce significantly different results. Consequently techniques are not interchangeable and patients must be measured by the same method on each occasion. Previous research supports this finding. There is a difference of 52° between the mean ranges of subtalar joint motion when the results of Viitasalo & Kvist (1983) and Alexander et al (1982) are compared. Interobserver reliability of measurement of the subtalar joint neutral position was poor. But intraobserver reliability was clinically acceptable. Interobserver determination of the neutral position by palpation of the talar head was also shown to be unreliable.

**The equipment.** The flexible electrogoniometer is known to be accurate, reliable and easy to use. However, the clinical application of the instrument allows errors to occur. Changes in standardisation of the measurement procedure should consider attempts to control the application of force when joints are manipulated and to prescribe a readily defined starting point before measurement commences.

**The practitioner(s).** Although the methods used were well defined it is difficult to standardise some subjective determinations. There could be subtle differences in positioning patients and differences in the amount of force used have already been mentioned. Differences were found between left and right inversion and eversion ratios, suggesting that observers are biased in the determination of measurements.

**The patient.** If patients are not able to relax completely the measured range of motion may be reduced because of muscle tone. It is also possible that repetition in movement of a joint through its full range could affect the repeatability of results. If periarticular structures become stretched greater ranges of motion might be possible.

## Conclusion

The exercise above has identified problems associated with clinical observations that are measured by many practitioners on a daily basis. Some suggestions of changes to the measurement techniques have been suggested which hopefully would reduce the margins of error.

Measurement of clinical observations is an essential part of clinical practice, but it is not a simple step-by-step process. The knowledge provided by research leads to continual improvements in standardisation of techniques and advancements in instrumentation. It is important that practitioners develop a scientific and systematic approach to clinical measurements and appreciate the value and limitations of their measurements. It is only by the diligent appli-

cation of measurement techniques that the body of scientific knowledge will increase and further improvements in the standards of clinical practice will occur.

## SUMMARY

Measurement may be conceptualised as being quantitative or qualitative in nature or a mixture of both. Data may be considered to have ordinal, nominal or graded (scores) properties which provide variable conclusions about the data collected from measurement. This chapter has attempted to highlight a number of the many pitfalls for the unwary which may lead to significant error. Ongoing research has identified many of the causes of error in measurement, particularly those associated with the subjective application of techniques to simple as well as sophisticated techniques. Error in measurement is affected by many influencing factors. Compensation for error is possible up to a point.

When using any sophisticated equipment it is essential that it is applicable to the purpose required, is calibrated and has known tolerances of error that can be accounted for. The terms 'validity', 'specificity', 'reliability' and 'repeatability' contribute to a better understanding from any type of equipment used. Results can be affected by different observers and therefore strict protocols in practice are essential to obtain the most helpful information.

The practitioner must therefore attempt, using the type of knowledge highlighted in this chapter, to minimise the potential for poor data collection and erroneous interpretation which could lead to false results.

## REFERENCES

Alexander R E, Battye C K, Goodwill C J, Walsh J B 1982 The ankle and subtalar joints 8: 703–711

Ball P, Johnson G R 1993 Reliability of hindfoot goniometry when using a flexible electrogoniometer. Clinical Biomechanics 8: 13–19

Boone D C, Stanley P A, Lin C M, Spence C, Baron C, Lee L 1978 Reliability of goniometric measurements. Physical Therapy 58: 1355–1360

Bovens A M P M, van Baak M A, Vrencken J G P M, Wijnen J A G, Verstappen F T J 1990 Variability and reliability of joint measurements. American Orthopaedic Society for Sports Medicine 18: 58–63

Bowling A 1991 Measuring health: a review of quality life measurement scales. Open University Press, Buckingham

Calnan J S 1989 Handling the original idea. In: Mathie R T, Taylor K M, Calnan J S (eds) Surgical research. Butterworth, London, p 14

Dainty D, Gagnon M, Lagasse P, Norman R, Robertson G, Sprigins 1987 Recommended procedures. In: Dainty & Norman (eds) Standardizing biomechanical testing in sport. Human Kinetics Publishers, Champaign, IL, p 87

Diamond J E, Mueller M J, Delitto A, Sinacore D R 1989 Reliability of a diabetic foot examination. Physical Therapy 69: 797–802

Drysdale J 1989 An investigation into the measurement of vibratory thresholds in the lower limb of normal subjects using the biothesiometer. Project report No 89/37. University of Westminster, London

Griffith C J 1988 An investigation of the repeatability, reliability and validity of clinical biomechanical measurements in the region of the foot and ankle. Project report No 88/25. University of Westminster, London

Hawes M R, Nachbauer W, Sovak D, Nigg B M 1992 Footprint parameters as a measure of arch height. Foot and Ankle 13: 22–26

Hughes J, Pratt L, Linge K, Clark P, Klenerman L 1991 Reliability of pressure measurements: the EMED F system. Clinical Biomechanics 6: 14–18

Johnson K W, Kassam M S 1985 Processing Doppler signals and analysis of peripheral arterial waveforms: problems and solutions. In: Bernstein E F (ed) Non invasive diagnostic techniques in vascular disease, 3rd edn. C V Mosby, St Louis, ch 7, p 55

Magee T R, Stanley P R, al Mufti R, Simpson L, Campell W B 1992 Should we palpate foot pulses? Annals of the Royal College of Surgeons of England 74: 166–168

Mooney J, 1987 A project to assess touch/pressure sensitivity of the sole of the normal, healthy, adult foot, using Semmes–Weinstein filaments. ACTUK Journal Spring: 7–9

Viitsalo J T, Kvist M, 1983 Some aspects of the foot and ankle in athletes with and without shin splints. American Journal of Sports Medicine 11: 125–130

Wade D T 1992 Measurement in neurological rehabilitation. Oxford Medical Publications, New York, p 20

## FURTHER READING

Edwards C R W 1990 The history and general principles governing physical examination. In: Munro J S, Edwards C R W (eds) Macleod's clinical examination. Churchill Livingstone, p 11

Munro J S, Edwards C R W 1990 McLeod's clinical examination. Churchill Livingstone, Edinburgh

Tollafield D R 1990 A reusable transducer system for measuring foot pressures. A study of reliability in a commercial pressure pad. Department of Health and Life Sciences, Coventry Polytechnic, Coventry, p 31–48

# Systems examination

# 5

# Medical and social history

*T. E. Kilmartin*

## INTRODUCTION

A patient's medical history, family history and current medication have a number of implications for the diagnosis and management of lower limb problems. Conditions affecting the lower limb may be caused by, or have implications for, the patient's general health and well being. Choice of treatment will be influenced by the patient's current health status, family and previous medical history. The medical and social history is concerned with the patient as a whole and not just the lower limb complaint with which the patient has presented. The approach outlined in this chapter forms the basis of a holistic approach to patient care.

## The purpose of the medical and social history assessment

History taking is as important as any diagnostic test or physical examination. Diseases or abnormalities of the lower limb often present with a history of signs and symptoms which can be recognised by the practitioner as a single diagnostic entity. Once a history has been taken, physical examination and diagnostic tests can then be employed to confirm the diagnosis and stage the severity of the condition. An example of a clinical diagnosis which can be obtained through history taking is Sever's disease of the heel, a common 'growing pain'. It will affect one or both heels just as the child approaches puberty. The onset of pain is abrupt; it is rarely provoked by any single incidence of trauma. Sever's disease is usually aggravated by field sports and relieved by rest and resolves with skeletal maturity. Recording the patient's age, site of discomfort and factors which aggravate and relieve the condition will in most cases suggest a diagnosis of Sever's disease. Diagnosis can then be confirmed by physical examination.

Comprehensive history taking helps the practitioner to formulate a diagnosis and develop and implement an effective management plan. An inadequate history of the patient's current medication and past and present health status may have the following consequences.

**1. The patient is placed at risk.** Performing nail surgery on a patient with a prosthetic joint may produce a bacteraemia which could infect and then loosen the joint replacement. Bacteraemia in patients with a history of infective endocarditis or rheumatic valvular disease may lead to bacterial growth on the previously damaged heart valves or endocardium (Anderson et al 1986). Invasive or operative treatment on haemophiliacs or patients taking anticoagulant therapy requires special consideration because of the likelihood of very slow blood clotting which could lead to severe blood loss.

Inadequate knowledge of the patient's existing medication could lead to adverse reactions with newly prescribed drugs. If drugs are prescribed in the absence of a detailed medical history an existing condition may be exacerbated. For example asthma attacks may be precipitated by aspirin or non-steroidal anti-inflammatory drugs.

**2. The practitioner is placed at risk.** Inadequate history taking may place the practitioner at risk when handling tissue products. A history of jaundice should alert the practitioner to the possibility of hepatitis while a history of haemophilia, blood transfusion, foreign travel or intravenous drug use may place the patient and thus the practitioner at risk of the human immunodeficiency virus (HIV) and hepatitis B.

**3. Treatment may fail or cause the patient's presenting condition to worsen** because inadequate history taking has prevented accurate diagnosis of the presenting foot complaint. Swelling on the top of the foot in a 39-year-old woman, which develops after an ankle sprain, may be nothing more than inflammation-related oedema. If the practitioner finds there is also a history of cigarette smoking, use of the contraceptive pill and recent immobilisation the differential diagnosis would include deep vein thrombosis, a potentially life-threatening condition that requires quite different management to an ankle sprain.

**4. Increased risk of clinical emergencies.** Individuals may be placed at risk by certain treatments, drugs or procedures which are normally considered routine. Adequate history taking will identify those patients who have previously developed adverse reactions. Hypersensitivity reactions to dressings, e.g. zinc oxide strapping, or medicaments, e.g. iodine, monochloroacetic acid or formaldehyde, may be known to the patient and should be noted.

# THE MEDICAL HISTORY AND SYSTEMS ENQUIRY

The medical history and systems enquiry is based upon the hospital assessment or clinical clerking system (Seymour 1984). Findings recorded with this system (Table 5.1) will indicate the patient's suitability for a range of treatments as well as determining the need for further clinical or laboratory investigation. Patients may be given a health questionnaire (see Appendix, pp. 73–74) to complete prior to seeing the practitioner. The use of questionnaires gives the patient time to consider his/her answers and reduces the amount of time spent during the consultation on taking a medical history.

## THE MEDICAL HISTORY
### Current health status

Before history taking begins the practitioner will gain some impressions about the patient's current health status from simple observation. Patients should be observed as they enter the consulting room. Diseases of nerves, muscle, bone and joints may all manifest in patients' gait

**Table 5.1**  The medical history and systems enquiry

*Part 1. The medical history*
Current health status
Current and past medication
Past medical history, including hospitalisations, operations and injuries

*Part 2. Family history of disease*
Including cause of death of immediate family members

*Part 3. Personal social history*
Home situation
Occupation—nature of work, special footwear requirements
Sports and hobbies
Foreign travel

*Part 4. The systems enquiry*
Cardiovascular system
Respiratory system
Alimentary system
Genitourinary system
Central nervous system
Locomotor system
Endocrine system

or posture. For example, upper and lower motor neurone lesions may create an ataxic gait where coordination and balance are impaired. Patients with acute foot or leg pain will walk with a limp as they try to 'guard' the injured part. Patients with chronic foot disorders will shuffle rather than stride because a propulsive gait will cause more forefoot pain. Gait disorders in children are best visualised as the child walks into the room to meet the practitioner. The patient's response to the exercise of walking into the consulting room may raise suspicions about cardiovascular or respiratory disease, e.g. shortness of breath. In these instances the patient's ability to talk as they first meet the practitioner may be impaired.

The consultation should begin with a handshake as considerable information can be gleaned from this simple contact. Wasting of the thenar eminence and intrinsic musculature of the hand occurs with rheumatoid arthritis and with some genetic disorders, e.g. Friedreich's ataxia and Charcot–Marie–Tooth disease. Patients with Dupuytren's contracture will only present the thumb, index and middle finger as the condition

causes flexion contracture of the ring and fifth finger. This condition of the hand may be associated with plantar aponeurosis of the foot. Disorders of skin and nails may manifest themselves in the hand, e.g. psoriasis and eczema may cause hypertrophy and anhidrosis of the skin, pulmonary or cyanotic heart disease may cause clubbed nails.

The patient's facial appearance and expression is also of interest to the practitioner. The tense tired face of those in chronic pain will appear similar to those suffering from depression. Parkinson's disease or long-term use of psychotropic drugs, e.g. chlorpromazine hydrochloride, will reduce facial expression while the thyrotoxic patient, with characteristic protruding eyes, will be striking for their 'angry' appearance. Patients on long-term steroid therapy will develop a fat round 'moon' face. Hypothyroidism will lead to loss of hair from the outer third of the eyebrows, baldness and coarse, thickened facial skin. Acromegaly, an excess of growth hormone due to a disorder of the pituitary gland, will give rise to a heavy 'lantern' jaw. Cyanotic blue lips are a sign of poor cardiac function. Small plaques of brown lipid under the eyes, seen with hyperlipidaemia, are associated with atherosclerosis.

Obvious weight abnormalities affect the lower limb and should be noted on first meeting the patient. Obesity is associated with recalcitrant heel pain and other postural symptoms. Seriously underweight patients may be suffering from a range of systemic conditions or may simply be poorly nourished due to alcohol, drug abuse or anorexia nervosa.

As discussed in Chapter 2 open and closed questions may be used when interviewing a patient. Closed questions are useful means for gaining specific information about the patient's current and past medical history. The use of a list of closed questions ensures that the practitioner has covered all relevant areas; they also prompt the patient to think about factors that have affected his/her general health.

In general, patients who are unwell are not good candidates for involved procedures or treatments which are likely to demand close compliance on their behalf. Fatigue and weight change are symptoms of many systemic illnesses and are always worthy of note, especially if weight change appears to be rapid (Case history 5.1). The following questions will reveal important information about the patient's general health:

- Are you feeling well?
- Do you sleep well at night?
- Do you feel tired during the day?
- Is your weight stable?

---

Case history 5.1

A 23-year-oid male commercial traveller attended clinic after developing a severe tinea pedis infection. The patient's weight had recently dropped dramatically. He had put that down to the worry of paying the mortgage on his new house. His sleep was disrupted most nights on account of feeling hot and sweating profusely. Severe body itching increasingly troubled him. He wondered whether this had anything to do with his athlete's foot. The dermatophyte infection was resistant to treatment. The practitioner queried the possibility of a systemic condition.

**Diagnosis**: Hodgkin's disease characterised by night sweats, weight loss and intense pruritus. A blood analysis confirmed the diagnosis.

---

## Current and past medication

Information about the patient's current and previous drug therapy can provide useful information about the patient's health. Patients should be asked if they are currently taking or have in the past taken any tablets or medicine or used any ointments or creams that have been prescribed by their doctor. It is not uncommon for a patient to have used prescribed drugs for many years with no clear understanding as to why he/she should take them. The practitioner should refer to the British National Formulary (BNF) or MIMS if unfamiliar with the drugs the patient is taking. Patients should also be asked if they are currently taking or have in the past taken any tablets or medicine or used any ointments or creams which they have purchased from the chemist.

Large doses or prolonged use of medication can be associated with significant side effects. Prednisolone, commonly used in the treatment of asthma, will reduce skin thickness and impair wound healing. Bendrofluazide, a useful diuretic for the treatment of cardiac failure or hypertension, can cause hyperuricaemia which may result in gout. Warfarin, an oral anticoagulant used for the treatment and prophylaxis of venous thrombosis and pulmonary embolism, increases clotting time. This has obvious implications if surgical treatment is planned. Other examples of adverse reactions to drug therapy can be found in Table 5.2. The dosage of prescribed drugs generally increases as a disease becomes chronic and/or the symptoms more severe. This can be seen with conditions such as parkinsonism, rheumatoid arthritis and diabetes.

Self-prescribed medication is of interest to the practitioner not least because the quantities used may be quite variable, with the possibility of chronic overdosing. For example, repeatedly exceeding the recommended daily dosage of vitamins A and D supplements may give rise to ectopic calcification in tendon, muscle and periarticular tissue.

**Table 5.2** Adverse drug reactions and their effects on the lower limb

| Drug | Adverse reaction |
|---|---|
| Beta-adrenoceptor blockers | Coldness of extremities |
| Calcium channel blockers | Ankle oedema |
| Salbutamol | Peripheral vasodilation |
| Contraceptive pill | Increased risk of thromboembolism |
| Propranolol | Paraesthesia |
| Chloramphenicol | Peripheral neuritis |
| Metronidazole, indomethacin, colchicine | Sensorimotor neuropathy |
| ACE inhibitors | Muscle cramps |
| 4-quinolone antibiotics | Damage to epiphyseal cartilage |
| Corticosteroids | Osteoporosis, joint pains, myalgia |
| Anticoagulants | Haemarthrosis |
| Aspirin | Purpura |
| Frusemide, nalidixic acid | Bullous eruptions |

The practitioner should be alert to the possibility of a patient developing an allergy or adverse reaction to medications used during treatment. In particular, details of any adverse reactions, either by the patient or any member of the patient's family, to previous local anaesthetic injections and other drugs (e.g. penicillin) should be sought and explored. A type I hypersensitivity reaction, which leads to anaphylactic shock, is of most concern. It is not known why some individuals are predisposed to anaphylaxis, though genetic mechanisms are certainly involved since there is a strong familial disposition. In some individuals contact with certain allergens will stimulate the production of an antibody of the IgE class, which has the ability to adhere to mast cells in tissues and basophils in the circulation. When an individual sensitised in this way is exposed on a second occasion to the allergen, the allergen combines with the IgE antibodies on the surface of the mast cells. This causes immediate destruction of the mast cell, which releases its contents, specifically histamine, serotonin, platelet-activating factor and slow-reacting substance. If the exposure to the allergen is systemic, hypotension, bronchiole constriction, laryngeal oedema, swelling of the tongue, urticaria, vomiting and diarrhoea may follow.

Fatal anaphylaxis is rare. When it does occur it usually follows entrance of an antigenic drug such as penicillin to the circulation of a sensitised individual. Insect stings are also an important cause of anaphylactic fatality. Of more concern to the practitioner is the overdose of local anaesthetics, which can lead to convulsions as a result of central nervous system stimulation. This may be followed by a profound drop in blood pressure and life-threatening cardiovascular system depression. In such circumstances oxygen must be administered to support the patient. The risk of such a clinical emergency can be minimised by adhering to the maximum safe dose values for the various local anaesthetic agents and always having oxygen available. A local type I hypersensitivity reaction may be caused by local anaesthetic agents. The skin around the area of the injection shows an immediate, localised inflammatory reaction.

Use of all recreational drugs should be recorded. Amphetamines, like many mood stimulants, will have a vasoconstrictive effect. The use of injectable drugs places the patient at risk of hepatitis and HIV. Long-term or heavy use of tobacco can affect wound healing due to the immediate vasoconstrictive effect of nicotine as well as the long-term effect of increased platelet adhesiveness and atherosclerosis. Tobacco smokers are also at greater risk of bronchitis, asthma and lung cancer.

Heavy alcohol consumption can affect peripheral sensation, immune response, post-operative healing and the metabolism of local anaesthetic, as well as having implications for treatment compliance (Victor & Adams 1953). Alcohol consumption is generally measured in units. One unit of alcohol is equivalent to one glass of wine, a single measure of spirits or half a pint of beer. More than four units of alcohol per day is noteworthy. Unfortunately, it is likely that those patients abusing alcohol are least likely to be forthcoming about their alcoholism. Where alcohol abuse is suspected, questions should be asked in a permissive manner:

- Although you may not be drinking a lot now, what about in the past?
- Was there ever a time when you were drinking more heavily?
- How much did you drink in the past—10 pints of beer a day?

Start with large volumes of alcohol and the patient will volunteer to amend the volume downwards. The patient should also be asked about dry retching in the morning, as this is a symptom of alcohol withdrawal. Drinking before 10 a.m. is an important finding as it is associated with chronic alcoholism.

## Past medical history

The past medical history consists of information about previous lower limb problems and the treatment received as well as details about any problems that have affected the patient's general health. The nature of previous podiatric treatment, the name of the practitioner, details of relevant investigations such as X-rays and the patient's view of the treatment success should be recorded. This information may prevent the repetition of tests or treatments which have previously been ineffective.

The patient should then be asked:

- Have you ever been off work for more than a week due to illness?
- Have you ever been admitted to hospital?
- Have you ever had an operation?
- Have you ever been under the care of a consultant or a hospital specialist?

Hospital records can provide this information but they are not always available. These questions will hopefully prompt the patient into recollecting any previous incidents of illness or surgery. Questioning should follow a sequence that moves from the patient's childhood to the present. It is particularly important to uncover a history of childhood rheumatic fever, which will have implications for any procedure that may create bacteraemia. Rheumatic fever is an acute inflammatory complication of streptococcal infection. It can cause transient arthritis, carditis, subcutaneous nodules, transient chorea and erythema of the skin. The most characteristic and potentially harmful complication is carditis, which can cause stenosis—shortening and thickening of the heart valves. The roughened damaged heart valves will subsequently provide a focus for infection. Bacteraemia occurring as a result of surgical manipulation of an infected part or from a postoperative infection is a particular risk to patients with heart valve damage. Prophylactic antibiotics should be taken prior to invasive surgery.

Hospitalisations for operations or injuries should be recorded and any complications noted. In females a particularly common procedure is hysterectomy. This has implications for the lower limb in that the effect on hormone balance can lead to premature osteoporosis. This may manifest clinically as vertebral collapse leading to spinal deformity and possibly causing referred neural compression symptoms. Injuries may often appear to be unrelated to the patient's presenting complaint but it must be remem-

bered that the lower limb functions as one unit and if one component of the unit is damaged, it can lead to compensations elsewhere in the lower limb.

If a patient is still under the care of a hospital consultant it is vital that the consultant is informed prior to any treatment.

## THE FAMILY HISTORY

A pedigree chart should record details of major illnesses and lower limb problems of the immediate family (Fig. 5.1). Many cardiovascular, alimentary, neurological and endocrine disorders can be inherited. Enquiring about the medical history of the immediate family may reveal a predisposition to a range of systemic diseases, e.g. non-insulin-dependent diabetes. It can also be of value to record the cause of death of immediate family. Certain lower limb pathologies can be inherited or appear to have a familial predisposition, e.g. Friedreich's ataxia

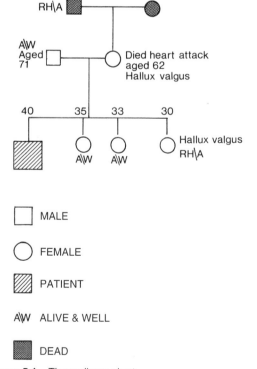

Figure 5.1  The pedigree chart.

and Charcot–Marie–Tooth disease. The diagnosis of a patient presenting with difficulties in walking will be affected by a positive family history of a condition such as these. All forms of spina bifida should be noted even if the problem has been labelled as spina bifida occulta. Impaired gait, pes cavus and plantar ulceration have been found to appear late in cases of spina bifida occulta (Anderson 1975, James et al 1962).

The ethnic origin of the patient should also be noted. Sickle cell anaemia will affect people of African or West Indian descent. Thalassaemia, another haemolytic anaemia, will affect patients from Mediterranean and South-East Asian regions.

The patient should be asked if anyone else in the family has suffered from leg or foot problems. This information will help to determine the inherited nature of any foot condition and in the case of pes cavus, hallux valgus and lesser digit deformity could indicate the degree of severity that the patient's presenting condition may eventually achieve.

## PERSONAL SOCIAL HISTORY

## Home situation

It is important to assess the patient's home situation. With some types of treatment patients are required to reduce their activity level to a minimum, change dressings or administer treatments at home. In the case of surgical treatment the practitioner must establish who is going to transport the patient to and from surgery and who is going to assist him/her through the immediate postoperative recovery period. Lack of home support may rule out certain forms of treatment.

## Occupation

A patient's occupation may be a contributory cause of the lower limb problem and may influence what treatment can be given (Case history 5.2). Some patients may experience particular difficulties in taking time from work to attend for treatment. The nature of the work

---

| Case history 5.2 |
| --- |

A male patient serviced amusement arcade betting machines. Over a 4-month period he had been suffering from increasing pain in his right foot. The pain was present every day during work but never occurred on rest days. The patient described the pain as radiating from the ball of his foot into his third and fourth toes. The pain was quite intense, sometimes nauseating, but could be relieved by removing his shoes and massaging his foot. He could not remember injuring his foot and found that changing his shoes had no effect. The pain would develop soon after starting work each day and become progressively worse throughout the day. The location and type of pain described was consistent with Morton's neuroma. But why should it affect him only at work? Closer questioning about the nature of his job revealed that as part of his job he had to collect money from a tray which was placed at waist height in the machine. To empty this tray the patient had to squat down on his toes.

**Diagnosis**: plantar foot strain related to the squatting position placing a stretch on the plantar structures of the foot. Stretching of the medial plantar nerve is thought to be a significant factor in the pathology of Morton's neuroma. A sitting position for emptying the machine was recommended and the pain completely abated with no further treatment.

---

should be determined and special footwear requirements should be noted. The types of surface that the patient stands and walks on during the day can be exciting factors. Bare concrete floors will exacerbate chilblains while patients whose occupation involves standing on ladders will often suffer from chronic medial longitudinal arch pain. If an occupationally related injury has occurred the practitioner should ask if any litigation is planned, as a full assessment report may be required by the patient's solicitor.

## Sports and hobbies

Active sportspeople may make the association between their sport and lower limb problem. Those who participate in occasional sporting activities and hobbies may not. Patients who participate in infrequent sporting activities may not think to inform the practitioner of these activities. However, these patients are often more prone to injury because they are not fit and do not follow a warm-up and warm-down regime. These patients are more likely to develop hamstring or calf muscle injury due to poor flexibility. Details of any sporting hobby should, therefore, be sought from the patient. The assessment of the sports injury patient is considered in detail in Chapter 15.

## Foreign travel

Details of foreign travel should be recorded in case the patient has acquired an infection. In particular, travel to tropical countries and any foot injuries sustained while walking barefoot should be recorded (Case history 5.3).

---

**Case history 5.3**

A 47-year-old male geography teacher presented with a large malodorous ulcer under his first metatarsophalangeal joint. History revealed that he had been treated in the Gambia, West Africa for schistosomiasis infection. While in Africa the condition had been nothing more than an itchy area on the plantar surface of his foot. On returning to England, however, he had been hospitalised for hepatic cirrhosis. His health had remained poor since. Examination of the lower limb revealed a sensory neuropathy affecting both legs. Blood tests were negative for diabetes.
  **Diagnosis**: suspected central nervous system damage due to parasitic invasion of the lower spinal cord, confirmed by analysis of cerebrospinal fluid which showed the presence of *Schistosoma japonicum*. Despite further antiparasitic drug therapy, the patient's condition continued to deteriorate with increasing motor neuropathy leading to gait ataxia.

---

## THE SYSTEMS ENQUIRY

The systems enquiry seeks to unearth any signs and symptoms which the patient has not complained of spontaneously and discover if there are any systemic conditions that may affect the patient's lower limb problem. All the body systems are worked through in a set order which can be remembered using the mnemonic 'GCRAGCLE' (Table 5.1). The systems enquiry involves asking questions that will seem, to the patient, to be quite unrelated to the lower limb problem. It is important, before the enquiry

begins, that patients are advised that the purpose of the questions is to ensure that there are no general health problems that may be causing the lower limb condition or that may influence the type of treatment considered. The first rule of any therapeutic intervention must be 'first do no harm'; the systems enquiry will help achieve this objective.

The systems enquiry may reveal significant symptomatology which the practitioner is inexperienced or unqualified to diagnose. In such circumstances the patient should be informed that a second opinion is recommended. The subsequent referral for a second opinion should be seen as part of the patient's overall treatment plan.

## Cardiovascular system

The status of the cardiovascular system has implications for foot health (Case history 5.4). To determine the presence of cardiac failure the patient should be asked:

- Are you suffering from shortness of breath?
- Are you bothered by chest or upper arm pain or palpitations?
- Do your ankles swell?

---

**Case history 5.4**

A 65-year-old female patient attended a podiatry clinic complaining of weak muscles in her legs. She had noticed the weakness for some time, complaining that if it continued to deteriorate she would have to give up her job as a school playground supervisor. Further questioning revealed that her weakness could be more accurately described as fatigue and heaviness of her legs after walking to and from work. The patient had also noticed that climbing stairs at school brought on a tight squeezing pain in her chest. She could relieve the pain by sitting down, but sitting was something she wished to avoid as it made her ankles swell.
  **Diagnosis**: congestive heart failure which can have a direct effect upon the ability of muscles to function under strain.

---

Shortness of breath may occur as a result of pulmonary oedema. In heart failure myocardial contraction becomes inadequate. To maintain a normal volume of cardiac output, first the heart rate and then the volume of blood filling the left ventricle increases. Because it takes longer to fill the left ventricle the pressure in the whole cardiac pulmonary system 'backs up', causing pulmonary congestion, reduced blood gas exchange and eventually pulmonary oedema. Pulmonary oedema and shortness of breath are, therefore, signs and symptoms of left-sided heart failure.

Right-sided heart failure is almost always associated with left-sided heart failure and gives rise to peripheral oedema. The right side of the heart can no longer deal with the volume of venous blood returning to the heart for transportation to the lungs and a similar 'back up' of pressure occurs in the systemic circulation resulting in transudation of fluid into the peripheral connective tissue. Gravity will force most of the transudate to collect in the feet and ankles. Initially the patient will notice that the swelling reduces at night when the legs are recumbent. In chronic right-sided heart failure the peripheral oedema will eventually be infiltrated by fibrous tissue that cannot be reduced.

Chest pain may originate from the heart, aorta, lungs, oesophagus or chest wall. Cardiac ischaemia can cause anything from the substernal chest pain of angina, which is precipitated by effort and relieved by rest, to the more generalised chest pain of myocardial infarction which will occur at rest and leave the patient pale, anxious and sweating profusely. This is a clinical emergency which requires immediate medical treatment. The pain of angina, on the other hand, can often be controlled by simply avoiding excessive exercise. Angina occurs as a result of atherosclerosis of the arteries to the myocardium and often coexists with atherosclerosis of the arteries to the lower limb.

While cardiac problems may affect lower limb perfusion, peripheral vascular disease can occur in the absence of cardiac symptoms. Assessment of the vascular status of the lower limb is covered in detail in Chapter 6.

Hypertension may be suspected if there is a history of dizziness, flushed face, headache, fatigue and nose bleeds. An increase in blood pressure will be asymptomatic until the condition has been present long enough to cause complications. About 25% of the estimated population of hypertensives do not realise they have the condition and will only become aware when they develop symptoms (transient ischaemic attacks) or routine screening discovers a diastolic blood pressure above 90 mmHg. An untreated hypertensive is at great risk of suffering left ventricular failure, myocardial infarction, cerebral vascular accident or renal failure. Practitioners should routinely take their patients' blood pressure, not least because the stress caused by treatment or examination may provoke a clinical emergency in an uncontrolled hypertensive.

While the general enquiry may have already revealed sleeping problems, the cardiovascular system investigation should determine whether sleep is disturbed by the shortness of breath associated with congestive heart failure or by cramp pain in the legs. Nocturnal cramps are a consequence of increased permeability of the microcirculation accompanying the warming of the legs under bedding. In the presence of any impairment of the venous system, toxic metabolites will accumulate, increasing carbon dioxide tension while lowering oxygen levels. Muscle ischaemia follows, manifesting as a painful tautness of muscle fibre.

Haematological disorders should be considered. Anaemia occurs when red blood cells or haemoglobin content decreases because of blood loss, impaired production or destruction of red blood cells. Tissue hypoxia results from anaemia and this in turn leads to cardiovascular and pulmonary compensations. Clinical symptoms depend upon the severity and duration of the anaemia. Severe anaemia is associated with weakness, vertigo, headaches, tiredness, gastrointestinal complaints and congestive heart failure.

Sickle cell disease affects those of African or West Indian descent. It is an inherited condition. Those who inherit the gene from both patients have more than a 75% chance of developing the condition. Sickle cell individuals are prone to ulceration around the malleoli, a complaint more characteristic of older people with venous insufficiency. In most cases patients will know whether they have sickle cell anaemia as from early childhood the digits of the hands and feet tend to swell and be very painful. The use of tourniquets is contraindicated. A tourniquet causes relative anoxia and this in turn causes occlusion in small vessels due to changes in the haemodynamic qualities of red blood cells. This may lead to small vessel infarction and possibly digital gangrene.

## Respiratory system

The respiratory system history should cover the following areas:

### 1. Chest pain related to breathing or exercise

Respiratory illness associated with pulmonary inflammation and pressure on the pleural surfaces will lead to chest pain. The pleura (the serous membrane covering of the lungs and thoracic cavity) is richly endowed with sensory nerve endings. Stimulation of these nerves will cause a knife-like pain which is intensified by deep breathing. Pulmonary hypertension and infection are commonly associated with such chest pain.

### 2. Shortness of breath

Dyspnoea or the subjective sensation of feeling breathless is one of the most common symptoms of respiratory disease. Table 5.3 indicates the causes of dyspnoea and the clinical implications.

### 3. Cough

Coughing is a protective mechanism employed to clear foreign material or mucus. The causes of coughing can be:

- mechanical, e.g. inhalation of dust
- inflammatory, e.g. mucous membrane oedema
- non-pulmonary, e.g. pulmonary embolism or transudate of fluid into the lung
- malignancy, e.g. dry cough
- drug-induced, e.g. ACE inhibitors.

Coughing may also be associated with the other major symptoms of respiratory illness, including:

- sputum production, a pulmonary secretion which can be infected in pneumonia and bronchitis; the sputum will have an offensive odour
- wheezing which occurs when a bronchiole is obstructed
- haemoptysis—the coughing up of bloody sputum is always considered an abnormal finding. It may result from a bacterial bronchitis. Massive haemoptysis is a life-threatening condition which follows pulmonary neoplasm, mitral stenosis, pulmonary hypertension or tuberculosis (Case history 5.5).

**Table 5.3** The clinical features and implications of respiratory diseases

| Disease | Clinical features | Clinical implications |
|---|---|---|
| Asthma | Dyspnoea, wheezing, cough | Attacks may be provoked by exercise, infection or stress. May be treated with long-term corticosteroid therapy |
| Chronic bronchitis | Cough with expectoration of sputum for at least 3 months in two successive years | Commonly a history of cigarette smoking carries an accompanying risk of peripheral atherosclerosis |
| Emphysema | Dyspnoea with varying degrees of exertion | Sufferer will have limited exercise potential; in time will lead to right-sided heart failure and peripheral oedema |
| Pulmonary embolism | Pleuritic chest pain and haemoptysis | A life-threatening condition which may follow prolonged postoperative bed rest |

Case history 5.5

A 46-year-old male presented with poor hygiene and ulcers on his toes. The ulcers arose from neglected chilblains. Social history revealed that he had been homeless since losing his job 3 years previously. A cough of 2 months' duration was noted. The sputum showed a yellow expectorate tinged with blood, indicating haemoptysis. This occurred several times daily.

**Diagnosis**: tuberculosis—a chest X-ray revealed a number of calcified granulomas and a small cavity consistent with tuberculosis infection.

## 4. Others

Past history of respiratory illness should be obtained after recording details of any existing complaints. Social and environmental history may also be relevant. The patient should be asked:

- Have you ever had asthma or an allergy to any airborne substances like house dust or pollen?
- Do you use any chemicals at work?
- Are you exposed to chemical vapours?
- Do you live or work with people who smoke cigarettes?

# Alimentary system

Gastrointestinal disorders are extremely common and have many implications for the lower limb and its treatment. Dental disease presents a bacteraemic risk, gastric ulcers will contraindicate non-steroidal anti-inflammatory drugs (NSAIDs) and analgesic preparations, while liver disease will impair metabolism and safe denaturation of many drugs, including local anaesthetics.

The enquiry should start with questions about the mouth and then progress to the stomach, intestines and bowel. The patient should be asked if he/she is currently suffering from toothache or gum disease. This question will establish the presence of any potential nidus of infection in the oral cavity. Information about previous dental care may reveal that the patient

has to take antibiotics before undergoing dental treatment. Patients who have prosthetic implants (e.g. hip or knee replacements) will also require prophylactic antibiotics prior to surgery.

A known side effect of the NSAID class of drugs is gastrointestinal irritation. This is significant when these drugs are used for prolonged periods. While the majority of people will suffer occasional indigestion, a history of dyspepsia provoked by small doses of alcohol or analgesics will indicate gastrointestinal sensitivity.

The character of the abdominal pain, its location, precipitating factors and pain radiation should be considered. The pain from gastritis is burning or gnawing in character and is localised to the epigastrium but may radiate to the back. Gastritis pain is precipitated by ingestion of alcohol, aspirin or fasting for long periods. Food consumption will rapidly relieve the pain. Chronic gastritis will eventually progress to peptic ulcerative disease. Pain arising from the biliary tract leads to a full or cramping sensation in the upper quadrant just behind the right rib cage. It will occasionally radiate to the right shoulder, will not be relieved by ingestion of food, and may be exacerbated by the ingestion of fatty food.

The commoner forms of liver disease are rarely accompanied by specific abdominal pain, although in most hepatic conditions the liver may be tender and enlarged on examination. A history of jaundice is common with most liver diseases. Jaundice is a syndrome characterised by deposition of yellow bile pigment in the skin, conjunctivae, mucous membranes and urine (Ch. 13). Liver disease is significant when the use of amide local anaesthetics (e.g. prilocaine, mepivacaine, bupivacaine) is being considered. If the liver is damaged and its function impaired by cirrhosis, first-pass metabolism will not operate effectively. First-pass metabolism refers to the removal of drugs from the portal circulation and their subsequent metabolism in the liver. Lignocaine, propranolol and morphine are all dealt with by first-pass metabolism. If first-pass metabolism is impeded an increase in circulating concentrations of the drug will follow. The maximum safe dose that can be administered will have to be reduced in these cases.

Chronic alcohol abuse can also increase the activity of the liver's mixed function oxidase enzymes which are responsible for the metabolism of drugs such as paracetamol, warfarin, barbiturates and benzodiazepines. This increase in enzyme activity and drug metabolism will significantly reduce the therapeutic effect of these drugs. Combined alcohol and drug ingestion, however, will have the immediate effect of enhancing the therapeutic effect of oral hypoglycaemics, benzodiazepines and tricyclic antidepressants. This could produce potentially life-threatening effects.

A history of regular nausea, vomiting or dysphagia (difficulty in swallowing) will always demand an explanation. These clinical features may be due to central nervous system problems (e.g. intracranial tumours, meningitis), endocrine disorders (e.g. myxoedema, diabetic ketoacidosis) or systemic or gastrointestinal tract infections. Constipation and diarrhoea are common complaints that are usually benign and self-limiting. Where there is an underlying disease the problem is usually accompanied by fever, severe pain and blood loss. Although not specifically relevant to the lower limb, a history of altered bowel habit is important when making an assessment of the patient's general health and can influence the type of drugs which may be used.

## Genitourinary system

The kidneys regulate the body's electrolyte and fluid balance. This has implications for lower limb circulation and oedema and can delay wound healing. For example, polyuria (excessive urination) is associated with diabetes, cardiac failure or cortisol deficiency, all of which will affect healing.

Patients should be asked if they have any problems with their kidneys or 'waterworks'. The practitioner should point to the renal angle (Fig. 5.2) and ask the patient if he/she suffers from pain in the small of the back. Renal pain is a symptom of gross structural disease of the kidney such as kidney stones or a blood clot

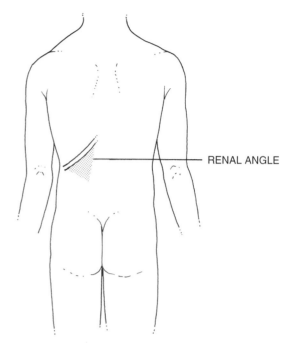

**Figure 5.2** The renal angle.

passing down the ureter. Infection or malignancy may also cause pain in the area of the renal angle as well as more anteriorly in the abdomen. Leg and ankle swelling is an important finding, which may be related to kidney disease and indeed could be the first clinical sign of a renal problem. Renal dysfunction that leads to a massive loss of protein into the urine will disrupt normal capillary haemodynamics, causing reduced transudation of fluid. Fluid will pool in the tissues rather than returning back into the capillary circulation. Oedema of the dependent limb will result, particularly around the ankles. However, it should be remembered that renal dysfunction is not the only cause of ankle oedema (see Ch. 17). Breathlessness on exertion, weight loss, nausea and vomiting also occur in renal failure and may further confuse the clinical picture. A symptom that is renal-specific is disturbed micturition. Frequency of urination is dependent upon fluid intake and specific drugs within food and drink. Most people urinate 4–6 times every 24 hours, mostly in the daytime. Table 5.4 lists the causes of abnormal micturition.

**Table 5.4** Causes of abnormal micturition

| Abnormality | Definition | Causes |
|---|---|---|
| Polyuria | Frequent micturition | Diabetes mellitus, diminution in bladder's effective filling capacity due to infection, foreign bodies, stones or tumour |
| Dysuria | Painful urination | Irritation and inflammation of bladder or urethra usually due to bacterial infection |
| Nocturia | Urination during the night | May reflect early renal disease. Decrease in concentrating capacity may be associated with cardiac or hepatic failure |
| Oliguria | Straining, decrease in force and calibre of urinary stream | Obstruction distal to the bladder. In men most commonly due to prostatic obstruction |
| Haematuria | Blood in urine | Haematuria without pain: renal or prostatic disease, bladder or kidney tumour. With pain: ureteral stone or bladder infection |

The patient should be asked if he/she experiences any pain or problems passing water and whether his/her sleep is disturbed by the need to pass water. A positive response to these questions requires further investigation as the kidneys may affect bone metabolism as well as blood pressure and water regulation (Case history 5.6)

---

**Case history 5.6**

A head waiter presented with a dull aching in his feet. He also had pain elsewhere, notably in his back and hands. His prime concern was his feet as he found it increasingly difficult to stand for long periods of time. Routine history revealed that he had been troubled, on at least three occasions, by kidney stones, making micturition difficult. Urine showed signs of haematuria. He had to strain to pass small volumes of water. Intense pain in the small of his back accompanied urination. Both problems resolved once the stone was passed. Physical examination was unremarkable.
  **Diagnosis**: Hyperparathyroidism—evidence from bilateral dorsoplantar X-rays showed coarsening (rotten gate sign) and a reduction in the number of trabeculae plus the resorption of the superficial layers of the cortex of his phalanges, indicating hyperparathyroidism.

---

*Sexually transmitted infections*

Reiter's disease, gonorrhoea, HIV and syphilis are all sexually transmitted infections. Practitioners investigating a lower limb complaint may find it difficult to enquire about sexually related problems. However, as these conditions can lead to an array of lower limb symptoms questions about them must be included in the systems enquiry (Table 5.5). After enquiring about the urinary system, the patient should be asked if he/she has ever had any sexually transmitted infections, skin problems or discharge.

# Central nervous system

Diseases of the nervous system may cause pain in the lower limb, deformity or gait abnormalities. Comprehensive history taking is essential

**Table 5.5** Lower limb signs and symptoms associated with sexually transmitted diseases

| Disease | Lower limb signs and symptoms |
|---|---|
| Reiter's | Asymmetric arthralgia of hip, knee, ankle and metatarsophalangeal joint. 'Sausage toe'. Keratoderma blenhorragica |
| HIV | Kaposi's sarcoma—a widespread skin or mucous membrane lesion appearing as a pink or red macule or violaceous plaques and nodules on the face, trunk and limbs. May appear wart-like |
| Gonococcal arthritis | Acute joint pain, swelling and stiffness. Usually accompanied by urethritis, dysuria and haemorrhagic vesicular skin lesions. Serious joint damage may result if the condition is not properly treated |

(Case history 5.7). Record details of injuries to the spine or head and family history of epilepsy or neuromuscular disease. The patient should be asked:

- Do you ever get shooting pains in your arms or legs?
- Do your hands or feet ever go numb?
- Have you ever noticed any weakness or sluggishness of your arms or legs?

---

**Case history 5.7**

An obese 50-year-old female complained of paraesthesia in the heel and arch of her right foot. The practitioner considered that her problem was weight-related and advised her to consult a dietician. Ultrasound therapy was administered to the heel. Although the practitioner had recorded that the patient had long-standing back problems, the history taking had failed to uncover that degenerative joint disease of her lumbosacral spine had led to chronic sciatica.
  **Diagnosis**: suspected proximal nerve impingement. The patient was referred to a rheumatologist.

---

Numbness and paraesthesia, loss of muscle bulk or weakness are significant findings. If the patient's response is positive, peripheral neuro-

**Table 5.6**  Causes of peripheral neuropathy

Nerve root compression of the sciatic or femoral nerve arising from L45, S123 and T12, L1234 respectively

Distal nerve compression of the popliteal, common peroneal and anterior tibial nerve

Hereditary neurological disease—Charcot–Marie–Tooth disease, Friedreich's ataxia

Endocrine—diabetes mellitus, hypothyroidism, hypocalcaemia

Chronic alcohol abuse

Nutritional disorders—pernicious anaemia, thiamine or vitamin $B_6$ deficiencies

Renal failure

Systemic disorders—rheumatoid arthritis, systemic lupus erythematosus, vasculitis, sarcoidosis, amyloidosis

Infections—tuberculosis, AIDS, leprosy, syphilis

Tumour—bronchogenic carcinoma, myeloma, lymphoma

Toxic agents—carbon monoxide, solvents, industrial poisons, lead

Medication—isoniazid, metronidazole, nitrofurantoin

pathy, which can result from a range of causes, should be considered (Table 5.6). It is essential to establish the course of the symptoms and consider them in the light of the patient's age. Slow progressive weakness of the limbs over a period of many years in a young person may point to muscular dystrophy whereas a more acute onset may indicate a demyelinating disorder or spinal cord compression (Case history 5.8). Neurological assessment of the lower limb is covered in detail in Chapter 7.

---

**Case history 5.8**

A 40-year-old policeman presented with weakness in his legs. History revealed that the weakness occurred intermittently, was sometimes particularly severe and was not related to exercise or activity. Further questioning revealed that 10 years earlier the patient had suffered from blurred vision in his right eye and some years previous to that he had suffered transient bouts of tingling in his left arm. He had not received an opinion on either of these neurological symptoms because he was concerned that it might affect his job prospects. The practitioner suspected that the patient's symptoms were related to a progressive central nervous system disease.
  **Diagnosis**: multiple sclerosis. The varied neurological signs and symptoms with obvious remissions and exacerbations were thought to be consistent with disseminated demyelinisation of the brain and spinal cord.

---

General neurological symptoms may be significant. The patient should be asked if he/she suffers from frequent headaches. While stress-related headaches, migraine and extracranial causes such as cervical spondylosis account for the majority of headaches, cranial arteritis is an important cause in the elderly. Brain tumour (slow onset) and subarachnoid bleeding (sudden onset) must be considered in severe headaches. Differential diagnosis can be arrived at from the clinical features of headaches (Table 5.7). Fainting, dizziness and visual disturbance may occur in association with headaches. The basis for most fainting episodes is inadequate blood supply to the brain and is commonly cardiac or cerebrovascular in origin. Anaemia, hypoglycaemia and emotional stress can also explain a temporary loss of consciousness.

**Table 5.7**  Causes of headaches and their associated clinical features

| Headache type | Location | Clinical features | Associated symptoms |
| --- | --- | --- | --- |
| Migraine | Forehead | Throbbing or dull ache, preceded by visual aura | Nausea, weakness or paraesthesia |
| Stress-related | Generalised or behind the eyebrows | Occurs in later afternoon, relieved by analgesics | Anxiety |
| Cranial arteritis | Deep within the head | Aching or burning occurs in the elderly | Loss of vision |
| Subarachnoid bleeding | Generalised | Intense pain, sudden onset | Stiffness of neck |
| Brain tumour | Variable | Variable frequency and intensity | Mood change, projectile vomiting |

The significance of some symptoms in the neurological enquiry will be very difficult to interpret because the enquiry relies on the patient's subjective account. However, inadequate assessment of the neurological basis of foot pathology can lead to inappropriate treatment through missed diagnosis (Case history 5.9).

## Locomotor system

The patient's account of spine or lower limb pain involving areas other than that of the presenting complaint should be obtained. The patient should be asked:

- Do you suffer from back, hip, knee, ankle or foot pain?
- Have you broken any bones in your legs or feet?
- Have you ever pulled or injured muscles in your legs?
- Do any of your joints swell or feel stiff?
- Do you experience pain during any specific activity?

The aim of the locomotor enquiry is to broaden the practitioner's outlook beyond the specific presenting complaint to a broader view of the locomotor system. Information from the locomotor enquiry will help to exclude conditions which may have a systemic origin (Case history

---

**Case history 5.9**

A 53-year-old female complained of a painful nail on her fourth toe and consequently underwent a total nail avulsion with phenolisation of the nail matrix. The pain was not resolved by the nail surgery so an excisional arthroplasty of the distal interphalangeal joint was performed as it was thought that the continued sensitivity was the result of apical weight bearing on the toe. Morton's neuroma was ruled out by traditional tests. Postoperatively the pain continued unchanged so the patient and practitioner agreed that amputation was probably the best course of action as the pain had become intractable. On amputating the digit a large neuroma was visualised at the base of the digit. Following this, her third operation, the patient reported that all the vague, shooting-type pain that used to radiate both proximally into her foot and distally into the third and fourth toes was relieved. She was no longer troubled by pressure-type sensations or numbness.
   **Diagnosis**: Morton's neuroma. The neuroma was not in the intermetatarsal space as would have been expected. It was placed more dorsally than in a typical plantar digital neuroma. Diagnosis confirmed by histopathology.

---

**Case history 5.10**

A 45-year-old female teacher presented with pain under both forefeet. She complained of feeling exhausted all the time and couldn't wait to leave school and return home to bed where she would stay until mid-evening, something that she had never done before. She described stiffness in her knees and hip joints. This was worse in the mornings but felt much better after a hot bath and an aspirin. The patient's metatarsophalangeal joints and knees were swollen. The polyarticular problems led the practitioner to suspect a systemic rather than local mechanical problem. The morning stiffness and fatigue was relieved by anti-inflammatory drugs.
   **Diagnosis**: rheumatoid arthritis. This was confirmed by a blood test which showed a raised erythrocyte sedimentation rate and rheumatoid factor.

5.10). Assessment of the locomotor system is considered in detail in Chapter 8.

## Endocrine system

Disorders of the endocrine system may be divided into those conditions which present relatively frequently and are of regular concern and those which are rare. In the assessment of the lower limb, diabetes, thyroid disease, growth disorders, obesity and problems associated with the menopause are particularly relevant. Routine questioning should begin with:

- Do you ever suffer from a thirst that you find hard to quench no matter how much you drink?
- Is your weight stable?

Diabetes is a disease of either insulin deficiency or peripheral resistance to insulin action. Insulin produced by the beta cells of the pancreas decreases blood glucose by inhibiting glycogen breakdown and facilitates entry of glucose into tissue cells. When peripheral tissues fail to utilise glucose, blood glucose levels rise and glucose is excreted in the urine. Because the body will continue to need a source of energy, homoeostasis provokes breakdown of body fat and muscle tissue. This process of 'accelerated starvation' can be quite abrupt in children, causing anorexia, nausea, coma and, if untreated, death. In older patients it is more gradual and indeed the first presenting symptom may be one of the complications of the disease.

Thirst, polyuria and weight loss are the three most common symptoms of diabetes. These three features may also occur with other conditions (Table 5.8). Although it is difficult to be precise as to what is excessive thirst, the patient is often aware that sleep is regularly disturbed by the need to urinate. A history of polyuria should always be followed up by glucose testing of the urine (Ch. 13). The thirst associated with diabetes is a result of the osmotic diuretic effect of glucose. Increased volume and frequency of urination will lead to a corresponding increase in fluid intake. While diabetics often believe that their decreasing weight is due to polyuria, it is

**Table 5.8** Causes of thirst and polyuria

| Cause | Physiological reason |
|---|---|
| Diabetes mellitus | Osmotic diuretic effect of glucose |
| Diabetes insipidus | Kidney disease prevents normal concentrating of urine or pituitary gland disorders cause a deficiency of antidiuretic hormone |
| Hypercalcaemia | Result of hyperparathyroidism where hypercalcaemia causes reversible impairment of renal concentrating mechanism |
| Hypocalcaemia | Often a side effect of diuretic therapy it leads to impaired concentrating ability in the kidney |
| Excess salt intake | Osmotic diuretic effect of increased sodium level |
| Renal failure | Normal concentrating function of kidney lost |

in fact a result of accelerated fat and protein catabolism.

The thyroid hormones tri- and tetra-iodothyronine ($T_3$ and $T_4$) are essential for normal growth and development and have many effects on body metabolism, the most obvious being to stimulate the basal metabolic rate. In thyroid disease there is either inadequate or excessive production of thyroid hormones. The clinical features of hyperthyroidism are shown in Table 5.9. Clinical features of hyperthyroidism such as muscle weakness, tachycardia, ptosis, weight loss and sleep disturbance may have already been picked up from the systems

**Table 5.9** Clinical features of hyperthyroidism

Weight loss (but appetite remains normal)
Sweating (heat Intolerance)
Fatigue
Cardiac palpitations
Irritability
Hand tremor (general restlessness)
Sleep disturbance
Generalised muscle weakness
Diarrhoea
Goitre
Bulging eyes

enquiry. Other features associated with the condition may not have been highlighted, e.g. heat intolerance, hand tremor and irritability. If hyperthyroidism is suspected the patient should be asked:

- Do you find that you cannot tolerate hot rooms or buildings?
- Have you noticed a change in your handwriting?
- Do your hands shake?
- Do your hands and feet get excessively sweaty?

Hyperthyroidism is an important systemic cause of hyperhidrosis of the feet and hands. Other lower limb signs and symptoms include infiltration of non-pitting mucinous ground substance on the anterior surface of the tibia, which causes intense itching and erythema. This so-called pretibial myxoedema (a confusing term since myxoedema suggests hypothyroidism) is more accurately described as an infiltrative dermopathy. Hyperthyroidism can cause tarsal tunnel syndrome and must be considered as a differential diagnosis for this condition, especially as the dermopathy will remain even after thyroid function is stabilised.

Inadequate levels of circulating thyroid hormone will lead to hypothyroidism. This condition may be discovered by asking the patient:

- Have you noticed any hair loss from your head or eyebrows?
- Are you troubled by dry scaly skin on your head or face?
- Have you noticed your hands or face getting puffy?
- Do you feel you have generally slowed down?
- Are you getting forgetful?
- Do you notice the cold?
- Has your weight increased?

In hypothyroidism the facial expression is dull and the features puffy with swelling around the eye sockets due to infiltration of mucopolysaccharides. The eyelids will droop due to decreased adrenergic drive and the skin and hair will be coarse and dry. The tongue may be enlarged, the voice hoarse and speech slow. Tarsal and carpal tunnel syndrome, caused by the infiltration of mucopolysaccharides, are common clinical features.

Either form of thyroid disease renders the patient a poor candidate for foot surgery because it reduces his/her ability to deal with stress. Cardiac arrhythmias or metabolic imbalance may occur in stressful situations. Screening for thyroid disease is therefore essential and the above enquiry should be included in any presurgery assessment.

Disorders of the adrenal gland should also be considered. The adrenal gland has two functionally distinct parts, the cortex and the medulla. The more important of the two, the adrenal cortex, is essential for life as it produces glucocorticoids and mineralocorticoids, which are essential for maintaining blood volume during stress. The patient should be asked:

- Do you ever feel faint or dizzy when standing up after sitting for some time?
- Have you noticed any coloured patches or streaks developing on your skin?
- Have you had any problems with increased facial hair?
- Do you bruise easily?

The adrenal cortex is susceptible to either hypo- or hyperfunction. Hypofunction or Addison's disease is an autoimmune condition; the majority of clinical features are due to deficiency in glucocorticoid and mineralocorticoid (Table 5.10). The most relevant aspect of Addison's disease is the reduction in the level of cortisol. This hormone is normally produced in response to stress. Cortisol deficiency will reduce resistance to infection and trauma.

Cushing's syndrome presents as an overproduction of glucocorticoids. High levels of cortisol increase carbohydrate production and leads to truncal obesity and development of a moon face. Purple striae or stretch marks will develop on the abdomen. An increased production of androgens may cause hirsutism (Table 5.10). Thinning of the skin and increased risk of infection are important lower limb features of Cushing's disease. Osteoporosis may occur as a

**Table 5.10** Clinical features associated with disorders of the adrenal glands

| Disorder | Clinical features |
|---|---|
| Adrenal undersecretion (e.g. Addison's disease) | *Common features:* Tiredness Generalised weakness Lethargy Anorexia Weight loss Dizziness and postural hypotension Pigmentation |
| | *Less comon features:* Hypoglycaemia Loss of body hair Depression |
| Adrenal oversecretion (Cushing's syndrome) | Truncal obesity (moon face, buffalo hump, protuberant abdomen) Thinning of skin Purple striae Excessive bruising Hirsutism Hypertension Glucose intolerance Muscle weakness and wasting, especially of proximal muscles Back pain (osteoporosis and vertebral collapse) Psychiatric disturbances |

sequel to disruption of normal kidney function. Secondary diabetes mellitus may also occur as a sequel to Cushing's disease.

Overactivity of the anterior pituitary gland will increase circulating levels of growth hormone, which results in excessive growth of feet, hands, jaw and soft tissue acromegaly (Case history 5.11). Excess growth hormone leads to glycogenesis: approximately 30% of acromegalics develop diabetes mellitus. Hypertension, due to inadequate renal clearance of phosphates, affects 30% of acromegalics. The majority of acromegalics suffer from constant headaches and joint pains.

---

**Case history 5.11**

A 40-year-old male steel worker sought the opinion of his practitioner when he began to suffer from corns on the dorsum of his fifth toe and dorsomedial aspect of his first metatarsophalangeal joint. The patient reported that he felt his industrial boots had suddenly stopped fitting him. He joked that he must be growing because his hard hat didn't feel right, neither did his heat-resistant gloves. Further questioning revealed a tendency to sweat a lot even when sitting quietly. This he believed had led to a return of teenage spots, while his wife had remarked that his facial features had become more 'rugged'. The patient also suffered from regular headaches, joint pain and pins and needles in his hands.
  **Diagnosis**: Acromegaly. A urine sample demonstrated traces of glucose and his blood pressure was elevated to 190/110 mmHg.

---

The condition, although rare, has significant foot health implications with a catalogue of signs and symptoms that will become apparent during virtually every stage of the functional enquiry.

## SUMMARY

Accurate diagnosis is the basis for effective treatment. A system for medical history taking has been presented which covers all aspects of the patient's current and past medical status (Fig. 5.3). It has been emphasised that the personal social history is as important as the medical history, since it enables an assessment to be made about aspects of the patient's lifestyle which could influence any proposed treatment. The approach outlined in this chapter will ensure that a broad range of factors are taken into consideration when making a diagnosis and drawing up a treatment plan.

**Current health status:**

Not sleeping well, appetite poor, 'nerves bad'.

**Current and past medication:**

Presently taking temazepam as required. Co-proxamol for foot pain. Uses purgatives once weekly. In past prescribed hormone replacement therapy, caused intolerable nausea and hot flushes. Also used amytal barbiturates for 2-year period. Current family doctor refused repeat prescription.

Smokes 20 per day, drinks rarely.

**Past medical history:**

'Nervous breakdown' 10 years ago after menopause. Bronchitis almost every winter requires antibiotics.

*Hospitalisations, operations, injuries*: Fell and broke wrist 2 years ago, required a plate subsequently removed. Patient now discharged from orthopaedic department.

**Family history:**

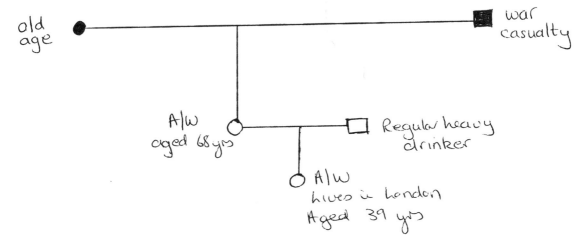

**Figure 5.3**  Specimen medical and social history and functional enquiry.

**Personal social history:**

Now retired previously factory operative—sedentary.

Lives with husband who appears to be a regular and heavy drinker. Owns terraced house. Uses public transport.

No foreign travel.

Daughter lives in London never visits. All friends have moved away few visitors.

**Systems enquiry:**

*Cardiovascular:* Chest pain only with bronchitis. Shortness of breath when walking fast or uphill. Ankles swell every day, feet always cold. No calf pain on walking.

*Respiratory:* Every morning productive cough, relieved by first cigarette. Occasionally blood-stained sputum.

*Gastrointestinal:* Still has lower teeth, top teeth all removed 1958. Regular indigestion, especially after vinegar or spicy food. Uses laxative to ease constipation.

*Genitourinary:* No dysuria, infections or discharge.

*Central nervous system:* No headache, no paraesthesia, vision fine, no fits or faints.

*Locomotor system:* Right hip painful ?arthritic. Painful bunions causing shoe-fitting problems.

*Endocrine:* No symptoms reported.

*Summary:* Depressed, lonely 68-year-old, generally run down though no specific health problems at present. In winter troubled by bronchitis probably related to heavy smoking.

## REFERENCES

Anderson F M 1975 Occult spinal dysraphism: a series of 73 cases. Paediatrics 55: 826–834

Anderson G, Katz J, Zier B 1986 Bacterial endocarditis, clinical considerations and prophylaxis. Journal of the American Podiatric Medicine Association 6: 332–335

James M, Lassman L 1962 Spinal dysraphism. Journal of Bone and Joint Surgery 828–840

Seymour C 1984 Introduction to clinical clerking. Cambridge University Press, Cambridge

Victor M, Adams R 1953 The effects of alcohol on the nervous system. Research publication of the Association for Research into Nervous and Mental Disorders 32: 526–573

## FURTHER READING

Berkow R (ed) 1987 The Merck manual, 15th edn. Merck Sharp & Dohme Research Laboratories

Bouchier I, Morris J 1982 Clinical skills. W B Saunders, London

Greenberger N, Hinthorn D 1993 History taking and physical examination: essentials and clinical correlates. Mosby Year Book Inc, St Louis, MO

Macleod J, French E, Munro J 1990 Introduction to clinical examination. Churchill Livingstone, Edinburgh

Miller S 1987 Morton's neuroma, a syndrome, in McGlammary (ed) A comprehensive textbook of foot surgery. Williams & Williams, Baltimore, MD

Royal College of Physicians 1987 The medical consequences of alcohol abuse. Tavistock Press, London

Zier B 1990 Essentials of internal medicine in clinical podiatry. W B Saunders, Philadelphia, PA

# Appendix: Medical Health Questionnaire

Please complete the health questionnaire in your own time. Take as long as you feel you need. If there are any areas of the form that you are not clear about, please ask the practitioner for help. It is important that we know about all aspects of your health as this may affect your legs and feet and may be important when deciding the best form of treatment.

What is your occupation?

Have you had any previous treatment for your feet? Yes/No
Who provided the treatment?

Were any X-rays taken? Yes/No
Were any blood samples taken? Yes/No
Are you generally well? Yes/No
Are you sleeping well? Yes/No
What is your weight?

Has your weight recently changed? No/Decreased/Increased
Are you taking any medication or tablets either prescribed by your doctor or purchased by yourself? Yes/No
Are you allergic to any of the following:
    Pollen Yes/No
    Animals Yes/No
    Certain types of food Yes/No
    Penicillin or any other tablets or medicines Yes/No
    Local anaesthetic injections Yes/No
Do you smoke? Yes/No
    If Yes, how many do you smoke per day?

Do you take any recreational drugs? Yes/No
Have you ever:
    Been off sick from work for more than a week? Yes/No
    Been admitted to hospital? Yes/No
    Undergone an operation? Yes/No
Have you ever been under the care of a hospital consultant/specialist? Yes/No
    If Yes, please give details:

Have you ever been injured at work? Yes/No
Do you participate in sporting activities? Yes/No

If Yes, please state which sports and how regularly do you participate.

Have you ever been in the services? Yes/No
    If Yes, when, and where were you stationed?

Did you have any childhood illnesses other than measles, chickenpox and mumps? Yes/No
    If Yes, please state which ones.

Does anyone in your family suffer from foot or leg problems? Yes/No
Please place a tick if a member of your family suffered from any of these illnesses:
    haemophilia
    sickle cell disease
    diabetes
    rheumatoid arthritis
    epilepsy
Have you ever had hepatitis or jaundice? Yes/No
Do you have a blood disorder, e.g. anaemia, sickle cell disease? Yes/No
Are you in a high risk group for blood-borne infections such as hepatitis B or AIDS? Yes/No
Do you have high blood pressure? Yes/No
Do you suffer from shortness of breath? Yes/No
Do you ever get pains in your chest, shoulders or upper arms? Yes/No
Do your ankles swell? Yes/No
Do you get cramp at night? Yes/No
Do you get muscle cramps while walking? Yes/No
Do you suffer from chilblains? Yes/No
Do your feet change colour if you get particularly cold? Yes/No
Have you ever had ankle ulcers? Yes/No
Have you ever had bronchitis or asthma? Yes/No
Have you ever had a cough for several months? Yes/No
Do you ever bring up blood when you cough? Yes/No
Are you troubled by toothache or gum swelling? Yes/No
Do you suffer from indigestion or stomach ache? Yes/No
Do painkillers like aspirin upset your stomach? Yes/No

Have you any bowel problems? Yes/No

Have you ever had any kidney problems or difficulties urinating? Yes/No

Is your sleep disturbed by the need to go to the toilet? Yes/No

Have you ever had any sexually transmitted infections? Yes/No

Have you ever injured your head? Yes/No

Have you ever injured your spine? Yes/No

Do you suffer from migraines or regular headaches? Yes/No
  If Yes, how frequently?

Do you ever get numbness, weakness, tingling, heaviness or shooting pains in your legs and feet? Yes/No

Do you ever get blackouts or feel faint? Yes/No

Are you always thirsty? Yes/No

Do you find that you can't bare hot rooms or buildings? Yes/No

Do your hands and feet get particularly sweaty? Yes/No

Are you particularly sensitive to cold? Yes/No

Do you bruise easily? Yes/No

Have you noticed any loss of hair from your head or eyebrows? Yes/No

Do you ever feel faint or dizzy when standing up after sitting down for some time? Yes/No

Do you ever get any aches and pains in your joints? Yes/No

Have you any arthritis or long standing muscle injuries? Yes/No

Thank you for completing this questionnaire. Please add any further information that you think may be of use.

# 6

# Vascular assessment

*J. McLeod-Roberts*

## INTRODUCTION

Assessment of the patient's vascular status is an essential part of the primary patient assessment. Davies & Horrocks (1992) noted that there has been an increase in the number of patients presenting with vascular disease. This chapter begins by explaining the purpose of a vascular assessment and then proceeds to provide an overview of the anatomy and physiology of the cardiovascular system. It continues by describing the necessary steps to be taken when assessing the cardiovascular and in particular the peripheral vascular status of the patient. Ranges of expected and abnormal values are included where appropriate. Simple, non-invasive tests are described which can be carried out by the practitioner using the minimum of equipment; hospital based tests are also briefly described.

## THE PURPOSE OF A VASCULAR ASSESSMENT

The vascular status of the lower limb bears a direct relationship to tissue viability; furthermore, the severity of vascular disease has been shown to be associated with an increase in morbidity and mortality (Howell et al 1989). It will be apparent from this that assessment of the vascular status performs a useful screening function by detecting previously unidentified vascular abnormalities.

Information gained from a vascular assessment can be used to achieve the following:

- identify whether the blood supply to and from the lower limb is adequate for normal function and tissue vitality.
- identify vascular problems which could compromise the state of the tissues. It is important to detect not only the presence of such abnormalities but also the functional site, e.g. is it an arterial or venous insufficiency or a combination of both? These patients require monitoring so that complications, e.g. necrosis, ulceration, infection, can be prevented or their effects reduced.
- identify whether there are any vascular abnormalities which could affect healing or the choice of treatment. These should be borne in mind when drawing up a treatment plan.
- identify those patients in whom vascular conditions require further investigation by referral to a specialist.

# OVERVIEW OF THE CARDIOVASCULAR SYSTEM

## ANATOMY OF THE CARDIOVASCULAR SYSTEM

The cardiovascular system (CVS) consists of a closed system of vessels through which blood and lymph are pumped around the body by means of the heart.

### The heart

The heart is constructed as a double pump in series, one pump comprising the left side of the heart and the other the right side (Fig. 6.1). Each pump has two chambers. Each upper chamber or atrium is a receiving vessel with a thin muscle wall (myocardium), whereas the lower chambers or ventricles are the dispersing vessels and therefore have much thicker muscle walls to generate strong propulsive forces (Fig. 6.2). The

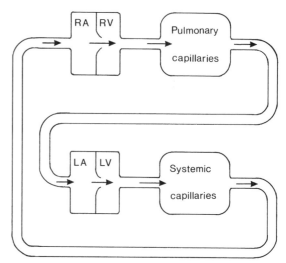

**Figure 6.1** The heart is a double pump in series. It serves two circulations, the low-pressure pulmonary and the high-pressure systemic circulation.

heart is lined by endocardium and surrounded by a tough, non-extensible pericardium. The endocardium forms the cusps of one-way valves, called the tricuspid and bicuspid valves, which control the flow of blood through the heart. It also forms semilunar valves, which control the entry of blood into the vessels leaving the heart. Closure of these valves is responsible for the two heart sounds, 'lub-dup', which can be heard through a stethoscope applied to the chest wall.

The heart serves two circulations. The right ventricle serves the pulmonary or minor circulation and sends deoxygenated blood via the pulmonary arteries to the lungs, whereas the left ventricle supplies the systemic or major circulation with oxygenated blood through the aorta to the body (Fig. 6.1). Oxygenated blood is returned from the lungs via the pulmonary veins into the left atrium and deoxygenated blood from the body flows through the superior and inferior vena cavae into the right atrium.

### Peripheral circulation

The blood flows through the two circulations via a system of vessels of varying diameters:

- Aorta—diameter 25 mm, thickness of wall 2 mm

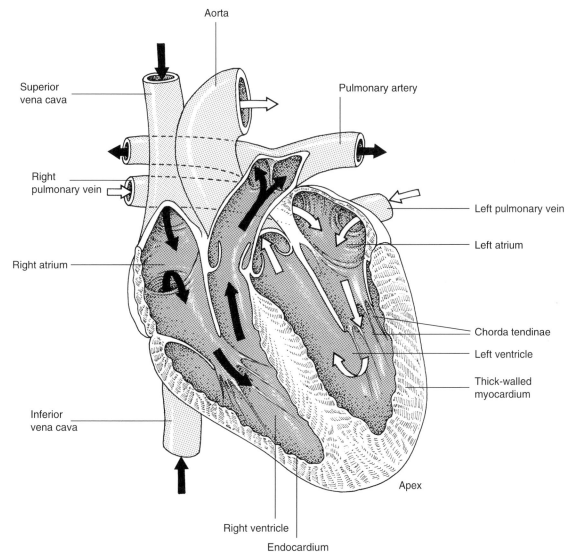

Aorta

Superior
vena cava

Pulmonary artery

Right
pulmonary vein

Left pulmonary vein

Left atrium

Right atrium

Chorda tendinae

Left ventricle

Thick-walled
myocardium

Inferior
vena cava

Apex

Right ventricle

Endocardium

**Figure 6.2**   Vertical section through the heart showing the valves, chorda tendinae, main vessels attached and the varying thickness of the myocardium. The direction of flow of oxygenated (non-shaded arrows) and deoxygenated (shaded arrows) blood is also shown.

- Artery—diameter 4 mm, thickness of wall 1 mm
- Arteriole—diameter 30 µm, thickness of wall 20 µm
- Capillary—diameter 6 µm, thickness of wall 1 µm
- Venule—diameter 20 µm, thickness of wall 2 µm
- Vein—diameter 5 mm, thickness of wall 500 µm

- Vena cava—diameter 30 mm, thickness of wall 1.5 mm.

### Arterial tree

The vessels which transport blood to the tissues are called arteries. These branch into consecutively smaller vessels called arterioles. The walls of arteries consist of three layers, the tunica intima, tunica media and tunica adventitia, all of

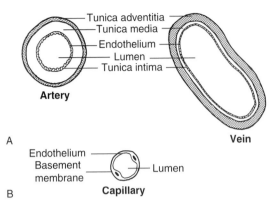

**Figure 6.3** **A.** Cross-section through an artery and vein showing tunica intima, media and adventitia. **B.** Cross-section through a capillary. Note the relative proportions of thickness in artery and vein and its absence in the capillary.

which are lined with vascular endothelium (Fig. 6.3A). All the vessels have some smooth muscle in the tunica media to enable them to change diameter, but arterioles have the greatest proportion. The arteries leaving the heart have a high proportion of elastic tissue in their walls, which enables them to act as secondary pumps, whereas the rest of the arterial tree consists of muscular distributing vessels.

*Venous tree*

Blood is drained from the tissue beds by small vessels called venules which join to form larger vessels called veins. The three layers seen in the arterial walls are again present but the proportions differ, as can be seen in Figure 6.3A. The vascular endothelium forms semilunar valves in the veins and venules to prevent backflow of blood. Veins are found either in the superficial fascia or deep in the muscle. Communicating veins link the two types so that blood can drain from the superficial veins to the deep ones.

*Capillary*

A third type of vessel, the capillary, links arterioles and venules. This is the smallest and most numerous vessel, having only a thin-walled endothelium (Fig. 6.3B). It permeates all the

tissue beds so that no tissue cell is far from a capillary. Flow of blood into individual capillaries is regulated by smooth muscle sphincters in vessels called metarterioles which are situated at the entrances to the capillaries. Capillaries can be bypassed by arteriovenous (A-V) anastomoses: these are vessels which form a direct link between an arteriole and a venule (Fig. 6.4A). In peripheral cutaneous sites exposed to extremes of temperature, such as the skin of fingertips, apices of toes, nose and earlobes, the A-V anastomoses are very numerous and form specialised structures under the nail beds called glomus bodies or Suquet–Hoyer canals (Fig. 6.4B).

*Microcirculation*

The smaller-diameter vessels collectively form the microcirculation.

*Collaterals*

Most microcirculations are served by more than one branch of the arterial tree. These parallel branches are called collaterals and may anastomose freely or hardly at all, the degree of communication varying from tissue to tissue (Fig. 6.5).

*Lymphatic tree*

Lymphatic vessels are very similar in structure to veins and capillaries, except that the smallest vessels are blind-ended. They drain the tissues and transport lymph through various lymph nodes, eventually rejoining the peripheral circulation through the thoracic duct (Fig. 6.6).

*Tissue fluid*

While capillaries bring blood close to all body cells, a diffusion medium is needed to enable nutrients, waste products and gases to be exchanged between the cells and the blood and lymph. This medium is tissue fluid, which is continuously forming from blood at capillary and postcapillary venular sites as a result of hydrostatic and oncotic pressures. Some tissue

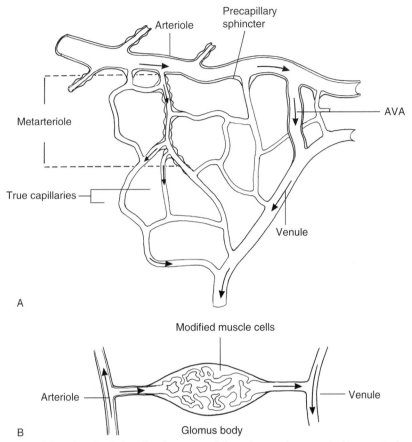

**Figure 6.4** **A.** Diagram of the microcirculation showing an arteriole and a venule connected by an arteriovenous anastomosis (AVA) and a capillary network.The arteriovenous anastomosis is a shorter, tortuous, muscular vessel of a larger calibre. The capillary network comprises of metarterioles, which have a muscular coat and the distal portion of the capillary network which consists solely of endothelial cells.  **B.** Diagram showing the specialised arteriovenous anastomosis under the nail bed (glomus body).

fluid is reabsorbed back into these vessels, the remainder draining into the lymphatic capillaries to be returned to the general circulation.

## NORMAL PHYSIOLOGY OF THE CARDIOVASCULAR SYSTEM

The essential function of the CVS is to ensure that there is sufficient perfusion pressure to maintain, under all circumstances, an adequate flow of blood to the vital organs, especially the brain. This is achieved by alteration of the rate and force of contraction of the myocardium and by varying the diameter throughout the peripheral circulation. In periods of increased demand, non-vital areas will have a reduced flow and this may very well affect the lower limb.

The heart contracts about once every 0.8 s in a healthy resting adult. The heart beat is divided into two phases; the relaxation phase or diastole and the contraction phase or systole. Systole is the shorter of the two phases, lasting about 0.3 s, though with increased heart rate, the period of diastole shortens.

The volume of blood ejected from each ventricle is the same and is called the stroke volume. In a healthy resting adult about 70 ml is ejected at each contraction of the ventricle. Since the normal resting heart rate is an average of 72 beats per minute, the volume ejected from each

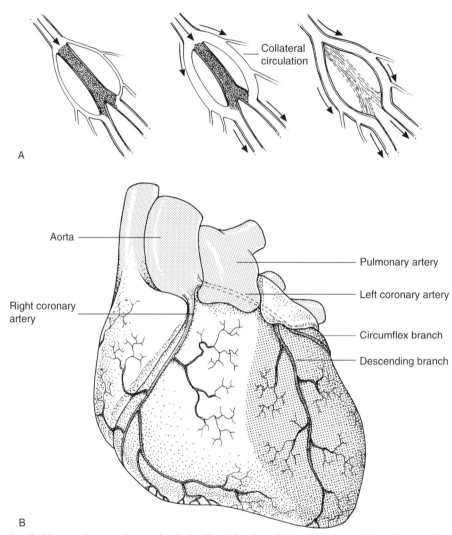

A

Collateral circulation

Aorta

Pulmonary artery

Left coronary artery

Right coronary artery

Circumflex branch

Descending branch

B

**Figure 6.5   A.** Small side vessels normally carry an insignificant fraction of blood into the peripheral tissues. Damage or occlusion of the major arteries alters pressure relationships to divert blood through the side vessels (collateral circulation). **B.** Anterior view of heart showing lack of anastomoses between arterial vessels supplying the myocardium. Left coronary artery supplies hatched area, right coronary artery supplies unhatched area.

ventricle in one minute is approximately 5 litres and is known as the cardiac output.

The myocardium has the ability to contract without nerve impulses. This property is called myogenicity and is due to the presence of specialised 'pacemaker' cells which generate spontaneous action potentials. The most important of these is the sinoatrial (SA) node, situated in the right atrium (Fig. 6.7). The action potential spreads rapidly through the other specialised conducting tissues and then out over the rest of the myocardium through gap junctions between the cells. This ensures that the cells can respond as a unit, producing a coordinated wave of contraction which pushes the blood in the desired direction. Apart from these specialised pathways, the septa that divide the four chambers of the heart consist of fibrous, non-conducting tissue.

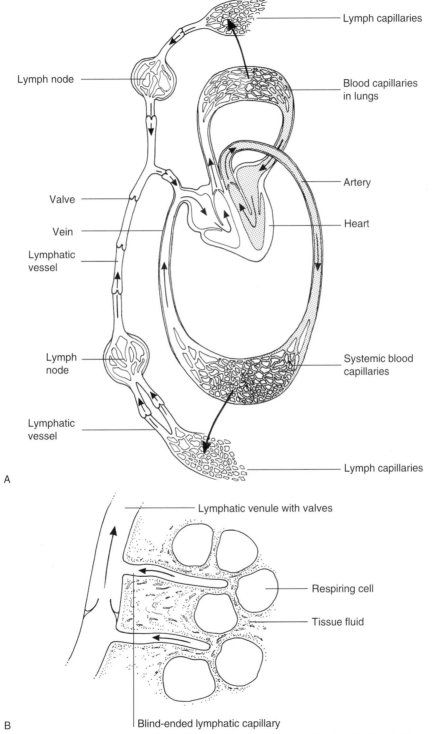

**Figure 6.6    A.** Diagram of lymphatic circulation    **B.** Diagram showing a blind-ended lymphatic capillary.

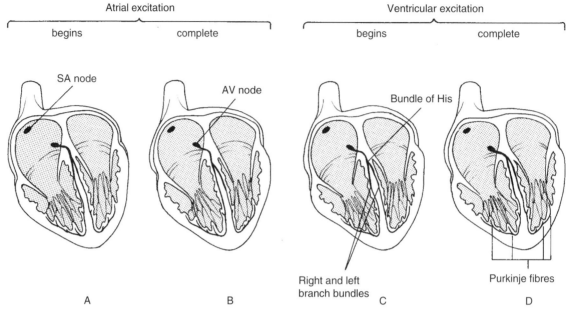

**Figure 6.7** Diagrams of the vertical outline of the heart, showing the SA node (**A**), AV node (**B**), bundle of His (**C**), Purkinje fibres (**D**) and spread of waves from the SA node (**A–D**).

While the heart can contract without nervous stimulation, it is essential that it can alter its activity according to the differing demands placed upon it as mentioned earlier. One way that this is achieved is via the autonomic system (ANS) (Ch. 7). The two branches of the ANS both send fibres to the SA node. The sympathetic nerve acts on the heart via specific receptors called beta₁ receptors, the action of which is to increase cardiac output by increasing both stroke volume (positive inotropy) and heart rate (positive chronotropy). The parasympathetic nerve (vagus) causes slowing of the heart rate (negative chronotropy), acting through cholinergic receptors.

At rest the parasympathetic nerve predominates, producing an average resting heart rate of 72 beats per minute. The rate is less in trained athletes and higher in children and is also affected by posture, increasing on a change from a supine to an upright position by approximately 10 beats per minute. The latter is due to compensation for the effects of gravity on blood in the peripheral vessels and is mediated through the baroreceptor reflex (Fig. 6.8). Baroreceptors are situated in both the arterial and venous sides of the systemic circulation, but the arterial baroreceptors in the aortic arch and carotid body are

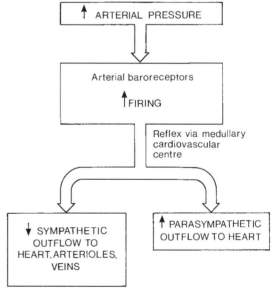

**Figure 6.8** Flow chart showing the arterial baroreceptor reflex. If arterial pressure decreased the arrows in the boxes would be reversed.

the more important for regulation of blood pressure. They continuously monitor the level and feed the information to the cardiovascular control centre in the brain stem. As a result of this information being integrated in the medulla, compensatory adjustments are made to the action of the heart and the diameter of the arterial tree through the sympathetic nerves, which act on the smooth muscle of the tunica media. Despite being very sensitive to changes in blood pressure, baroreceptors show a rapid adaptation to a sustained change, so that in hypertension they are triggered by a higher than normal 'operating' range.

All vessels except capillaries are subject to some sympathetic influence or 'tone'. The greater the sympathetic tone, the more vasoconstriction is achieved, with vasodilation being produced by a reduction in this tone. This in turn produces a change in resistance to flow, a change in the pressure exerted on the blood and a change in the work the heart has to do (afterload). The greatest effect is produced in the arterioles, called the resistance vessels, which as mentioned previously have the largest proportion of smooth muscle in their walls. They allow the CVS to control distribution of blood and, together with the heart, are the effector organs for the homeostatic control of blood pressure. A similar reflex exists to regulate blood volume, which in addition involves, to a greater extent, the low pressure baroreceptors in the right atrium and where the effector organs include the kidney as well as the CVS.

The aorta and pulmonary arteries are the elastic arteries, having a large proportion of elastic tissue in their walls. This distends as the bolus of blood is received from the ventricles and acts as a secondary pump during diastole when the elastic recoil propels the blood forward. The rebound causes a shock wave to travel rapidly through the blood in the arterial tree and it can be felt as a pulse wave at certain points called pressure points.

The overall purpose then of all the vessels within the systemic circulation, except the capillaries, is to deliver blood with its dissolved nutrients, oxygen and hormones to the tissues and to remove metabolic waste such as carbon dioxide and urea. This transportation must meet the demands of the different tissues, which will vary in need according to their nature and level of activity. Heat is also distributed from areas such as active muscles and the liver to the rest of the body. The skin is an important organ for controlling heat loss, involving the superficial papillary loops and the specialised glomus bodies which can reroute blood towards or away from the skin surface. The purpose of such redirection is either to control heat loss or to ensure that superficial tissues do not suffer from ischaemia caused by cold-induced vasoconstriction.

The function of the capillaries is the exchange of the substances transported to the tissues by the blood. It is here that tissue fluid plays its essential role of intermediary between blood and tissues mentioned earlier, being the ideal candidate since it bathes every cell. There is a large pressure drop across the capillary beds so that blood flowing in the venules and veins is at low pressure and needs help to get back to the heart, in the form of semilunar valves, venoconstriction and the pumping action of surrounding skeletal muscle on the deep veins. The volume of blood returning to the heart is termed the venous return or preload. It is essential that ventricular output exactly matches this venous return to avoid a transfer of blood from one circulation to the other. In addition to returning blood to the heart, veins, because of their distensibility, act as capacitance vessels, normally holding three-fifths of the total volume of blood in the body. This can boost the circulation when necessary.

The purpose of the pulmonary circulation is to deliver blood containing carbon dioxide to the lungs and exchange it via the alveolar capillaries for oxygen. Having two separate circulations also allows each to operate at a different pressure.

Red blood cells contain the pigment haemoglobin, which picks up oxygen in the lungs in a stepwise manner and releases it in the tissues. Presence or absence of oxygen causes a change in shape of the haemoglobin molecule and with it a change in colour, so that oxygenated blood is bright red and deoxygenated blood is bluish-red.

Red blood cells are formed from stem cells in the red bone marrow and mature under the influence of kidney hormones or erythropoietins. Various factors are needed, such as iron, folic acid and vitamin $B_{12}$ for formation of the mature erythrocyte. The red blood cell circulates for 120 days before being broken down in the liver by phagocytic Kupffer cells. Anaemias, reduction in the oxygen carrying capacity of blood, can result from a defect in any part of this process. For example, damage to the bone marrow by radiation can damage the stem cells or the young red blood cells, resulting in aplastic anaemia. An autoimmune disease can destroy the parietal cells in the stomach, leading to lack of intrinsic factor of Castle and this causes an inability to absorb vitamin $B_{12}$ and, after some delay, results in pernicious anaemia.

## THE VASCULAR ASSESSMENT

Assessment of the vascular status of the patient consists of a general overview of the cardiovascular system and a detailed assessment of the peripheral vascular system. The peripheral vascular system can be subdivided into arteries, veins and lymphatics.

The assessment of each part of the vascular tree involves:

- Past history and current medication
- Symptoms
- Observable signs
- Clinical tests
- Hospital tests.

Accurate diagnosis can often be achieved by simple observation. Research which compared diagnoses made by practitioners using observation with diagnoses arrived at with the aid of hospital tests found that the former method was almost as reliable as the latter.

## GENERAL OVERVIEW OF THE CARDIOVASCULAR SYSTEM

Central problems can have a bearing on the diagnosis and management of lower limb prob-

**Table 6.1** Cardiac conditions which may affect lower limb perfusion

| |
|---|
| Heart failure: left- and/or right-sided |
| Ischaemic heart disease: angina or myocardial infarction |
| Rheumatic fever |
| Myocarditis |
| Valve disorders:<br>  mitral stenosis<br>  aortic stenosis<br>  mitral regurgitation<br>  tricuspid regurgitation |
| Infective endocarditis |
| Congenital heart disease:<br>  septal defects<br>  valve defects<br>  coarction of the aorta<br>  Fallot's tetralogy |

lems and so must be taken into consideration (Table 6.1). Full investigation of such problems are beyond the scope of this textbook.

## Past history and current medication

This was discussed in Chapter 5. Coronary artery disease is often linked to atherosclerosis of arteries of the lower limb. The medical history should reveal conditions which indicate coronary artery disease such as angina of effort or previous myocardial infarctions. The presence of risk factors for atherosclerosis should also be noted, such as the habit of smoking, the presence of diabetes mellitus, hypertension or hyperlipidaemia (Case history 6.1).

Antihypertensives such as diuretics, beta-blockers, ACE inhibitors and calcium antagonists all indicate a vascular problem. Diuretics act on various parts of the kidney nephron to reduce water and salt reabsorption and so reduce preload and cardiac output and as a consequence, blood pressure. Beta-blockers prevent the stimulatory action of endogenous catecholamines on the heart, again reducing cardiac output and blood pressure. ACE (angiotensin converting enzyme) inhibitors interfere with the production of angiotensin 2 which is both a powerful vasoconstrictor and triggers release of the hormone aldosterone from the adrenal cortex. As aldos-

---

Case history 6.1

A male Caucasian first presented to the clinic when 74 years old, complaining of hard skin on the balls of his feet and on the ends of his toes. He was finding it difficult to focus and so had sought chiropody treatment. His medical and social history revealed that he was a smoker and that he had had an aortic aneurysm resected when aged 73. He was taking bendrofluazide. A preliminary vascular assessment showed telangiectases and haemosiderosis superimposed on a normal skin colour in both lower limbs. Varicose veins were present in the right leg, hair was absent from legs and feet and the skin was dry. Nails were long but otherwise unremarkable. The feet felt cold but capillary filling time was less than 1 *second*. All four pedal pulses were palpable and demonstrated arrhythmias. Brachial BP was 110/60 mmHg.

When examined 3 years later, the patient's feet were cyanotic with the right foot being worse than the left. His toenails were thickened and crumbly, capillary filling time was 6 *seconds* and oedema was present in both ankles. Pedal pulses were barely palpable. He had suffered a myocardial infarction and a stroke when 76 and his medication had been changed to digoxin and frusemide.

When the patient first presented at the clinic, the condition of the skin, nails and general tissue viability were unremarkable for someone of his age. 3 years later he had suffered a myocardial infarction and a stroke, which suggests possible atherosclerosis in coronary and cerebral arteries. The likelihood of the lower limb arteries also being involved is considerable and would account for the barely palpable pedal pulses. Smoking is a risk factor for atherosclerosis and for strokes. The peripheral oedema and cyanosis were likely to be consequences of cardiac insufficiency following the myocardial infarction, although the asymmetry also suggests that some peripheral factor may have been contributing, such as venous incompetency.

---

terone promotes water and salt reabsorption from the kidney, drugs that inhibit its release will again reduce preload and cardiac output, so that ACE inhibitors promote a two-pronged attack on blood pressure. Calcium antagonists act by interfering with the process of vascular smooth muscle contraction, which in turn reduces peripheral resistance and so reduces blood pressure.

## Symptoms

### Angina and myocardial infarction

Pain in the chest on exercise or other stress indicates inadequate blood supply to the myocardium. Angina may occur as the result of a previous myocardial infarction (MI). The pain of angina can vary from a mild discomfort to an intense crushing sensation, or a feeling as if the chest is being gripped by a steel band. It may radiate into the left arm, to the back and the throat or even down the right arm. It may settle into a predictable pattern so that the patient will be able to describe the trigger factors and the intensity, duration and frequency of the attacks. More seriously, the attacks may increase in frequency or intensity, when it is termed unstable angina and may be prodromal to an acute heart attack (Berkow 1987). It is important to recognise such situations should they develop as prompt action is essential.

The chief distinguishing feature of an acute myocardial infarction as opposed to an angina pectoris attack is that the latter lasts only minutes and is usually relieved within 5 minutes by rest or by sublingual nitroglycerine. Any chest pain that does not ameliorate after both these procedures must be viewed with concern. If after administration of further nitroglycerine the patient still does not obtain relief, emergency services should be called.

There are many other causes of chest pain, though few closely mimic angina. However, indigestion and other gastrointestinal disorders are often confused with angina (Ch. 5).

### Breathlessness (dyspnoea)

While the most common cause of dyspnoea is physical exertion, it can be associated with cardiac problems (Berkow 1987). It should be established whether the patient is a smoker or not, since there is a close correlation between smoking and cardiovascular problems. The early stages of heart failure results in metabolic acidosis which causes compensatory hyperventilation. In later stages the lungs are congested and ventilatory effort is increased. Difficulty in breathing when supine (orthopnoea) accompanies left ventricular failure.

### Lassitude and pallor

The main symptoms associated with anaemia are lassitude and pallor, with other specific symptoms associated with particular types of anaemia.

## Observation

The practitioner should initially take a general overview of the cardiovascular system, looking for indications of central problems such as oedema or central cyanosis.

### Oedema

Any factor which interferes with the normal process of tissue fluid formation and reabsorption may cause fluid to accumulate in the tissues. This will cause swelling which is referred to as oedema. It can be due to central factors such as congestive heart failure, where the failure of the left ventricle to produce an adequate cardiac output causes backward pressure through the CVS, in time causing right ventricular failure. Just as left ventricular failure produces oedema in the pulmonary circulation, right ventricular failure results in peripheral oedema, especially noticeable in the lower limbs. An important exacerbating factor is the renin–angiotensin–aldosterone system which is triggered by the low cardiac output and causes renal retention of salt and water, thus imposing an even greater load on the failing heart.

### Cyanosis

Central cyanosis is the bluish discoloration of lips, tongue and mucous membranes and indicates that arterial blood is inadequately oxygenated. It may be due either to deficiencies in the pump, such as a congenital hole in the heart, or deficiencies in ventilation, such as chronic obstructive airways disease.

### Spoon shaped nails (koilonychia)

Lack of iron results in iron-deficiency anaemia, which causes koilonychia of the finger nails and a red tongue.

### Clubbing of the nails (hippocratic nails)

Clubbing of the finger nails may be due to sub-acute infective endocarditis and cyanotic heart disease. It is also associated with a variety of other, primarily respiratory, causes, e.g. bronchial carcinoma.

## Clinical tests

### Heart rate

This is normally assessed by taking the pulse at the wrist. Arrhythmias are abnormal heart rates and can be physiological or pathological, depending on the cause. Heart rates of less than 60 beats per minute are classified as bradycardia and those over 100 beats per minute as tachycardia. An example of a physiological bradycardia is that seen in trained athletes whereas the bradycardia due to a complete heart block in the atrioventricular septum is pathological. Physiological arrhythmia may also be associated with respiration and is called sinus arrhythmia, appearing as a tachycardia on inspiration and a bradycardia on expiration. It is more noticeable in young people and is thought to be due to fluctuations in the parasympathetic output to the heart (Ganong 1991).

Beta$_1$-blockers such as atenolol will induce a bradycardia and thus reduce cardiac output and blood pressure. Such drugs are therefore given as antihypertensives. In contrast, thyroid hormones, if present in excess, increase the affinity of beta$_1$-receptors to catecholamines and so induce tachycardia as seen in hyperthyroidism. The tachycardia of exercise illustrates the relationship between heart rate and efficiency, since with up to approximately 180 beats per minute cardiac output also rises; however, at rates greater than this the diastolic period is so short that the heart cannot fill properly and cardiac output falls.

The quality of the pulse should also be noted. Is it irregular, bounding or feeble? The pulse can be graded on a score of 0–4, with 0 representing no pulse and 4 representing a bounding, strong pulse. Irregular or abnormal pulses (arrhythmias) may be physiological (e.g. due to exertion, anxiety, training or age) or may be due to some underlying systemic condition such as thyroid disorders or medication such as beta blockers. Similarly, a bounding pulse can be due to response to stress, a sign of pyrexia, or can be seen in pathological conditions such as thyrotoxicosis, or in a hypoglycaemic diabetic. Irregular pulses, i.e. bradycardia, tachycardia or absent pulses, with no apparent explanation should be investigated with Doppler apparatus.

*Blood pressure*

Hypertension is usually asymptomatic unless very severe. Symptoms usually indicate the presence of complications and include headache, nose bleeds and dizziness. Hypertension is a risk factor for many serious conditions such as myocardial infarction, left ventricular failure and renal failure. There is a direct correlation between the degree of hypertension and the likelihood of a stroke, so blood pressure values can be one of the most reliable indicators for prognosis of life span, it is therefore, one of the most useful screening exercises which can be done in the clinic. Simple non-pharmacological intervention is usually tried as a first-line method of treatment, unless the condition is severe, with drugs being used only if the situation does not respond or worsens.

The pressure in the large arteries will vary during the cardiac cycle. The highest pressure will be at ventricular systole when blood is being forced into the arteries. The pressure at this point is called the systolic blood pressure. The lowest point is when the heart is relaxed, just before it begins its next contraction. This is called the diastolic pressure. The blood pressure is always written as systolic pressure/diastolic pressure. The value for a healthy adult is 120/80 mmHg (17/11 kPa). Pulse pressure is the difference between the systolic and diastolic pressures and will widen or reduce as either or both pressures change. The value of the systolic and the pulse pressures rises with age due to loss of compliance in the arterial tunica media.

The taking of blood pressures by the auscultatory method is a simple technique but requires practice and attention to detail in the procedure (Fig. 6.9). Other methods such as the palpatory method are not considered to be as sensitive. The sphygmomanometer is a tube filled with mercury, connected to a rubber hand pump with a valve and an inflatable cuff. Other manometers such as an aneroid manometer could be used instead.

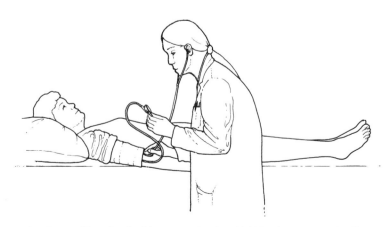

**Figure 6.9** Diagram showing position of patient for measuring brachial blood pressure using the auscultatory method.

The following procedure should be adopted.

- The patient should be seated comfortably with one arm flexed at the elbow and resting at heart level on a flat surface.
- The brachial pulse should be palpated.
- The cuff should be wrapped around the selected arm of the patient, well clear of the brachial pulse point.
- The pressure cuff should be inflated until the brachial pulse can no longer be palpated. The value of this pressure should be noted and the pressure released rapidly.
- The diaphragm of the stethoscope should be placed on the pulse point and the pressure cuff re-inflated to the same value as previously obtained. Nothing will be heard at this stage. All vessels will be occluded so that no blood can flow through the artery.
- The pressure should be released slowly and steadily, watching the mercury level fall. As the pressure falls to the level of the patient's systolic blood pressure a knocking sound will be heard in the stethoscope. At this stage the pressure in the cuff is sufficient to prevent flow of blood during diastole, but not during systole, so that the systolic flow can be heard. The reading of the manometer when the sound is first heard should be noted; this corresponds to the value of systolic blood pressure.
- The pressure should continue to be released. The sounds will first increase then decrease in intensity and finally disappear. At this stage the pressure in the cuff is insufficient to occlude the artery at any stage in the cardiac cycle and this point is taken as the value for the diastolic blood pressure.
- The practitioner should ensure that the cuff is deflated completely.

The first person to describe this method was Korotkoff and the sounds heard are called Korotkoff sounds. Practice makes perfect! If the readings are not consistent, there are a number of ways in which errors may have been introduced.

- The tubes may be dirty so that the mercury clings to the glass.

- The rubber may be perished.
- The valve may be faulty.
- The cuff may be the wrong size for the diameter of the limb.
- The arm may not be at heart level.
- The practitioner may not read the values correctly. The height of the mercury meniscus should be read at eye level. If in doubt, or if the values are not as expected, the exercise should be repeated, after the patient has had time to relax.

Blood pressure values show a Gaussian distribution curve, so the values used to indicate hypertension are somewhat arbitrary. In this country hypertension for adults is taken as any systolic value over 160 mmHg and any diastolic value over 95 mmHg. Ideally, readings should be taken on three separate occasions since stress can cause a temporary rise in blood pressure. The most effective way of measuring blood pressure is by a self-monitoring technique. Patients measure their blood pressures at regular intervals throughout the day and an average value is obtained. The upper normal limit is lower in children and higher in the elderly.

## Hospital tests

These are performed both to confirm diagnosis and to identify the exact site of a problem so that accurate surgical therapy can be performed.

### Non-invasive

**Electrocardiogram:** The electrical activity of the heart is recorded using limb and chest leads attached to the skin. Many pathologies of the heart, such as myocardial infarction or ventricular enlargement in a failing heart, will alter the normal PQRS wave form. Exercise may be used to highlight problems not apparent at rest.

**Chest X-ray:** A standard radiograph of the chest will show such pathologies as enlargement of the heart, calcification of coronary arteries and malignant masses.

**Echocardiography:** This uses ultrasound at a frequency of 2.5 MHz to visualise both the heart and the coronary arteries. It can visualise movement of ventricular walls, septum and heart valves (Kapoor & Singh 1993, p. 131).

### Invasive techniques

**Blood analysis:** Diagnosis of anaemia can be easily confirmed with a full blood count, where the number and volume of the red blood cell is calculated, as is the oxygen content (Ch. 13). Where aplastic anaemia is suspected, a sample of bone marrow is analysed, usually from the sternum. During unstable angina or episodes of myocardial infarction the ischaemic myocardial cells produce increased amounts of particular enzymes and metabolites, which peak 24 hours after the attack, so that quantitative analysis of these substances aids diagnosis.

**Coronary angiography:** This involves introduction of a diagnostic catheter through the femoral artery into the left ventricle and associated vessels (Kapoor & Singh 1993, p. 131). Injection of a radio-opaque dye occurs at the site to be investigated.

**Myocardial perfusion scintigraphy (radionuclide perfusion imaging):** This is a very sensitive test using exercise thallium-201 or technetium-99m imaging to detect coronary artery disease (Kapoor & Singh 1993, pp. 130–1, 145).

## PERIPHERAL VASCULAR SYSTEM

It is important to distinguish between an impoverished arterial supply, reduced venous drainage and impaired lymphatic drainage, though of course more than one impairment may coexist.

## ARTERIAL INSUFFICIENCY

Conditions which can affect the arterial supply to the lower limb can be divided into those that lead to acute and those that lead to chronic problems (Table 6.2). Most arterial problems affecting the lower limb are chronic in nature, resulting in poor tissue viability. Inadequate blood supply to the lower limb leads to a range of signs and symptoms; these are known as the six Ps:

**Table 6.2** Causes of arterial insufficiency

| | |
|---|---|
| Acute | Extrinsic:<br>    tight clothing<br>    tourniquet<br>    plaster cast<br>    trauma<br>    frostbite<br>    immersion foot<br>Intrinsic:<br>    thrombosis<br>    embolus (from a mural thrombosis)<br>    ruptured aneurysm<br>    oedema |
| Transient | (usually lead to acute problems but may progress to chronic)<br>Raynaud's phenomenon<br>Chilblains<br>Hereditary cold fingers |
| Chronic | Arteriosclerosis (macro- and microangiopathy)<br>Atherosclerosis<br>Vasculitis (e.g. rheumatoid arthritis)<br>Thromboangiitis obliterans (Buerger's disease) |

- Pain
- Pallor
- Pulselessness
- Paraesthesia
- Paralysis
- Perishing cold.

## Medical history

Any history of previous myocardial infarction, stroke or transient ischaemic attacks suggests the presence of atherosclerosis which, in addition to affecting the coronary and cerebral arteries, may also be affecting the arterial supply to the lower limb. A past history of vascular surgery such as coronary or femoropopliteal bypass grafting is also a good indicator that atherosclerosis may be present. A history of cryovascular disorders (e.g. chilblains, Raynaud's phenomenon) should be noted.

## Symptoms

Pain is usually associated with arterial insufficiency. It is important that the site, nature, duration and aggravating factors of the pain are recorded. This information can be very helpful when assessing the prognosis of diseases affecting the arterial supply. Inadequate blood supply to respiring tissues may be an acute situation, producing a characteristic range of signs and symptoms including pain, pallor and lack of pulses. When the deficiency is prolonged, the tissues eventually suffer irreversible damage and this stage can be recognised by mottling, muscle tenderness, motor or sensory deficit and necrosis. Continuation of the condition will lead to a chronic state of insufficiency, accompanied by pain on exercise, or even at rest if very severe, and necrosis and ulceration. The following types of ischaemic pain may be noted.

### Intermittent claudication

Just as angina pectoris indicates insufficient blood supply to the myocardium, so intermittent claudication indicates inadequate blood supply to the periphery. When the blood supply is in-adequate, the deficiency will be accentuated on exercise. The exercising muscles have to respire anaerobically and produce metabolites which are not cleared by the blood. These cause is-chaemic pain which forces the patient to stop the activity. Resting for a few minutes reduces the amount of metabolites produced and allows the patient to continue walking for a further period. The distance walked before onset of the pain is called the ischaemic or claudication distance and is a good indication of the severity of the condition. The exercise should be stan-dardised, e.g. 4 min at 0% incline at 4 km\h (Lainge & Greenhalgh 1980). The site of the is-chaemic pain is an indication of the site of the occlusion. It should be borne in mind, however, that patients with neuropathy may not complain of intermittent claudication.

### Night cramps

If the blood supply is more severely com-promised, the patient will experience night cramps, which are alleviated by dangling the legs over the side of the bed or walking on a cool floor. The warmth of the bedclothes increases the metabolic rate of the tissues and so increases their demand for oxygen; this cannot be met and produces ischaemic pain. Using gravity to aid flow and cool the limb helps to reduce metabolic activity.

### Rest pain

This is the most severe condition. Here the blood supply is inadequate even at rest, walking is impossible and the only way that the peripheral tissues can obtain any blood is by gravity. The legs must always lie below the level of the heart, either by raising the head of the bed or by sleeping in a chair. Even the contact of the bed-clothes on the limbs may be too painful. Cages are sometimes used to protect the limbs.

## Observation

A great deal of information about the vascular status of the patient can be gained by simple observation. The patient should be seated on a couch in a comfortably warm room.

### Colour

Skin may appear pink, white, blue, red or dusky pink. In the lower limbs of a person with no vascular problems, the skin should be a healthy pink colour; this indicates blood supply to the skin is satisfactory.

A pale skin may be simply due to vasocon-striction of the superficial capillary loops, in an effort to reduce heat loss due to a low ambient temperature. The skin may also appear pale if the patient is anaemic. A very cold and white skin below a definite line is a very grave sign, indicating that the arterial supply is severely compromised due to vascular occlusion, and is a pregangrenous condition. The most common cause of peripheral arterial insufficiency is arteriosclerosis obliterans.

A blue colour (cyanosis) means that the blood in the area is deoxygenated. This can again be due to the cold, causing vasoconstriction and consequent stagnation of blood in the skin capillaries and loss of oxygen. Where it affects the hands and feet it is called peripheral cyanosis and is most noticeable under the nails.

A red skin (erythema) can indicate simply that the patient is hot due to a high ambient temperature or previous exercise, where peripheral cutaneous vasodilation is attempting to increase heat loss. Vasodilation also occurs in cold weather in the extremities, as an intermittent flushing of the skin due to regular contractions of the specialised arteriovenous anastomoses or Glomus bodies that exist in the exposed regions of the skin (Fig. 6.4). The flushing is called 'cold-induced vasodilation' or 'the hunting phenomenon' and protects the tissues from conditions such as frostbite. Erythema is also one of the cardinal signs of inflammation and may indicate either a local or a systemic inflammatory condition. It is also possible for the skin to appear red in an extremely cold environment. Here the blood has again stagnated but, because of the very low ambient temperature, the blood does not lose its oxygen and so stays bright red. Blood flow is very slow. This can be seen especially in exposed areas such as the fingers, toes, cheeks and nose. The skin will feel very cold. This situation should not be allowed to continue as the tissues are unable to get oxygen.

A patient with polycythaemia vera will have a flushed appearance due to the raised red blood cell count, but this could be masking an associated ischaemia due to microembolism caused by the increased blood viscosity. A dusky red colour is also serious and usually indicates that the supply to the area is very inadequate. It suggests obstruction or reduction in blood supply to the periphery, as is seen in peripheral vascular disease such as atherosclerosis obliterans of large vessels, or Buerger's disease of the smaller vessels.

Vasospastic disorders such as chilblains or Raynaud's disease are usually associated with colour change that can be white, blue or red, according to the stage of the condition (Case history 6.2).

### Tissue vitality

A poor blood supply will mean that the skin and other soft tissues will be receiving inadequate nourishment. If chronic, it will result in thin,

---

**Case history 6.2**

A 67-year-old female Caucasian first presented to the clinic when aged 63, complaining of broken skin on the toes. The patient lived in a community home and had a history of poor circulation to both hands and feet. Footwear was inadequate for winter and foot hygiene was poor. Examination of the lower limb revealed pale skin and cold feet. The lesser toes were held in flexion deformities. No hairs were present. The nail on the left fifth toe was black. The skin was dry, scaly and fissured. There were painful ulcers on the apices of toes and fingers. All ulcers showed signs of infection. Pedal pulses were palpable but feeble. Popliteal pulses were stronger. Capillary filling time was 6 seconds.

A diagnosis of Raynaud's phenomenon was made. The condition was exacerbated by personal and social factors. The repeated breakdown of lesions, as evidenced by the patient's long history of attendance at the clinic, was due to the underlying vasospastic disorder which was exacerbated by cold weather and self-neglect. Current treatment was successful in healing the lesions but without continued patient compliance the overall prognosis is poor.

---

dry, shiny skin with absent hairs (Plate 1). However, the practitioner should bear in mind that absence of hairs on the lower limb could be due to the use of a depilatory or in males due to the effects of socks rubbing off the hairs. In chronic situations atrophy (wastage) of soft tissue, including muscle, will also be present. This is especially noticeable on the plantar surface of the foot.

An impaired peripheral circulation can also cause delayed healing of skin lesions and ulcers. The characteristics of the latter can assist in diagnosis of the circulatory problem, since ulcers caused by ischaemia differ in many respects from those caused by other deficiencies such as poor drainage or neuropathy (Ch. 17). Ischaemic ulcers are caused by trauma and are usually very painful, unless there is neuropathy present as for example in some diabetic patients. There is lack of granulation tissue and slough is often present. The borders are well demarcated and they may have a 'punched out' appearance (Plate 2). They often occur first under the toenails or on the apices of the toes or on the heels. Leg elevation can exacerbate the pain whereas lowering the leg into dependency can improve the blood supply and ease the pain. Ulcers of any type are less likely to heal if the patient is on medication which reduces cardiac output, e.g. beta-blockers.

### Nails

Poor blood supply will affect the nails. These may be crumbly, discoloured or thickened. They are prone to fungal infection and pitting. The latter should be differentially diagnosed from dermatological conditions such as psoriasis (Ch. 9).

### Gangrene

Severe ischaemia, if unrelieved, will progress to gangrene, with the most distal regions being affected first. If the cause of the ischaemia is arteriosclerosis obliterans, it usually results in dry gangrene (Plate 3).

### Oedema

Oedema is not usually associated with poor peripheral arterial supply. Presence of oedema may suggest some central problem such as congestive heart failure.

## Clinical tests

The following tests should be repeated for both lower limbs and require none or very simple apparatus of the type usually found in a practitioner's clinical environment.

### Temperature gradient

The back of the practitioner's hand should be used to stroke the anterior surface of the patient's lower limb from the knee to the toes. The proximal part of the leg should feel warm to the touch, with a gradual cooling as the feet are approached. On a cold day the toes can feel very cold; this is quite normal but a sharp temperature drop on a comfortably warm day will suggest an inadequate blood supply, with possibly an obstruction occurring at the level of the sudden change.

Remember too, that the temperature felt is relative to the temperature of the hand of the practitioner. This problem can be overcome by measuring skin temperature with a simple probe thermocouple attached to a hand-held digital display unit.

### Capillary filling time

To be strictly accurate, it is not the capillaries but the subpapillary venous plexus which is responsible for colour in the skin and is blanched by digital pressure. Using a thumb, the practitioner should apply sufficient pressure to the apices of the patient's toes to blanch the skin. As the practitioner removes the pressure, counting in seconds should begin and the time taken for the normal colour to be restored should be noted. Several areas of the feet should be tested. Normal colour should return within 2–3 seconds on a warm day and within 5 seconds on a cold day. A delayed capillary filling time suggests an inadequate supply through the capillaries producing a compromised microcirculation. It is perfectly possible to observe a good arterial supply but for there to be a poor capillary filling time due to microangiopathy. Absence of blanching in a cyanotic foot is a poor sign, since it shows that the tissues are devitalised. Gangrene is likely to develop.

### Buerger's elevation/dependency test

The leg should be elevated until all the veins in the dorsal arch of the foot have emptied. The plantar surface of the foot will appear pale as blood will have drained out of all superficial vessels due to the effects of gravity. The blood can be stroked from the raised limb to accelerate the gravitational effects. A mild pallor should then be seen within 1 minute. A severe, widespread pallor suggests arterial insufficiency. The limb should be lowered into dependency and the time taken for the plantar surface to return to the colour of the other limb should be noted. If the blood supply is adequate, the plantar surface of the foot should regain its normal colour within 15 seconds. A delayed time of 20 seconds or more suggests that blood supply is inadequate, with severe ischaemia being likely if the delay is 40 seconds or more. If the colour on dependency is a dusky red, this is a serious sign, indicating that the blood supply is severely compromised. Buerger's test has been shown to be a useful adjunct to routine vascular assessment and can be an indicator of more severe ischaemia with distal limb artery involvement (Insall et al 1989).

### Allen's test

This can be used to detect occlusion distal to the ankle. One leg of the patient is elevated and the dorsalis pedis artery is compressed with the practitioner's thumb. Maintaining pressure on the artery, the leg is lowered into dependency. If the tibialis posterior artery is patent, the foot should return rapidly to its normal colour. The patency of the dorsalis pedis artery can be tested in a similar manner, by compressing the tibialis posterior artery.

### Pedal pulses

Each time the heart contracts, blood is ejected into the aorta from the left ventricle. Because the aorta has a large amount of elastic tissue in its walls, the walls will be distended by the blood. At diastole, as the heart relaxes, the pressure on the walls drops and the elastic recoil of the walls causes them to spring back, pushing the blood on and acting as a secondary pump. The recoil causes a pressure wave which travels rapidly through the blood in the arterial tree. It travels much faster than the actual velocity of the blood, rather as ripples can travel rapidly over the surface of a slow-moving stream. It is called a pulse (wave) and can be palpated wherever the arterial tree comes close to the skin surface, e.g. wrist. The main pressure points in the lower limb are indicated in Figure 6.10. These places are called pulse points or pressure points. The frequency of the pulse wave will be the same as

the frequency of the heart beat, or the ventricular systole.

The practitioner should place the thumb or second, third and fourth digits on the dorsalis pedis pulse point; the number of shock waves in 1 minute should be counted. This procedure should be repeated at the posterior tibial pulse point and for the other leg. When the practitioner is familiar with this technique, the time can be reduced to 30 or 15 seconds, with the score being doubled or quadrupled appropriately. This is slightly less accurate than taking the pulse for 1 minute.

If the arteries are all patent and there is no vascular problem, then the values should be identical at each site. If they are not, the pulses should be checked again. If the pulse appears to be absent, it may suggest that there is some occlusion in the artery, proximal to the pulse point. This will either produce a faint pulse or an absent one. The site which is immediately proximal to the absent pulse should be tried to see if the approximate area of obstruction can be located. However, it should be noted that the dorsalis pedis pulse is absent in 10% of the population and the posterior tibial pulse is absent in 2%, but only 0.5% have both absent in the same foot.

A large pulsatile mass behind the knee or in the inguinal area suggests the presence of an arterial aneurysm. 10% of aneurysms occur in the popliteal fossa. They should be differentiated from popliteal cysts. Aneurysms are liable to rupture or stagnate in the area, which may lead to thrombus formation.

### Bruits

These are abnormal sounds which can be heard, using a stethoscope, in the arterial part of the cardiovascular system. Normal flow is laminar and is silent. Bruits are due to turbulence in arteries caused either by an increased velocity or an obstruction. Nicholson et al 1993 consider that clinical examination for bruits has good accuracy (78%) and may be of clinical value in the early detection of patients who are suitable for percutaneous angioplasty.

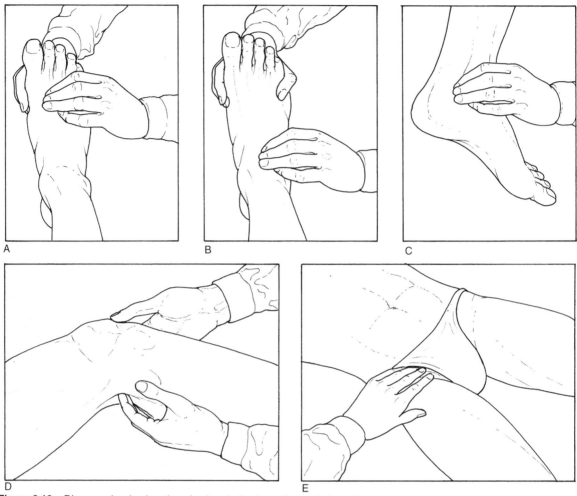

**Figure 6.10**  Diagram showing location of pulses in the lower limb  **A.** Dorsalis pedis  **B.** Anterior tibial  **C.** Posterior tibial  **D.** Popliteal  **E.** Femoral.

## Doppler ultrasound

The Doppler ultrasound machine enables the pulse to be heard much more clearly. The machine consists of two piezoelectric quartz crystals, one of which emits sound waves of very high frequency (2–10 MHz). The degree of penetration of the wave is inversely proportional to its frequency. The waves are reflected off moving objects such as blood cells and received back by the second crystal. The difference in frequency between the emitted and reflected waves is emitted as a sound, the fre-quency of which is proportional to the velocity of the moving object. Alternatively, the output may be fed to a chart recorder to produce a visible tracing. To protect the head of the probe, a coupling gel must always be used on the skin surface. For best results the pulse should be palpated and a blob of gel placed on the site. The probe should be placed at an angle of 45° to the skin surface and gently moved until an artery is located.

The arterial pulse is unmistakeable as three clear sounds, a triphasic response, the first being louder and of a higher pitch. This is due to the ventricular bolus being ejected from the heart during systole. The second and third sounds are the diastolic sounds, due to the reversal of flow caused by the elastic distension in the arteries. They correspond to the 'dichroitic notch' seen on Doppler traces. A diphasic response can be seen in the elderly or it may indicate disease of the arteries. A monophasic response always indicates disease, but care must be taken first to ensure that the technique is not at fault. Patients with bradycardia will have a weak triphasic sound and patients with tachycardia will show only a biphasic sound as the heart is beating too rapidly for reverse flow to occur. More sophisticated uses of the Doppler apparatus are described under hospital tests.

## Claudication distance

If the patient complains of intermittent claudication or if pedal pulses seem weak or absent, this test can be used to give an indication of the severity of the arterial occlusion. The patient is exercised, preferably on a treadmill, as the exercise should be standardised, and the distance the patient walks before the onset of pain is noted. The treadmill should be at 0% incline and at a speed of 4 km/h. No patient should be exercised if there is a history of angina and it is recommended that a full resuscitation kit should always be present for any exercise test.

## Ankle–brachial pressure index (ABPI)

This was first described by Yao in the 1960s. The ankle–brachial index provides a good indication of the presence of ischaemia in the lower limb. It can be used quantitatively since it also correlates well with the patient's symptoms, walking distance and angiography. It can be used to determine the optimum level of amputation and prognoses for grafts (Ameli et al 1989, Davies 1992).

The ankle–brachial pressure index is arrived at by recording the systolic pressure at the brachial artery and at the posterior tibial artery (ankle). Practitioners may find Doppler easier to use than a stethoscope when trying to take a reading of the systolic pressure in lower limb arteries. The reading obtained for the ankle is then divided by the brachial systolic reading and is expressed as a ratio. The value obtained at the ankle will depend on the position of the patient. If the person is supine and the legs are at the same horizontal level as the heart the ratio should be 1. If the person is sitting or standing, the pressure in the artery at the ankle will be greater than in the arm, because of the vertical column of blood between heart and ankle. As a rule of thumb the ankle systolic pressure will be 1 mmHg higher for every inch below the heart. Thus the ratio will be greater than 1. Average values for healthy adults in the sitting position are 0.98–1.31 (Davies 1992).

A ratio which is greater than 1 does not always mean that all is well. Diabetics are prone to calcification of the artery wall (Mönckeberg's sclerosis): this leads to incompressibility of the artery, so giving an artificially high reading of the ankle systolic pressure (Fig. 6.11). Nevertheless, 'the measurement of ankle pressure using Doppler is the single most valuable adjunct to the assessment of the blood supply to the foot' (Faris 1991).

Any value below 1 should be checked again. Values less than 0.8 suggest some obstruction in the more proximal part of the artery to the lower limb, although it is possible to find good capillary filling time and no associated lesions in such patients. Values of 0.75 or less indicate severe problems and at values below 0.5, healing is unlikely to take place, the leg being in a pregangrenous state. Ischaemic ulcers may be present.

Since mild to moderate atherosclerotic change may not affect the ankle–brachial pressure index the effects of exercise on the index is often observed (Davies 1992). Again a standardised treadmill exercise should be used (4 km/h, 0% incline, 4 min). In a healthy adult, unless exercise is severe, the index will show no change or will rise but rapidly returns to resting value once exercise has stopped. In a person suffering from peripheral vascular disease, the index will not rise and may fall, taking a long time to return to resting values. Heavy exercise may produce a

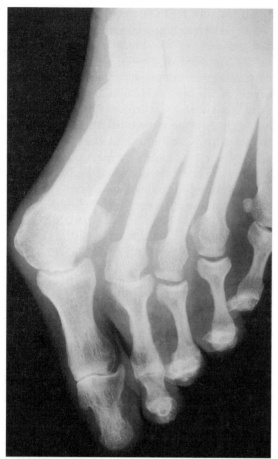

**Figure 6.11** X-ray showing Mönckeberg's sclerosis of the dorsalis pedis artery.

systolic blood pressure and so raise the value of the ABPI, but will quickly return to normal values. In a patient with peripheral vascular disease the narrowed arteries will be unable to respond to the vasodilatory effects of the metabolites, either because they are unable to dilate or because the occlusion prevents an increased flow, so that the ABPI will either stay the same or fall.

If a low ankle–brachial index is recorded the index should be calculated at progressively higher positions up the leg, to ascertain the site of the occlusion. When using the ankle–brachial pressure index it is also important to remember that the value obtained for the ankle cannot accurately predict the healing of lesions in the forefoot. In these instances the blood supply to the ankle may be adequate but the supply distal to the ankle may be affected. Digital cuffs can be used to assess the systolic reading in toes.

## Hospital tests

If an ischaemic limb has been identified, further investigation may be required to assess:

- suitability for reconstructive surgery
- the prognosis for the healing of ulcers
- the level at which amputations should be performed.

### Non-invasive

**Photoelectric plethysmography:** This method is used to measure skin blood pressure. A light-emitting diode is placed on the skin and a photocell is used to detect the emitted light, which is proportional to the amount of haemoglobin in the tissues. A sphygmomanometer cuff is used to blanch the skin. The cuff is then slowly deflated and the pressure point at which a flow signal returns is taken to be the skin perfusion pressure. A similar piece of apparatus is used to measure oxygen percentage saturation of the blood in pulse oximetry (Coull 1988). The laser Doppler can be used in a similar way.

**Duplex ultrasound:** This combines B mode ultrasound and Doppler to give both an image

fall in the index in healthy subjects due to shunting of blood from the distal arteries to the exercising muscles.

If the patient cannot be exercised, the hyperaemic test can be used. A second occlusion cuff is placed proximal to the first and inflated to above the systolic pressure for 2 minutes. It is then deflated and the systolic blood pressure is immediately taken. The second cuff occludes the arterial supply. Since venous drainage is also temporarily interrupted, metabolites will accumulate in the area. These have a vasodilatory effect on the blood vessels, so that in a healthy person, on releasing the second cuff, blood will rush into the area producing a temporary hyperaemia. This will cause a slight rise in of the artery under investigation and the flow within that artery. It takes time and requires a level of expertise, but using Doppler and pulse generation run off (PGR) provides a complete non-invasive assessment of lower limb. Duplex can also be used to ascertain the long saphenous vein suitability for femoral bypass grafting.

**Transcutaneous oxygen tension (TcPO₂):** The skin is heated to arterialise the capillaries and the partial pressure of oxygen which diffuses to the surface of the skin is measured by an electrode. This is not a routine test but can be used as a predictor of level of amputation. Faris 1991 (p. 145) suggests that the $TcPO_2$ values are affected by both macro- and microangiopathy.

**Magnetic resonance imaging (MRI) and positron emission tomography (PET) scanning:** These are expensive new procedures which can be used to visualise the various parts of the circulation, but doubts have been raised as to the value of such procedures in the absence of evidence to suggest any improvement in patient outcome (Kapoor & Singh 1993, pp. 4, 11, 423).

*Invasive*

**Isotope clearance:** This method is used to measure skin perfusion pressure (SPP) and skin vascular resistance (SVR) in the compromised foot in order to ascertain the likelihood of the healing of ischaemic ulcers. The SVR can be calculated from the graph of clearance values and applied pressure. A straight-line relationship exists between the two and the SVR is the reciprocal of the slope. Faris (1991) considered the level of SVR to be an independent indicator of the presence of microangiopathy, increasing in the presence of the latter. A small volume of the radioisotope technetium-99m, together with a vasodilator such as histamine, is injected into the skin and the rate of clearance of the isotope is recorded. The pressure from a sphygmomanometer cuff just necessary to prevent the radioisotope from leaving the area is taken as the SPP. This value reflects large artery disease. A value of 30 mmHg or more is needed to ensure healing. Radionuclide imaging as performed for investigation of coronary arteries can also be used to

estimate blood flow in the foot and to detect the presence of osteomyelitis (Faris 1991, p. 150).

**Angiography (arteriography):** This can be used to locate occlusions and stenotic vessels and to determine whether a collateral circulation has been established. It is unlikely that a collateral circulation will be established below the knee. A needle is inserted into the artery, just proximal to the occlusion and a radio-opaque dye is injected.

## VENOUS DRAINAGE

Venous problems may arise in the superficial and/or deep veins (Table 6.3). These problems affect the return of blood to the heart causing pooling of blood, exacerbated by the effects of gravity, around the ankles. The arterial supply to the lower limb may be adequate but if the venous return is poor, tissue viability will be adversely affected, particularly around the malleoli (Case history 6.3). Conversely it may well be that there is an inadequate arterial supply as well as poor venous return.

## Past history

The patient should be asked if he/she has previously suffered with any venous problems, e.g. deep vein thrombosis (DVT). Women of childbearing age may have experienced a deep vein thrombosis during, or more probably shortly after, childbirth. Although this may have occurred some years ago it may be the underlying cause

**Table 6.3** Causes of venous insufficiency

| | |
|---|---|
| Superficial | Varicose veins:<br>    primary—idiopathic<br>    secondary—backflow from deep to<br>    superficial vein |
| | Thrombophlebitis |
| | Phlebangioma (swelling of vein, congenital) |
| | Phlebectasia (dilated vein, congenital) |
| Deep | Deep vein thrombosis due to:<br>    abnormalities affecting blood flow<br>    abnormalities of clotting<br>    abnormalities of the vein wall<br>    idiopathic |
| | Thrombophlebitis |

---

### Case history 6.3

A 79-year-old female Caucasian presented to the clinic with an ulcer by the medial malleolus of the right ankle. The skin around the right ankle was reddish-brown (haemosiderosis) with white plaques (atrophie blanche). The patient complained that the skin had been itchy prior to the ulcers occurring. Oedema was present in the right leg but not the left. The ulcer was shallow, approximately 5 cm in diameter, with an irregular border, and there was a clear discharge. Peripheral vascular assessment showed there was an adequate blood supply to both legs; bounding pulse of 70 beats per minute, capillary filling time 2 seconds and no evidence of trophic changes to the skin of the feet. An ischaemic index test was not undertaken on the right leg because of the ulceration around the ankle. Ischaemic index for the left leg was 1.2.

Assessment of venous drainage showed impairment in the right leg but not the left. In the right leg there was evidence of pitting oedema, gravitational eczema, haemosiderosis, atrophie blanche and the characteristic features of venous ulceration.

The past medical history revealed the patient had developed a deep vein thrombosis while recuperating from a major abdominal operation when 20 years old. The thrombosis had been treated effectively at the time but the patient had noticed some 10 years after the thrombosis that her right leg, after periods of standing, began to feel very heavy and ache. When she was 40 years old her ankle started to swell towards the end of the day and by the time she was 50 the skin around the area had become discoloured and itchy. The patient thought the ulcer had developed after she had knocked her right ankle against a chair. The ulcer had been present for a year and despite a range of treatments had not shown any signs of healing.

A diagnosis of venous ulceration, as a result of poor venous drainage exacerbated by trauma was made. These ulcers are notoriously difficult to heal: they account for the most common cause of ulceration in the lower limb.

---

of current deep vein problems. Varicose veins tend to have a familial predisposition; it is therefore important to ask the patient if anyone else in the family suffers from this condition.

## Symptoms

### Varicose-related pain

A bursting or aching sensation associated with ankle oedema suggests problems with venous drainage. The pain and oedema are often alleviated by leg elevation. Varicosities may be apparent, especially on standing. Unilateral presentation suggests a peripheral venous cause, whereas symmetrical presentation is more likely to be due to congestive heart failure. The onset of deep vein thrombosis (DVT) is often associated with severe pain and tenderness in the calf, which increases when the foot is dorsiflexed or when the calf muscles are squeezed (Homan's sign). However, this is not generally thought to be a very reliable diagnostic test for deep vein thrombosis.

## Observation

### Hosiery

The wearing of elastic or support stockings or bandages suggests some problem with venous drainage. The extra compression provided by the stocking aids venous blood flow and reduces peripheral oedema.

### Colour

Telangiectases around the medial malleoli can indicate poor drainage (Plate 4). A mottled cyanosis may often appear in the lower third of the lower limb due to stagnation of blood in the veins as a result of poor drainage. Atrophie blanche, white patches on the skin around the ankles, occurs due to strangled microcirculation and leads to fibrotic and sclerotic changes in the skin (Plate 5).

Haemosiderosis can also indicate poor drainage (Plate 6). Back pressure in the veins produces leakage from superficial vessels causing brown deposits of the iron complex haemosiderin in the skin. Differential diagnoses with haemosiderosis are erythema ab igne, common in the elderly, and necrobiosis lipoidica diabeticorum, a condition associated with diabetes, where yellowish patches are seen on the shins and the skin appears very transparent, so that superficial blood vessels can be seen.

### Temperature

In venous insufficiency the skin often feels warm, which suggests that the arterial supply is satisfactory. However, it should be borne in mind that recent thrombosis may result in inflammation in the veins (phlebitis) due to the presence of the thrombosis.

## Varicose veins

These may be due to incompetent valves in the superficial veins alone or as a consequence of DVT. Back pressure due to an obstruction in the deep veins will accumulate through the communicating veins to the superficial veins. This causes the superficial veins to become incompetent and forward flow of blood is deficient. These veins are very extensible with non-uniform areas of weakness and have little support in the superficial tissues. They therefore bulge unevenly due to the pressure of blood, giving the knotted appearance of varicose veins. Poor tissue vitality results which may lead to cellulitis or superficial phlebitis, where the vein will be cord-like and painful.

## Tissue vitality

Poor drainage results in the accumulation of waste products. As a result tissue viability is adversely affected. The skin may eventually become indurated. Atrophy, venous eczema and venous ulcers may result.

## Gravitational eczema

Signs of discoloration and pigmentation, scaly and lichenified skin, in the presence of oedema, haemosiderosis and atrophie blanche suggest a diagnosis of gravitational eczema (Plate 6). The area can be very itchy; scratching may lead to the development of ulcers. Patients with gravitational eczema often find that they become sensitised to topical antibiotics and to preservatives in other topical medicaments and bandages.

## Venous ulcers

These account for 85% of all leg ulcers and are more common in women than men. They are commonly found around the malleoli, in particular the medial malleolus, but can often spread completely around the leg. Venous ulcers are associated with gravitational eczema. They are usually shallow with irregular borders and have either a healthy or slightly sloughy base unless infected (Plate 7). Trauma is not always the initiating factor. They are usually only painful if they become infected. The pain can be alleviated by leg elevation. Bacterial infection is very common in long-standing ulcers.

These ulcers are notoriously indolent. It is not unusual for a patient to have suffered a venous ulcer for many years which, despite daily attention, refuses to heal. In some cases malignant change, squamous cell carcinoma, may occur. It is important the practitioner regularly monitors these ulcers for signs of rolled edges and a hyperplastic base.

## Oedema

Oedema may be associated with venous problems (Plate 7). It may occur as part of the sequelae to deep vein thrombosis (DVT). The increased hydrostatic pressure causes leakage of tissue fluid so that oedema results. Where the tissue fluid is an exudate, it will contain plasma proteins, including fibrinogen, and will become organised. Transudate will not become organised unless it is very long-standing. Once the oedema is organised it cannot be squeezed by digital pressure and so is called non-pitting. The oedema due to deep vein thrombosis usually demonstrates pitting unless it is very long-standing. There will often be an outline of the patient's hosiery or footwear impressed on the skin.

Oedema may result in ischaemia around the ankle. In these instances moist gangrene may occur if the occlusion of arteries is very severe. The different types of oedema which can occur in the lower limb and their differential diagnosis are covered in detail in Chapter 17.

## Leg shape

Patients with chronic venous ulceration and oedema may develop characteristic 'champagne legs', also known as 'inverted bottle legs'.

## Clinical tests

### Pitting/non-pitting oedema

Digital pressure is firmly applied to the area for a period of 3–5 seconds. If an imprint of the fingers remains, the oedema is described as pitting.

### Buerger's elevation/dependency test

The observation for competency of venous drainage can be done simultaneously with the observation for adequacy of arterial supply. If the veins are competent they should refill within 15 seconds. A delay of 40 seconds or more suggests venous incompetency. Backflow will cause stagnation and a bluish colour to result.

### Perthes test

This test can also be used to test the competency of leg veins. With the leg dependent, an occlusion cuff is inflated at mid-thigh level. The superficial veins will become prominent as they fill. The patient is then asked to walk for 5 minutes. If the veins are healthy, the prominence will reduce due to drainage into the deep veins. If the superficial veins are incompetent, the prominence will remain and if this is accompanied by a dusky rubor it suggests that the deep veins are incompetent.

### Doppler

In contrast to the pulsating sounds of arteries, veins sound like wind sighing down a chimney, because of the effects of respiration on the flow of venous blood in the thorax. However, if there is excessive fluid in the lower limbs, as in congestive heart failure, the veins may give a pulsatile sound.

## Hospital tests

### Non-invasive

**Plethysmography.** A range of methods can be used—impedance or air plethysmography, phleborheoplethysmography and mercury strain-gauge plethysmography. These instruments can be used to diagnose thrombotic obstruction of major proximal veins of the extremities. They are not useful for detecting calf vein thrombosis.

### Invasive

**Venous angiography.** A radio-opaque dye is injected into the affected vein to show valvular incompetence and the presence of an obstruction.

## LYMPHATIC DRAINAGE

As previously described the lymphatics play an important part in draining tissue fluid back, via the thoracic duct, to the heart. If lymphatic drainage is adversely affected it results in oedema (lymphoedema). Lymphoedema can be congenital where it is classified as primary, or acquired, where it is classified as secondary lymphoedema. The causes of primary and secondary lymphoedema are outlined in Table 6.4.

## Medical history and symptoms

A history of permanent oedema, usually confined to the lower limbs, suggests primary lymphoedema, especially if there is a family history of the disease as one form is an autosomal dominant condition (Milroy's disease). Onset is either early in life (lymphoedema praecox) or after the age of about 35 years (lymphoedema tarda). It affects females more than males. Un-

**Table 6.4** Causes of lymphoedema

| | |
|---|---|
| Primary (congenital) | Milroy's disease |
| | Idiopathic |
| Secondary (acquired) | Intrinsic: |
| | malignant neoplasia |
| | radiotherapy |
| | surgical excision of lymph nodes |
| | filariasis |
| | infection |
| | Extrinsic: |
| | trauma |
| | plaster cast |

like venous oedema, once it is organised, it will not be alleviated by leg elevation. In contrast, secondary lymphoedema will arise as a result of some trauma to the lymphatic system such as obstruction or damage due to radiotherapy, malignant disease, surgery, pregnancy ('white leg'), or certain tropical infections (filariasis).

## Observation

### Oedema

In primary lymphoedema the oedema begins as a soft, pitting form but becomes harder and non-pitting with time. The condition can be unilateral or bilateral. Secondary lymphoedema is usually unilateral and considerable fibrosis may occur (Case history 6.4).

---

**Case history 6.4**

A 40-year-old male Caucasian attended clinic complaining of difficulty in undertaking routine footcare of the left foot. An assessment of the vascular status revealed that the left leg was considerably larger than the right and the skin was thickened, dry and coarse. The nails on the left leg were very thickened, distorted and discoloured. Examination of the left leg showed the presence of non-pitting oedema. The patient said the left leg had become very swollen and the skin thickened and dry after an operation on his groin.

The past medical history revealed that the patient had had testicular cancer. This had been treated by surgical removal of the testicles and radiotherapy. His problems with the left leg had resulted after the course of radiotherapy.

A diagnosis of secondary lymphoedema was made. It is likely that the radiotherapy damaged the left-side inguinal lymph nodes and as a result lymphatic drainage of the left leg was adversely affected, resulting in lymphoedema.

---

### Tissue vitality

The tissue fluid stagnation will interfere with diffusion of gases and nutrients and removal of waste products and as a result impair tissue vitality. It may be associated with troublesome cellulitis and usually leads to a thickening and

scaling of the skin which can lead to an 'elephantiasis-like' appearance: an oedematous leg with skin that resembles elephant skin.

### Yellow nail syndrome

The nail appears yellow in colour, thickened but smooth and there is an increase in lateral curvature. The rate of growth of the nail is reduced. The condition is associated with chronic lymphoedema.

## Clinical tests

It is not usual to carry out any clinical tests for lymphoedema apart from those which will distinguish it from other types of oedema, such as whether it is pitting or non-pitting.

## Hospital tests

Angiography for lymphatic vessels (lymphangiography) can be carried out in the same manner as for venography. In primary lymphoedema X-rays may show hypoplasia of the lymphatic system, with the lymphatic channel appearing scanty and spidery.

## SUMMARY

This chapter has outlined an assessment process from which practitioners can arrive at a diagnosis of the vascular status of a patient. This information can be used to make a diagnosis and to formulate an appropriate treatment plan. Case studies have been included to illustrate the effects of vascular problems.

The information gained from the vascular assessment can be used to draw up an effective treatment plan. It is important to establish if tissue perfusion falls within an acceptable range in relation to the patient's age. If it does, the patient, as long as no other problems exist, can receive treatment as for any other non-risk patient. If vascular problems are present or there is a distinct possibility they will occur in the future then it is important to give prophylactic advice and treatment. Choice of treatment, e.g.

surgery, will be affected by the presence of vascular problems as wound healing will be impaired and the patient is at greater risk of developing infections.

REFERENCES

Ameli F M, Stein M, Provan J L, Aro L, Prosser R, St Louis E L 1989 Comparison between transcutaneous oximetry and ankle–brachial pressure ratio in predicting run off and outcome in patients who undergo aortofemoral bypass. Canadian Journal of Surgery 32(6): 428–432

Berkow R (ed) 1987 The Merck manual, 15th edn. Merck Sharp & Dohme Research Laboratories, NJ

Coull A 1988 Making sense of pulse oximetry. Nursing Times 32: 42–43

Davies C S 1992 A comparative investigation of ankle:brachial pressure indices within an age variable population. British Journal of Podiatric Medicine 48(2): 21–24

Davies A H, Horrocks M 1992 Vascular assessment and the ischaemic foot. Foot 2(1): 1–6

Faris I 1991 The management of the diabetic foot, 2nd ed. Churchill Livingstone, Edinburgh, ch 9

Ganong W F 1991 Review of medical physiology, 15th ed.

Lange, London, p 510

Howell M A, Colgan M P, Seeger R W, Ramsey D E, Sumner D S 1989 Relationship of severity of lower limb peripheral vascular disease to mortality and morbidity: a six year follow-up study. Journal of Vascular Surgery 9(5): 691–696, discussion 697

Insall R L, Davies R J, Prout W G 1989 Significance of Buerger's test in the assessment of lower limb ischaemia. Journal of the Royal Society of Medicine 82(12): 729–731

Kapoor A S, Singh B N 1993 Prognosis and risk assessment in cardiovascular disease. Churchill Livingstone, New York

Lainge S P, Greenhalgh R M 1980 Standard exercise test to assess peripheral arterial disease. British Medical Journal 280: 13–16

Nicholson M L, Byrne R L, Steele G A, Callum K G 1993 Predictive value of bruits and Doppler pressure measurements in detecting lower limb arterial stenosis. European Journal of Vascular Surgery 7: 59–62

FURTHER READING

Bardwell J 1993 Arterial assessment. Community Outlook Mar: 34–35

Berne R M, Levy M N 1992 Cardiovascular physiology, 6th ed. Mosby/Year Book, St Louis, MO

Walker W E 1991 A colour atlas of peripheral vascular diseases. Wolfe Medical, London

Wilkerson D K, Keller I, Mezrich R, Zatina M A 1991 The comparative evaluation of three-dimensional magnetic resonance for carotid artery disease. Journal of Vascular Surgery 14(6): 803–809, discussion 809–811

Yao S T 1970 Haemodynamic studies in peripheral arterial disease. British Journal of Surgery 57: 761–766

# 7

# Neurological assessment

*J. McLeod-Roberts*

There are many conditions affecting the nervous system which modify lower limb function (Table 7.1). The purpose of this chapter is to enable the practitioner to detect the presence of these conditions. The chapter begins with an outline of the histology, organisation and function of the nervous system. Reflexes are dealt with as a separate topic as they form the basis of so much neurological behaviour. A detailed description of the assessment of each part of the neurological system is then presented.

## Why undertake an assessment of the patient's neurological status?

It is important to undertake an assessment of the neurological status in order to identify whether the patient has an intact and normally functioning neurological system. The purpose of the assessment is to:

- establish which, if any, part of the nervous system is functioning abnormally
- identify the extent of dysfunction
- where possible, arrive at a specific diagnosis
- draw up a treatment plan which takes account of the above information.

It is important to establish which part or parts of the nervous system are affected. For example, an ataxic (uncoordinated) gait may be due to a disorder of the cerebellum or a lack of proprioceptive information. The practitioner may be in a position to identify early changes in neurological function, e.g. initial clinical features

**Table 7.1** Neurological conditions that may affect the lower limb

| Condition | Description |
| --- | --- |
| Cerebral vascular accident (CVA) | Due to haemorrhage, embolus or thrombosis of the cerebral arteries |
| Parkinsonism | Degeneration of dopaminergic receptors. Usually idiopathic but can be drug-induced |
| Friedreich's ataxia | Hereditary, autosomal dominant condition which affects children. Death from heart failure common by 40 |
| Multiple sclerosis | Patchy demyelination of the CNS. Shows relapses and remissions. Onset 20+ |
| Poliomyelitis | Virus that affects LMNs |
| Syringomyelia | Progressive destruction of the spinal cord due to blockage of central canal, e.g. tumour |
| Tabes dorsalis | Occurs with tertiary stage syphilis |
| Spina bifida | Defective closure of vertebral column. Congenital |
| Motor neurone disease | Degeneration of neurones and tracts. Idiopathic |
| Subacute combined degeneration of the spine | Due to lack of vitamin $B_{12}$ |
| Charcot–Marie–Tooth disease | Hereditary disorder, usually autosomal dominant. Affects peroneal nerve |
| Guillain–Barré syndrome | Autoimmune disorder that affects peripheral nerves and results in loss of function of motor, sensory and autonomic systems |
| Neurofibromatosis | Autosomal dominant condition that leads to tumours of nerves and compression of spinal cord |
| Peripheral neuropathy | Occurs due to a variety of causes, e.g. alcoholism, injury, diabetes mellitus |
| Myasthenia gravis | Autoimmune disease that affects the neuromuscular junction and leads to severe fatigue and weakness/paralysis |

associated with multiple sclerosis: double vision, falling over, tingling sensations, loss of function. If an appropriate treatment plan is to be drawn up, knowledge of the presence of any condition and its specific effects on the lower limb is essential. For example, sufferers of Guillain–Barré syndrome are predisposed to foot ulcers and so the treatment plan should include preventative measures and a monitoring programme as 10% of patients may show incomplete recovery.

# OVERVIEW OF THE HISTOLOGY, ORGANISATION AND FUNCTION OF THE NERVOUS SYSTEM

## HISTOLOGY

There are two types of cell that make up the tissue of the nervous system: glial cells and neurones.

## Glial cells

There are four types of glial cell (Fig. 7.1):

- ependymal
- oligodendrocytes (brain) and Schwann cells (periphery)
- astrocytes
- microglial.

Ependymal cells are involved in the secretion and absorption of cerebrospinal fluid (CSF), which acts as an interstitial fluid, bathing the cells of the brain and spinal cord. Oligodendrocytes in the brain and what are known as Schwann cells in the periphery are responsible for the manufacture of a fatty (myelin) sheath around the axons of the neurones, which improves the speed of nerve conduction. They also play a role in the development and repair of nervous tissue, helping to guide the growing axons to their correct destinations. Astrocytes have a buffering

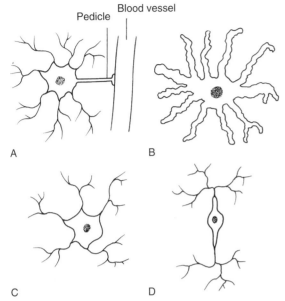

A

B

C

D

**Figure 7.1**  Neuroglia  **A.** Fibrous astrocyte
**B.** Ependymal cell  **C.** Oligodendrocyte  **D.** Microglial cell.

Pedicle  Blood vessel

function, ensuring that the K$^+$ concentration of the CSF is constant. This is essential for the correct functioning of the neurones. These cells may also have a nutritive role, they are phagocytic and they take up certain neurotransmitters. Microglial cells are also phagocytic and remove debris. Since glial cells outnumber the neurones by a factor of at least 10 to 1, their sheer bulk means that they provide structural support, there being no connective tissue within the nervous tissue.

## Neurones

Despite being in the minority, a mere 10$^{12}$ in the brain, it is these cells which have the very special function of rapid communication, transmitting signals or nerve impulses from one neurone to the next, or to other excitable tissue such as muscle. Like other highly specialised cells neu-

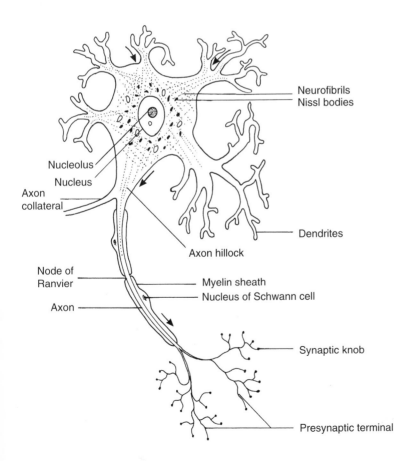

Neurofibrils
Nissl bodies
Nucleolus
Nucleus
Axon collateral
Axon hillock
Dendrites
Node of Ranvier
Myelin sheath
Nucleus of Schwann cell
Axon
Synaptic knob
Presynaptic terminal

**Figure 7.2**  A single neurone (not to scale) illustrating the four parts: cell body, dendrites, axon, presynaptic terminals. Note that in the CNS some neurones may have no axons.

rones lose the ability to mitose soon after birth and so once the cell body is destroyed, it cannot be replaced; damage results in permanent changes.

A neurone consists of four main parts (Fig. 7.2).

**1. Cell body.** This contains the nucleus and other organelles and is the site of synthesis of chemicals (neurotransmitters) for the transmission of impulses.

**2. Dendrites.** These fine branches from the cell body are the chief receptive area for impulses from other neurones or for the reception of other stimuli.

**3. Axon.** This is the conducting portion and can be up to 1 m in length. It conducts electrical impulses and is also involved in the transport of various substances to and from the cell body. It may be myelinated as shown but if less than 1 μm in diameter it will be unmyelinated.

**4. Presynaptic terminals.** These are fine branches of the axon and are responsible for the release of neurotransmitters to enable the impulse to pass from one neurone to the next or on to a muscle or gland.

The gap or synapse between one neurone and the next is an area of physical discontinuity (Fig. 7.3).

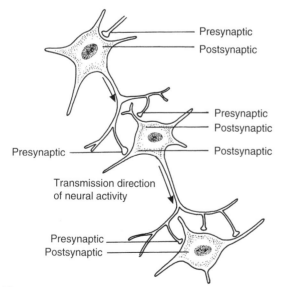

**Figure 7.3** Diagram of synapses, identifying pre- and postsynaptic membranes (adapted from Vander et al 1990).

# ORGANISATION

The nervous system can be divided in a number of ways to identify its different parts, based on both anatomical and functional classifications (Fig. 7.4).

## Anatomical classification

### Central nervous system (CNS)

This contains all the structures lying within the central axis of the body; the brain and spinal cord. It consists of neurones and glial cells.

The brain can be divided into fore-, mid- and hindbrain and is covered by the three meninges and protected by the cranium (Fig. 7.5). The cerebral cortex consists of two hemispheres (right and left), each of which is divided into four lobes by deep grooves or sulci. The four lobes are frontal, parietal, temporal and occipital. The cortex is highly convoluted, which increases its surface area and therefore the number of neurones it contains. It overshadows other structures in the forebrain such as the thalamus and basal ganglia.

The cerebellum consists of two hemispheres which are primarily composed of the anterior and posterior lobes. These are phylogenetically younger than the flocculonodular lobe and the midline structure called the vermis. The brain stem consists of the medulla, pons and midbrain. It contains a diffuse network of neurones called the reticular formation and discrete clusters of neurones called nuclei. The parts of the brain and their main functions are listed in Table 7.2.

The spinal cord is surrounded by the 32 vertebrae of the spinal column; the cell bodies of the neurones form the so-called 'grey matter' and their axons form the 'white matter' because of the presence of myelin. Cerebrospinal fluid (CSF) circulates through and over the brain and spinal cord. During development a difference in growth rates between the spinal cord and the surrounding vertebrae means that the spinal cord ends at the upper border of the second lumbar vertebra (Fig. 7.6). The dura mater and the subarachnoid space, with CSF, continue to the level of the second sacral vertebra, so that lumbar punctures

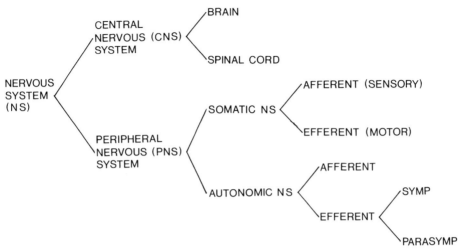

**Figure 7. 4**    Flow diagram of the organisation of the nervous system.

can be performed at the level of L3 or L4 to withdraw a sample of CSF without damaging the spinal cord.

### Peripheral nervous system (PNS)

This comprises those nerves that lie outside the spinal cord and brain. These can be subdivided into:

- afferent nerve fibres, which carry impulses towards the CNS from receptors such as warmth receptors

- efferent nerve fibres, which carry impulses away from the CNS to effectors such as sweat glands.

The nerve processes form 12 pairs of cranial nerves originating from the brain stem and 31 pairs of spinal nerves. The spinal nerves emerge from the spinal cord as two roots, a dorsal (posterior) and a ventral (anterior) root, which then join to form the peripheral mixed spinal nerve, which emerges between two adjacent vertebrae (Fig. 7.7). The dorsal root contains the cell bodies of afferent fibres in a swelling called

**Table 7.2**    Areas of the brain and their function

| Area | | Function |
|---|---|---|
| Forebrain | Cerebral cortex | Frontal lobe: abstract thought, conscious action, speech<br>Parietal lobe: general senses, verbal understanding<br>Temporal lobe: hearing, taste, smell, emotions<br>Occipital lobe: vision |
| | Diencephalon | Thalamus: sensory relay station<br>Hypothalamus: emotions, endocrine system, ANS<br>Limbic system: motivation and emotions<br>Basal ganglia: movement |
| Midbrain | Corpora quadrigemina | Superior colliculi: visual orientation |
| | | Inferior colliculi: auditory orientation |
| Hindbrain | Pons | Modification of respiration |
| | Cerebellum | Modification of movement |
| | Medulla oblongata | Vital control centres |

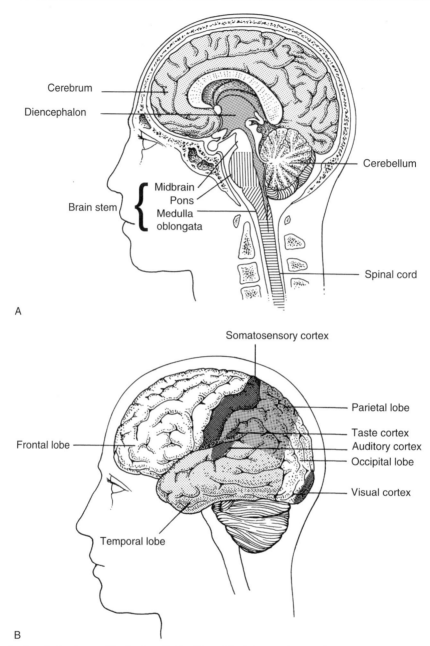

**Figure 7.5** The brain **A.** Anatomy of the brain **B.** Position of the lobes and cortex (adapted from Vander et al 1990).

the dorsal root ganglion. The central process of each afferent neurone travels into the area of grey matter of the spinal cord called the dorsal horn. The ventral root contains mainly efferent fibres, the cell bodies of which lie within the ventral and lateral horns of the spinal grey matter.

The spinal nerves are mixed as they contain both afferent and efferent fibres, from both the somatic and the autonomic nervous system (see below). This is why damage to a spinal nerve may affect autonomic function (e.g. loss of bladder control) as well as motor and sensory function, depending upon the site of damage.

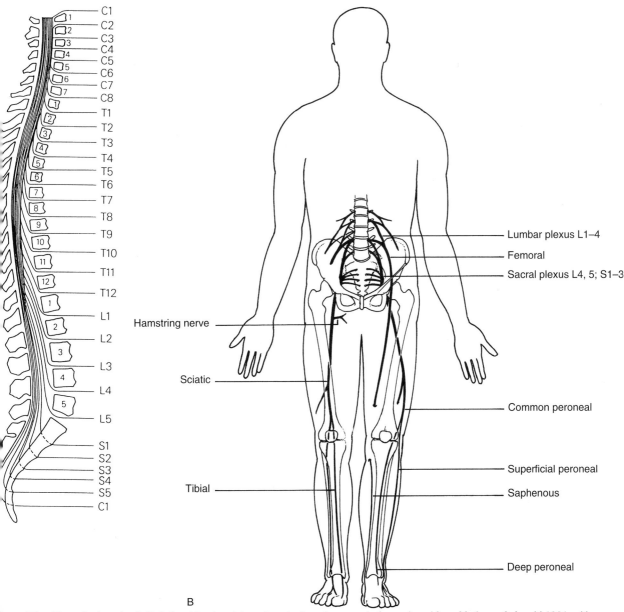

C1
C2
C3
C4
C5
C6
C7
C8
T1
T2
T3
T4
T5
T6
T7
T8
T9
T10
T11
T12
L1
L2
L3
L4
L5
S1
S2
S3
S4
S5
C1

Hamstring nerve

Sciatic

Tibial

Lumbar plexus L1–4

Femoral

Sacral plexus L4, 5; S1–3

Common peroneal

Superficial peroneal

Saphenous

Deep peroneal

B

**jure 7.6**   The spinal cord   **A.** Relationship of vertebrae to spinal cord segments (reproduced from Mathews & Arnold 1991, with rmission)   **B.** Organisation of the lumbar and sacral plexi and innervation of the lower limb (adapted from McClintic 1980).

Again, the unequal growth rates of spinal cord and vertebral column mean that the spinal nerves from L2 onwards have to travel some way posteriorly before emerging at the appropriate level between the vertebrae. This results in the formation of the 'cauda equina'.

A *dermatome* is defined as an area of skin supplied by a single nerve's dorsal root. It also implies that muscles are innervated in a similar segmental pattern. Dermatomes overlap each other by up to 30%, so if a spinal nerve is damaged there will not be a total loss of sensation in that

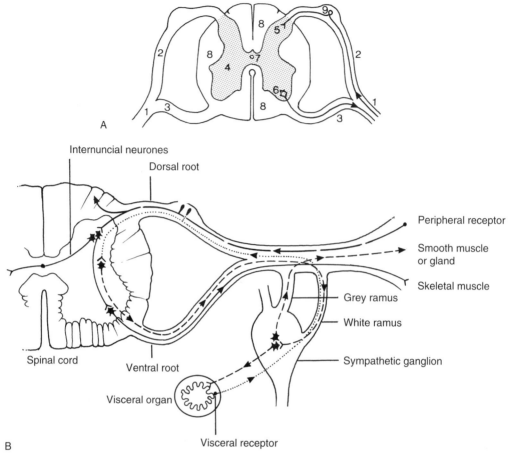

**Figure 7.7** **A.** Transverse section through the spinal cord showing mixed spinal nerve roots: 1) the paired mixed spinal nerves; 2) dorsal (posterior) root; 3) ventral (anterior) root; 4) central grey matter; 5) dorsal horn; 6) ventral horn; 7) central canal; 8) surrounding white matter; 9) dorsal root ganglion **B.** Connection between sensory and motor neurone to the spinal cord (adapted from McClintic 1980).

area as adjacent dermatomes will respond to stimuli. The dermatomes of the lower limb are outlined in Figure 7.8.

## Functional classification

### Somatic nervous system

This includes all parts of the nervous system that deal with the conscious perception of stimuli and conscious action. The afferent nerves can also be called sensory nerves and the efferent nerves can be called motor nerves. The receptors detect changes in the external environment and the effectors bring about movement of the skeleton.

### Autonomic nervous system (ANS)

This is the part of the nervous system that deals with the internal organs. The terms sensory and motor are not used here, as these terms imply consciousness and the information coming from the viscera rarely reaches consciousness; likewise the movements of the viscera are rarely voluntary movements. The afferent neurones are similar in arrangement to those of the somatic system, with cell bodies in the dorsal root ganglion, although the receptors are situated in internal organs such as the baroreceptors of the carotid sinus. The efferent branches of the ANS differ from those in the somatic system in that

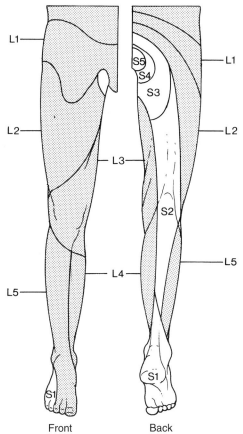

L1

S5
S4
S3

L1

L2

L2

L3

S2

L4

L5

L5

S1

S1

Front                    Back

**Figure 7.8**   The lower limb sensory dermatomes and their nerve roots (adapted from Epstein et al 1992).

there are two neurones in the pathway. The cell body of the first neurone is in the CNS but those of the second are found in the autonomic ganglia outside the CNS. This divides the efferent neurones into pre- and postganglionic neurones. This efferent outflow can be further divided into the sympathetic and parasympathetic systems (Fig. 7.9).

**Parasympathetic nervous system.** This is the efferent part of the autonomic nervous system which restores the 'status quo' and allows emptying actions. The cell bodies of the preganglionic neurones are situated in the brain stem and sacral region of the spinal cord (craniosacral outflow). The postganglionic cell bodies are found in ganglia close to or within the effector organ being innervated, so that the majority of the

efferent pathway is preganglionic. The neurotransmitter released at both the pre- and post-ganglionic endings is called acetylcholine.

**Sympathetic nervous system.** This is the efferent branch of the autonomic nervous system, which prepares the body for action; the fight or flight response. The cell bodies of the preganglionic neurones are found in the lumbar and thoracic regions of the spinal cord and the sympathetic ganglia form a chain alongside the spinal cord, so that the majority of the efferent pathway is postganglionic (Fig. 7.7B). The neurotransmitter released at the preganglionic endings is again acetylcholine, but the postganglionic endings mostly release noradrenaline.

Where an effector organ receives dual innervation, the two branches usually act antagonistically, in a push–pull or accelerator–brake fashion, to regulate the activity of the effector organ. For example, the vagus nerve (tenth cranial nerve) slows the heart rate down and the sympathetic nerve speeds it up. However, the parasympathetic nerves do not innervate structures outside the central axis and so only sympathetic nerves innervate the skin and blood vessels. Sympathetic activity causes peripheral vasoconstriction and a reduction in this activity or 'tone' causes vasodilation.

## FUNCTION

As with all systems within the body, the prime function of the nervous system is to ensure that the internal environment which bathes the cells is maintained within acceptable limits (homoeostasis). The particular role of the nervous system is to ensure that the collection of cells and tissues that constitute our bodies can act as an organised whole. This can only be achieved if the cells can communicate with one another. The nervous system has evolved as the system of rapid communication, usually producing short-term effects. It evolved with, and works alongside, the generally slower endocrine system, which tends to have long-term effects.

### The nerve impulse

Neurones use two types of signal to achieve

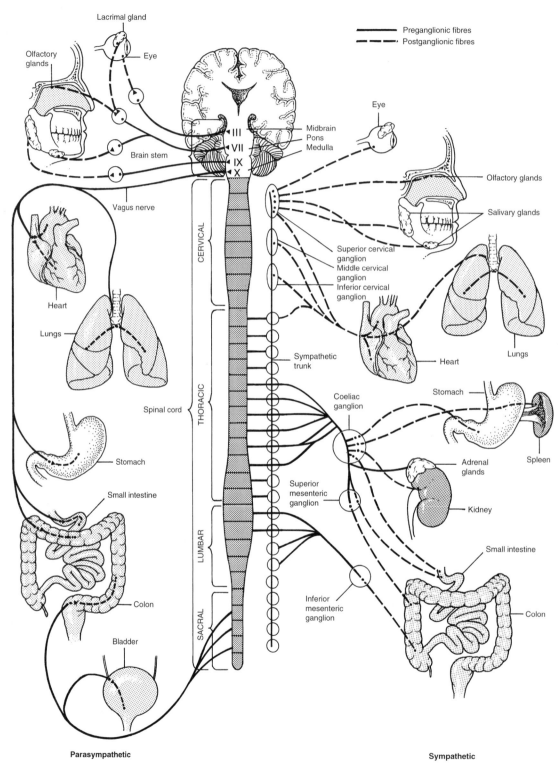

**Figure 7.9** Autonomic outflow (adapted from Vander et al 1990).

intercellular communication—graded and action potentials. Both types of signals are dependent upon the movement of ions across the cell membrane and through protein ion channels, but they also show many differences.

## Action potential

This is used by the neurone to transmit an impulse over long distances along its fine cytoplasmic processes, the dendrites and axons (Fig. 7.2). The action potential is initiated by a voltage change which causes sodium channels to open, allowing the influx of sodium. The entry of these positively charged ions causes a reversal of the resting membrane potential or a 'depolarisation'. Provided the initial voltage change is large enough and of sufficient duration, a threshold value of depolarisation will be reached and a positive feedback cycle will be established, causing further opening of sodium channels and depolarisation. The magnitude of this depolarisation will be dependent on the number of ion channels present in the plasma membrane and is therefore fixed for a particular neurone. Provided threshold is reached, the resulting action potential will always have the same value for that neurone. This is known as the 'all or nothing law'. Since the ion channels are operated by a voltage change, they are described as voltage gated channels.

The depolarisation is reversed when the sodium channels close and potassium channels open, allowing an efflux of potassium ions. This renders the interior of the neurone more and more negative, and the membrane is now 'repolarised'. At the same time the sodium pump, present in all plasma membranes, actively pumps out the sodium which has recently entered and claws back the escaped potassium. Due to a time lag in the closing of the potassium channels, the inside of the neurone actually becomes briefly more negative than when at rest, and this phase is described as 'hyperpolarisation' (Fig. 7.10).

The opening and closing of the ion channels is triggered by the initial voltage change, but because this opening and closing operates at different rates, the ions move in the sequence

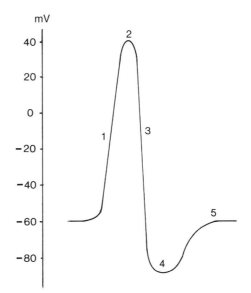

**Figure 7.10**   Diagrammatic representation of an action potential. 1 = $Na^+$ enters axon; 2 = $Na^+$ channels close, $K^+$ leaves; 3 = $Na^+/K^+$ pump begins; 4 = $K^+$ channels close; 5 = resting potential restored.

just described. Finally the distribution of ions is restored to their pre-action-potential level and the membrane is at resting potential once more. All this activity is ultimately dependent upon energy being expended by the sodium/potassium ATPase pump, hence the term 'action potential'. Due to the establishment of local current flow, the initial depolarisation triggers an identical action potential at adjacent sites and this is propagated along the axon without any attenuation of the impulse. If the axon is unmyelinated, this sequence of events will be repeated at every point along the axon, spreading out in both directions away from the initial stimulus.

Presence of myelin speeds up the passage of the impulse since it enables the local current to spread further, up to 1 mm, along the axon before another action potential needs to be generated. Hence the sodium channels need only be situated at 1 mm intervals, at the so-called 'nodes of Ranvier' with a myelin coat in between. Since local current flow is faster than the generation of an action potential, the impulse appears to jump or leap from node to node, hence the term 'saltatory conduction' from the Latin word *saltare* meaning 'to leap'. In multiple sclerosis there is a loss of the myelin coat and the nerve impulse is adversely affected, leading to the clinical features associated with this condition.

### Graded potential

When the action potential reaches the terminals of the neurone there has to be some mechanism by which the impulse can cross the synaptic gap, reach the next neurone in the pathway and generate an action potential in this neurone. This is achieved by means of release of a chemical or 'neurotransmitter' from the presynaptic terminals, which diffuses across the gap and combines with receptors on the postsynaptic membrane (Fig. 7.3). The postsynaptic membrane is usually the dendrite of the next neurone, but can be an axon or the cell body itself.

The release of the neurotransmitter from the presynaptic membrane is triggered by the arrival of the action potential, which opens calcium channels in the plasma membrane. Influx of calcium causes the movement and exocytosis of vesicles laden with neurotransmitter. The latter is referred to as the first messenger. The consequence of combination of the neurotransmitter with postsynaptic receptors is a conformational change in proteins of the plasma membrane, resulting either in a direct effect on proteins to open or close ion channels or, much more commonly, in activation of an enzyme such as adenyl cyclase. This catalyses the production of cyclic AMP from ATP. Cyclic AMP acts as a second messenger, triggering a cascade of internal events that finally results in the opening of ion channels, allowing depolarisation of the post-synaptic membrane, the so-called 'graded potential'. Since the ion channels are opened by chemicals they are called chemically-gated channels. In parkinsonism there is a loss of the neurotransmitter dopamine and with myasthenia gravis there is a loss of cholinergic receptors; both these conditions adversely affect the normal functioning of the graded potential.

Synapses are not the only site for graded potentials. They also occur at receptors where the ion channels may be triggered by mechanical

**Table 7.3**  Differences between action and graded potentials

| Action potentials | Graded potentials |
|---|---|
| Voltage-gated ion channels | Chemically/mechanically/light-gated ion channels |
| Threshold must be reached before an action potential is generated | No threshold, all triggers will generate graded potentials |
| Fixed magnitude (all or nothing) | Magnitude proportional to size of trigger |
| Large potentials | Small potentials |
| Do not summate | Summate |
| Do not attenuate | Rapidly attenuate |
| Used for long-distance signalling | Used for local signals |

or light changes as well as chemicals. Graded potentials rapidly dissipate and so can only travel over very small distances. Since they are small, they must summate to produce an action potential. This is initiated within a short distance of the postsynaptic membrane.

Synapses slow down the passage of impulses due to the time taken for the neurotransmitter to be released, but this disadvantage is more than outweighed by the variability or plasticity which synapses confer on the system. They are also responsible for converting the pathways into one-way systems, essential if chaos is not to reign.

The differences between action and graded potentials are summarised in Table 7.3.

## Sensory pathways

The various changes in the internal and external environments are detected by receptors. Receptors may be found within specialised organs, such as the rods and cones of the eye, or they may be distributed throughout the body, such as the pain receptors of the skin and gut. The first type give rise to the special senses of sight, hearing, balance, taste and smell, whereas the second type give rise to the general senses of pressure, touch, temperature, pain and position sense, the so-called somatic receptors (Table 7.4). Again,

**Table 7.4**   Classification of the somatic receptors

| Category | Sense | Receptor |
|---|---|---|
| Mechanoreceptor | Touch, pressure | Encapsulated and free nerve endings |
| Thermoreceptor | Warmth, cold | Free nerve endings |
| Nociceptor | Pain | Free nerve endings |
| Proprioceptor | Position | Encapsulated nerve endings |

the use of the word 'sense' implies awareness of the stimulus, i.e. it reaches the conscious cortex.

Those receptors situated in the skin can also be referred to as exteroceptors. There are also stimuli which do not usually reach consciousness but go to different areas of the brain; these originate within the internal organs and are called interoceptors. Examples of these are the baroreceptors in the aorta, which monitor changes in blood pressure, and the osmoreceptors in the hypothalamus, which monitor the osmolarity of the extracellular fluid. Receptors in the muscles, tendons and joints that register position sense, tension and degree of stretch are called proprioceptors. They send impulses both to the cerebellum, which is part of the unconscious brain, and to the part of the conscious brain called the somatosensory cortex.

The area served by a sensory unit (afferent nerve, its branches and the attached receptors) is called the receptive field. Receptor fields may overlap and the density of receptors may vary in different regions of the body. The precision with which a stimulus can be located and differentiated depends on the size of the receptive field and the density. For example, fingers and thumbs are very good at detecting stimuli from the external environment because the receptive fields are small and dense.

The peripheral afferent (sensory) pathway is the name given to the pathway from a receptor to the CNS. As explained earlier the cell body of the afferent neurone is usually situated along this pathway, near to, but not in, the spinal cord. The central process then travels into the spinal cord where it may synapse with one or more neurones in the dorsal horn or continue on its path up the spinal cord to the brain stem. The grey matter is divided into layers or laminae of Rexed and the neurones in the various layers

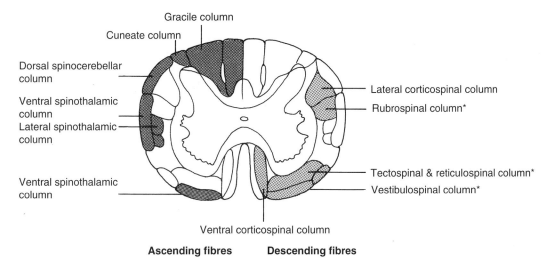

Figure 7.11   Transverse section of the spinal cord showing ascending and descending pathways  (adapted from McClintic 1980). *Multineuronal tract.

differ in size and functions. Stimuli detected in the periphery will initially be conveyed by afferent neurones to the spinal cord, but if further integration and interpretation is to occur, the information must reach the appropriate part of the brain. The information travels to these higher centres in ascending tracts or columns of the white matter of the spinal cord (Fig. 7.11).

All information from a particular receptor type, such as pressure, travels together in the same ascending tract. The ascending tract is joined, at each spinal segment on its upward journey, by neurones which are carrying information from pressure receptors in other dermatomes. The organisation continues in the brain, so that discrete areas of the cortex receive the information from the various parts of the body (Fig. 7.12). This is called somatotopic organisation.

There are two main ascending systems (Budd 1984):

• the rapid, highly organised oligo- (few) synaptic pathways

• the less well organised multisynaptic pathways.

Most of the tracts are named according to their origin and destination: e.g. the lateral spino-thalamic tract carrying pain information runs from the lateral region of the spinal cord up to the thalamus, an important sensory relay station in the brain. The spinocerebellar tracts do not reach consciousness but instead carry proprioceptive information to the ipsilateral lobes of the cerebellum, in the hindbrain.

The oligosynaptic pathway consists of two tracts:

• the dorsal (posterior) columns
• the neospinothalamic tracts (part of the anterolateral tract).

The multisynaptic pathways also travel via two ascending tracts. One of these tracts, the fasciculi proprii, runs as a central chain of neurones through the spinal cord and ascending reticular activating system (RAS) of the brain

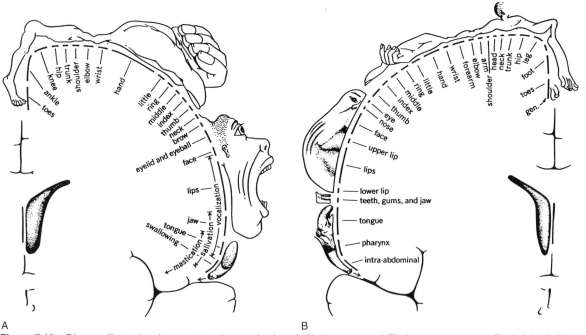

A                                    B

**Figure 7.12** Diagram illustrating the somatotopic organisation of (**A**) the motor and (**B**) the sensory cortex. The left half of the body is represented by the right hemisphere of the brain and the right half of the body by the left hemisphere (reproduced from Ross & Wilson 1990, with permission).

stem to the central areas of the thalamus, before projecting to the limbic system and the hypo-thalamus. These pathways do not cross and can be activated by more than one stimulus. The other multisynaptic pathway is the palaeospino-thalamic tract, which follows the same course as the neospinothalamic tract until it reaches the brain stem, where it diverges, to make further synaptic connections with the RAS and central thalamus before travelling on to the limbic system. The information is interpreted in a less precise manner but with emotional overtones, such as the sensation of a deep, burning abdominal pain.

The division into tracts of differing modalities is not hard and fast, however, since the nervous system demonstrates the phenomenon of redun-dancy, which means that if one tract is damaged another is usually able to take over the function, albeit in a slightly altered form. For example, impulses conveying information about touch travel in both the dorsal column and the ventro-spinothalamic tract though the nature of the information differs, as the dorsal column deals with detailed localisation of the touch sensation and the spinothalamic tract with gross tactile sensations.

Some of the pathways, the pain pathways in particular, carry information about a single type of stimulus. These are described as specific path-ways, since they are interpreted as well localised, precise sensations by the somatosensory cortex —e.g. the sharp sensation of a pinprick.

The majority of these ascending tracts cross over to the opposite side at some stage, either in the spinal cord or in the brain stem, synapsing with contralateral areas of the thalamus before continuing to the conscious cortex. This arrangement explains why a stroke affecting a particular part of the sensory cortex produces numbness or paraesthesia in a specific part of the body on the opposite or contralateral side. Neurological damage to the spinal cord may produce numbness on either the contra-lateral side, if the site of damage is before the tracts cross, or the ipsilateral (same) side, if the site of damage occurs after the tracts have crossed.

# Motor pathways

Just as all conscious stimuli are interpreted in the cortex, so all conscious actions originate there. The whole area is known as the sensori-motor cortex; one part is called the primary motor cortex and initiates conscious action (Fig. 7.12). It too shows somatotopic organisation, so that damage to this region produces precise effects on particular actions on the contralateral side of the body. Close to this area is the pre-motor cortex, which is involved in the planning of actions. Since the actions produced by these neurones are the conscious movements of the body, the muscles involved will be skeletal and the neurones will be part of the somatic motor system.

Neurones in the brain which are responsible for initiating the commands are called upper motor neurones (UMNs). They do not send impulses directly to the muscles but exert their influence via neurones in the ventral (anterior) horn of the spinal cord called lower motor neurones (LMNs). The latter send impulses to the skeletal muscles via their axons which form the peripheral efferent pathways within spinal nerves.

The descending pathways from brain to spinal cord can be divided into two main tracts: the corticospinal tract and the multineuronal tract (Fig. 7.11).

**The corticospinal tract** is a rapid pathway and is mainly responsible for the skilled movements of small, distal limb muscles such as those used in scalpel work. Most of the fibres cross over in the brain stem and descend in the white matter of the spinal cord as the lateral corticospinal tract. The uncrossed fibres descend as the ventral (anterior) corticospinal tract. At the appropriate level in the spinal cord they enter the ventral horn of the grey matter to synapse with a lower motor neurone. Because the corticospinal tract forms a rough pyramid shape as it passes through the brain stem, it is also called the pyramidal tract.

**The multineuronal tract** also runs from upper to lower motor neurones but by a slower, more diffuse route, since it makes many more synaptic connections on the way, particularly in the descending reticular system and the nuclei of the brain stem. From here the tracts emerge to travel through the spinal cord as the vestibulospinal, tectospinal and reticulospinal tracts. The tracts enter the ventral horn of the grey matter to influence the appropriate lower motor neurone.

These tracts do not form part of the pyramids in the medulla and so are also called the extra-(outside) pyramidal pathways. They mainly influence the large, proximal limb muscles and the axial muscles of posture, and have a predominately inhibitory effect on the ventral horn cells. They are responsible for the antigravity reflexes which keep our knees extended and head erect in order to maintain upright posture.

The division of the descending tracts is not clearcut, as they also demonstrate redundancy, there being much overlap and interaction between the two. Other areas of the brain also have strong modifying influences, such as the cerebellum and clusters of neurones in the fore- and midbrain known collectively as the basal ganglia.

The last stage in the production of a conscious action is the excitation of a LMN in the ventral (anterior) horn of the spinal cord and the passage of an impulse along its axon in the spinal nerve to the skeletal muscle. The LMN will be subject to influences from many neurones, not only from descending tracts but also from spinal neurones. As many as 10–15 000 synapses, both excitatory and inhibitory, can occur on one lower motor neurone. If the sum of these influences is excitatory, the LMN will be stimulated to discharge an impulse along its axon and the skeletal muscle will contract. This peripheral pathway from LMN to skeletal muscle is called the final common pathway (Fig. 7.13).

## Cerebellum

The actions of the cerebellum are unconscious and are very important in postural reflexes. The cerebellum has no direct descending pathways to the spinal cord; instead it has a rich afferent input and sends modifying influences to the sensorimotor cortex, the reticular formation and the brain-stem nuclei. Thus symptoms of cerebellar defects may be due to lesions in the ascending spinocerebellar tracts, in the cerebellum itself or in efferent pathways going to other parts of the brain.

The cerebellum receives all information about position sense. The vestibular apparatus of the ear projects via the vestibular nuclei of the brain stem to the flocculonodular lobe. The spinocerebellar tracts carry proprioceptive information from the muscles, tendons, joints and cutaneous pressure receptors which project to the vermis and anterior lobes. The cerebral cortex gives information about the actions decided upon and

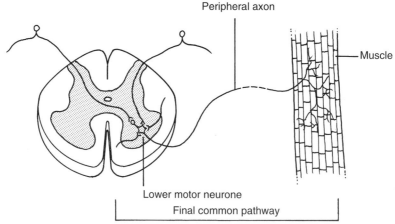

Peripheral axon

Muscle

Lower motor neurone
Final common pathway

**Figure 7.13** The final common pathway.

projects to the posterior lobes via pontine nuclei. The cerebellum integrates the information received from all these areas and compares it with the information on intended actions received from the cerebral cortex. It then sends modifying influences back to the motor cortex and brain stem, so that descending instructions to the LMNs can be altered where necessary.

## Basal ganglia

At present the precise functions of the basal ganglia in movement are unknown, but they are thought to enable abstract thought (ideas) to be converted into voluntary action (Ganong 1991). Like the cerebellum they function at an unconscious level and have no direct pathway to LMNs but influence the sensorimotor cortex and the descending reticular formation. Because the main action of the basal ganglia is on the descending extrapyramidal tracts, they have become known as the extrapyramidal system and conditions affecting them are referred to as extrapyramidal syndromes.

## REFLEXES

Reflex actions are automatic responses to particular stimuli and form the basis of much of our behaviour, from the simple knee jerk to driving a car. They are also very important in posture, balance and gait. Reflexes can be inborn (inherited, innate, instinctive) or acquired (learned). Examples of the former are eye blink, pupil dilation/constriction, change in heart rate, knee jerk (stretch) reflex, pain withdrawal and sweat secretion. Examples of the latter are swimming, walking, driving, debriding callus. They can involve any subdivisions of the nervous system and any type of effector organ. We may be aware of them or they may never reach consciousness. It is here that the close association between the nervous and endocrine systems is best illustrated, since both can contribute to the same reflex arc. For example, when the retina of the eye detects a threatening situation, this information will be carried by the optic nerve to the brain and one of the responses will be the release of the hormone

adrenaline from the adrenal medulla, to prepare the body for action.

In all cases, the pathway allows the body to respond rapidly to a given stimulus. Generally, inborn reflexes produce stereotypic responses which are usually protective reflexes or those needed for posture and balance. Acquired reflexes are more complex, involving the conscious cortex and many different effectors, so that the response is more easily modified. Try standing upright and leaning backwards as far as you can. What happens to your arms and knees? Can you prevent their movement? Compare this with the ease with which you can change from a walking to a running gait.

## Reflex arcs

The pathway between detector and effector is called a reflex arc and always involves the CNS, though not necessarily the brain (Table 7.5). There are three reflexes that are of particular importance to the functioning of the lower limb:

- pain withdrawal reflex
- crossed extensor reflex
- stretch reflex.

**Pain withdrawal reflex.** Injured cells produce local chemical mediators, including prostaglandins, that sensitise the nociceptors to other mediators. Graded impulses, proportional to the damage done, are generated and trigger action potentials in the afferent pathways. The action

**Table 7.5**   Essential elements of a reflex arc

1. A detector to detect the change (stimulus) in either the internal or external environment

2. Afferent neurones that send the information into the CNS along the afferent pathways

3. An integrating centre to match the appropriate response to the stimulus. This will be in the brain or spinal cord. Different parts of the CNS communicate with one another via ascending and descending pathways

4. Efferent neurones that carry instructions from the CNS via efferent pathways to the effectors (skeletal, smooth or cardiac muscle or gland)

5. An effector to carry out the necessary response

potential travels to the CNS (in this case the spinal cord) via the afferent neurone and synapses within the grey matter of the dorsal horn, in either Rexed's laminae II and III (the substantia gelatinosa) or in laminae V. It is here that the pain gating mechanism is thought to take place. This mechanism was first described by Melzack & Wall in the 1960s to explain pain inhibition by such techniques as rubbing the painful area. From here the impulse is transmitted to a LMN in the ventral horn of the spinal cord. Excitation of this neurone results in an action potential reaching the motor end-plate. The neurotransmitter acetylcholine is released and its combination with receptors in the muscle membrane results in a graded potential that will be transmitted to the interior of the muscle as an action potential and cause contraction of skeletal muscle fibres (Fig. 7.14). The number of fibres contracting depends on the number of muscle fibres innervated by that neurone, i.e. the size of the motor unit. Thus the limb suffering damage is removed from the deleterious cause. The presence of more than one synapse in the reflex arc means that the arc is described as polysynaptic. In addition to this reflex arc, the first order neurones will synapse in the dorsal horn with neurones which transmit impulses up to neurones in the brain, via the ascending anterolateral tracts. However, the cortex is not needed for the withdrawal reflex to occur.

**The crossed extensor reflex** is often super-imposed on the pain withdrawal reflex and is a postural reflex, enabling an injured lower limb to be withdrawn while the remaining limb bears weight. In order for this to occur, many LMNs must be excited and their antagonists inhibited (Fig. 7.15). This ensures that the flexors of the injured limb contract while the extensors relax, whereas in the contralateral limb the flexors are inhibited and the extensors contract to provide a rigid support. This reflex occurs not only when a lower limb is injured, but at each step in walking, when one limb is in the swing phase and the other is weightbearing.

**The stretch reflex** is a very important reflex for all motor activity, especially when new actions are being learnt. It can be demonstrated by the patellar and Achilles tendon reflexes and exists to supply the cerebellum with information about the state of contraction in muscle.

The receptors are stretch receptors in specialised muscle fibres called intrafusal fibres. These receptors lie within swellings of the intrafusal fibres called muscle spindles. Whenever the ordinary muscle fibres (extrafusal fibres) are stretched, as when the patellar tendon is hit by the hammer, the receptors will generate graded potentials. These will in turn trigger action potentials which will travel rapidly into the spinal cord, to synapse directly with the alpha LMNs. Efferent impulses will travel out to the extrafusal fibres, causing contraction of the muscle. The stretch receptors are of two types,

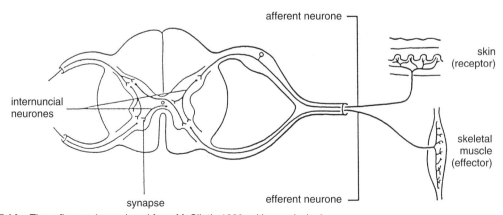

**Figure 7.14** The reflex arc (reproduced from McClintic 1980, with permission).

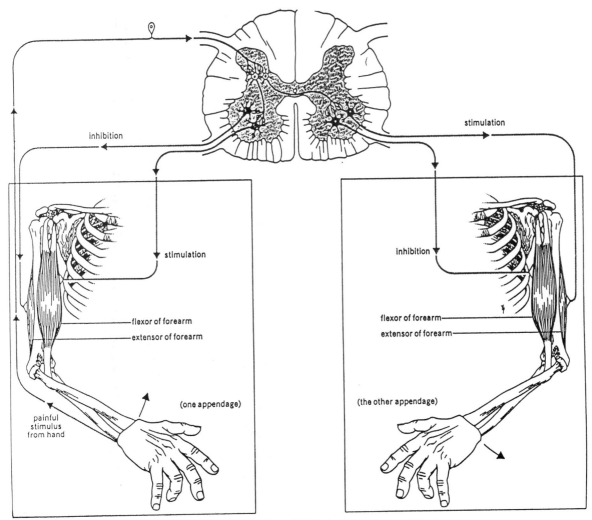

**Figure 7.15**   The crossed extensor reflex (reproduced from McClintic 1980 with permission).

**Table 7.6**   Role of CNS in posture, balance and coordination

| Action | Site | Function |
| --- | --- | --- |
| Motor coordination | Premotor cortex | Plans actions |
| | Sensorimotor cortex | Initiates action |
| | Basal ganglia | Converts thought into action |
| | Cerebellum | Modifies action. Compares actual and intended action, smooths action |
| | Brain stem (extrapyramidal) (pyramidal) | Modifies action Corrects position Skilled work |
| Posture and balance | Cerebellum | Rich input, miniprogrammes |
| Gait | All of above | |

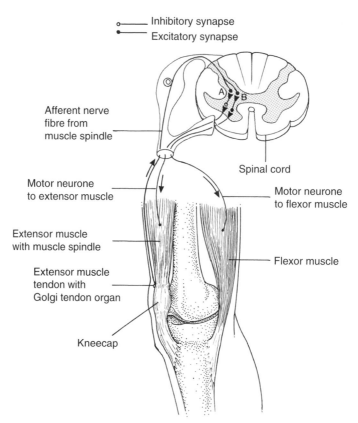

o———— Inhibitory synapse
•———— Excitatory synapse

Afferent nerve
fibre from
muscle spindle

Spinal cord

Motor neurone
to extensor muscle

Motor neurone
to flexor muscle

Extensor muscle
with muscle spindle

Flexor muscle

Extensor muscle
tendon with
Golgi tendon organ

Kneecap

**Figure 7.16** The stretch reflex. Contraction of the extensor muscle causes stretch in the muscle spindle and increases the firing rate of action potentials. This information is conveyed to the spinal cord and results in inhibition of the extensor muscle's motor neurone and excitation of the flexor muscle's motor neurone (adapted from Vander et al 1990).

one conveying information about the degree of stretch (static) and the other about the rate of change of stretch (dynamic). This information is sent along the spinocerebellar pathway to the cerebellum as part of the rich input that the cerebellum needs to be able to compile a precise 'picture' of what is happening in the muscles (Fig. 7.16). The reflex contraction of the muscle switches off the muscle spindle and deprives the cerebellum of information. This does not matter if the action being carried out by the muscle is a well-learned one, but if it is still being learned the cerebellum needs this information and can switch the spindle back on. This is achieved by a system of alpha–gamma coactivation, whereby small gamma LMNs are activated. These go to the poles of the muscle spindle and, by contracting the poles, the spindle continues to fire.

## COORDINATION AND POSTURE

It is now possible to summarise the various parts of the nervous system which are involved in posture, balance, gait and coordination of motor activity (Table 7.6).

## THE NEUROLOGICAL ASSESSMENT

Once the organisation and function of the nervous system is understood, it is often possible to diagnose the site of a lesion by careful history taking, observation and simple tests. Neurological disorders may be caused by the following factors:

• heredity, e.g. Huntington's chorea

- developmental defect, e.g. spina bifida
- trauma, e.g. severing of a spinal nerve
- ischaemia, e.g. cerebral vascular accident
- tumours, e.g. tumour of the cerebellum
- infection, e.g. HIV.

The effects of any lesion in the nervous system will depend on the area involved. For example, occlusion of the posterior cerebral artery, which feeds the occipital lobe of the brain (striate cortex), may result in visual disturbances, occlusion of a cerebellar artery may result in ataxia, and occlusion of the vasa nervosum of a peripheral nerve may result in a 'glove and stocking' paraesthesia.

Nerve function deficit is called neuropathy and is classified according to the numbers and types of nerves involved and the site of the lesion (Table 7.7).

The assessment process involves a general overview of neurological function followed by assessment of:

- levels of consciousness
- motor function
- sensory function
- posture and coordination
- autonomic function.

Many neurological conditions present with multiple signs and symptoms because more than one part of the nervous system is affected. It is important to bear this in mind when assessing each of the above parts in order that information from all the assessments can be put together to produce a definitive diagnosis. For example, multiple (disseminating) sclerosis is a progressive disease where repeated patchy demyelination of nerve sheaths occurs, leading to temporary loss of function. The nerve axons most often affected are the optic nerves, the cerebellar nerves and those of the lower spinal cord, leading to blurring of vision (diplopia), unsteady gait, weakness in the lower limbs and/or disturbances of micturition.

# GENERAL OVERVIEW OF NEUROLOGICAL FUNCTION

## History

It is important to undertake a thorough medical and social history (Ch. 5). In particular the following should be borne in mind.

### Presenting problem

Onset and duration may provide vital clues as to the cause of a problem. For example, Guillain–Barré syndrome has a sudden, postviral onset. The type of pain and its distribution can help to establish whether the problem affects a nerve pathway or is referred pain from entrapment of a spinal nerve. The patient should be asked if his/her limbs feel weak or sluggish (paresis): a slow, progressive onset of muscular weakness suggests muscular dystrophy, whereas an acute onset suggests a demyelinating disease.

The history of the problem and the type of onset may facilitate a diagnosis. For example, pain, numbness, a sensation of heaviness or a 'pins and needles' sensation in the arm could be due to compression of nerve roots in the spine, as seen in cervical spondylosis, or to an attack of angina pectoris. The sensation is likely to be spasmodic and associated with exercise or some other stress in the latter case, and of a more continuous nature in the former.

A history of frequent falls with no loss of consciousness suggests a lesion in one of the areas of the brain dealing with balance and posture, such as the cerebellum or basal ganglia. Such episodes can be seen in patients with Parkinson's disease or in multiple (disseminated) sclerosis. Where loss of consciousness has occurred, the

**Table 7.7** Classification of neuropathies

| Type of neuropathy | Description |
| --- | --- |
| Mononeuropathy | Abnormality of a single nerve |
| Mononeuritis multiplex | Asymmetrical abnormality of several individual nerves |
| Radiculopathy | Abnormality of a nerve root |
| Polyneuropathy | Widespread, symmetrical abnormality of many nerves, usually characterised as sensory/motor/autonomic 'glove and stocking' distribution |

period of unconsciousness and the age of the patient should be taken into account when making a diagnosis.

The presence of a severe headache is an important sign, since it may indicate one of several underlying causes, e.g. brain tumour, subarachnoid haemorrhage or migraine. Again, the onset, nature and duration of the headache should be established.

### Social habits

Smoking and alcohol consumption should be noted. Smoking is a risk factor for certain conditions such as atherosclerosis and therefore CVAs. Chronic alcoholism can affect both motor coordination and memory (Korsakoff syndrome). Patients suffer from damage to the limbic system due to thiamine deficiency (Fuller 1993). They appear alert and fully conscious, but recent memory of time and place is severely impaired. The patient denies any loss of memory and frequently attempts to disguise the deficit by confabulation (McLeod & Lance 1989). Similarly, indications of a lifestyle that increases the risk of contracting the HIV virus, such as intravenous drug abuse, may explain a neurological deficit, since the infection can produce a progressive encephalopathy.

### Gender

Some conditions occur much more frequently in one sex than the other. For example, myasthenia gravis affects females more than men whereas Duchenne's muscular dystrophy is seen much more in males.

### Age

There is a general slowing in the passage of impulses throughout the nervous system with age, as shown by nerve conduction tests. In addition, many conditions affecting the nervous system have typical onsets at particular ages. For example, shingles (herpes zoster), parkinsonism and CVAs are all associated with the over-60 age group whereas Charcot–Marie–Tooth disease usually manifests itself in people in their twenties and some forms of spina bifida have observable effects from birth. However, where two or more systemic conditions coexist the picture may be altered—for example, patients with diabetes mellitus or sickle cell anaemia are predisposed to earlier onset of CVAs. Coexisting chronic disease can also be helpful in diagnosing the cause—for example, atherosclerosis and hypertension are major risk factors for strokes (Macleod & Lance 1989).

## Observation

The patient should be observed while walking, sitting and speaking as well as while performing particular tasks. A change in the level of consciousness, inability to follow simple instructions and deficits in voluntary movement or sensation, including the presence of pain, all provide important clues. Important points to note are:

- the affected areas of the body, their distribution and whether one or more modalities are involved
- whether the effect is uni- or bilateral
- if affecting movement, whether it causes weakness or complete paralysis
- whether it involves particular muscles or particular actions
- whether it produces any change in muscle tone and bulk
- if the deficit is affecting sensation, whether the sensation is altered (paraesthesia) or lost (anaesthesia)
- the presence of a deformity, e.g. a cavoid-type foot and clawed toes are often seen with spina bifida occulta
- presence of tremors. Tremors can have a physiological cause or be associated with a neurological deficit. The exact nature of the tremor should be noted, when it appears/disappears, area of body involved, etc. The causes of tremor are summarised in Table 7.8.

**Table 7.8**  Classification of tremors and their likely causes

| Type of tremor | Condition |
| --- | --- |
| Physiological | Maintenance of posture is accompanied by a tremor (10 Hz). This may be exacerbated by anxiety, fatigue, thyrotoxicosis |
| Age (senile) | With age the normal physiological tremor slows to 6–7 Hz. As a result the tremor becomes more noticeable especially when undertaking a slow motion such as picking up a cup to drink from |
| Resting | Tremor that is present during rest (4–5 Hz), seen in parkinsonism |
| Intention | Tremor that increases as the individual tries to undertake a coordinated movement, seen with cerebellar dysfunction |
| Essential | Postural tremor similar to a physiological tremor but of much greater amplitude, usually hereditary |
| Drug-induced | Tremor similar to an essential tremor may occur in 40% of patients treated with barbiturates |

## ASSESSMENT OF THE LEVEL OF CONSCIOUSNESS

The cerebral cortex and the reticular formation of the brain stem are the two areas of the brain most concerned with maintaining consciousness. The general level of the patient's awareness, ability to answer questions and follow instructions can all give indications of the level of consciousness.

## History

Any history of loss of consciousness should always be questioned further, to try to establish whether the cause was:

- a simple faint
- transient ischaemic attack (TIA)
- an epileptic episode
- a metabolic disorder such as a hypoglycaemic coma.

Simple faints (syncope) are always due to a temporary interruption of blood supply to the brain, which is rapidly restored by the prostrate position of the patient. This may be caused by:

- benign causes, such as emotional shock, causing vasovagal syncope
- autonomic neuropathy if the fainting episode is associated with a change to an upright posture
- serious causes such as haemorrhage or anaphylactic shock.

TIAs are a temporary interruption in the vascular supply to the brain and like strokes and cardiovascular attacks usually occur in the older person (60+). Both strokes and TIAs are primarily caused (80% of cases) by thrombosis resulting from atheromatous plaques in cerebral vessels, haemorrhage being the cause of the remainder (McLeod & Lance 1989). TIAs usually last from 1–30 minutes and always less than 24 hours.

Epileptic attacks can occur at any age and are due to unusual electrical activity in the cortex, which could be caused by a lesion or a tumour.

## Observation

TIAs may be accompanied by disorders of speech (dysphasia), vision, movement (dyskinesia) or swallowing (dysphagia), depending on the area of brain involved. However, a full recovery is usual. CVAs can result in permanent neurological deficits, though partial or total recovery is possible depending on the extent and site of damage to the brain.

Epileptic attacks can involve the whole brain (global) and result in a brief loss of consciousness (petit mal) which may not show any other symptoms or may last much longer, being accompanied by tonic-clonic jerks (grand mal). Such an attack is often preceded by an 'aura' and the patient may cry out. Attacks can also be focal, as in a Jacksonian attack, which affects only the primary motor cortex and in which different parts of the body show jerks as the attack spreads over the motor cortex.

## Clinical tests

In the clinic the following can be used to establish the level of consciousness:

**Table 7.9**  Assessment of the level of consciousness (McLeod & Lance 1989)

| Level | Observable effects |
|---|---|
| Alert wakefulness | Patient is fully aware of environment and self and responds to stimuli |
| Confusion | Patient shows lack of attentiveness, cannot concentrate and has impaired memory |
| Delirium | Patient is anxious, excited, agitated and may be hallucinating |
| Lethargy | Patient is drowsy but responds to verbal stimuli |
| Stupor | Patient is unconscious but responds to pain |
| Coma | Patient cannot be roused |

- the patient's response to a question and answer schedule
- whether the patient can follow instructions
- the patient's response to stimuli.

Levels of consciousness can be graded as shown in Table 7.9.

## Hospital tests

The following is a brief summary of some of the hospital tests that may be undertaken if a patient shows an altered level of consciousness.

**Duplex Doppler ultrasound.** This technique uses sound waves of 4–8 MHz, which are beyond the range of human hearing. The transmitted beams are reflected from their interface with tissues in amounts proportional to the density of the tissues. The difference between transmitted and reflected beams is proportional to the density of the tissues and is used to create an acoustic image. In this particular technique, two-dimensional B-mode scanning is used, which gives greater resolution than the M-mode scanning of conventional Doppler. Duplex Doppler may reveal stenosis or occlusion of the carotid arteries, a possible cause of a CVA or a TIA, and is often used prior to an angiogram.

**Angiography.** Interarterial angiography with injection of a radio-opaque dye into the suspected artery will show atherosclerotic plaques in cerebral vessels, which are a common cause of embolitic strokes.

**Brain scans.** Computed tomography (CT) or magnetic resonance imaging (MRI) can be used to confirm TIAs, full blown CVAs, neoplastic mass or epileptic foci. Both techniques produce digitised images that can be numerically graded according to the pixel value of the matrix. This can then be converted to a grey–white scale. CT uses X-rays to scan the brain. MRI uses radio-frequency pulses that excite the protons of tissue.

**Electro-encephalogram (EEG).** EEGs, or 'brain waves', are traces which show the electrical activity of the cortex, as measured by scalp electrodes. EEGs are normally used to confirm a clinical diagnosis and locate the focus of epilepsy.

## ASSESSMENT OF LOWER LIMB SENSORY FUNCTION

It is important that the sensory system is intact in order that a person can respond to his/her external and internal environment. Failure to respond, especially to noxious stimuli, can lead to serious pathological changes and may even be life-threatening. Some patients may be unaware that sensory loss has occurred; it is therefore essential that the practitioner assesses the functioning of the sensory system.

Assessment involves checking whether sensory units are functioning normally and, if not, the extent of damage and the possible cause. Sensory deficits may arise as a result of damage to:

- parietal cortex
- ascending pathways
- receptors.

Conditions which may cause sensory deficits are outlined in Table 7.10.

The most important area of the brain for somatic sensory perception is the parietal cortex (Fig. 7.12). Any damage to this area, whatever the cause, will produce a contralateral sensory deficit in the appropriate part of the body. Damage to the occipital lobe (striate cortex) will produce visual disturbances. The most common

**Table 7.10** Causes of sensory deficits

- Diabetes mellitus
- Subacute combined degeneration of the spinal cord (vitamin $B_{12}$ deficiency)
- Congenital absence of particular sensory neurones
- Spina bifida
- Syringomyelia
- Tabes dorsalis
- Nerve injuries
- Guillain–Barré syndrome
- Multiple sclerosis
- Cord compression/lesion, e.g. tumour (Brown–Séquard syndrome)
- Chronic alcoholism

cause of such neurological deficits is an occlusion or haemorrhage of one of the cerebral arteries.

Damage to the ascending tracts in the spinal cord will produce either ipsi- or contralateral effects, depending on the site of the lesion in relation to the point of crossover of the tracts. This is well illustrated in the Brown–Séquard syndrome, where damage to one side of the spinal cord results in:

- ipsilateral loss of touch, position sense, two-point discrimination and vibration sense below the level of the lesion, due to dorsal column injury
- contralateral loss of pain and temperature sensation below the level of the lesion, due to damage to the anterolateral tracts.

The exact effect of peripheral nerve damage depends on the site and the nature of the damage, since this dictates the repair process (Table 7.11).

**Table 7.11** Classification of nerve damage

| Type | Damage |
| --- | --- |
| Neuropraxia | Mild trauma or compression causing local demyelination and leading to temporary loss of function. Full recovery within days or weeks |
| Axonotmesis | Crush injuries causing degeneration of axon and myelin sheath (wallerian degeneration) Neurolemma sheaths intact and reinnervated |
| Neurotmesis | Whole nerve axon severed. Surgical repair needed to ensure reinnervation of distal trunk |

## History

The nature and distribution of any sensory deficit can be an important aid in diagnosing the underlying cause. This may take the form of complete anaesthesia (total lack of sensation) or paraesthesia (an altered sensation). Examples of paraesthesia are pins and needles, burning, pricking, shooting pain and dull ache. Patients should be asked if they experience any abnormal sensations.

An unusual phenomenon that arises from amputation of a limb is that of 'phantom limb', where the patient has the very real sensation of the amputated limb still being present and behaving just like a normal limb. The most unpleasant effect is the sensation of pain which is said to occur in 70% of amputees (Melzack 1992). The traditional explanation, that this is due to the growth of neuromas in the nerve stumps which continue to generate impulses, cannot be the entire explanation since cutting the afferent pathways from such nerves does not abolish the pain. Melzack has suggested that the phantom sensations are due to learned circuits in the brain that are capable of generating impulses in the absence of sensory inputs.

Injury to the viscera often produces pain in a somatic structure some distance away. This is called referred pain. For example, a myocardial infarction can produce pain in the left arm, both the heart and the skin of the left arm having developed from the same dermatomal segment. However, the exact mechanism is still not clearly understood although both convergence and facilitation are thought to play a role (Ganong 1991). Damage to a spinal nerve may result in referred pain which is experienced around the heel; this occurs if there is damage to S1.

## Clinical tests

Simple apparatus is all that is needed to undertake an assessment of sensory function: cotton wool, a graded compass or a pair of blunt-ended orange sticks, a 128 Hz tuning fork, neurothesiometer, the sharp end of the patellar hammer and two small metal test-tubes, metal being a better

**Table 7.12** Sensory testing

| Sense | Method | Pathway |
|---|---|---|
| Light touch | Cotton wool/brush | Dorsal columns (ipsilateral) |
| Two-point discrimination | Two orange sticks/compass | |
| Vibration (pressure) | Tuning fork (128 Hz) | |
| Temperature | Hot and cold test-tubes | Anterolateral columns (contralateral) |
| Pain | Sharp object (end of hammer) | |
| Proprioception | Dorsi/plantarflexion of hallux | Dorsal columns (ipsilateral) |

conductor of heat than glass. The tests examine the integrity of the afferent pathways that involve the ipsilateral dorsal columns and the contralateral anterolateral columns (Table 7.12). It is important to remember when undertaking sensory testing that, where possible, the patient should have his/her eyes closed in order that the results cannot be influenced by him/her seeing what is being done. A deficit may not always be due to pathological causes: factors such as overlying callus render the skin less sensitive and the normal slowing of conduction rates associated with ageing results in a reduction in sensation. It is important that the tests involve more than one dermatome (Fig. 7.8).

**Light touch.** The patient's eyes should be shut. The skin of the foot is then stroked lightly with a wisp of cotton wool. The patient is asked to indicate the site. The sense of touch will be reduced in the elderly and in calloused skin (due to thickened skin). The patient may incorrectly distinguish between the lesser toes in this test, but this is normal and is due to the particular innervation of the lesser digits.

**Two-point discrimination.** The plantar surface of the foot is usually tested. The patient is asked, with eyes shut, to state how many points can be felt when the tips of a compass lightly press the skin surface simultaneously. The distance between the tips of the compass that allows the patient to detect two points rather than one should be noted. Usually the distance, on the foot of a healthy young adult, is 2 cm. It will increase with age and if the skin is calloused. The receptors responsible for identifying two-point discrimination are also essential for stereognosis—the

ability to recognise objects by touch—and are therefore very important for readers of Braille.

**Vibration.** The vibrating tuning fork is placed on the skin above a bony prominence such as the malleolus or the first MTPJ and the patient is asked to describe what is felt. Most patients describe the sensation as a 'buzzing'. The receptors involved are the pacinian corpuscles which are found deep in the hypodermis of the skin. Because they are rapidly adapting receptors they respond to high-frequency changes in pressure such as are produced by a tuning fork, but the layered connective tissue capsule around the nerve ending absorbs constant pressure or low-frequency changes.

**Neurothesiometers** provide an alternative method of assessing vibration. The neurothesiometer is basically a vibrator that delivers vibrations of increasing strength, measured in volts per micrometre. It is powered by rechargeable batteries to meet Health and Safety requirements. The neurothesiometer is positioned on a bony prominence and the strength of the vibrations is increased until the patient can detect a 'buzzing' sensation. Up to 12 readings can be stored in the memory of the apparatus. Since vibration is one of the first sensations to be affected by sensory neuropathy this is a very useful tool, though limited by the fact that it is not possible to apply the head at a standard pressure.

**Temperature.** This mainly tests the integrity of the anterior part of the anterolateral columns. One test-tube is filled with cold water and the other with warm water. Each in turn is placed on the same site of the foot, e.g. the dorsum or the instep. Cutaneous receptors detect changes in temperature, rather than absolute values. If the receptors are functioning normally the test-tube with warm water should feel warmer than the one with cold water.

**Pain.** This tests the integrity of the sharp pain pathway, in the contralateral anterolateral columns. It can be combined with the plantar reflex test. A relatively sharp instrument can be used (sharp end of a patellar hammer) for this test, but not one sharp enough to draw blood. The instrument should be drawn firmly and swiftly across the skin. The patient usually shows the flexion (pain withdrawal) reflex in response to this. It is important to remember that neuropathy does not always mean absence of pain, as is witnessed by diabetic patients with neuropathy, who can experience a period of intense pain (Faris 1991). Fortunately in these instances the area eventually does become analgesic.

**Tinel's sign.** This helps in the diagnosis of nerve compression. Palpating the nerve, or tapping it with a patellar hammer, at the site of compression will often elicit an abnormal sensation distally, but it can also follow the proximal distribution of the nerve. Usually the sensation is paraesthesia (tingling, burning) or is like an electric shock. Tinel's sign can be used to assess for compression of the medial nerve at the wrist or the posterior tibial nerve at the ankle (carpal and tarsal tunnel syndromes).

**Referred pain.** Entrapment of a spinal nerve may lead to paraesthesia, pain and weakness of muscles in the lower limb. Normally when pressure is applied to a site of pain the pain becomes worse. However, with referred pain the level of pain stays about the same. A suspected entrapment of the sciatic nerve usually leads to pain when the affected leg is raised while the patient lies in a supine position.

## Hospital tests

**Nerve conduction test.** Sensory nerve conduction velocities are measured by placing stimulating electrodes on the skin over the nerve to be tested. Recording electrodes, either skin or needle electrodes, are placed either proximally for orthodromic stimulation or distally for antidromic

stimulation. The latter gives more consistent results. The lower limit of normal sensory conduction velocities in the lower limb is around 35 m/s. Values are less than those for the upper limb. A slowing of conduction velocity may be due to a variety of causes (Matthews & Arnold 1991):

- ageing
- damage to the cell body as in herpes zoster (shingles) or poliomyelitis
- nerve axon damage as in compression due to a spinal tumour, a slipped disc or tarsal/carpal tunnel syndrome
- demyelinisation as seen in muscular sclerosis.

## ASSESSMENT OF LOWER LIMB MOTOR FUNCTION

If the motor system is functioning normally muscles should display a resting tone, show good muscle power on active contraction and be able to move against resistance (Ch. 8).

The lower limb reflexes, patella and Achilles, should also show a normal response.

**The patellar reflex** tests the integrity of the spinal reflex pathway (L3, L4) and demonstrates descending influences on the ventral horn cell. It is important that the limb being tested is as relaxed as possible. The patient should sit sideways on the examination couch with the feet clearing the ground. The practitioner can gently push the leg to be tested which should swing freely in response. A gentle tap on the patellar tendon with the hammer should elicit a knee jerk. If the leg is not relaxed, the patient should clasp both hands around the other knee and pull (Jedrassik manoeuvre). This releases spinal influence and allows the leg to relax. The test should be undertaken on both legs.

**The Achilles reflex** tests the spinal reflex pathway (S1, S2). The response is best elicited if the foot of the patient is slightly dorsiflexed by applying gentle pressure to the plantar surface of the forefoot with one hand and tapping the Achilles tendon while the pressure is maintained. In a healthy young adult the forefoot will gently plantarflex. In an elderly person no visible movement may be seen, but a very slight plantarflexion will be felt against the practitioner's hand.

Lower limb motor dysfunction can occur as a result of damage to upper motor neurones or lower motor neurones.

# Upper motor neurone lesions

Upper motor neurone (UMN) lesions are due to damage occurring anywhere between the cortex and L1 in the spinal cord. Since the spinal cord ends at level L1, lesions below this level will not produce UMN signs. Conditions which can lead to UMN lesions are listed in Table 7.13.

Although a specific area of the frontal lobes (precentral gyrus) is designated the primary motor cortex (Fig. 7.12), many neurones from other areas of the cortex are also involved in planning and initiating conscious movement and so can also be called upper motor neurones. This includes neurones of both descending tracts. Damage to the descending tracts will produce the same effects as damage to the neurones themselves. The effects on the body are absence of movement (plegia) or weakness of action (paresis).

## Observation

Damage to the corticospinal neurones and tracts will result in contralateral loss of skilled movements. Lack of movement will in turn eventually lead to a form of muscle atrophy known as disuse atrophy. Damage to the multineuronal pathway causes release of inhibition on the LMNs in the spinal cord, especially those which innervate the antigravity muscles, producing the effect most commonly associated with UMN lesions, that of spasticity or stiffness in the limbs.

**Gait.** Observation of the patient's gait is an important part of the assessment for UMN lesions. In the lower limb the effect is extension at the hip and knee, with plantarflexion and inversion of the foot. If the effect is unilateral, the person is described as hemiplegic. The inability to flex the knee and hip leads to a circumductory gait, with the lateral border of the forefoot and toes often scraping the ground. If both sides are affected the person is paraplegic and the gait is described as a scissor gait, with the knees adducted and feet abducted. Walking aids such as Zimmer frames are essential.

## Clinical tests

**Clasp knife spasticity.** The affected limb will be initially stiff to passive stretch, but if gentle stretch is continued, the limb may suddenly relax, rather like the opening of a clasp-knife. This is due to a length-dependent inhibition of the stretch reflex (Fig. 7.16).

**Tendon reflexes.** Due to the reduced inhibition by the multineuronal tracts, the alpha LMNs responsible for the contraction of extrafusal fibres are hyperexcited. This results in exaggerated patella and ankle tendon reflexes and clonus—increased rhythmic contractions elicited at the ankle or patella by causing brisk stretch of the muscles. More than three contractions as a result of testing the patella or Achilles reflex is indicative of UMN damage (Fuller 1993).

**Plantar reflex.** Damage to the corticospinal neurones or their axons has another effect that is clinically detectable, the so-called plantar reflex or Babinski sign. It has been suggested that the abnormal reflex, a dorsiflexing big toe, is due to release of a spinal inhibitory reflex (Van Gijn 1975). The plantar surface of the foot is stroked firmly and briskly from the posterolateral border of the heel to the hallux as shown in Figure 7.17. The normal response is a slight plantarflexion of the hallux and lesser toes,

**Table 7.13** Conditions associated with UMN signs

- Cerebral palsy due to anoxia at birth
- Cerebral vascular accidents
- Brain injury
- Friedreich's ataxia
- Spinal injury
- Brain or spinal tumours
- Amyotrophic lateral sclerosis (motor neurone disease)
- Vitamin $B_{12}$ deficiency
- Multiple (disseminated) sclerosis
- Later stages of syringomyelia

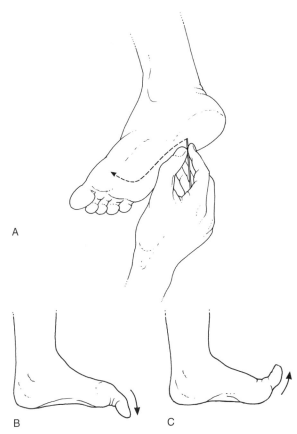

A

B          C

**Figure 7.17**   The Babinski response   **A.** Eliciting the response   **B.** Flexor response (normal response)—toes plantarflex   **C.** Extensor response (positive Babinski sign)—toes dorsiflex.

although no response is also often seen, especially in the elderly. In patients with corticospinal tract dysfunction, the hallux will extend (dorsiflexion of the hallux) and the lesser toes may fan out. This is the extensor response, sometimes referred to as a positive Babinski response. However, it should be remembered that the normal response does not become established until the person has learnt to walk and so an extensor response is quite normal in babies.

**Muscle tone.** Due to the release of spinal inhibition in UMN conditions, the LMNs will be in a hyperexcited state and so will be firing more frequently. This will result in greater muscle 'tone' and the affected muscle will feel very firm or tense.

Any condition which causes damage to the UMNs or their descending tracts can produce UMN signs. If the cortex is affected, the effects will occur on the contralateral side of the body, and if the lesion(s) is in the spinal cord, the effects will be on the same side, below the level of the lesion (Case history 7.1).

---

**Case history 7.1**

A 70-year-old female Caucasian presented to the clinic complaining of excessive wear on the lateral border of the left shoe and a corn on the dorsum of the fifth toe. The patient walked with a stick and had a slow, circumducted gait; the left arm was held in a flexed position.

Neurological assessment revealed normal tendon reflexes and muscle power in the right leg but exaggerated tendon reflexes and an extensor plantar response (positive Babinski sign), clonic spasm of the muscles and signs of muscle atrophy in the left leg.

**Diagnosis**: History taking revealed the patient had suffered a major CVA, which had affected the right cortex. The clinical features were consistent with the history. Fortunately for the patient she was right-handed so her speech was not affected and she was still able to feed herself and write.

---

*Hospital tests*

**Nerve conduction.** To measure motor conduction velocities the stimulating electrode is placed along the path of the nerve and the recording electrode is placed over the belly of the muscle. The lower limit of normal conduction velocities is 40 m/s.

The use of other tests will vary according to the suspected cause. For example, brain scans are indicated if a CVA is suspected whereas a spinal radiograph would be used if a tumour of the spine was suspected.

## Lower motor neurone lesions

Since LMNs or their spinal nerves exit at all segments of the spinal cord, LMN symptoms can be seen as a result of damage to any segment from C1 to S5. However, due to the anatomy of the spinal cord any damage to the cord from L2 will only result in a LMN lesion. It is possible to see a combination of UMN and

**Table 7.14**  Conditions associated with lower motor neurone lesions

* Poliomyelitis
* Injury to lower motor neurone and/or peripheral nerve
* Motor neurone disease
* Syringomyelia
* Vitamin $B_{12}$ deficiency
* Cord compression/lesion (Brown–Séquard syndrome)
* Spina bifida
* Charcot–Marie–Tooth disease

LMN symptoms, if the lesion is between C1 and L1, e.g. syringomyelia. The conditions that can lead to lower motor neurone lesions are listed in Table 7.14.

## Observation

If the pathway is interrupted or damaged in any way, either at the level of the cell body or along its axon, then the impulse cannot reach the muscle. The result will be weakness (paresis) or flaccid paralysis, depending on the site and extent of the damage. The sites of damage may involve:

* lower motor neurone, e.g. poliomyelitis virus (Case history 7.2)

---

Case history 7.2

A 54-year-old male Caucasian first presented to the clinic complaining of corns and callus under the metatarsal heads of both feet. He was unable to bend down to cut his toenails.

A vascular assessment revealed weak pulses in both feet, with the right foot being cold. A neurological assessment revealed diminished reflexes in the right leg and absence of vibration sense in the right foot. Two-point discrimination was 2 cm in the left foot and 10 cm in the right foot. Orthopaedic examination showed a leg length discrepancy of 2.5 cm, the right leg being the shorter and having developed a functional equinus at the ankle. Muscle wastage was apparent in the lower limb of the right side. The patient walked with a limp.

**Diagnosis**: The signs and symptoms are all consistent with poliomyelitis. The patient had contacted the virus when a child. The lower motor neurones of the right side of the spinal cord at the level of the lumbar plexi had been affected.

---

* peripheral axon, e.g. diabetes mellitus
* cholinergic receptors of the skeletal muscle, e.g. myasthenia gravis.

In contrast to UMN lesions, which affect particular movements, LMN lesions affect particular muscles (Case history 7.3). For example, if the tibialis anterior is affected there will be a slapping gait.

---

Case history 7.3

A 52-year-old Caucasian female presented to the clinic with plantar callus and fissuring, which had arisen following plantar fasciotomy to correct 'clubbed feet'. The patient stated that she had been born with normal feet, but by the time she was 6 years old she could not run or jump properly and by the time she was an adolescent her feet had become high-arched and inverted.

She had noticed a gradual weakness in her arms and legs and on one occasion, when 41 years old, she had almost dropped a baby while working as a nursing auxiliary. This incident had caused her to be sent for a neurological examination which revealed slowed motor nerve conduction velocities. She had a recent history of several falls, with her ankle 'going over'. She also complained of aching joints in the feet, knees and hips. Her 27-year-old son was similarly affected.

Neurological examination showed all sensory perception except vibration to be normal, but reflexes were absent. Muscle power was reduced in all limbs and muscle wasting of hands, feet and calf muscles was noted. Orthopaedic examination showed reduced dorsiflexion and eversion, with a pes-cavus-type foot and a high-stepping gait.

**Diagnosis**: The patient suffered from Charcot–Marie–Tooth disease, also known as peroneal muscle atrophy. It is an inherited peripheral neuropathy and exists in more than one form, the two most common forms being autosomal dominant.

---

Nerve impulses are essential to the health of the muscle, so that lack of impulses leads to rapid atrophy of muscle, skin and other soft tissue. This is known as denervation atrophy. In addition the denervated muscle becomes highly sensitive to very small amounts of neurotransmitter (acetylcholine), possibly due to upregulation of receptors. This results in a quivering of the muscle (fasciculation), seen on an electromyogram as fibrillation.

## Clinical tests

**Muscle power.** The patient is asked to push his/her foot against resistance such as the practitioner's hand. A reduced strength of contraction suggests paresis or paralysis.

**Muscle tone.** In the skeletal muscles of a healthy person there will always be some motor units firing, which means that the muscle will feel firm. This is referred to as the 'tone' of the muscle. In LMN damage, the muscle will feel flabby, because of loss of this tone.

**Tendon reflexes.** Reflexes will be weak or absent, because of interruption of the final common pathway. A single reduced or absent reflex suggests mononeuropathy or radiculopathy. A reduction or absence of all reflexes suggests peripheral polyneuropathy.

## Hospital tests

**Electromyographs.** These use a needle electrode inserted into the muscle to show the electrical activity of the muscle in response to an electrical stimulus. Abnormal results are detected in myopathies such as Charcot–Marie–Tooth disease or in dysfunction of the motor nerve (Matthews & Arnold 1991).

Tests may be performed that are specific to particular conditions, such as detection of the presence of antibodies to cholinergic receptors in myasthenia gravis.

The differences between UMN and LMN lesions are summarised in Table 7.15.

# ASSESSMENT OF COORDINATION/PROPRIOCEPTION FUNCTION

The receptors in the muscles, joints and tendons all feed position sense information to the cerebellum and cortex. In turn the cerebellum and the cortex bring about vital postural reflexes and reflexes necessary for accurate movement. The basal ganglia also plays an important part in the coordination of movement. Damage to these parts of the nervous system may have an effect on gait and coordination. Conditions that may affect coordination and proprioception function are listed in Table 7.16.

## Observation

Careful observation of motor activity can give an indication of a deficit in posture, balance or coordination; for example, a stamping gait may be due to loss of proprioception as occurs in tabes dorsalis, where the ascending tracts in the dorsal columns degenerate. The patient will not know where his body is in space and so lifts his legs much higher than necessary to clear the ground. The patient will also be unaware of when his foot is about to make ground contact and so stamps the foot down. This has the advantage of stimulating pressure receptors proximally, as vibrations from the foot travel up the leg and so provide much needed information to the brain.

The cerebellum has modifying influences on the UMNs in the cortex and on brain-stem nuclei.

**Table 7.15**  Differences between upper motor neurone and lower motor neurone lesions

| Upper motor neurone | Lower motor neurone |
| --- | --- |
| Exaggerated tendon reflexes | Loss of tendon reflexes |
| Extensor plantar response (positive Babinski sign) Loss of abdominal reflex | Flexor plantar response (negative Babinski sign) Normal abdominal reflex |
| Normal electrical excitability of muscle | Fasciculation (fibrillation seen on EMG) |
| Some muscle wasting over a period of time due to lack of use | Marked muscle wasting occurs relatively quickly |
| Increase in muscle tone (clonus) | Flaccid muscles (lack of tone) |
| Whole limb affected | Certain muscle groups affected depending on site of damage; deformity due to contracture of antagonists |

**Table 7.16** Conditions that may result in poor coordination

| Part | Conditions |
|---|---|
| Cerebellum | Tumour |
| | Multiple sclerosis |
| | Arnold–Chiari malformation |
| | Friedreich's ataxia |
| | Other hereditary spinocerebellar ataxias |
| | Hypothyroidism |
| | Repeated head trauma as in boxing |
| Basal ganglia | Parkinsonism |
| | Huntington's chorea |
| | Wilson's disease |
| | Sydenham's chorea |
| Ascending pathways | Subacute combined degeneration of the spinal cord |
| | Guillain–Barré syndrome |
| | Tabes dorsalis |
| | Alcoholism |

It receives rich proprioceptive information and adjusts the activity of the UMNs to ensure that the actual action and intended action are matched. The cerebellum is essential for smooth, accurate movement and posture and balance. Dysfunction of the cerebellum or of its afferent and efferent tracts produces characteristic effects that are easily observable.

**Dysarthria.** Here cerebellar dysfunction affects the speech muscles and produces a scanning speech, with inappropriate syllabic stress and volume.

**Dysdiadochokinesia.** This is where actions are no longer smooth, continuous movements, but are broken down into their component parts, producing clumsy, jerky actions.

**Tremor.** The tremor associated with cerebellar defect is due to the dysfunction of the stretch reflex and is an intention tremor, i.e. one which increases in amplitude as the person tries to carry out any tasks with the affected limb. The tremor disappears at rest.

**Gait.** If maintenance of balance is upset, the patient will feel unsteady and adopt a wide base of gait. As voluntary movement is also affected, the gait will be clumsy or staggering, as if drunk. Such gait is described as ataxic. The patient may complain of deviating to one side, which suggests the dysfunction is limited to that

hemisphere.

Although the basal ganglia also have a modifying role on voluntary movement, the effects of their dysfunction is quite different from that of the cerebellum. Damage to the basal ganglia produces either a poverty of movement (hypo/bradykinesia) as seen in Parkinson's disease, or jerky writhing movements (choreo-athetosis) as seen in the inherited disease of Huntington's chorea or the benign and brief effects of Sydenham's chorea, associated with rheumatic fever (Case history 7.4).

---

**Case history 7.4**

A 30-year-old Caucasian male attended the clinic complaining of sore corns. Questioning revealed that he was mentally handicapped. Examination showed warm, hyperhidrotic feet with a poor skin condition and fibrous lesions on the plantar aspect of the feet. The left foot had a marked pes cavus deformity. The gait revealed limping and shuffling with excessive arm movement in order to maintain balance.

Over a period of a few years further mental and physical deterioration became apparent. The patient's brother was similarly affected and so apparently had been their father.

**Diagnosis**: A diagnosis of Huntington's chorea was made. This disease is inherited as an autosomal condition with complete penetration and late onset, and is characterised by progressive chorea and dementia.

---

## Clinical tests

**Proprioception in joints.** To test proprioception, the practitioner holds the sides of the hallux between forefinger and thumb. While the patient's eyes are shut, the toe is moved up and down and the patient should be able to state the final position of the toe. This information travels up to the cerebellum in the ipsilateral spinocerebellar tracts and to the conscious cortex in the dorsal columns. A positive result shows that the pathway to the cortex is intact. An inability to give the correct responses would be seen in conditions such as tabes dorsalis.

**Romberg's sign.** This test can be used to confirm proprioceptive dorsal column disturbance (Berkow 1987). The patient is observed standing with eyes open and then closed. Deprivation of visual information means the brain has to rely on proprioceptive input and if this is not being transmitted then the patient will sway and find it difficult to keep balance. This can be exacerbated by giving the patient a gentle push, but the practitioner must be prepared to catch him/her.

**Nystagmus.** This is rapid eye movements due to vestibular dysfunction and can be elicited by asking the patient to make a sudden rapid head movement. Its presence indicates a cerebellar lesion.

**Heel–shin test.** The patient is asked to slide the heel of one leg straight down the shin of the other. Patients with cerebellar dysfunction are often unable to do this because of lack of co-ordination and the heel will follow a wavy path down the other leg.

**Heel–toe test.** The patient is asked to walk in a straight line heel to toe. Patients with cerebellar dysfunction will stagger about the midline, but it must be remembered that there are many other causes of an unsteady gait, especially in the elderly.

**Finger–nose test.** The patient is asked to stand comfortably and then, with eyes shut and one arm outstretched, to bring his/her fingertip to the nose. Repeat for other arm. Cerebellar dysfunction will cause the patient to overshoot (hypermetria) or undershoot (hypometria) and miss the nose.

**Muscle tone.** This will be reduced in the affected limbs.

**Tendon reflexes.** These may be unusually sustained, because of the oscillations of an abnormal stretch reflex, but should not be exaggerated or diminished in amplitude.

## Parkinson's disease

This is the commonest extrapyramidal disease and is due to depletion of dopaminergic neurones in the substantia nigra, which project to the caudate nucleus. The most troublesome effect is hypo/bradykinesia, which results in the patient having great difficulty initiating or stopping movement (Case history 7.5). Rest tremor and

rigidity are also features. If the hand is affected, the tremor may cause the patient to move index finger and thumb in a 'pill-rolling' movement. The patient may show a mask-like face, and speak in a soft voice. Micrographia (small handwriting) is also a characteristic.

---

Case history 7.5

A 65-year-old female Caucasian presented to the clinic requesting nail care. On examination her nails were found to be long, thickened and mycotic and a variety of dorsal, apical and interdigital lesions were present.

The patient could appreciate temperature, light touch and pressure and reflexes were normal, but she was very confused and nervous, so that communication was difficult. A full orthopaedic assessment could not be carried out because of the patient's inability to relax her legs and feet. Ankle dorsiflexion was limited and the feet adopted a varus position. Most of the toes showed retraction deformities. Movements were hypokinetic and gait was stooped and shuffling. There was a minor rest tremor in the right arm.

**Diagnosis**: The symptoms are consistent with Parkinson's disease. This is a progressive idiopathic condition which gradually affects all limbs. Mental confusion/dementia is not always present.

---

The antigravity muscles are affected, producing a stooped posture with knees flexed, so that the patient's centre of gravity is no longer over the base of gait. This causes the festination seen in gait, where the patient has to move more and more quickly to avoid falling forward. Gait also tends to be shuffling, with poor heel–ground contact—'marche à petits pied'.

The tendon reflexes are unaffected. There is a general resistance to passive stretch, described as 'lead-pipe rigidity'. It may show a superimposed intermittent release of the resistance, producing a series of jerks, the so-called 'cogwheel' effect.

In a patient with Parkinson's disease, there is no habituation with the glabellar tap reflex. The glabellar tap reflex involves the practitioner gently, slowly and repeatedly tapping the forehead of the patient between his/her eyes. In a healthy person, the first tap or two will elicit the eye-blink reflex, but this will rapidly habituate.

The frequency of the tremor may be measured via hospital tests but usually the above clinical tests and a positive response to drug therapy will be sufficient to confirm the diagnosis of Parkinson's disease.

## ASSESSMENT OF AUTONOMIC FUNCTION

As explained earlier, the autonomic nerves innervate the viscera and internal structures such as blood vessels, since they enable the nervous system to maintain homoeostasis (Fig. 7.9). Medical history may reveal abnormalities of bowel and bladder function.

### Observation

There will be various signs which would suggest autonomic neuropathy such as abnormal sudomotor responses in the skin and abnormal cardiovascular responses in the functioning of the heart and peripheral blood vessels (Faris 1991). Sudomotor neuropathy usually leads to an absence of sweating and a dry skin, although it may produce hyperhidrosis. Vasomotor neuropathy usually produces a warm red skin and an absence of vasoconstriction in response to cold although it may occasionally produce a prolonged vasoconstriction. It may also lead to postural hypotension. Neuropathy of nerves to the cardiac pacemaker tissue may lead to failure of the heart to respond appropriately to the demands of the body, e.g. an absence of tachycardia in response to exercise.

### Clinical tests

**Heart rate.** The pulse is taken while the patient is in a supine position and repeated when he/she adopts an upright posture. The normal response is an increase in heart rate of greater than 11 beats per minute. A loss of response suggests parasympathetic abnormality.

**Blood pressure.** Repeat the above test measuring blood pressure in the two positions. The systolic blood pressure should fall on standing by approximately 30 mmHg and the diastolic pressure by about 15 mmHg. An increased drop suggests sympathetic abnormality.

**Valsalva manoeuvre.** The patient is asked to take a deep breath and exhale against a closed glottis for 10–15 seconds and then breathe normally. The pulse rate is taken during the Valsalva manoeuvre and on release. Heart rate should increase during the manoeuvre and fall on release. No increase during the manoeuvre suggests sympathetic abnormality and no decrease on release suggests parasympathetic abnormality.

The condition commonly associated with autonomic neuropathy is diabetes mellitus, where the foot will often appear red and feel dry and warm. It is quite usual to find neuropathy of other small fibres such as pain and temperature fibres (A delta and C), giving rise to the typical picture of a neuropathic foot (Ch. 17). Less common conditions are Guillain–Barré syndrome, amyloidosis and congenital autonomic failure. It should be remembered that other conditions, such as infection and anaemia, and certain drugs, such as beta-blockers, can also affect the cardiovascular system and may give a false positive result.

## SUMMARY

This chapter has considered the assessment of the various components on the nervous system. However, as stated earlier, it is important to remember that a number of conditions affect more than one part. Those conditions that result in damage to more than one part of the nervous system are summarised in Table 7.17. It is essential that all parts of the nervous system are assessed in order that the practitioner may acquire a full picture of neurological function (Case history 7.6).

**Table 7.17**   Conditions that affect more than one part of the nervous system

| Condition | Parts affected |
| --- | --- |
| Diabetes mellitus | Sensory, motor (LMN) and autonomic |
| Motor neurone disease | LMN and UMN |
| Spina bifida | LMN and sensory |
| Syringomyelia | Sensory, LMN and UMN |
| Vitamin $B_{12}$ deficiency | Sensory, LMN and UMN |
| Multiple sclerosis | Sensory and UMN |
| Cord compression/lesion | Sensory, LMN and UMN |
| Guillain–Barré syndrome | LMN, sensory and autonomic |
| Charcot–Marie–Tooth disease | Mainly LMN but possible sensory |
| Nerve injuries | Depends upon site, may result in LMN, UMN, sensory or autonomic |

**Case history 7.6**

A 47-year-old male Caucasian was referred to the clinic with a small ulcer which had existed for 6 months beneath his right heel. When 29 years old, he had visited Nigeria where he had contracted schistosomiasis with resultant paraparesis from his lower abdomen downwards. Since then he had suffered repeated ulceration of both feet. The present ulcer was covered with dense callus which when debrided revealed a lesion 15 mm in diameter and 8 mm deep. Its border was surrounded by macerated callus.

A vascular assessment showed no remarkable features, all tests indicating a good blood supply to the foot. The neurological assessment revealed absent reflexes, lack of appreciation of all senses and a constant 'pins and needles' sensation around his hips and legs. The skin of the feet was dry. The patient used a walking stick to support his right leg and walked with an abductory gait to achieve ground clearance as the right foot could not dorsiflex. The right leg showed wasting of the triceps surae.

**Diagnosis**: A diagnosis was made of neuropathic ulcer associated with peripheral sensory, motor and autonomic neuropathy due to damage in the spinal cord caused by the parasitic blood fluke *Schistosoma haematobium*.

## REFERENCES

Berkow R (ed) 1987 The Merck manual, 15th edn. Merck Sharp & Dohme Research Laboratories, NJ
Budd K 1984 Pain. Update Postgraduate Centre Series. Update, Guildford
Epstein O, Perkin G, de Bono D, Cookson J 1992 Clinical examination. Gower Medical, London
Faris I 1991 The management of the diabetic foot. Churchill Livingstone, Edinburgh
Fuller G 1993 Neurological examination made easy. Churchill Livingstone, Edinburgh
Ganong W 1991 Reviews of medical physiology. Lange, London
McClintic, J R 1980 Basic anatomy and physiology of the human body. John Wiley, New York
McLeod J, Lance J 1989 Introductory neurology. Blackwell, Oxford
Matthews P, Arnold D 1991 (eds) Diagnostic tests in neurology. Churchill Livingstone, Edinburgh
Melzack R 1992 Phantom limbs. Scientific American, April: 90
Vander A J, Sherman J H, Luciano D S 1990 Human Physiology, 5th edn. McGraw Hill, New York
Van Gijn J 1975 The Babinski response: stimulus and effector. Journal of Neurology, Neurosurgery and Psychology 38: 180–186
Wilson K J W 1990 Ross & Wilson Anatomy and physiology in health and illness. Churchill Livingstone, Edinburgh

## FURTHER READING

Hendry B 1981 Membrane physiology and cell excitation. Croom Helm, London
Kandel E, Jessel, Schwartz J 1991 The principles of neural science. Elsevier, New York

# 8

# Assessment of the locomotor system

*D. R. Tollafield*
*L. Merriman*

## INTRODUCTION

Locomotion is the act of moving from one place to another due to the interaction between the musculoskeletal and the nervous system. The musculoskeletal system provides the framework for the body and comprises bones, joints and ligaments, and muscles. This chapter concentrates on the assessment of the musculoskeletal system. Details of the neurological basis of movement and assessment of the nervous system are covered in Chapter 7.

The assessment process is based upon an approach which involves look, feel and move (Apley & Solomon 1988). Qualitative, semi-quantitative and quantitative measurement techniques are used. The practitioner should be aware of the likely errors that can ensue from such measurements and take these into consideration when interpreting and analysing data from the assessment (see Ch. 4). The chapter concentrates on the assessment of the lower limb: details regarding the upper part of the body and spine have been excluded but can be found in other text.

## WHY ASSESS THE LOCOMOTOR SYSTEM?

Normal locomotion should be pain-free and energy-efficient. The main purpose of the assessment is to identify whether the system is functioning within the boundaries of 'normality'. Normal function can be affected by one or more of the following:

- hereditary/congenital problems, e.g. Charcot–Marie–Tooth disease, talipes equinovarus
- acute/chronic injury causing pain, e.g. ankle sprain, repeated stubbing of toes in ill-fitting footwear
- abnormal alignment, e.g. internal femoral torsion, genu valgum
- infections, e.g. tuberculosis
- neurological disorders, e.g. CVA
- footwear, e.g. high heels
- muscle disorders, e.g. Duchenne's muscular dystrophy
- neoplasia, e.g. osteosarcoma
- systemic disease, e.g. autoimmune (rheumatoid arthritis), bone disease (Paget's disease)
- degenerative processes, e.g. osteoarthritis
- psychological factors, e.g. attention seeking.

The effects of the above can vary from relatively minor to profound and may result in:

- secondary problems, e.g. mechanically induced skin lesions such as corns and callus, acquired deformities
- physiological effects, e.g. kyphosis may produce breathing difficulties and alimentary dysfunction (Rasch & Burke 1978)
- fatigue due to increased energy expenditure
- socioeconomic problems, e.g. inability to work
- psychological problems, e.g. isolation, stress.

When assessing the locomotor system it is important to remember that a problem that affects one part of the system can lead to problems elsewhere in the system. This is because the locomotor system functions as one mechanical unit; as a result a problem in one part has to be compensated for in another part of the system. Compensation is a change in structure, position or function of one part in an attempt to adjust to an abnormal structure, position or function in another part. For example, a scoliosis of the spine may lead to an apparent leg-length discrepancy which will affect foot function. Conversely, a problem affecting the foot, e.g. an uncompensated rearfoot varus, may lead to discomfort/pain at the knee.

Taking the above into account the purpose of an assessment of the locomotor system can be summarised as follows:

- identify the site of the primary problem, e.g. foot, leg, hip
- identify any secondary problems and relate them to the primary problem, e.g. lesion patterns, pronation due to leg-length discrepancy
- identify the cause of the problem, e.g. abnormal alignment
- utilise the data from the assessment to produce an effective management plan
- utilise the data from the assessment to monitor the progress of the condition.

## TERMS OF REFERENCE

The body is divided into three cardinal planes: sagittal, frontal (coronal) and transverse (Fig. 8.1). These planes form the reference points from which to describe:

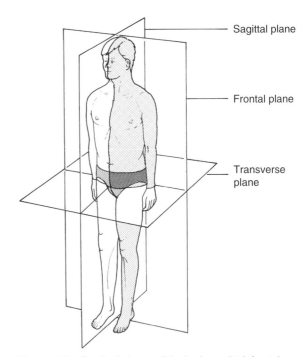

**Figure 8.1** Cardinal planes of the body: sagittal, frontal and transverse. Sagittal divides the body into right and left halves, frontal divides the body into front and back and transverse divides the body into upper and lower sections. The diagram shows midplanes but the terms refer to any plane parallel to the appropriate midplane.

- position of a part of the body
- joint motion
- position of a joint
- deformity of a part of the body.

## Position of a part of the body

The cardinal body planes are used as reference points to describe positions within the body. *Anterior* (to the front of) and *posterior* (to the rear of) describe positions in the frontal plane, e.g. the patella lies anterior to the knee joint. *Distal* (away from the centre) and *proximal* (towards the centre) describe positions in the transverse plane, e.g. the interphalangeal joints (IPJs) lie distal to the metatarsophalangeal joints (MTPJs). *Medial* (towards the midline of the body) and *lateral* (away from the midline of the body) describe positions in the sagittal plane, e.g. the navicular lies on the medial side of the foot and the cuboid on the lateral side. In the foot, *dorsal* is used to refer to the top of the foot and *plantar* to the sole of the foot.

## Joint motion

### Sagittal plane

Motion in the sagittal plane produces *extension* and *flexion*. The term *flexion* denotes the bending

of a joint whereas extension denotes the opposite, straightening of a joint. The terms used to describe sagittal plane motion in the foot are slightly different from those used to describe such motion at the hip and knee (extension and flexion). At the ankle (Fig. 8.2), subtalar (STJ), midtarsal (MTJ), metatarsophalangeal (MTPJ), interphalangeal (IPJ) and first and fifth rays, sagittal plane motion is termed *dorsiflexion* and *plantarflexion*. Dorsiflexion denotes a raising of the whole or part of the foot towards the leg whereas extension denotes the movement of the dorsal aspect of the foot away from the leg.

### Frontal (coronal) plane

Motion in the frontal plane produces *abduction* and *adduction* of the thigh and leg and *inversion* and *eversion* of the foot. This is because the foot lies at right angles to the leg, so the terminology used to describe movements of the foot differ from that for the leg and thigh. Abduction is when the distal segment moves away from the midline of the body and adduction when it moves towards the midline. For example, in order to do the 'splits' gymnasts must abduct their legs.

Inversion of the foot is when the plantar aspect of the foot is tilted so as to move towards

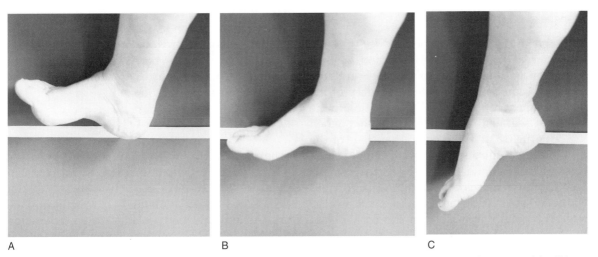

A                                    B                                    C

**Figure 8.2**  Sagittal plane motion at the ankle  **A.** Dorsiflexion: movement of the foot toward the anterior aspect of the tibia **B.** Neutral position  **C.** Plantarflexion: movement of the foot away from the tibia.

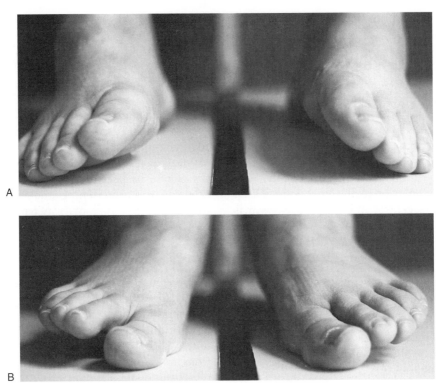

A

B

**Figure 8.3** Frontal plane motion in relation to the midline of the body (black line) **A.** Inversion: the foot is lifted up and away from the line **B.** Eversion: the foot is moved down and towards the line.

the midline of the body. Eversion is when the plantar aspect of the foot is tilted so as to face away from the midline of the body (Fig. 8.3).

### Transverse plane

Motion in the transverse plane produces internal and external rotation of the thigh and leg and adduction and abduction of the foot. Internal rotation occurs when the anterior surface of the distal segment rotates medially in relation to the proximal segment and external rotation when the opposite occurs—the anterior surface of the distal segment moves laterally in relation to the proximal segment (Fig. 8.4).

In the foot the use of the terms adduction and abduction is dependent upon the site of the reference point: the midline of the body or the midline of the foot. Functionally, the midline of the body is usually used as the reference point: abduction of the foot is where the distal part of

the foot moves away from the midline of the body and adduction when the distal part of the foot moves towards the midline of the body (Fig. 8.4). Anatomically the midline of the foot is commonly used as the reference point, for example, adductor hallucis is inserted into the lateral side of the proximal phalanx of the hallux and is so termed because it brings about adduction of the hallux, movement of the hallux towards the midline of the foot.

### Triplanar motion

The position of the joint axis together with the shape of the articulating surfaces can result in joint motion in more than one plane. If a joint axis is positioned at an angle of less than 90° to all the cardinal body planes triplanar motion occurs—pronation and supination. Pronation is the collective term for dorsiflexion, eversion and abduction and supination for plantarflexion,

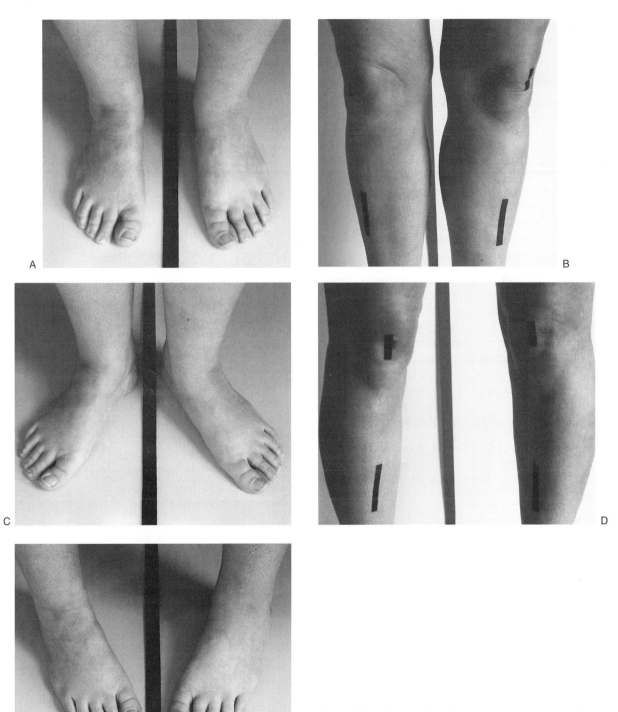

**Figure 8.4**   Relationship between transverse plane motion in the leg and transverse plane motion in the foot   **A.** The feet are mildly abducted; this is the normal standing position **B.** The legs are externally (laterally) rotated, which results in abduction of the feet (**C**)   **D.** The legs are internally rotated (medially), which results in the adduction of the feet (**E**).

inversion and adduction. In the foot the subtalar and midtarsal joints produce triplanar motion.

## Position of a joint

To describe the position of a joint the suffix -ed is used:

- *Sagittal plane*—extended and flexed (thigh and leg); dorsiflexed and plantarflexed (foot)
- *Transverse plane*—internally and externally rotated (thigh and leg); adducted and abducted (foot)
- *Frontal plane*—abducted and adducted (thigh and leg); inverted and everted (foot)
- *Triplanar*—pronated and supinated (foot).

It is important that a distinction is made between joint motion and position; a joint moves in the opposite direction to the position it is in. For example, at heel-strike the foot is slightly supinated (position) but as soon as the heel contacts the ground pronation (motion) occurs at the subtalar joint in order to absorb shock from ground contact.

## Deformity of a part of the body

The term 'deformity' is used to describe a fixed position adopted by a part of the body. Terms used to denote deformity usually have the suffix -us:

- *Sagittal plane*—equinus when the foot or part of the foot is plantarflexed, e.g. ankle equinus, and extensus when the foot or part of the foot is dorsiflexed, e.g. hallux extensus. Calcaneus, although rarely seen, is used to describe the calcaneus when it is in fixed dorsiflexion, e.g. talipes calcaneovalgus
- *Frontal plane*—varus and valgus (Fig. 8.5)
- *Transverse plane*—adductus or abductus.

## AN OVERVIEW OF FUNCTIONAL ANATOMY AND BASIC BIOMECHANICS

The musculoskeletal system is primarily composed of collagen arranged in different physical states: bone, muscle, ligament, cartilage. The

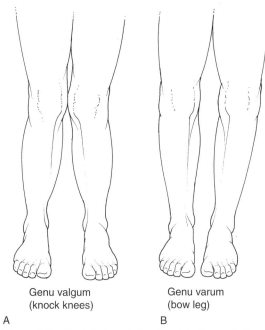

Genu valgum (knock knees)    Genu varum (bow leg)

A    B

**Figure 8.5** Frontal plane deformity of the legs    **A.** Genu valgum (knock knees): the knees are close together and the medial malleoli are far apart    **B.** Genu varum (bow legs): the knees are far apart and the medial malleoli are close together.

skeletal architecture protects vital organs, especially the heart, lungs and brain. The shape and alignment of the vertebral column (axial skeleton) is important for the normal transmission of forces through the pelvis to the foot via the hip, knee and ankle joint. Disruption of the alignment and shape of the skeletal framework can affect the biomechanics of the lower limb. Biomechanics is defined as the application of mechanical laws to the body.

The skeleton is composed of long and short bones and has a non-uniform cross-section. This offers greater strength under compression than square or round cross-sections. Even the smaller metatarsal bones and phalanges conform to this geometry. The smaller (short) bones which make up the tarsus of foot have a thinner cortical structure than the shafts (diaphyses) of the long bones. A cortex made up of compact bone cells (osteocytes) with calcium salts surrounds a lighter open matrix of cancellous spongy bone. The composite properties of cortical and cancellous bone offer lightness and strength. The internal structure of long bones is filled with marrow which is vital for haemopoietic activity.

Sesamoids and accessory bones are an interesting feature of the skeletal structure; they are found in tendons. The most important sesamoids in the lower limb are the patella (knee) and the first metatarsal sesamoids. The principal function of sesamoids is to aid the direction and efficiency of tendon pull. The quadriceps muscle exerts a pull on the anterior surface of the tibia via the ligamentum patellae. The presence of the patella enables the leg to be extended at the knee with less effort than if it was not present. The efficiency of this mechanical effect is dependent upon the position of the patella. The metatarsal sesamoids are constant after the age of 8–10. They ensure that flexor hallucis brevis plantarflexes the proximal phalanx during the 'toe-off' (propulsive) part of the gait cycle. Sesamoid bones can give rise to pathology, e.g. fracture, as well as affecting normal function, e.g. because of displacement. Unfortunately, pain arising in sesamoids has been found to be difficult to treat (Campbell et al 1993).

A joint is the junction between two bones and can be classified as follows:

- fibrous (syndesmotic joints)
- cartilaginous
- synovial.

The majority of joints in the lower limb are synovial. Synovial joints are classified by the shape of their articulating surfaces and the motion they produce (Table 8.1). Anatomical variation in the shape of the articulating surfaces and the position of the joint axis will have a significant effect on the motion produced (Tollafield 1988) (Fig. 8.6).

Joints are supported by a joint capsule and ligaments. Some have ligaments that lie within the joint in order to provide greater stability to the joint, e.g. the cruciate ligaments of the knee, ligamentum teres of the hip and the interosseous talocalcaneal ligament of the subtalar joint.

Bone ends are made up of layers of cartilage cells (chondrocytes). Cartilage has a semi-lubricant function and will deform under stress, losing fluid from its matrix (Radin et al 1992). This deformation is vital in coping with increased loads and helps to spread the synovial fluid through the joint, which prevents interposing surfaces from being damaged. Synovial fluid bathes the chondrocytes. Most joints have only a small amount. An increase in synovial fluid leads to a swollen joint; in such instances pathological changes should be suspected, e.g. rheumatoid arthritis. The nature of cartilage is complex. In very young people it is thought to have limited power to regenerate, but in adults this is not the case: damage to cartilage is irreversible.

Muscles are important for posture as well as movement. Postural muscles such as soleus and gluteus maximus are slow-acting but tend to fatigue less readily. They are known as red muscles on account of their high myohaemo-

**Table 8.1** Classification of synovial joints in the foot and leg

| Joint | Example | Axis/motion |
|---|---|---|
| Plane simple | Base of intermetatarsals with cuneiforms and cuboid | Uniaxial, sliding |
| Hinge (ginglymus) | Interphalangeal joints | Uniaxial, sagittal |
| Condylar | Knee joint (tibiofemoral) | Biaxial, mainly sagittal |
| Ellipsoid | Metatarsophalangeal joints | Biaxial, sagittal and frontal |
| Sellar | Talocrural (ankle)<br>Calcaneocuboid | Uniaxial, triplanar<br>Uniaxial, triplanar |
| Ball and socket | Talonavicular (part of midtarsal)<br>Hip | Uniaxial, triplanar<br>Triaxial, triplanar |
| Spiral/twisting action | Subtalar | Uniaxial, triplanar |

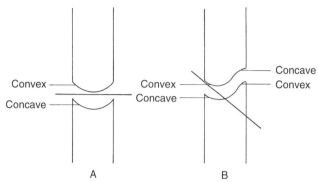

**Figure 8.6** Theoretical joint structures **A.** Simple convex–concave joint with a uniplanar axis, which produces motion in the plane perpendicular to the axis **B.** Compound joint structure that alters the axis to a biplanar or triplanar axis; motion occurs in more than one plane because the axis lies in more than one plane.

globin content. Prime movers such as gastrocnemius and tibialis anterior move rapidly but fatigue quickly. These are known as white muscles and consequently have less myohaemoglobin content. Normal muscle innervation ensures that a healthy tone exists. Muscles bring about joint motion in relation to the joint axis and have a pulley effect over bones. Bursae and synovial sheaths facilitate efficiency of the pull of tendons.

Effective locomotion involves smoothing out the vertical displacement of the centre of gravity (Saunders et al 1953). Without the existence of a well articulated and coordinated vertebral–pelvic link human movement would use energy inefficiently. For example, stiffness in lower limb joints can cause a shift in the centre of gravity, which causes alteration to the normal gait pattern. Table 8.2 provides a summary of the determinants of gait. Motion during gait can be described as *translatory* and *rotary*.

Torque conversion is the means by which motion of the thigh and leg influences the foot; the subtalar joint (STJ) is the interface between the leg and foot and is where torque conversion takes place. Internal rotation of the leg is transferred into pronation of the foot and external rotation of the leg is transferred into supination

**Table 8.2** Summary of the determinants of gait

| Determinant | Description |
| --- | --- |
| 1. Pelvic rotation | Movement forward and back about a vertical axis at pelvis<br>Effect: reduces the angle of hip flexion |
| 2. Pelvic list | Movement in frontal plane<br>Effect: lowers the centre of mass oscillation, assisted by action abductors of hip |
| 3. Knee flexion | Relates to stance phase from heel contact<br>Effect: flattens out vertical oscillation with 1 and 2 by shortening the leg and keeping translatory motion between hip and knee smooth |
| 4. Ankle mechanism | Effect: reduces the length of the leg but improves action of knee flexion, preventing abrupt movement |
| 5. Combined foot involvement | Effect: provides a rocker motion which acts as a stable base, spreading out the load from the lower limb, movement is aided by torque conversion |
| 6. Lateral shift | Effect: relates to sideways shift of the body. Each stride will involve 4–5 cm of lateral displacement. This is dependent upon the width of the base of gait and distance between the knees. A wide base, for instance, would increase the lateral shift |

of the foot. During gait the leg rotates internally and externally in order to bring about pronation, required for shock absorption, and supination, required for stability of the foot during propulsion. However, a variety of factors may affect torque conversion and lead to abnormal pronation and supination occurring in the foot. For example, variation in the position of the STJ axis, e.g. high STJ axis, can alter the amount of internal and external leg rotation.

It is important to remember walking style changes with age. Tachdjian (1985) cites Sutherland who has provided much in the way of studies on the effects of changing cadence (steps per minute) from the first to sixth year of life. After 6 years of age, the adult features of gait are discernable.

## THE ASSESSMENT PROCESS

When undertaking an assessment of the locomotor system it is essential that the system is observed weightbearing (dynamic and static) and non-weightbearing. Differences between the two can help to determine whether compensation has occurred. For example, non-weightbearing assessment may identify the presence of a forefoot varus, observation of the patient's gait may show this problem has been fully compensated through abnormal pronation at the subtalar joint. Conversely, information from the non-weightbearing assessment may explain the cause of a gait abnormality, e.g. a patient may have a bouncy gait due to an early heel lift, non-weightbearing assessment of the ankle joint may reveal that the cause is an ankle equinus due to a short gastrocnemius muscle.

In order to gain a full and detailed picture of the function of the locomotor system the following must be assessed:

- gait
- alignment and position of the lower limb
- joint motion
- muscle action.

Practitioners vary as to the sequence in which they assess the above. There is no one correct sequence, practitioners should adopt the sequence and approach they feel most comfortable with. However, it is essential a systematic approach is adopted in order to ensure vital pieces of data are not missed. For the purposes of this chapter the following sequence has been adopted:

1. Gait analysis. This will focus on the position and alignment of the body and foot–ground contact
2. Non-weightbearing. This will focus on the assessment of joints and muscles
3. Static weightbearing. This will focus on the position and alignment of the body and the relationship of the foot to the ground during stance.

In order to achieve a successful assessment it is important the patient is at his/her ease, cooperates with and has confidence in the practitioner. The practitioner should always be sensitive to the patient's needs and explain what he/she is about to do, and why, prior to undertaking the assessment. Measurement should be undertaken where possible, but the data must be meaningful and reproducible if it is to be of any use in assessing improvement or deterioration. Various measuring devices may be used; their use will be discussed in the appropriate sections.

## GAIT ANALYSIS

Gait can be affected by a variety of factors:
- Neurological dysfunction, which may involve one or a combination of the following parts of the CNS and/or PNS:
  — motor, e.g. CVA
  — sensory, e.g. tabes dorsalis
  — cerebellum, e.g. Friedreich's ataxia
  — basal ganglia, e.g. Parkinson's disease

- Joint disease, e.g. rheumatoid arthritis, osteoarthritis
- Muscle disease, e.g. Duchenne's muscular dystrophy
- Pain (antalgic gait), e.g. ankle sprain
- Bone disease, e.g. rickets

- Alignment disorders, e.g. rearfoot varus, genu varus
- Sensory defect, e.g. blindness.

The effects of the above may lead to gross or relatively minor changes to gait. Gross disorders are readily observed whereas those that lead to relatively minor changes, e.g. rearfoot varus, may not be so obvious. Gait can be adequately assessed with few aids, providing that sufficient room is available; ideally there should be a walkway 1.1 m wide and 6 m long. A treadmill may be used; this facilitates the observation of a sufficient number of strides without the patient having to make frequent turns and is especially appropriate if there is not enough room for a 6 m walkway. It is important that the patient is appropriately attired (ideally shorts and T-shirt) so that key parts can be observed; these are summarised in Table 8.3.

This section concentrates on the observation of gait. Methods of analysing gait are discussed in Chapter 12; these can provide a very useful adjunct to information obtained from observation and are particularly useful in the monitoring of gait changes.

**Table 8.3** Anatomical and functional features to observe during gait

- Head position
- Shoulders
- Arm swing
- Pelvic tilt
- Thigh segment
- Anterior knee—tibial tubercle/patella
- Lateral knee
- Tibial shank
- Ankle motion
- Heel position
- Navicular point
- Midtarsal position/movement
- Metatarsals (lateral and anterior view)
- Digital position
- Foot position
- Muscle activity
- Swing phase

**Table 8.4** Questions the practitioner should consider when assessing the patient's gait

- Does the patient lurch or look uncoordinated? This suggests ataxia and requires examination of the cerebellum and nervous system.
- Does the patient have any postural problem? Is the posture abnormal?
- Does the spine appear curved?
- Does one leg/foot lead, followed by the other without obvious asymmetry or alteration in cadence?
- Does the face shows signs of pain or anxiety? Could this be an antalgic gait?
- Does the patient appear to be overweight in relation to his/her height?
- Does the whole foot contact the ground when shod?
- Does the foot look straight, adducted or abducted?

The patient's gait must be observed from the posterior, anterior and lateral views in order that movement in all three body planes can be assessed. Gait should be observed with the patient both barefoot and wearing shoes.

Gait analysis commences with the patient entering the room. At this point the patient is less conscious of being observed and is less likely to act unnaturally. The practitioner's eye should run from the patient's head to ground level, observing foot–ground contact. At this stage there are some key points the practitioner should address about the patient's gait (Table 8.4).

Gait is divided into a *swing phase* and a *stance phase*; stance phase relates to the period of the gait cycle when the foot is in contact with the ground and swing phase to when it is not. Stance phase is easier to visualise than swing phase; it consists of the contact, midstance and propulsive stages (Fig. 8.7). Contact phase starts when the heel makes ground contact; this is followed by the rest of the foot. During contact phase the foot pronates in order to absorb shock from the effects of ground reaction. Midstance starts when all the foot is in ground contact and ends with heel lift. During midstance the foot starts to re-supinate ready for propulsion. Propulsion starts at heel lift and ends when the hallux leaves the ground. During propulsion the foot continues to supinate; the fifth metatarsal

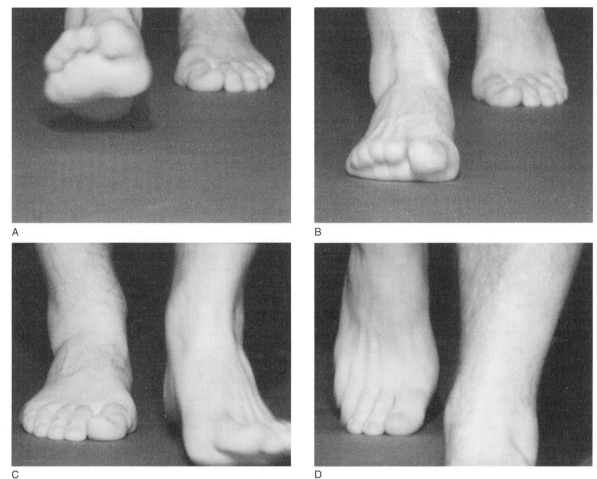

A

B

C

D

**Figure 8.7**    Series of photographs taken at 400 frames per second    **A.** The right heel contacts the ground; forefoot motion is decelerated by the extensor muscles    **B.** The metatarsal heads have contacted the ground but the toes are still dorsiflexed    **C.** The right foot completes forefoot contact and the left heel is about to leave the ground (heel lift)    **D.** Propulsion: the fifth and fourth toes are no longer in ground contact and the third, second and first are about to follow in that order.

head is the first to leave the ground, followed in sequence by the others. The hallux should be the last to leave the ground. Assessment of foot–ground contact and swing phase can be facilitated by high-quality video recording and playback with freeze frame. The movement and relationship of both limbs during gait is summarised in Table 8.5.

The following section considers each of the specific pointers listed in Table 8.3.

**Head.** The head should not show excessive movement. Altered positions may include twisting (torticollis), due to muscle contracture, or tilting on one side as a result of pain or limb-length inequality (LLI).

**Shoulders.** Both shoulders should be level. Unilateral tilting may be due to LLI or scoliosis. Fixed deformities should be distinguished from flexible vertebral deformities (see static weight-bearing examination).

**Arm swing.** The arms should swing to even out leg movement. While arm swing is not mentioned in the determinants of gait (Table 8.2), it is difficult to exclude arm swing as a feature of normal forward progression. The upper torso will act to decelerate lower limb

**Table 8.5** Stance phase of gait showing 'normal' movement of the left and right limbs

| Left knee/hip | Left foot | Right knee/hip | Right foot |
| --- | --- | --- | --- |
| Knee extended<br>Hip flexed | Heel contact | Knee and hip extended | Heel lift |
| Knee flexed<br>Hip extending | Foot flat (forefoot loading) | Knee and hip flexing to max | Toe-off |
| Knee extended<br>Hip extended | Midstance | Knee starts to extend from maximum flexion<br>Hip flexed | Midswing |
| Knee and hip extended | Heel lift | Knee extended<br>Hip flexed | Heel contact |
| Knee and hip flexing to max | Toe-off | Knee flexed<br>Hip extending | Foot flat (forefoot loading) |

motion. Some subjects fail to swing their arms; this alone is not abnormal but can affect spine position during walking: there is a tendency to lean either forward or back as the arms do not swing. Arm and hand position may point to signs of injury or motor disability and should be recorded, for example flexed position of arm and hand held close to the body suggests a CVA.

**Pelvic tilt.** This forms the pivot of lower limb function. The pelvis moves in all three cardinal planes in order to provide smooth up and down (sinusoidal) motion. Tilting may arise from neurological problems, spinal deformity, LLI, osteoarthritis of the hip and injury.

**Thigh segment.** Thigh movement is a reflection of the transfer of pelvic motion through the hip joint. Excessive transverse plane rotation (internal and external rotation) should be noted; this may be due to a variety of factors, e.g. abnormal femoral torsion or version.

**Anterior knee (tibial tubercle/patella).** As long as the patella proves to have normal alignment then it can be used as a reference point to determine the extent of transverse plane motion of the leg. Alternatively, if the patella has an abnormal alignment, a bisection line drawn through the tibial tubercle with a black felt marker may assist observation of transverse plane motion. The amount of transverse plane rotation at the knee should be slightly greater than at the hip and may therefore be easier to observe than at the thigh. At heel contact the leg should internally rotate (patellae face inward);

throughout midstance and most of propulsion the leg should externally rotate (patellae face outward) (Fig. 8.4). Excessive internal or external rotation should be noted; it may be due to proximal or distal abnormality.

**Lateral knee.** Sagittal plane motion of the knee joint during gait is outlined in Table 8.5. Alteration in sagittal plane knee motion will affect the third determinant of gait. If the knee does not flex it causes the hip to lift further and allows greater height on that side. To swing the leg from stance through swing back to stance again, the pelvis has to rotate more and has a vertical displacement which should appear obvious. Excessive extension of the knee (genu recurvatum) should be noted if it occurs during gait.

**Tibial shank.** Frontal plane problems (genu valgus/varum) can be identified from observing the tibia. The normal tibial outline shows a slight genu varum because muscle distribution results in lateral bulk. Bowing of the legs (genu varum) or knock knees (genu valgum) should be noted (Fig. 8.5). Valgum of the hip (coxa) can produce the effect of a genu varum and conversely coxa vara can produce a genu valgum. If a genu varum or valgum is present it should be noted if it is bi- or unilateral. A unilateral deformity may suggest injury, infection or growth disturbance at the epiphysis in earlier life. Tumours are a rare cause but should always be considered.

**Ankle.** The ankle complex provides smooth transference of weight from heel to toe. A minimum of 10° dorsiflexion is required to allow the leg to pass over the foot during midstance. Equinus is the term used to indicate loss of dorsiflexion. Toe walking and/or an early heel lift may indicate an ankle equinus but non-weightbearing examination of the ankle joint must be carried out before a definitive diagnosis can be made. Unstable ankles may have frontal plane instability, which shows as tilting hesitations. The subtalar joint works in concert with the ankle (talocrural) joint. Inman (1976) regarded the talocrural (TCJ) and subtalar (STJ) as the 'ankle joint' because they have a symbiotic relationship. The TCJ provides predominantly sagittal plane motion and the STJ frontal and transverse plane motion. If one of these joints is unable to produce motion, e.g. after surgical arthrodesis (joint in fixed position), then the other compensates.

**Heel position.** The posterior position of the heel should be observed. The heel contacts the ground in a slightly inverted position. As a result of ground contact the calcaneus everts, without the need for active muscle contraction, in order to bring the medial tubercle of the calcaneus into ground contact. The position of the heel moves very quickly from an inverted to an everted position; it is therefore often easy to miss subtle changes. At the end of midstance the heel lifts off the ground in order to prepare the foot for propulsion (Case comment 8.1). An early heel lift or a heel that makes no ground contact suggests a neurological problem, an ankle equinus or hamstring tightness.

---

Case comment 8.1

Given that the average time of contact is between 650 and 750 ms, information has to be rapidly absorbed by the observer. Practitioners may think there is an ankle equinus as a result of gait analysis only to find that on video replay the timing of heel lift is in correct sequence with the opposite foot.

---

**Navicular point.** At heel contact the foot pronates in order to absorb shock from ground contact. During pronation the talar head adducts against the navicular and as a result the distance between the ground and the navicular reduces. As the foot progresses into midstance and then toe off the foot re-supinates (talus abducts); at this point the distance between the navicular and the ground increases. If the talonavicular prominence is visible for more than a moment, or if the extent of the displacement is abnormal, careful examination of the cause must be considered during the non-weightbearing examination.

**Midtarsal (MTJ) joint.** During midstance and propulsion the MTJ plays an important role in maintaining foot stability in order to withstand the forces on the foot generated by uneven surfaces and particularly during propulsion. Functioning of the MTJ is difficult to observe during gait. However, if there is abnormal pronation at the subtalar joint the forefoot will appear abducted on the rearfoot at the site of the MTJ; this is an important sign of dysfunction which may result in forefoot deformity (Fig. 8.8).

**The metatarsals.** Forefoot loading during the contact phase should be observed from the anterior viewpoint (Fig. 8.7A–C). The fifth metatarsal head makes ground contact first followed in sequence by the other metatarsals; the first metatarsal head is the last to make ground contact. At propulsion the reverse should happen; the fifth is the first to leave the ground, followed in sequence by the others with the first being the last to leave ground contact (Fig. 8.7D). During propulsion motion at the first MTPJ should be observed from the lateral side; ideally the MTPJ should dorsiflex to approximately 70°.

**Digital position.** Toes should be dorsiflexed at contact (Fig. 8.7A–B). Once the first metatarsal has contacted the ground on the medial side, all toes should be plantigrade (Fig. 8.7C). At propulsion the hallux should be the last to leave the ground. Any change in normal digital position should be noted. The position of the digits during the stance phase is influenced by the intrinsic muscles (lumbricals and interossei) and the long and short flexors and extensors. The role of the intrinsic muscles is to provide transverse plane stability at the distal and proximal

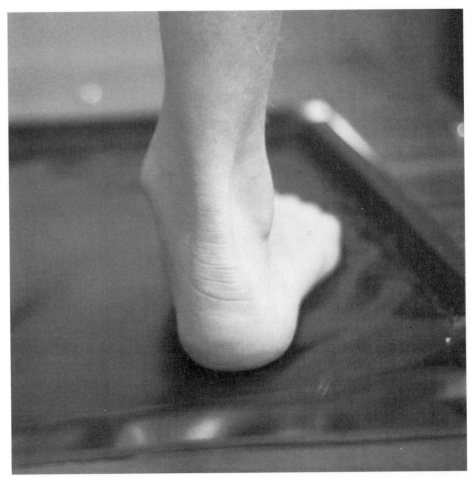

**Figure 8.8** The foot should be viewed from the posterior aspect to determine subtalar joint and midtarsal joint position during midstance. The midtarsal joint offers a useful gauge to determine deformity due to abnormal pronation leading to a medial shift in the talonavicular relationship. The lateral border may be very apparent as the foot pronates abnormally. The photograph shows moderate pronation with abduction at the midtarsal joint.

IPJs and prevent the toes from buckling under the effects of contraction of the extensors and/or flexors. Clawing of toes during gait can occur if the flexors have a mechanical advantage over the intrinsic and extensor muscles. Conversely, clawing can also occur if there is extensor muscle activity prior to heel lift.

**Foot position.** When all the foot is in contact with the ground the position of the foot in relation to the midline of the body should be observed. Normally the foot should be slightly abducted (approximately 13°). If the foot is adducted (in-toeing) or excessively abducted (out-toeing) this should be noted together with whether the problem is bi- or unilateral.

**Muscle activity.** The anterior view allows muscle activity to be observed (Fig. 8.9). Normal 'decelerator' muscle activity can be observed. Deceleration implies that the muscle resists joint movement by eccentric contraction; extensor tendons on the dorsum of the foot are active at contact because they decelerate the foot, prevent foot slap and allow the sole to contact the ground smoothly (Fig. 8.7A–B). Paralysis of the anterior muscle group will lead to a rapid collapse of the foot on to the ground and an

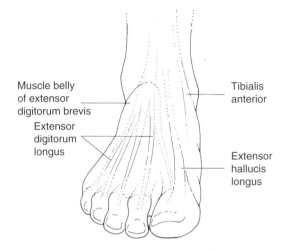

Muscle belly of extensor digitorum brevis

Extensor digitorum longus

Tibialis anterior

Extensor hallucis longus

**Figure 8.9** Muscles on the dorsal aspect of the foot. It is important to observe muscle activity during gait. The contraction of the extensor and tibialis anterior muscles should be clearly seen (Fig. 8.7A–B).

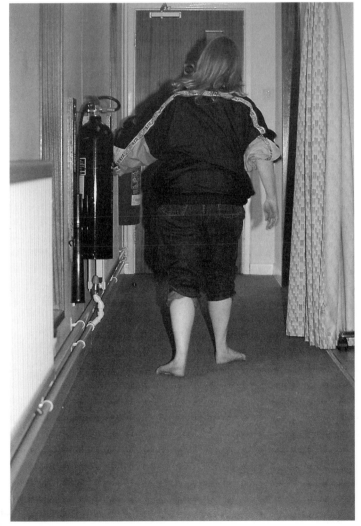

**Figure 8.10** The flat-footed and abducted gait has been brought about by muscle paresis (weakness) in the lower leg. Extensive tests have shown no obvious diagnosis. The gait shows shuffle-waddling. There is marked abduction with bilateral ground contact for most of the stance phase. The left foot shows medial roll off as the leg prepares to move into swing.

audible slap. An example of a severe form of muscle group weakness is shown in Figure 8.10. The peronei, longus and brevis, are difficult to identify during gait unless they show spasm. When this happens, and it is not common, the tendons stand out around the lateral malleolus (peroneus longus) and lateral foot (peroneus brevis).

**Swing phase.** The foot pronates during early swing because the STJ provides additional dorsiflexion with pronation to aid ground clearance. Some neuromuscular conditions may prevent this from occurring and lead to the toes dragging across the ground, e.g. poliomyelitis. Signs of skin lesions over the digits may provide a clue that this is happening.

## Abnormal gait patterns

Gait can be affected in a variety of ways leading to abnormal gait patterns. Below some of the commonly encountered patterns are described.

**Apropulsive gait.** During the propulsive stage of gait the MTPJs should dorsiflex to approximately 70° and the hallux should be the last digit to leave the ground; if this does not occur the gait is said to be *apropulsive*. An apropulsive gait may occur due to a variety of factors, e.g. hallux limitus/rigidus, abnormal pronation, unusual metatarsal formula, excessive internal rotation of the leg. The foot may compensate for lack of propulsion by rolling off its medial border (Fig. 8.10), by propelling from a hyper-extended (dorsiflexion) first IPJ rather than MTPJ or by an abductory twist. This is when the distal part of the foot twists outwards during propulsion. Whatever the cause, the foot is prevented from re-supinating during the later stages of midstance. However, once the heel lifts off the ground the effect of ground reaction, which prevented the re-supination, is reduced and the forefoot twists outwards in order to bring the foot into a more medial position for toe-off.

**Abnormal pronation.** Abnormal pronation can be classified as excessive pronation and/or pronation occurring when the foot should be supinating. Signs of abnormal pronation during gait are excessive/prolonged internal rotation of the leg, eversion of the calcaneus, abduction at the midtarsal joint, an apropulsive gait and abnormal phasic activity of the muscles.

**Early heel lift.** This may vary from the heel making no contact with the ground (toe walking) to a relatively normal heel contact but an early heel lift. Heel lift should normally occur at the end of midstance prior to propulsion. An early heel lift can give rise to a bouncy gait. The most common cause is an ankle equinus.

**Leg-length inequality (LLI).** One shoulder is usually lower than the other, and there may be a functional scoliosis. The determinants of gait are affected and the gait appears uneven. The foot of the shorter leg is usually in a supinated position and the foot of the longer leg abnormal pronates. Early heel lift may occur in the shorter leg.

**Circumducted gait.** A CVA victim has the characteristic features of unilateral limb weakness and will circumduct (rotate the leg in an arc) and flex the elbow and hand towards the body. Movements are made slowly to maintain balance. Jerky movements suggest muscle coordination problems; the nature of upper and lower motor neurone deficits are described in Chapter 7.

## NON-WEIGHTBEARING EXAMINATION

The prime purpose of the non-weightbearing examination is to undertake an assessment of the joints and muscles of the lower limb. Information from this part of the examination may explain the cause of a gait abnormality or the patient's presenting problem. For example, a foot may in-toe as a result of an osseous and/or soft tissue problem of the leg; the purpose of the non-weightbearing examination is to establish which is most likely.

A flat couch is required for the patient to lie on. The patient should feel comfortable and relaxed and should not wear restrictive clothing.

Non-weightbearing examination involves an assessment of the following:

* Hip
* Knee

- Ankle complex (talocrural, subtalar and midtarsal)
- Rays (metatarsals)
- Metatarsophalangeal joints (MTPJs)
- Digits (proximal and distal interphalangeal joints—IPJs)
- Alignment of the lower limb.

Prior to describing the assessment process in detail some general points regarding the assessment of joints and muscles are outlined below.

## Assessment of joints

Joints should be assessed for:

- signs of inflammation
- pain
- range of motion (ROM)
- direction of motion (DOM)
- quality of motion (QOM)
- symmetry of motion (SOM)
- dislocation and subluxation.

Features of an inflamed joint are redness, heat, pain, swelling and loss of function. Inflammation of a joint may be due to a range of factors: trauma, infection, loose body (osteochondritis desiccans). Examination of the joint, information from the medical and social history and results from X-ray and lab tests will enable a diagnosis to be made. If a patient complains of a painful joint the characteristic features of the pain should be recorded (Ch. 3).

Prior to assessing a joint it is important that the joint is warmed up (moved through its range of motion); this relaxes the ligaments and muscles and also reduces the viscosity of the synovial fluid.

Rand of motion (ROM) is the amount of motion at a joint and is usually measured in degrees. The ROM at a joint can be compared to the expected ROM for that joint; e.g. if only 20° of motion is found at the first MTPJ when the expected norm is 70° (28% of the normal ROM) it can be concluded that the ability of this joint to carry out normal function is impaired (hallux limitus). Often a guestimate of the amount of joint motion is made from observation. Pro-

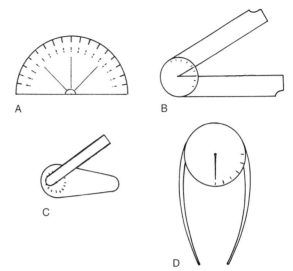

**Figure 8.11**   Devices used to measure joints
**A.** Protractor   **B.** Tractograph   **C.** Finger goniometer
**D.** Gravity goniometer.

tractors, tractographs and goniometers can be used to quantify joint motion (Fig. 8.11).

A joint may show a normal ROM but the direction of the motion (DOM) may be abnormal. It is, therefore, important to note the direction as well as the range. For example, the total ROM of transverse plane rotation at the hip is 90°; 45° internal rotation and 45° external rotation. If the ROM is 90° but there is 70° of external rotation and 20° of internal rotation then the ROM would be normal but the DOM would be abnormal.

Normal joint motion should occur without crepitus, pain or resistance (quality of motion). The ROM and DOM of motion of a joint, e.g. hip, should be the same for both limbs (symmetry of motion). The presence of asymmetry of motion should always be noted. Joint motion can be affected by the ligaments around the joint. It is important as part of joint assessment to identify any dysfunction of the ligaments, e.g. ligament tear or contracture of a ligament.

Finally, joints should be assessed as to whether they are subluxated or dislocated. Dislocation occurs where there is no contact between articulating surfaces of the joint and subluxation where there is only partial contact.

# Assessment of muscles

Muscles bring about motion at joints. In order to identify the cause of joint dysfunction and/or pain it is important to differentiate between muscle, ligament and joint abnormality. As a number of muscles may affect any one joint it is important to neutralise the effects of other muscles prior to testing the muscle in question. One way in which a muscle can be neutralised is by flexing the joint which the muscle crosses so that tension is removed.

Muscles should be tested for:

- strength
- tone
- spasm
- bulk.

## Strength

The Medical Research Council (MRC) system is commonly used for grading muscle strength (Crawford Adams & Hamblen 1990):

0 = no contraction
1 = a flicker from muscle fasciculi
2 = slight movement with gravitational effects removed
3 = muscle can move part against gravity
4 = muscle can move part against gravity + resistance
5 = normal power.

Muscle strength can be assessed by the patient bringing about the motion (active) or by the practitioner moving the part (passive). Active motion can be tested against resistance, i.e. the practitioner attempts to prevent active motion.

## Tone

All muscles should show tone. Tone denotes that a muscle is in a state of partial contraction without full movement being necessary. Asking the patient to undertake isometric contraction of a muscle is a useful means of identifying tonal quality. For example, the tone of the quadriceps can be assessed by asking the patient to contract the muscle while the knee is in an extended position. During contraction muscles should feel firm as well as appearing taut. Flaccid muscles lack tone; this is common with lower motor neurone disorders. Absence of tone in young males could be due to Duchenne's muscular dystrophy.

## Spasm

Muscles may present in spasm and as a result affect joint motion. There are two types of muscle spasm; tonic and clonic. Tonic spasm usually occurs as an attempt by the muscles to stop movement at a painful joint; clonic spasm is associated with neurological (upper motor neurone) deficit and is involuntary. Information from the neurological assessment, medical history and presenting problem should enable identification of the type of spasm.

## Bulk

Muscle bulk should be observed and comparisons made between the lower limbs. Atrophy of muscle can result in a loss of muscle bulk and may be due to a number of factors, e.g. lack of use, lower motor neurone lesion (Case comment 8.2). Hypertrophic muscles that show normal tone and symmetrical distribution are considered normal and are usually due to the effects of exercise. Unilateral atrophy/hypertrophy can be assessed by observation and measuring the girth of both limbs with a tape measure (Fig. 8.12).

---

Case comment 8.2

Be mindful of diabetics who inject themselves with insulin. The quadriceps and abdominal muscles are often used and will show patchy loss of fat and muscle.

---

# Neutral position

A number of the tests described below require the foot to be put into its neutral position. This is defined as the foot being neither pronated or supinated. To put the foot into the neutral

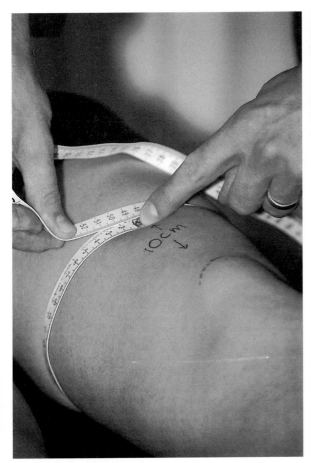

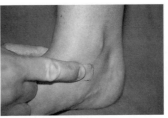
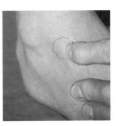

A                                                    B

**Figure 8.13** Finding subtalar joint neutral **A.** Locating the talar head on the medial side **B.** Locating the talar head on the lateral side. It is easier to palpate the talar head on the lateral side than it is on the medial side.

**Figure 8.12** Assessment of muscle bulk (quadriceps) using a tape measure.

position the practitioner should feel on the dorsum of the foot for the talar head. The foot should be moved into pronation and supination; while the foot is pronating the talar head can be felt protruding on the medial side of the talonavicular joint and while the foot is supinating it can be felt protruding on the lateral side of the talonavicular joint (Fig. 8.13). Neutral position is achieved when the talar head cannot be palpated on either side. If the foot is non-weightbearing it is also necessary to 'lock' the midtarsal joint in order to reproduce the position the foot would adopt if it were weightbearing. In order to lock the midtarsal joint the talar head should be held in its neutral position and a slight dorsiflexing force applied to the fourth

and fifth met heads until the foot is at 90° to the leg. The neutral position of the foot acts as a reference point from which joint motion and the position of parts of the foot can be assessed.

## NON-WEIGHTBEARING EXAMINATION—HIP

It is not usually necessary to examine every patient's hip. The hip should only be examined if the patient complains of discomfort or pain in the area and/or gait analysis reveals an abnormality which affects normal pelvis and thigh/leg motion.

Hip pain (coxodynia) is felt deep in the groin and not on the outside of the femur. The main cause of hip pain is osteoarthritis, a particularly common condition in the elderly. X-ray of the hip should be considered if confirmation of a disease process is necessary or diagnosis unclear, e.g. osteoarthrosis, Perthes disease.

### Joint motion

The hip's ball and socket joint provides free movement.

#### Sagittal plane

In order to ensure forward progression during gait sagittal plane motion at the hip is necessary. Ideally there should be approximately 120–140° of flexion and 5–20° of extension, although not

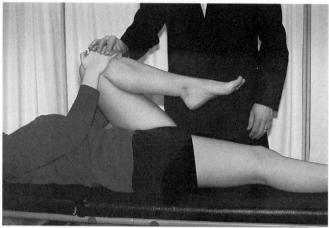

**Figure 8.14** The patient should be asked to draw the leg towards the stomach as depicted in the photograph. The hip is flexed to its limit against the abdomen. Thomas's test should be considered at the same time by looking for contralateral lifting.

all of this is necessary for gait. To assess hip flexion the patient is placed supine (back to the couch) on a firm, flat couch. The practitioner holds the leg firmly and flexes the hip by pushing the leg towards the body until resistance is met (Fig. 8.14). To assess extension the patient is turned over on to the stomach (prone). The practitioner places one hand on the posterior superior iliac crest to stabilise the pelvis while the other hand holds the opposite leg just above the anterior knee and moves the leg towards the body to the point of resistance.

Loss of sagittal plane motion may be due to pain, femoral nerve entrapment or effusion in the hip joint as the anterior ligaments (iliofemoral and pubofemoral) will be under greater tension and resistance than usual. Any asymmetry should be noted.

### Frontal plane

To assess abduction and adduction at the hip the patient lies supine and the practitioner holds the leg just below the anterior knee. The leg with the knee extended is moved across the opposite leg (adduction) and then brought back and abducted. The pelvis should not move during this assessment. There should be less adduction than abduction at the hip. Tightness of the adductors on abduction can lead to a scissors-type gait: this is when one or both legs have a tendency to cross over during gait and can be seen with cerebral palsy.

### Transverse plane

Internal and external rotation of the lower limb is essential for normal gait. Ideally the total range of transverse plane motion in an adult should be 90°, comprising 45° internal and 45° external rotation. Females tend to show more internal rotation than males (Svenningsen et al 1990). The range of transverse plane motion at the hip decreases with age and the DOM changes from symmetry to more external than internal rotation.

To assess transverse plane rotation the patient lies in a supine position. The hip and knees are flexed and the leg is moved medially and laterally as one would the arms of a clock. A gravity goniometer can be used to assess the range of motion (Fig. 8.15). Asymmetry in the DOM should be noted. For example, a patient who shows 70° internal rotation and only 20° external rotation has an internally rotated femur which will affect normal lower limb function and may result in abnormal pronation at the subtalar joint.

The test can be repeated with the patient in the same position but with the hip and knees

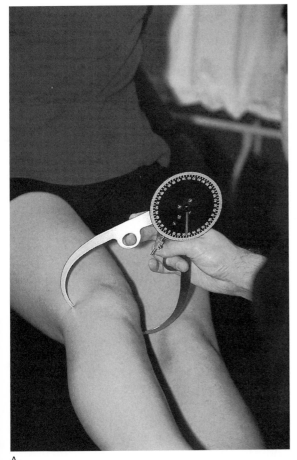

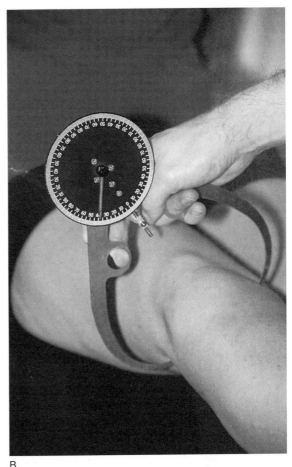

A                                                        B

**Figure 8.15** The hips are in a flexed position    **A.** A gravity goniometer is used to assess the amount of internal femoral rotation    **B.** A gravity goniometer is used to assess the amount of external femoral rotation.

extended. The practitioner may note a difference in the ROM and DOM at the hip when the knees are flexed compared to when they are extended. It was thought that this technique could be used to detect the presence of torsion (bone influence) or version (soft-tissue influence). Torsion was said to exist if there was no difference between the ROM and DOM at the hip with the knees flexed and extended and version if there was a greater ROM when the knees were flexed. It was considered important to make a distinction as torsion cannot be treated conservatively while version can. This concept, while plausible, is not consistent with bone torsion measurement and is open to misdiagnosis. However, it is important

when undertaking an assessment of the muscles around the hip to see if there are any soft-tissue contractures, which may be responsible for limiting motion.

### Scouring

This assesses QOM and joint congruency. The hip is flexed and adducted and the practitioner rotates the hip to test for any crepitations. A posterolateral force is then placed on the hip in order to test the posterior and lateral hip capsule. Fabere's test involves stressing the medial hip capsule by placing an anteromedial force on the hip; this also assesses for sacroiliac discomfort.

Another way is for the practitioner to place his/her hands on either side of the pelvis and press it together.

## Muscle action

### Young's test

A taut tensor fasciae latae causes the knee and hip to flex. By abducting the lower limb, tension on the tensor fasciae latae is reduced and any flexion deformity should disappear. A tight tensor fasciae latae may be the cause of an apparent limb length discrepancy.

---

**Case comment 8.3**

Thomas's test: while the patient flexes the hip, the practitioner must observe the opposite (contralateral) thigh for any sign of elevation. The lumbar spine must lie flat. If the iliopsoas muscles are tight, the contralateral hip will rise as the ipsilateral hip will force the lumbar spine against the couch. Fixed flexion will cause an apparent LLI.

---

### Iliopsoas

This group of muscles—psoas major, psoas minor and iliacus—are the prime flexors of the hip. Thomas's test will rule out the presence of iliopsoas contracture: if a flexion deformity exists the affected leg will flex at the knee (Fig. 8.14) (Case comment 8.3). Furthermore, the femoral nerve can be irritated by a taut iliopsoas group. Damage to the nerve will lead to weakness of the quadriceps, as well as loss of sensation on the anterior and medial aspects of the leg (Case comment 8.4).

---

**Case comment 8.4**

The obturator nerve arises in the psoas major and crosses the hip joint, exiting through the obturator foramen. If this nerve is injured in the hip region, e.g. due to a slipped capita femoris epiphysis, knee pain may result. Where knee pain exists, hip pathology must always be ruled out.

---

### Iliotibial band

Ober's test is designed to test for iliotibial contraction or tightness. The patient lies on his/her side and the outer limb with the knee extended is moved anteriorly and then adducted towards the couch (Fig. 8.16A). This stretches the lateral structures, primarily the iliotibial band. A modified form of the test separately tests the short fibres of the knee; this is achieved by flexing the knee and repeating the manoeuvre.

### External rotators

The smaller hip rotators can be examined by rotating the hip while in a flexed position. However, if the patient is placed on his/her side the external rotators of the free side can be tested. The piriformis muscle can be put on tension (Fig. 8.16B).

### Adductors

These have their insertion on the medial side of the femur along the linea aspera. The adductor muscles are important during the swing phase, stabilising the contralateral side of the hip against the pelvis as the leg swings forward. Adductor strength can be tested as in Figure 8.16C. Gracilis, a partial adductor, rotates the femur on the hip. As it shares some of the function of the adductors, it can be examined with them. However, this muscle crosses the knee and lies between the sartorius and semi-tendinosus on the medial aspect of the knee. The knee should be extended to include the action of gracilis, but flexed to remove its influence.

### Abductors

The abductors include the gluteus medius and minimus as well as the tensor fasciae latae, acting through the iliotibial tract. Abductor strength is best assessed when the subject lies on his/her side. The patient should raise the upper leg away from the couch against gravity and resistance. When a patient stands on one leg, the pelvis should tilt upwards on the side of the

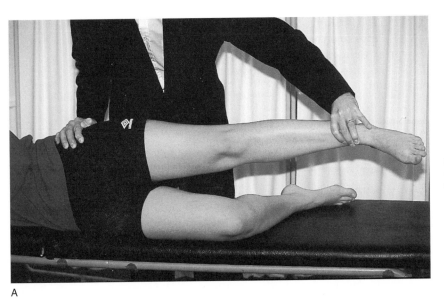

A

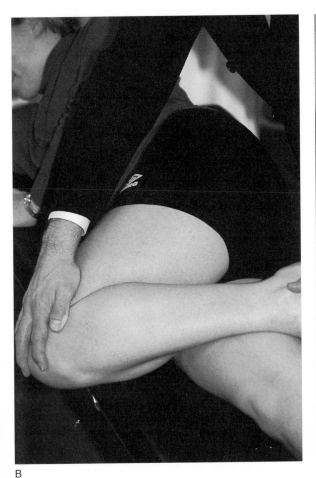

B

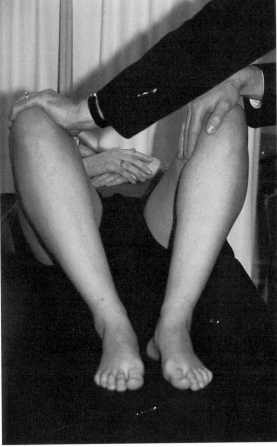

C

**Figure 8.16    A.** Ober test identifies resistance in the tensor fascia/iliotibial tract
**B.** Assessment of the external rotators. Muscle strength can be gauged by resisting external rotation    **C.** The patient is asked to bring the knees together against resistance. This tests adductor strength.

lifted leg (*Trendelenburg's test*). A positive Trendelenburg sign occurs when the reverse happens: the pelvis tilts downwards, indicating weak glutei. Osteoarthritis of the hip can produce a positive Trendelenburg sign.

## NON-WEIGHTBEARING EXAMINATION—KNEE

The knee should be examined if dysfunction is observed during gait and/or the patient complains of knee discomfort/pain. It is important that the practitioner establishes whether knee pain/discomfort is due to a primary problem affecting the knee, e.g. meniscus tear, or is due to compensation for a problem elsewhere, e.g. abnormal pronation causing instability and damage to the knee.

Figure 8.17 illustrates the anatomy of the knee joint and the knee joint margin. The knee joint can be compared to a boiled egg lying on a plate; the configuration of an oval femoral surface on a flat tibial plateau allows great mobility. During gait it is important that the knee is stable; the cruciate and collateral ligaments, the menisci and the iliotibial band and sartorius muscles provide most of the stability.

The patella forms part of the knee joint; it articulates with the anterior surface of the inferior end of the femur. It acts as a sesamoid as described earlier and provides a key mechanical advantage, increasing the moments of force applied through the ligamentum patellae on to the tibial tubercle.

The presence and site of swelling in the knee should be noted (Case comment 8.5). Swelling of an extreme nature can be associated with bursitis, acute synovitis, tearing of the menisci, rheumatoid arthritis (*Baker's cyst*) or osteoarthritis. Spontaneous swelling is usually caused by cruciate or meniscus injury.

## Joint motion

Any examination of joint motion at the knee must involve an assessment of the capsular and intracapsular ligaments.

---

| Case comment 8.5 |
| --- |
| A 10-year-old male developed a tender area on the anterior aspect of his knee during activity. The site of the tibial tubercle was shown to have been damaged by force from the traction of ligamentum patellae, leaving clinically a hot swollen prominence. The condition was Osgood–Schlatter's disease, a common example of a traction apophysitis. Examination may reveal an old unilateral or bilateral condition typified by an enlarged tubercle. |

### Sagittal plane

The main motion at the knee occurs in the sagittal plane; this is important for forward progression during gait. Ideally the knee should

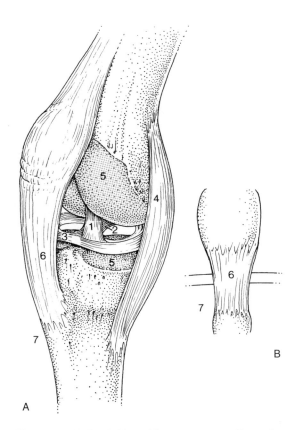

**Figure 8.17 A, B   A.** Normal knee anatomy:   **1)** anterior cruciate   **2)** posterior cruciate   **3)** meniscus   **4)** collateral ligament   **5)** cartilage   **6)** ligamentum patellae surrounding patella   **7)** tibia tubercle   **B.** Diagrammatic representation of the joint margin. (Fig. 8.17C on next page).

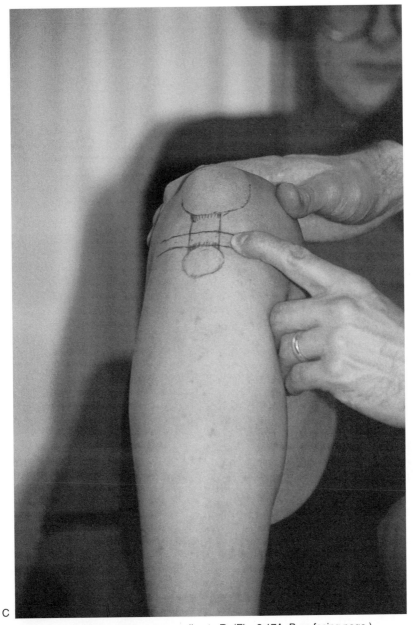

**Figure 8.17   C.** Photograph of the joint margin corresponding to **B**. (Fig. 8.17A, B on facing page.)

flex to approximately 135°; the thigh muscles restrict further motion. The amount of sagittal plane motion can be measured with a protractor or tractograph. The amount of extension available is minimal (0–10°). The knee should extend and lock without pain, with the patella in the centre of the knee. Postural extension beyond

10° is known as genu recurvatum and is indicative of lower limb dysfunction.

*Frontal plane*

There should be no or limited frontal plane motion at the knee. Frontal plane motion is normally only available to a child under 6 years of age.

## Collateral ligaments

A lateral stress test is used to assess the collateral ligaments. With the patient supine the knee is flexed to 30°. The practitioner places one hand on the medial side of the lower end of the femur and the other on the lateral side of the upper end of the tibia. The practitioner then pushes with both hands in an attempt to 'break' the knee by stressing the lateral collateral ligament. The medial collateral ligament can then be stressed by placing the hands in the opposite position. Motion at the knee during these tests indicates weak collaterals and poor knee stability.

## Cruciate ligament

There are two cruciate ligaments within the knee joint; posterior and anterior. Their purpose is to prevent the knee joint from 'opening up'. To assess the anterior cruciate ligament the patient lies supine with the knee flexed to 45° and the foot flat on the couch. The practitioner grasps the upper end of the tibia and pulls it forward to stress the anterior cruciate ligament. The posterior cruciate is examined by reversing the manoeuvre. This test is known as the drawer test because the action is like opening and shutting a drawer (Fig. 8.18A). More than 2–3 cm displacement of the tibia is considered abnormal and may be painful; excessive movement suggests tearing of these structures. *Lachman's test* specifically tests the anterior cruciate ligaments. The knee is flexed to 25° and the tibia is pulled forward while the knee is externally rotated. If there is displacement of the tibia this is indicative of a weak anterior cruciate ligament.

## McMurray's test

This is used to detect meniscus tears. The medial meniscus is most likely to tear because it has less flexibility as it is attached to the capsule. The

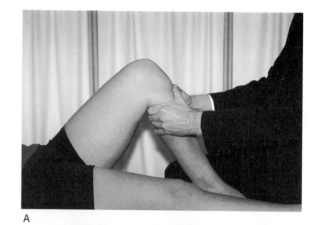

A

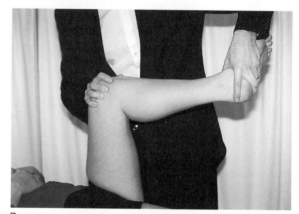

B

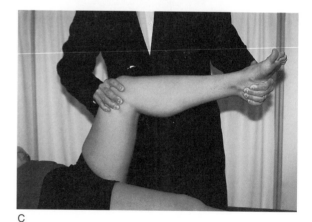

C

**Figure 8.18** Knee joint examination **A.** Drawer test requires the tibia to be push–pulled against the femur **B.** McMurray's rotation test with the knee flexed and the leg externally rotated **C.** McMurray's rotation test with the knee flexed and the leg internally rotated.

McMurray test is also designed to seek out any loose bodies by detecting crepitations and clicking (Fig. 8.18B–C). There may be a history of knee locking due to tonic spasm of the hamstrings in order to protect the joint. The patient lies supine with the knee and hip flexed to 90°. The practitioner grasps the sole of the foot with one hand; the other should be placed around the knee so that the joint line can be palpated. By moving the foot the tibia is externally rotated and a valgus stress is applied. A positive test will elicit a 'popping' or 'snapping' sound or sensation. The test is repeated with internal rotation and a varus stress for the lateral meniscus. Ensure that snapping and clicks due to normal tendon movement over prominences are not misdiagnosed as pathological lesions.

### Apley's compression test

The patient lies prone and the knee is flexed and the foot grasped. The practitioner creates a compression at the knee joint while producing a rotation movement. A noisy and painful response suggests meniscus damage.

### Clarke's test

This used to be a popular test for the diagnosis of chondromalacia patellae. However, chondromalacia patella can only really be diagnosed on arthroscopic examination. Clarke's test is useful to detect anterior knee pain. The patient lies supine and the practitioner places one hand over the patella and asks the patient to contract the quadriceps.

### Ballottement test

This is used to assess the presence of fluid around the suprapatellar pouch. This test involves the practitioner placing one hand on the patella and, if fluid is present at the knee, forcing fluid from one side to the other.

### Laboratory tests

X-rays may be requested in order to gain a full picture of the extent of damage and to rule out loose bodies or a fragmented patella. Assessment of joint aspirate will rule out haemorrhage, in, e.g. haemophilia, or pus, in, e.g. infective arthritis. Arthroscopy can be combined with surgical exploration of the joint.

## Muscle examination

### Quadriceps

The practitioner should inspect the tone of the quadriceps. Wasting of the medial vastus in particular may occur as a result of knee dysfunction. A tape measure can be used to assess muscle bulk in this area and monitor any change as a result of treatment (Fig. 8.12). The circumference of both legs should be measured at a standard distance above the tibial tubercle.

The rectus femoris muscle is a weak flexor of the hip but a powerful extensor of the knee. As part of the quadriceps group of muscles, rectus femoris is an important stabiliser of the knee, in conjunction with the vasti, and is needed to swing the leg forward in gait. Pain at its insertion (anterior inferior iliac spine) can arise with a strong kicking action. Examination of the rectus femoris muscle is undertaken with the patient sitting on the edge of the couch with the knees flexed. To assess the strength of this muscle the patient is asked to extend the knee while the practitioner attempts to resist this active motion (Fig. 8.19).

### Q angle

The 'Q angle' is the position the patella adopts in relation to the direction of pull of the quadriceps tendon. A line is drawn from the ASIS to a line bisecting the patella. If the angle of this line to the bisection of the patella is greater than 15° the patient is said to have a high Q angle. This suggests medial displacement of the patella and is often associated with greater than normal internal rotation and anterior knee pain.

### Hamstrings

The 90:90 test is used to identify tightness and contracture of the hamstring muscle group.

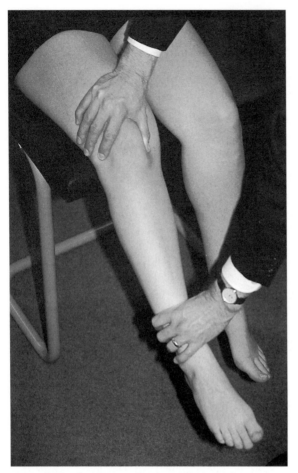

**Figure 8.19** Rectus femoris is tested by extending the knee against resistance.

Tight hamstrings may cause knee flexion, creating an inefficient antagonist action with the quadriceps and a functional equinus at the ankle joint. The 90:90 test is performed with the patient supine. The knee and hip are flexed to 90°. The practitioner holds the leg and extends the knee until resistance is met. If the knee can be fully straightened or to within 10°, then the hamstrings are within normal limits. If the leg can only be partially extended it indicates tight hamstrings.

Any asymmetry should be noted. In order to assess whether this is due to a tight biceps femoris or semitendinosus, stretch can be placed on the biceps femoris muscle by medially rotating the extended leg and on the semitendinosus by laterally rotating the leg (Fig. 8.20).

## NON-WEIGHTBEARING EXAMINATION—ANKLE COMPLEX

Inman (1976) regards the ankle as a two-joint system comprising the subtalar (STJ) and the talocrural joint (TCJ). Motion of the foot is primarily controlled through this joint complex, but the whole proximal segment also relies upon the TCJ and STJ working in concert. Elftman (1960) considered the midtarsal joint to be the third member of the ankle complex. Each of these joints will be considered separately for examination purposes but functionally they should be considered together.

Coalitions between the joints making up the ankle complex may be present. The two most common involve the talocalcaneal (medial and posterior facets) and the calcaneonavicular. Other types may occur but are quite rare. The coalition may be fibrous, cartilaginous or osseous. Fibrous coalitions permit some motion whereas cartilaginous and osseous coalitions produce little motion but more symptoms. Tonic spasm of the peronei is a common finding with tarsal coalitions. X-rays are necessary to diagnose a synostosis (osseous coalition).

## TALOCRURAL JOINT

The trochlear surface of the talus articulates with the inferior surface of the tibia to form the talocrural joint. The talocrural joint is a triplanar joint but because of the position of its axis and the shape of the joint surfaces its main motion is in the sagittal plane. The lateral curvature and radius of the trochlear surface of the talus has been found to be variable—the longer its radius, the less dorsiflexion (Barnett & Napier 1952). During midstance there should be at least 10° of dorsiflexion at the ankle in order to allow the leg to move over the foot.

The body compensates for a lack of ankle dorsiflexion at the knee and/or subtalar and

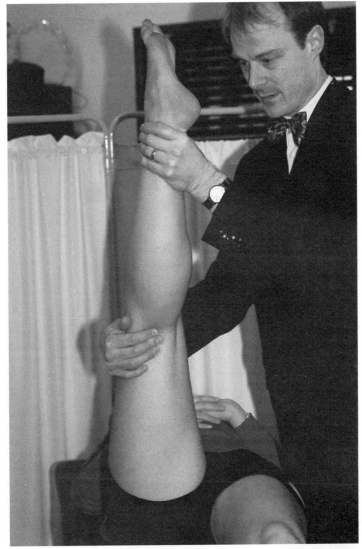

**Figure 8.20**   90:90 test. The leg can be laterally and medially rotated to identify specific areas of tightness. The photograph shows the leg laterally rotated to identify tight medial hamstrings.

midtarsal joints. The STJ has less available sagittal plane motion than the TCJ, but if necessary the STJ will increase the amount available if there is insufficient motion at the TCJ. In addition the knee can hyperextend (genu recurvatum) as a way of compensating for an ankle equinus.

## Joint motion

Assessment of the stability of the ankle joint and the presence of an ankle equinus are important parts of the ankle joint assessment.

### Sagittal plane

Ankle equinus is traditionally defined as less than 10° of dorsiflexion at the ankle, although some practitioners suggest less than 5° dorsiflexion leads to abnormal compensation. It may arise from soft tissue or bone abnormalities of an acquired or congenital nature.

Assessing sagittal plane motion at the TCJ is difficult. It can be assessed either weightbearing or non-weightbearing. If assessed non-weight-bearing the patient should lie in a prone or supine position with the knee extended and the foot and ankle free of the end of the couch. The practitioner holds the foot in a neutral position with one hand, places the other hand on the sole of the foot and dorsiflexes the ankle (Fig. 8.21A). The force applied by the practitioner to produce ankle dorsiflexion can vary; this will have an effect on the result. A tractograph can be used to assess the range of motion but the practitioner may find it difficult to use, while at the same time keeping the foot in a neutral position (Fig. 8.21B).

A tight soleus and/or gastrocnemius may prevent ankle dorsiflexion. In order to differentiate between the two the amount of dorsiflexion with the knee extended and flexed should be measured. With the knee flexed the tendons of gastrocnemius which cross the knee are released from tension and as a result a tight gastrocnemius should not effect ankle dorsiflexion. If the amount of dorsiflexion is still reduced when the knee is flexed the cause is likely to be soleus (Fig. 8.21C).

More consistent results have been achieved when sagittal plane motion is assessed with the patient weightbearing. The patient stands facing a wall with a distance of approximately 0.5 m between the patient and the wall. One leg, with the knee in a flexed position, is placed in front, approximately 30 cm from the wall. The other leg is placed behind the forward foot with the knee extended and the foot held in a neutral position. The patient leans towards and places both hands on the wall and is asked to move his/her body towards the wall. In order to do this the patient must dorsiflex the ankle of the limb furthest from the wall. The amount of dorsiflexion can be measured with a tractograph (Fig. 8.21D).

### Stability

By moving the TCJ in all three planes the ligaments can be stressed and any tenderness noted. There should be little or no displacement in the frontal plane and the patient should find the movement pain-free. Tenderness from the lateral ligaments (calcaneofibular and talofibular) should be noted before stressing the joint at the extreme

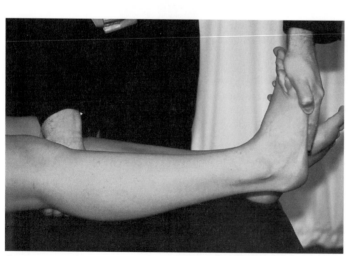

A

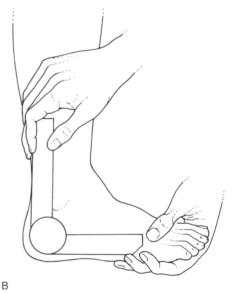

B

**Figure 8.21 A, B** Ankle joint dorsiflexion  **A.** Non-weightbearing assessment of ankle joint dorsiflexion with the knee extended and the foot in the neutral position. Restriction of motion may be due to tight gastrocnemius, soleus or bony block **B.** A tractograph is used to measure the amount of dorsiflexion. (Fig. 8.21 C, D on facing page).

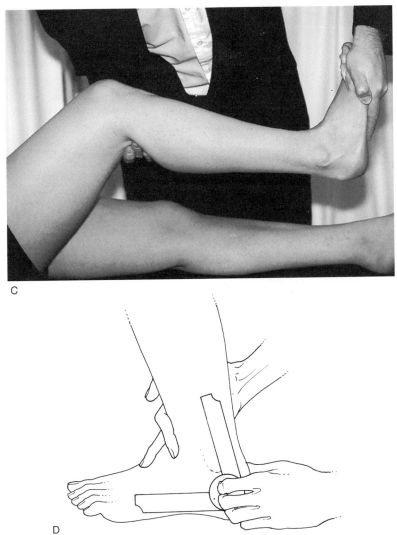

C

D

**Figure 8.21 C, D  C.** Non-weightbearing assessment of ankle joint dorsiflexion with the knee flexed and the foot in a neutral position. Restriction with the knee flexed due to a bony block or tight soleus   **D.** Assessment of ankle joint dorsiflexion weightbearing. (Fig. 8.21 A, B on facing page).

ends of inversion and eversion. The anterior joint line should be pressed upon firmly at the tibial plafond. The talus may have less stability if the inferior transverse tibiofibular ligament is affected as this holds the distal end of the tibia and fibular within the ankle mortise.

Stability in the sagittal plane can be tested by applying a forward and then a backward push on the ankle while the knee is flexed and the foot is in contact with the examining couch. This is the drawer test and should reveal minimal

positional change and no discomfort. The posterior aspect of the talus should be palpated while the ankle is in a plantarflexed position. Stieda's process may become irritated, or fracture if extra-long, or may appear as a separate bone (os trigonum) and become transiently irritated. The pain is deeper than with soft-tissue problems such as a tender Achilles tendon.

Stress X-rays using a German system known as TELOS allows the ankles to be compared (Fig. 8.22). Anterior–posterior shift and lateral stress

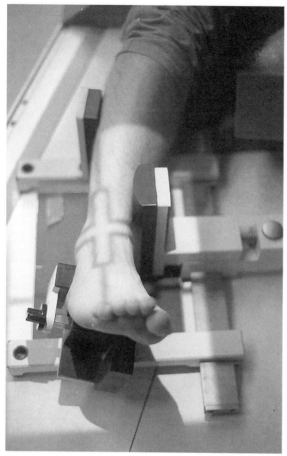

**Figure 8.22** Telos: lateral ankle stress test under local anaesthesia (reproduced by courtesy of Fifth Avenue Hospital, Seattle).

views can be taken. The procedure is performed under local anaesthesia using a common peroneal nerve block; it provides a reproducible method to determine ankle stability.

## SUBTALAR JOINT

The inferior surface of the talus articulates with the superior surface of the calcaneus at three facets. The largest facet forms the posterior joint, which is separated from the others by the interosseous talocalcaneal ligament, which lies in the sinus tarsi. Pain may arise from damage to the sinus tarsi. The STJ produces triplanar motion. Because of the position of its axis—42° from the transverse plane, 45° from the frontal

plane and 16° from the sagittal plane—little movement is produced in the sagittal plane but motion does occur in the frontal and transverse plane (1:3:3). Alteration of the axis can favour motion in one direction at the expense of motion in another. The knee and foot are affected by the axial position of the STJ (Green & Carol 1984).

## Joint motion

In order to measure triplanar motion at this joint one would have to measure the motion produced in each plane; this is impossible to achieve clinically. The amount of frontal plane motion at the STJ can be measured, and this is used as an indicator of the ROM at the STJ. It is important that there is an adequate ROM and appropriate DOM at the STJ for normal pronation and supination of the foot.

In order to assess frontal plane STJ motion the patient lies prone with the ankle and foot hanging over the edge of the couch. The distal third of the leg is bisected, this line is used as a reference point for measuring the ROM and DOM. The calcaneus is moved into its maximally inverted position and the posterior surface of the calcaneus is bisected (Fig. 8.23A). A tractograph is used to measure the angle between the bisection of the leg and the bisection of the posterior surface of the calcaneus. The calcaneus is placed in its maximum everted position and a reading is taken of the angle between the bisection of the leg and the bisection of the posterior surface of the calcaneus (Fig. 8.23B). This technique is helpful but should not be considered accurate; 272 male infantry recruits were examined and an error in excess of 20% was identified (Milgrom et al 1985). There is normally twice as much inversion as eversion (2:1 ratio). Many patients appear to have a 3:1 ratio of inversion to eversion without any abnormal sequelae arising.

## Subtalar varus

Subtalar varus implies that the neutral position of the calcaneus is varus (inverted). Subtalar varus or rearfoot varus (discussed under static observation) can affect the function of the rear-

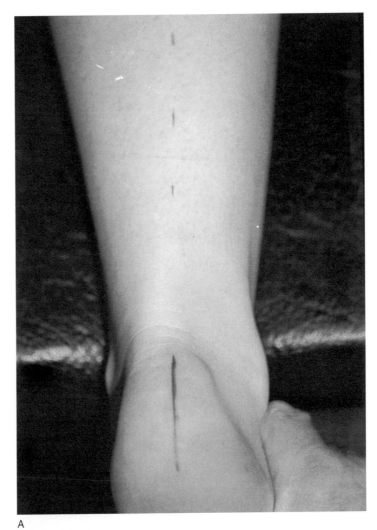

A

**Figure 8.23** Assessing frontal plane motion at the STJ **A.** The distal third of the leg is bisected and a line is drawn at the bisection point. The posterior surface of the calcaneus is moved into its maximally everted position and the angle between the bisection of the leg and the bisection of the calcaneus is measured. (Fig. 8.23B overleaf.)

foot during gait and may lead to excessive pronation of the foot and delay re-supination of the foot during gait. The presence of a subtalar varus can be calculated from the measurements obtained for the ROM and DOM of frontal plane motion at the STJ (Table 8.6).

## MIDTARSAL JOINT

The MTJ is made of two synovial joint complexes: talonavicular and calcaneocuboid. The MTJ is also

known as the transtarsal or Chopart's joint, and is an articulation between the rearfoot and forefoot. The MTJ has two axes; longitudinal and oblique. The longitudinal axis provides frontal plane motion facilitated by the ball and socket fit of the talonavicular articulation. The oblique axis involves both calcaneocuboid and calcaneo-talonavicular joints and primarily produces transverse and sagittal plane motion. A high oblique axis causes excessive pronation and is more difficult to control with orthoses (Hice 1984).

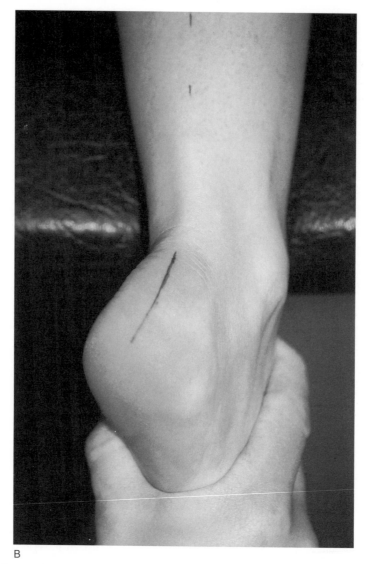

B

**Figure 8.23** **B.** The calcaneus is moved into its maximally inverted position and the angle between the bisection of the leg and the bisection of the calcaneus is measured.

The MTJ assists in reducing impact forces and helps to prepare the foot for propulsion. It can also accommodate walking on uneven terrain without affecting the rearfoot. This means that the forefoot might invert while the heel remains vertical; the converse does not occur.

## Joint motion

In order to assess the motion at the MTJ the practitioner must stabilise the STJ and prevent any motion occurring at this joint by firmly holding the heel with one hand and holding the foot just distal to the midtarsal joint with the other. The MTJ should then be moved in the sagittal, transverse and frontal planes. There should be most motion in the sagittal and transverse planes and minimal motion in the frontal. The position of the axes will affect the amount of motion at the MTJ, for example a high (vertical) oblique axis will result in an increase in transverse plane motion but a reduction in sagittal plane motion.

**Table 8.6**  How to calculate the subtalar joint's neutral position (Root et al 1971)

| | |
|---|---|
| Normal neutral | 30° inversion with supination<br>15° eversion with pronation<br>Total range of motion equals 45°<br><br>Assuming a ratio of 2:1 (2 + 1 = 3)<br>45° ÷ 3 (thirds) = 15°<br><br>Expected eversion would be 1 × 15 = 15<br>Expected inversion would be 2 × 15 = 30<br><br>As these are the same values taking the calculated away from the measured angles gives 0°. This means that neutral is 0°. |
| STJ varus | 25° inversion with supination<br>8° eversion with pronation<br>Total range of motion would equal 33°<br><br>Assuming ratio of 2:1 again<br>33° ÷ 3 = 11°<br><br>Expected eversion would be 1 × 11 = 11<br>Expected inversion would be 2 × 11 = 22<br><br>Calculated from measured inversion (25 − 22 = 3°)<br>Calculated from measured eversion (8 − 11 = −3°)<br><br>These values are not zero. The neutral position would be 3°, but which direction? The easiest way of determining the direction is identifying which ratio has the greatest direction, i.e. more than expected. In this case it would be inversion, which has already been calculated as being expected as 22°. The 3° of inversion means that a subtalar joint varus of 3° exists. |
| STJ valgus | 15° inversion with supination<br>15° eversion with pronation<br>Total range would be equal to 30°<br><br>Assuming ratio of 2:1 again<br>30 ÷ 3 = 10°<br><br>Expected eversion would be 1 × 10 = 10<br>Expected inversion would be 2 × 10 = 20<br><br>Calculated from measured inversion (15 − 20 = − 5°)<br>Calculated from measured eversion (15 − 10 = 5°)<br><br>In this example, eversion is 5° more than expected from calculation and neutral is given as 5° of subtalar joint valgus |

# EXAMINATION OF MUSCLES AFFECTING THE ANKLE COMPLEX

## Plantarflexors

The posterior group of muscles plantarflex the foot at the ankle but may also restrict the amount of dorsiflexion at the ankle. The patient should be asked to plantarflex the foot with and without resistance in order to test muscle strength. Rupture or partial rupture of the tendo achillis should be ruled out. If the tendo achillis is functioning normally the foot should plantarflex when the calf muscle is squeezed. Plantaris is a small muscle that is not present in everyone. Spontaneous rupture of plantaris may occur; it shows as a painful medial swelling over the posterior aspect of the calcaneus at its insertion near the tendo achillis.

## Invertors

Tibialis posterior and anterior are the main invertors of the foot. These extrinsic muscles play an important role in re-supinating the foot during midstance and propulsion. To assess the strength of these muscles the patient should be asked to move his/her foot into supination against resistance.

## Dorsiflexors

The main dorsiflexors of the foot are the long extensors and tibialis anterior. In order to assess the strength of the anterior muscles the patient should be asked to dorsiflex the ankle with the foot in inversion against resistance. Weakness of the anterior group is often linked to neurological problems, e.g. poliomyelitis. The plantarflexors have a work capacity 4.5 times that of the dorsiflexors. If the dorsiflexors are weak the foot is held in a plantarflexed position as the plantarflexors have a mechanical advantage.

*Evertors*

The evertors of the foot are the peronei. To assess the strength of the peronei the patient should be asked to evert the foot against resistance. The evertors are not as powerful as the invertors and in the case of neurological problems and/or muscle imbalance the invertors have a mechanical advantage over the evertors and the foot is held in an inverted position. Tonic spasm of the peroneal muscles can occur; this is noted particularly with tarsal coalitions. A local anaesthetic can be administered in order to differentiate between a muscle spasm and a tarsal coalition.

# NON-WEIGHTBEARING EXAMINATION—FOOT

## RAYS (METATARSALS)

Each ray consists of a metatarsal. The first and fifth have independent axes of motion and produce triplanar motion. The second ray is firmly anchored to the intermediate cuneiform and has least motion; the third has less motion than the fourth ray. While the first and fifth rays provide triplanar motion, the central three only move in the sagittal plane. The ability of the first ray to plantarflex is important in order that the medial side of the foot makes ground contact during gait and the first MTPJ can dorsiflex during propulsion. Patients commonly present with cutaneous changes associated with dysfunction of the rays; especially the first and fifth. The position of the rays can affect gait and foot mechanics.

## Joint examination

Clinical assessment of the motion of the first and fifth ray can only be satisfactorily undertaken in the sagittal plane. Unlike most joints, motion at the first and fifth rays is measured in millimetres, not degrees. In order to assess sagittal plane motion the patient can be in a supine or prone position. The feet must be allowed to hang free of the couch. The practitioner places one hand, with the thumb to the plantar surface, around the lateral side of the forefoot including the second metatarsal while maintaining the foot in its neutral position. The other hand, again with the thumb to the plantar surface, is placed around the first metatarsal. The first ray is moved into maximum dorsiflexion and plantarflexion. It is usual to find approximately 10 mm in each direction (Fig. 8.24A–B). Lack of plantarflexion of the first ray is known as metatarsus primus elevatus. The amount of motion can be assessed using the thumb technique (Fig. 8.24A–B). A 'sagittal raynger' provides an alternate means of assessing first ray motion (Fig. 8.24C–D) (Kilmartin et al 1991). Sagittal plane motion of the fifth ray can be undertaken using the same approach.

Deformity of the rays is said to occur when the ROM or DOM of one or more rays is asymmetrical or the metatarsal heads do not lie in the same plane. Table 8.7 refers to the various positions and terms associated with the deformities affecting the rays; these may be congenital or acquired. It is not unusual for a problem affecting the rays to be unilateral.

## METATARSOPHALANGEAL JOINTS (MTPJs)

The MTPJs are the joints between the metatarsals and the proximal phalanges; they produce motion in the sagittal plane. During the propulsive period of gait it is important that dorsiflexion occurs at these joints in order to facilitate toe-off.

## Joint examination

The ROM and DOM in the sagittal plane should

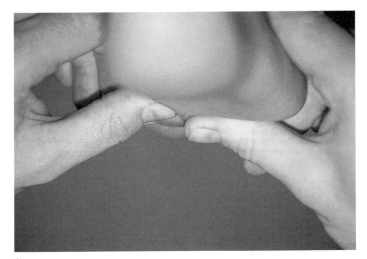

A

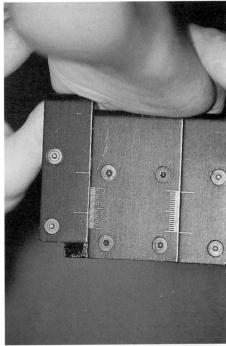

C

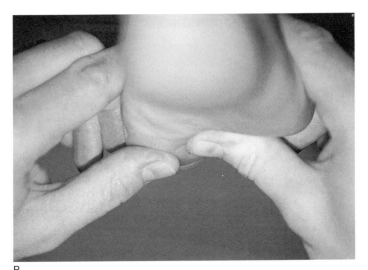

B

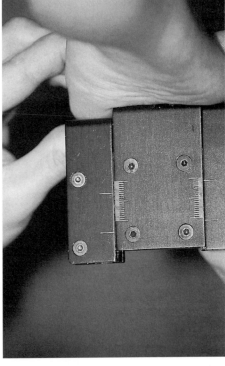

D

**Figure 8.24**  Assessment of motion at the first ray    **A.** Measurement of dorsiflexion of the first ray using the thumb test    **B.** Measurement of plantarflexion of the first ray using the thumb test    **C.** Dorsiflexion of the first ray measured with a Sagittal Raynger (reproduced by courtesy of Nova Instruments)    **D.** Plantarflexion of the first ray measured with a Sagittal Raynger (reproduced by courtesy of Nova Instruments).

**Table 8.7** Abnormal positions of the metatarsals (rays)

| Position | Description |
| --- | --- |
| Normal position | The first and fifth metatarsals (rays) exhibit equal motion above and below the second/fourth metatarsal of 10–20 mm (5–10 mm in each direction) |
| Metatarsus primus elevatus (dorsiflexed first ray) | Reduces ability of first metatarsal to weight bear and overloads central rays. Differential diagnosis forefoot varus. Shows limited plantarflexion and cannot be reduced below level of second metatarsal |
| Flexible plantarflexed first ray | The first metatarsal may appear pronounced on the plantar surface of the foot with a cleft between the first and second metatarsal heads. Most of the movement is in the plantar direction. Loading the metatarsal head produces reduction of the position |
| Rigid plantarflexed first ray | The first metatarsal cannot be reduced at all from its plantarflexed position. The forefoot tends to rotate in inversion when on the ground; this affects the function of the hindfoot |
| Partially plantarflexed first ray | The first metatarsal adopts a position which is partially reducible, being neither rigid nor flexible but adopting more plantarflexion then dorsiflexion |

be assessed for all MTPJs; they should have a free range of motion without pain or restriction (Fig. 8.25). The first MTPJ has the greatest range of motion: approximately 70–90° dorsiflexion and 20° plantarflexion. The ROM and DOM at the first MTPJ can be assessed with a tractograph or finger goniometer. The practitioner should appreciate that the declined angle of the first ray accounts for at least 15° of dorsiflexion at rest.

A lack of dorsiflexion at the first MTPJ is known as hallux limitus, and a complete absence as hallux rigidus. The presence of either of these conditions, but particularly hallux rigidus, will affect toe-off and can lead to an apropulsive gait and overloading of one or more of the other metatarsal heads. Hallux flexus is not so common; this is where the proximal phalanx adopts a plantarflexed position.

Restriction of movement at MTPJs could be due to osteophytes, loose bodies or articular damage, e.g. osteochondritis dessicans. The effects of Freiberg's disease may be to produce an enlargement of the metatarsal head and early osteoarthritic changes; this usually affects the second or third metatarsal. In some patients, particularly younger ones, the clinical appearance of the joint may appear normal and X-rays may reveal no abnormalities. It is essential in these cases that spasm of flexor hallucis brevis and/or abductor hallucis is ruled out via the use of local anaesthetic blocks.

## INTERPHALANGEAL JOINTS (IPJs)

Toes have considerably less functional movement than fingers. The practitioner should note any restriction or fixed deformity affecting either the proximal (PIPJs) or distal (DIPJs) joints.

## Joint examination

The PIPJs can plantarflex (approximately 35°) but cannot dorsiflex (Fig. 8.26A). The DIPJs can dorsiflex to 30° and plantarflex up to 60° (Fig. 8.26B–C). The patient may be unable to actively move the toes to assess the function of the intrinsic muscles. However, plantarflexion can be assessed by placing the fingers under the apices of the toes and asking the patient to claw the toes around them.

## NON-WEIGHTBEARING ALIGNMENT OF THE LEG AND FOOT

While the patient is lying on the couch the following should be assessed:

• presence of genu varum/valgum
• malleolar torsion
• rearfoot to forefoot alignment
• arch height
• metatarsal formula
• digital position
• foot length.

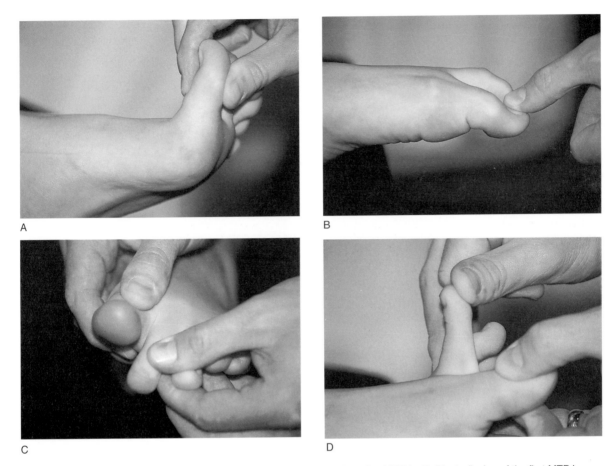

**Figure 8.25**    Assessment of motion at the MTPJs    **A.** Dorsiflexion of the first MTPJ    **B.** Plantarflexion of the first MTPJ
**C.** Dorsiflexion of the second MTPJ    **D.** Plantarflexion of the second MTPJ. In both cases (first and second MTPJ) dorsiflexion
is greater due to the shape of the articular surfaces.

### Genu varum/valgum

In order to assess the presence of lower limb
varus or valgus the patient lies supine with the
knees extended. The practitioner takes hold of
the ankles and brings the legs together. If there
is a difference of more than 5 cm between the
knees genu valgum is suspected; if it is impossible
to bring the malleoli together a genu varum is
present. Obesity may prevent the knees and
malleoli being brought together. Marked bowing
as illustrated in Figure 8.27 cannot be missed.

### Malleolar torsion

Torsion of the leg can affect the position of the
foot; adducted (in-toe) and abducted (out-toe),

as well as the position of the patellae. Assessing
the amount of tibial torsion clinically is impossible, but it is suggested in the literature that
assessing the relationship of the tibia and fibula
malleoli to each other gives an indication of
torsion in the leg (Hutter & Scott 1949). To
measure malleolar torsion the patient lies in a
supine position with the knees flexed and the
soles of the feet on the couch. The practitioner
holds the foot and moves the leg until the knee
is flexed to 90° and rotates the leg until the knee
joint is parallel to the couch. The practitioner
bends down until his/her eye is level with the
malleoli and observes the relationship of the
malleoli to each other. The amount of malleolar
torsion can be measured in three ways:

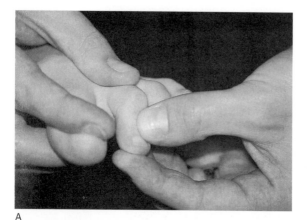

A

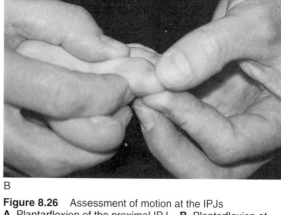

B

**Figure 8.26** Assessment of motion at the IPJs
**A.** Plantarflexion of the proximal IPJ **B.** Plantarflexion at
the distal IPJ **C.** Dorsiflexion at the distal IPJ.

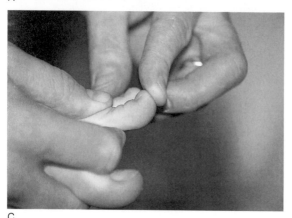

C

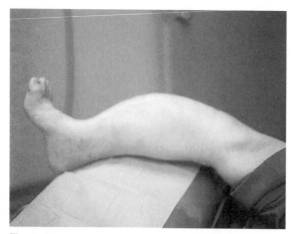

**Figure 8.27** Patient with severe bowing associated with
Paget's disease, 'sabre tibia' affecting patients in the
sixth/seventh decade of life. Deformity occurs in the sagittal
as well as the frontal plane.

- Guestimate from observation
- *Tractograph.* The protractor end of the
  tractograph should be held on the fibula side,
  one arm of the tractograph is placed parallel
  to the couch and the other arm is moved until
  it bisects the malleolus
- *Gravity goniometer.* The ends of the arms of
  the gravity goniometer are placed on the
  malleoli and the goniometer is held vertical
  (Fig. 8.28).

When the techniques were examined, the
gravity goniometer fared best (Hayles & Lang
1987). 13–18° of torsion is considered normal.
Malleolar torsion is considered to be 5° less than
tibial torsion, therefore normal tibial torsion is
18–25°.

### Forefoot to rearfoot alignment

The plantar plane of the forefoot should lie
parallel to the plantar plane of the rearfoot (Fig.

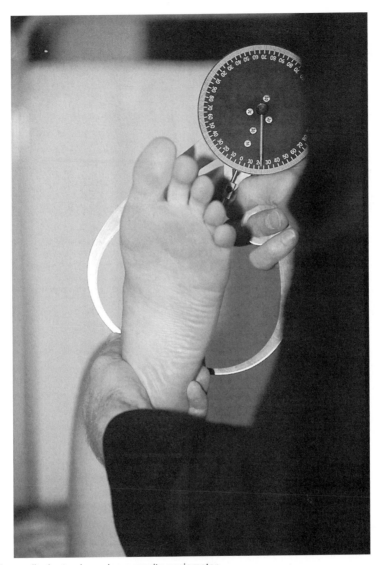

**Figure 8.28** Assessing malleolar torsion using a gravity goniometer.

8.29A). The relationship of the forefoot to the rearfoot is assessed by placing the foot in its neutral position; the patient may be either supine or prone but it is important that the foot hangs free of the couch. A tractograph or a forefoot-measuring device can be used to measure any deviation of the forefoot to the rearfoot in the frontal plane; the forefoot may be inverted or everted to the rearfoot (Fig. 8.29B–C). Minor differences between the forefoot and rearfoot are usually insignificant and are often due to examiner error, but quite high angles of discrepancy can exist in excess of 15°.

The appearance of an inverted or everted foot can be complicated by the position of the first and fifth rays. An inverted forefoot may be due to:

- *True forefoot varus*: bony abnormality due to lack of declination of the talar head. The presence of a true forefoot varus is said to lead to a very flat foot with no longitudinal arch (Grumbine 1987).

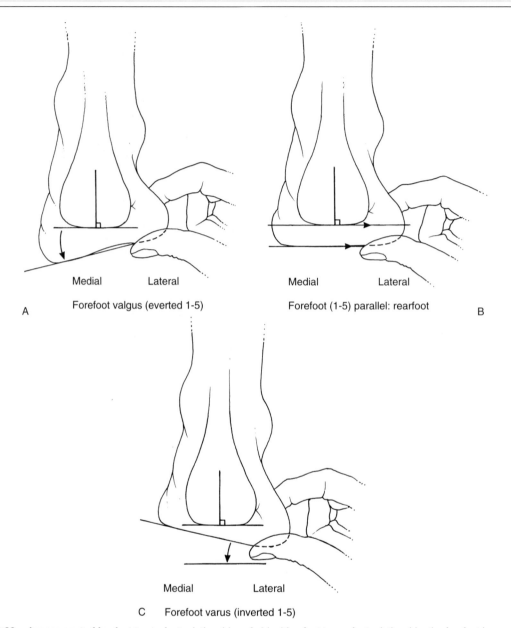

A    Forefoot valgus (everted 1-5)

B    Forefoot (1-5) parallel: rearfoot

C    Forefoot varus (inverted 1-5)

**Figure 8.29**   Assessment of forefoot to rearfoot relationship   **A.** Ideal forefoot to rearfoot relationship: the forefoot is parallel to the rearfoot   **B.** Inverted forefoot: the forefoot is inverted to the rearfoot   **C.** Everted forefoot: the forefoot is everted to the rearfoot.

- *Forefoot supinatus*: soft-tissue deformity due to abnormal pronation of the rearfoot. The forefoot is held in an inverted position because of soft-tissue contraction. This condition can be reduced with treatment. It can be difficult to differentiate between a forefoot supinatus and forefoot varus.

Various techniques are suggested. One is to get the patient to stand; the foot is put into its neutral position. With both conditions the medial side of the foot should not be in ground contact. Pressure is applied to the dorsum of the first MTPJ, with a supinatus there should be some give and the first ray should plantarflex, with forefoot varus any pressure on the dorsum of the first ray should cause the foot to tilt inwards and the fifth ray to leave ground contact.

- *Dorsiflexed first ray (metatarsus primus elevatus)*: may be a fixed or flexible deformity.
- *Plantarflexed fifth ray*: as with the first ray this may be a fixed or flexible deformity, dependent upon the cause treatment may reduce the deformity.

An everted forefoot may be due to:

- *Forefoot valgus*: bony abnormality due to excessive declination of the talar head which holds the forefoot in a fixed everted position that cannot be reduced with treatment.
- *Plantarflexed first ray*: a common cause of an everted forefoot position that may be due to a fixed or flexible deformity.
- *Dorsiflexed fifth ray*: as with the first ray this may be a fixed or flexible deformity.

The incidence of metatarsus primus elevatus and plantarflexed first ray is thought to be greater than that of forefoot varus and valgus.

There may also be malalignment between the forefoot and the rearfoot in the sagittal and transverse planes. The forefoot may appear plantarflexed in relation to the rearfoot or vice versa. This may be a flexible or fixed deformity and may lead to a pes-cavus-type foot. The forefoot may appear adducted on the rearfoot; this may be due to a metatarsus adductus or metatarsus primus adductus; non-weightbearing the lateral border of the foot appears banana-shaped with a metatarsus adductus.

### Arch height

The shape and height of the longitudinal arch should be observed and compared to its position when weightbearing. Creasing of the skin in the arch of the non-weightbearing foot usually indicates that the foot is mobile and excessively pronates on weightbearing.

### Metatarsal formula

The metatarsal formula refers to the apparent length of the metatarsals. The second metatarsal is usually the longest and the fifth the shortest. A typical metatarsal formula is $2 > 1 > 3 > 4 > 5$ or $2 > 3 > 1 > 4 > 5$. It is important that the first metatarsal is shorter than the second in order to allow normal function during propulsion. When the first MTPJ dorsiflexes the first ray plantarflexes on to the sesamoids; if the first metatarsal is as long as the second this cannot occur and as a result the first MTPJ is not able to dorsiflex, resulting in overloading of the other metatarsal heads, commonly the second. The practitioner should look at the shoe crease to observe the normal oblique angle afforded by the typical $2 > 1 > 3 > 4 > 5$ formula. A rare but well-recognised formula is when the fourth metatarsal is congenitally short, known as brachymetatarsia (Tachdjian 1985). In this case the formula would be $2 > 1 > 3 > 5 > 4$. The metatarsal formula is important for normal digital function. Abnormalities of the formula may affect forefoot pressure distribution. Short first metatarsals do not necessarily cause symptoms in the foot (Harris & Beath 1949); a correlation between long first metatarsals and the incident of hallux abductus has been reported (Duke et al 1982). Minor changes in metatarsal length may not adversely affect forefoot function and weight distribution.

### Digital position

The position the toes adopt non-weightbearing should be noted and compared with the position they adopt weightbearing. It is common to observe flexed deformities of the toes while the patient is sitting (Fig. 8.30). Depending upon the effects of muscle pull and ground reaction, the extent of the deformity may reduce or increase on weightbearing. The toes may appear retracted (apices of toes not in ground contact) and be fixed rather than flexible.

### Foot length

The length and width of the foot should be measured non-weightbearing and compared with weightbearing measurements. Foot length

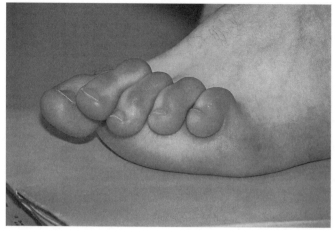

**Figure 8.30**   Flexed deformity of toes (28-year-old male) due to extensor substitution present on non weight bearing and weight bearing.

and width should increase by a small amount when weightbearing; usually there is up to one or one and a half shoe size difference. However, noticeable differences in foot length (two to three shoe sizes) indicates a mobile foot which excessively pronates during gait. No difference between the two is indicative of a rigid foot.

## STATIC EXAMINATION (WEIGHTBEARING)

In order to complete the assessment the patient should be observed standing. Information from this part of the assessment should help to complete the picture of lower limb alignment, give an indication of whether compensation is occurring at the STJ and enable deformities of the forefoot to be observed. It may be helpful to ask the patient to walk on the spot for a few minutes and then tell him/her to stop. The position the patient adopts on stopping can be accepted as the normal angle and base of gait. As with gait analysis the patient should be observed from head to toe. The following should be noted:

• Head
• Shoulders

• Spine
• Pelvis
• Angle and base of gait
• Relaxed and neutral calcaneal stance position
• Longitudinal arch
• Digits
• Foot width and length.

Points related to the position of the head, shoulders and pelvis are the same as those made for gait analysis. Any abnormality may be indicative of a LLI, neurological or spinal problem. The shape of the lower limb and distribution of muscle bulk should be noted. There should be symmetry of muscle bulk, although there may be slight variation between the dominant and recessive side of the body. This is particularly true where one side, arm and/or leg engages in a greater level of activity than the other.

### Spine

The position of the vertebrae should be observed for the presence of kyphosis, lordosis or scoliosis. A true scoliosis can be differentiated from a functional scoliosis by asking the patient to bend forward. If the spine is still deviated when the hips are flexed a true scoliosis exists; if vertebrae alignment improves it is likely to be a functional scoliosis.

## Angle and base of gait

A normal angle and base of gait is when the feet are slightly abducted (approximately 13° from the midline of the body) and the distance between the malleoli is approximately 5 cm (Fig. 8.4A). Frontal plane deformity of the legs—genu valgum or varum—may be very noticeable when the patient stands and will affect the base of gait, i.e. the gap between the malleoli will be greater (genu valgum) or less (genu varum) (Fig. 8.5). The angle of gait will be affected by torsional problems affecting the leg. Excessive internal torsion will lead to an adducted base of gait and squinting patellae whereas excessive external rotation will lead to an abducted base of gait (greater than 13°) (Fig. 8.4B–D). Torsional problems may be due to bony or soft-tissue problems; the true cause should be identified from the non-weightbearing assessment.

## Relaxed (RCSP) and neutral (NCSP) calcaneal stance position

The relaxed calcaneal position is an indicator of STJ motion when weightbearing. This position can be used to assess whether compensation for any proximal (e.g. tibial varum) or distal (e.g. forefoot varus) deformities has taken place at the STJ.

The RCSP is measured by bisecting the posterior surface of the calcaneus; the angle this line makes with the ground is measured (Fig. 8.31A). The amount of calcaneal eversion or inversion can be measured. Values greater than 4° eversion indicate the presence of abnormal pronation:

- 0–4°: normal limits
- 4–7°: moderate pronation requiring treatment if symptomatic or a cause for concern
- 8° and above: marked pronation.

The causes of an abnormal everted RCSP are numerous, e.g. compensated forefoot varus, compensated ankle equinus, tibial valgum and varum, internal and external torsion of the leg.

If the calcaneus does not have an everted position during RCSP it does not mean that abnormal pronation is not occurring. Compensation for a rearfoot varus involves excessive STJ pronation in order to bring the medial tubercle of the heel into ground contact and provide shock absorption during the contact

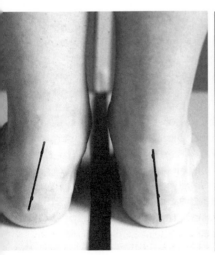
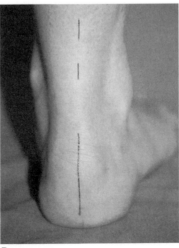
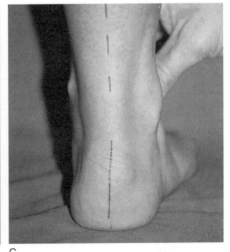

B        C

**Figure 8.31** Assessment of RCSP and NCSP   **A.** Feet in relaxed calcaneal stance position (RCSP)   **B.** Bisection of the posterior surface of the calcaneus and the distal third of the leg   **C.** Foot held in the neutral position in order to assess neutral calcaneal stance position.

phase of gait. A 10° rearfoot varus will require 10° of pronation in order to bring the heel into a vertical position. Although excessive pronation has occurred the RCSP will appear vertical and not everted.

An inverted RCSP may be due to a neurological problem, an uncompensated varus deformity affecting the rear or forefoot, subtalar joint damage, tonic spasm of the invertors of the foot or the presence of a plantarflexed first ray.

The NCSP is measured by placing the foot into its neutral position while in ground contact and bisecting the calcaneus (Fig. 8.31C). The angle between the bisection of the posterior surface of the calcaneus and the ground should be measured; usually the calcaneus is in a slight inverted position. This is known as rearfoot varus and may be due to the presence of a subtalar varus (see non-weight-bearing assessment of the STJ) and/or tibial varum.

The presence of a tibial varum can be assessed during assessment of the NCSP. While the foot is in NCSP a bisection of the posterior surface of the leg should be compared to the ground. Ideally the bisection of the leg should be vertical to the ground (Fig. 8.31B). An angle of less than 90° when measured from the medial side of the bisection of the leg indicates a tibial valgum and an angle greater than 90° indicates a tibial varum. It was thought that the NCSP position was a composite of the STJ plus the tibial position. For example, a value of 7° rearfoot varus might be deemed to be made from 4° STJ varus and 3° tibial varum. A tibial valgum would conversely have a negative effect upon the presence of a STJ varus. Because of the inaccuracy and error in measuring these values, however, this concept is questionable.

It is important to note the difference between the RCSP and NCSP in order to assess the compensation that occurs for proximal or distal problems (Fig. 8.31A & C). It is normal for there to be a difference of up to 6° between RCSP and NCSP; this is because most people have a slight subtalar varus and need to pronate to provide shock absorption.

## Longitudinal arch

Arch shape is affected by the rearfoot and forefoot position, the declination angles of the metatarsals, the inclination angle of the calcaneus and the tone and activity of intrinsic and extrinsic muscles. In the past flat-footed people were rejected from the army as it was considered that their feet would not cope with the demands of army life. However, there is rather more to foot function and mechanics than the height and shape of the longitudinal arch.

The patient should be asked to stand on tiptoe and the position of the foot arch should be noted. With rigid flat feet the arch height does not increase when the patient stands on tip toe, with a flexible flat foot the arch height increases. Rigid flat feet may be due to bony coalitions (synostoses), contractures due to muscle imbalance or neurological paralysis with subsequent soft-tissue contractures. The shape and size of the arch can be captured by taking a footprint; this can be used to monitor changes.

## Digits

Hallux abductus and hallux abductovalgus are common complex deformities affecting the first MTPJ (Fig. 8.32). Slight abduction of the hallux is considered normal, up to 15°. Deviation of the hallux can be measured with a finger goniometer; the value should be recorded so that deterioration of the condition can be monitored.

The fifth ray may frequently be abducted: tailor's bunion or digiti quinti varus may be associated with hallux abductus, giving a splayed and therefore broad forefoot appearance. Changes in forefoot shape due to hallux abductus and digiti quinti varus can be monitored by taking photographs or ink prints of the foot on a regular (twice-yearly) basis. It is also useful to draw around the foot at regular intervals to gain a visual representation of foot shape and to monitor changes.

Digital formulae should be noted; usually the first toe is longest or the first and the second are of equal length—1 > 2 > 3 > 4 > 5, 1 = 2 > 3 > 4 > 5. An excessively long toe, e.g. the fourth, may be

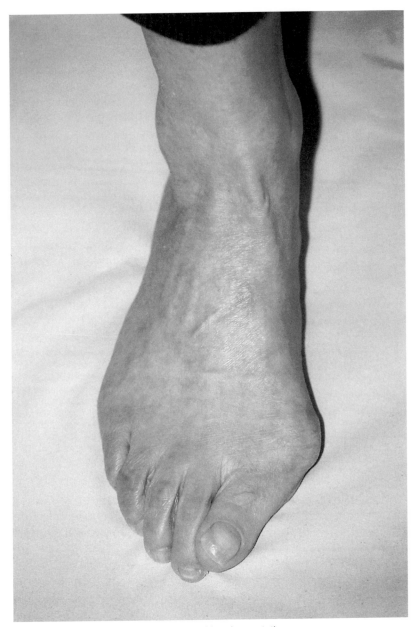

**Figure 8.32**    Hallux abductovalgus: abduction of the hallux with valgus rotation.

impacted in footwear resulting in toe deformity and secondary lesions.

Deformities of the lesser digits (toes 2–5) can be described in various ways; unfortunately there is no commonly agreed set of definitions. When assessing and recording the presence of digital deformities the best approach is to describe the plane that the deformity is in, e.g. sagittal, and whether the deformity is fixed or mobile. A fixed deformity implies that there is no motion at the joint due to soft-tissue changes and possible bony ankylosis; such deformities can only be corrected by surgery. Table 8.8 lists and defines the main digital deformities.

**Table 8.8** Classification of digital deformities

| Digital deformity | Description |
| --- | --- |
| Hallux abductus | Hallux abducted more than 15° from the midline of the body |
| Hallux abductovalgus | As above but the hallux is also rotated so that the hallux nail faces towards the midline of the body |
| Hallux limitus | Reduced dorsiflexion at the first MTPJ |
| Hallux rigidus | Complete lack of dorsiflexion at the first MTPJ |
| Hallux flexus | Plantarflexion of the hallux at the first MTPJ |
| Hyperextended hallux | Distal phalanx of the hallux dorsiflexed |
| Hammer toe | Dorsiflexion at the MTPJ, plantarflexion at the proximal IPJ and either normal position or dorsiflexion at the distal IPJ |
| Claw toe | Dorsiflexion at the MTPJ, plantarflexion at the proximal and distal IPJs |
| Retracted toe | Claw toe where the apex of the toe is not in ground contact |
| Mallet toe | Plantarflexion at the distal IPJ |
| Adductovarus fifth | Fifth toe rotated so that nail is facing away from the midline of the body and the toe is adducted (moved towards the midline of the body) |
| Dorsally displaced | One or more digits is in a dorsiflexed position in comparison to the other digits |

## OTHER ASSESSMENTS

### Limb length inequality

Assessment of the locomotor system is complete once gait analysis, non-weightbearing and static weightbearing examinations have been completed. Below are specific details of how to assess for leg-length inequality and abnormal pronation.

A LLI can have profound effects on the locomotor system affecting the spine, sacroiliac and hip joints as well as the foot. A difference of greater than 1 cm affects normal body alignment.

In a sedentary person a small discrepancy may have a negligible effect upon posture, but if a person increases his/her level of physical activity, the effects of any imbalance become amplified.

A leg-length discrepancy may be real or apparent. A real leg-length discrepancy is due to a difference in the length of the femurs or the tibiae and is common after a hip replacement. An apparent leg-length discrepancy may be due to a number of factors, e.g. osteoarthritis of the hip or a scoliosis. It is important to identify the difference in length between the limbs and to differentiate between a real and apparent discrepancy prior to commencing treatment. It should be noted that a real and an apparent leg-length inequality may coexist. The possible effects of treatment should be considered prior to commencing treatment (Case comment 8.6).

---

**Case comment 8.6**

It should be remembered that a patient who has had a discrepancy for years will have compensated by altering his/her body posture. If any raise under the heel is considered, this must only be for a proportion of the difference. Heel raises used alone may cause unwanted plantar flexion, especially when the deformity is greater than 2.5 cm. The adaptation to footwear should affect the whole sole in this case.

---

The presence of a limb length discrepancy can be observed during gait analysis:

• Shoulder tilt to one side
• Unequal arm swing
• Pelvic tilt
• Foot supinated on the short side
• Foot pronated on the long side
• Knee flexed on the long side
• Ankle plantarflexed on the short side.

To assess for the presence of a LLI the patient lies supine on a flat couch with the hips and knees extended. The practitioner places his/her hands around the heels and exerts a slight pull on the legs, at the same time bringing the legs together so that the knees and malleoli are touching. The knees and malleoli should be

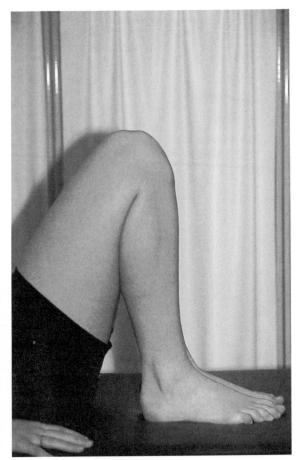

**Figure 8.33**    Assessment of leg-length inequality. The knees are flexed so that the position of the knees and ankles can be compared.

level. A difference indicates an inequality at the femur or tibia. To identify which bone is affected the knees should be flexed and the heels pushed flush against the buttocks (Fig. 8.33). If the tibiae are of equal length the tibial tubercles will be at the same level. This is a relatively crude method of assessment and does not quantify the extent of the difference.

A flexible non-stretch tape measure with a metal end can be used to measure leg length. With the patient supine the distance between the anterior superior iliac spine (ASIS) and the medial malleolus is measured (Crawford Adams & Hamblen 1990). The metal end of the tape fits snugly in front of the ASIS as shown in Figure

8.34A. The practitioner may use any part of the medial malleolus as a reference point, but it is important that the same point is used for repeat measurements. An error of up to 10% should be allowed for because the tape measure may wrap around asymmetrical muscle bulk or, more commonly, the patient's pelvis may not be properly aligned.

Radiological measurement is only used when surgical correction is planned as it is expensive and, unless the results are going to be used for surgery, exposes the patient to needless radiation.

Distinction between a real or actual difference can be achieved by measuring each limb from a common reference point above the pelvis; the xiphisternum is usually used. The metal end of the tape is placed on the xiphisternum and the distance from the xiphisternum to each malleolus is measured (Fig. 8.34B). If values are the same then the LLI is likely to be apparent. The cause usually lies at the hip or pelvis, where a fixed deformity makes the limbs appear unequal so that the body compensates by tilting laterally.

An alternate method can be used with the patient weightbearing:

- The patient stands in the RCSP position (Fig. 8.31A)
- The position of the ASISs is assessed to see if they are level
- The feet are then placed in the NCSP (Fig. 8.31C)
- The position of the ASISs is assessed to see if they are level
- If the ASISs are not level in either the RCSP and NCSP, and the extent of the discrepancy remains the same in RCSP and NCSP, a true LLI should be suspected. If the ASISs are on the same level in the NCSP but differ for the RCSP, an apparent LLI should be suspected.

## Abnormal pronation

Abnormal pronation, i.e. excessive STJ pronation during contact phase and/or STJ pronation occurring when the STJ should be supinating during midstance and propulsion, is one of the most common disorders of the lower limb. It gives rise to forefoot pathology, ankle dysfunction

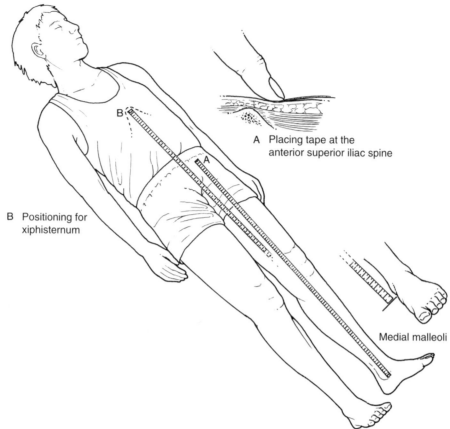

A   Placing tape at the
    anterior superior iliac spine

B   Positioning for
    xiphisternum

Medial malleoli

**Figure 8.34**   Assessment of a true and apparent leg-length inequality   **A.** Measurement from the anterior superior iliac spine (ASIS) to the medial malleolus   **B.** Measurement from the xiphisternum to the medial malleolus.

and can affect knees, hips and spine; lower back and sacroiliac pain may be due to uncontrolled pronation.

The presence of four or more of the following indicates abnormal pronation:

- More than 6° between the RCSP and NCSP
- Medial bulging of the talar head
- More than 4° eversion of the calcaneus
- Helbing's sign (medial bowing of the tendo achillis)
- Abduction of the forefoot at the MTJ
- Apropulsive gait.

Numerous conditions arising in the lower limb may lead to abnormal pronation; many of them

have been highlighted in this chapter (the list is not exhaustive):

- Internal or external torsion of the leg/thigh
- Tibial (genu) valgum/varum
- Coxa vara/valga
- Ankle equinus
- Rearfoot varus
- Inverted forefoot
- Everted forefoot.

In order for treatment to be effective it is important that the cause and the extent of the abnormal pronation are correctly identified, otherwise only symptomatic treatment on a trial and error basis can be provided.

# SUMMARY

Assessment of the locomotor system is complex and time-consuming. It can be compared to doing a jigsaw—all the pieces have to be put together in order to produce the picture. Because the locomotor system functions as one mechanical unit, it is important that the practitioner differentiates between primary and any secondary problems. However, it is not always necessary to examine every part of the locomotor system. The practitioner should weigh up the necessity for a head to toe examination against assessing isolated parts of the anatomy. This decision will be informed by information from the patient's presenting problem, a brief gait analysis and information from other parts of the assessment process.

## REFERENCES

Apley A G, Solomon L 1988 Concise system of orthopaedics and fractures. Butterworths, London

Barnett C H, Napier J R 1952 The axis of rotation at the ankle joint in man. Its influence upon the form of the talus and the mobility of the fibula. Journal of Anatomy 86: 1–9

Campbell A C, McBride D J, Anderson E G 1993 Surgical treatment in disorders of the sesamoids of flexor hallucis brevis. Foot 3: 43–45

Crawford Adams J, Hamblen D L 1990 Outline of orthopaedics, 11th edn. Churchill Livingstone, Edinburgh, p 280–283, 353

Duke H, Newman L M, Bruskoff B L, Daniels R 1982 Relative metatarsal length patterns in hallux abductovalgus. Journal of the American Podiatry Association 72: 1–5

Elftman H 1960 The transverse tarsal joint and its control. Clinical Orthopaedics 16

Green D R, Carol A 1984 Planal dominance. Journal of the American Podiatry Association 74: 98–103

Grumbine N A 1987 The varus components of the forefoot in flatfoot deformities. Journal of the American Podiatric Medical Association 77: 14–20

Harris R I, Beath T 1949 The short first metatarsal its incidence and clinical significance. Journal of Bone and Joint Surgery 31A, 4: 553–565

Hayles M, Lang L 1987 Measuring tibial torsion: comparison of measurement techniques. ACTUK Journal Spring: 17–20

Hice G A 1984 Orthotic treatment of feet having a high oblique midtarsal joint axis. Journal of the American Podiatry Association 74: 577–582

Hutter C G, Scott W 1949 Tibial torsion. Journal of Bone and Joint Surgery 31A: 511–518

Inman V T 1976 The joints of the ankle. Williams & Wilkins, Baltimore, MD

Inman V T, Ralston H J, Todd F 1981 Human walking. Williams & Wilkins, Baltimore, MD

Kilmartin T E, Wallace A, Hill T W 1991 First metatarsal position in juvenile hallux abductovalgus—a significant clinical measurement? British Journal of Podiatric Medicine 46: 43–45

Milgrom C, Giladi M, Simkin A, Kashtan H, Matgulies J, Steinberg R, Aharonson Z 1985 The normal range of subtalar inversion and eversion in young males as measured by three different techniques. Foot and Ankle 5: 143–145

Radin E L, Rose R M, Blaha J D, Litsky A S 1992 Practical biomechanics for the orthopedic surgeon, 2nd edn. Churchill Livingstone, New York, p 152–158

Rasch P J, Burke R K 1978 Kinesiology and applied anatomy, 6th edn. Lea & Febiger, Philadelphia, PA, p 363–364

Root M L, Orien W P, Weed J H, Hughes R J 1971 Biomechanical examination of the foot. Clinical Biomechanics Incorporation, Los Angeles

Root M L, Weed J H, Sgarlato T E, Bluth D R 1966 Axis of motion of the subtalar joint. An anatomical study. Journal of the American Podiatry Association 56: 149–155

Saunders J B, Dec M, Inman V T, Eberhart H D 1953 The major determinants in normal and pathological gait. Journal of Bone and Joint Surgery 35A, 3: 543–558

Svenningsen S, Terjesen T, Auflem M, Berg V 1990 Hip rotation and in-toeing gait. A study of normal subjects from four years until adult age. Clinical Orthopaedics and Related Research 251: 177–182

Tachdjian M O 1985 The child's foot. W B Saunders, Philadelphia, PA

Tollafield D R 1988 The objectives of joint examination in the foot and lower limb. Chiropodist 43: 171–173

Tollafield D R, Price M 1985 Hallux metatarsophalangeal joint survey. Chiropodist 40: 284–288

## FURTHER READING

Altman M I 1968 Sagittal plane angles of the talus and calcaneus in the developing foot. Journal of American Podiatry Association 58: 463–470

American Academy of Orthopaedic Surgeons 1965 Joint motion. Method of measuring and recording.

Anderson J A D, Sweetman B J 1975 A combined flexirule/hydrogoniometer for measurement of lumbar spine and its sagittal movement. Rheumatology and Rehabilitation 14: 173–179

Bailey D S, Perillo J T, Forman M 1984 Subtalar joint neutral. A study using tomography. Journal of the American Podiatry Association 74: 59–64

Bartlett, M D, Wolf L S et al 1985 Hip Flexion Contracture Measurements. Archives of Physical and Medical Rehabilitation 66: 620–625

Bland J M, Altman D G 1986 Statistical methods for assessing agreement between two methods of clinical measurement. Lancet February: 307–310

Cochran G, Van B 1982 A primer of orthopaedic biomechanics. Churchill Livingstone, New York

D'Amico J C, Schuster R O 1979 Motion of the first ray clarification through investigation. Journal of American Podiatry Association 69: 17–23

Ebesui J M 1968 The first ray axis and first metatarsophalangeal joint. An anatomical and pathological study. Journal of American Podiatry Association 58: 160–167

Fabry G, Leuven, Belgium G, MacEwan D M, Shands A R 1973 Torsion of the femur. A follow up study in normal and abnormnal conditions. Journal of Bone and Joint Surgery 55A: 1726–1738

Fairbank J C T, Pynsent P B, van Poortvliet J, Phillips H 1984 Mechanical factors in the incidence of knee pain in adolescents and young adults. Journal of Bone and Joint Surgery 66B: 685–692

Green D R, Whitney A K, Walters P 1979 Subtalar joint motion. A simplified view. Journal of the American Podiatry Association 69: 83–91

Gould J A, Davis G J (eds) 1985 Orthopaedics and sports. Physical Therapy

Helal B, Gibb P 1987 Freiberg's disease: A suggested pattern of management. Foot and ankle 8(2): 94–102

Henry A P J, Waugh W 1975 The use of footprints in assessing the results of operations for hallux valgus—a comparison of Keller's operation and arthrodesis. Journal of Bone and Joint Surgery 57-B: 478–481

Hicks J H 1953 I The joints. The mechanics of the foot. Journal of Anatomy 87

Holden M K et al 1984 Clinical gait assessment in the neurologically impaired. Reliability and meaningfulness. Physical Therapy 64: 35–41

Jiminez A L, McGlamry E D, Green D R 1987 Lesser ray deformities. In: McGlamry E D (ed) Comprehensive textbook of foot surgery, vol 1. Williams & Wilkins, Baltimore, MD

Kelso S F, Richie D H, Cohen I R, Weed J H, Root M L 1982 The direction and range of the first ray. Journal of the American Podiatry Association 72: 600–605

Manter J T 1941 Movement of the subtalar and transverse tarsal joints. Anatomy Records 80: 397–410

McRae R 1990 Clinical orthopaedic examination, 3rd edn. Churchill Livingstone, Edinburgh

Mann R, Inman V T 1964 Phasic activity of intrinsic muscles of the foot. Journal of Bone and Joint Surgery 46A: 469–481

Myerson M S, Shereff M J 1989 The pathological anatomy of claw and hammer toes. Journal of Bone and Joint Surgery 71A: 45–49

Neale D, Adams I M 1989 Common foot disorders, 3rd edn. Churchill Livingstone, Edinburgh

Scott J H in Harris N 1983 Leg length inequality, a postgraduate textbook of clinical orthopaedics. Blackwell, Oxford, p 282–291

Sgarlato T E 1973 A compendium of podiatric biomechanics. California College of Podiatric Medicine

Subotnick S I 1979 Cures for common running injuries. Anderson World Inc, California

Sussman R E, Piccora R 1985 The metatarsal sesamoid and first metatarsophalangeal joint. Journal of American Podiatric Medical Association 75: 327–330

Tollafield D R 1984 A podiatric perspective in evaluating limb length discrepancy. Journal of the Podiatry Association Jul/Aug: 6–8

Warwick R, Williams P L (eds) 1989 Gray's anatomy, 36th edn. Churchill Livingstone, Edinburgh

Welton E A 1992 The Harris and Beath footprint: interpretation and clinical value. Foot and Ankle 13: 462–468

Whittle M 1991 Gait analysis. An introduction. Butterworth Heinemann, Oxford

# 9

# Assessment of the skin and its appendages

*K. Springett*
*L. Merriman*

# INTRODUCTION

Disorders of the skin and its appendages result from a number of factors (Table 9.1). These disorders can have far-reaching social and psychological consequences for the patient, quite out of proportion to the condition seen (Burge 1989). This chapter looks at why the skin and its appendages should be assessed. An overview of the anatomy, histology, physiology and function of the skin is presented. This is followed by a description of the assessment process. The chapter concludes by highlighting the clinical features associated with skin and nail conditions which may affect the lower limb.

Data from an assessment of the skin provides a plethora of information which the practitioner

Table 9.1 Causes of skin conditions

| Cause | Examples |
|---|---|
| Hereditary/congenital | Port wine stain, ichthyosis |
| Mechanical | Blisters, corns, ulcers |
| Infection | Folliculitis, tinea pedis, plantar warts |
| Infestation | Scabies, lice |
| Autoimmune | Vasculitis in rheumatoid arthritis |
| Allergy | Contact dermatitis |
| Cutaneous signs of systemic condition | Striae tensae with pregnancy, necrobiosis lipoidica or ulceration with diabetes, malnutrition |
| Cutaneous signs of a peripheral condition | Ulceration due to incompetent venous drainage, dry fissures with poor arterial supply |
| Idiopathic (causes not yet known) | Psoriasis, pompholyx |

must collate and form into something workable; a diagnosis or differential diagnosis. A diagnosis is made from a review of the clinical features, history of the condition and the general health status of the patient; this information is then matched against the practitioner's knowledge of skin disorders.

## Why undertake an assessment of skin and nails?

The purpose of the assessment is to:

- identify whether the condition is localised or systemic
- identify, where possible, the cause of the problem
- arrive at a diagnosis
- provide a baseline to monitor the progress of the condition
- identify whether advice and treatment are required
- provide a prognosis.

If the skin is disordered problems occur due to changes in the structure and function of the skin (morphology). The main morphological changes that occur are outlined in Table 9.2.

It is important to determine whether the changes are due to a localised or generalised (systemic) cause as this information will affect treatment. Skin, nails, hair and glands can act as cutaneous indicators of systemic disease, e.g. granuloma annulare can affect the skin of patients with diabetes mellitus. Erythema ab igne (reddish-brown discoloration of the legs due to deposits of haemosiderin in the skin that occur as a result of the effects of heat on cutaneous blood vessels) may suggest that the patient sits huddled over a fire trying to keep warm because of a systemic complaint such as myxoedema or because of poor living conditions. The skin, nails and hair also provide an indicator of deficiency due either to inadequate blood supply or lack of nutrient intake, e.g. vitamin C. Localised skin infections, e.g. tinea pedis (athlete's foot) and verrucae (plantar warts), can sometimes be associated with the patient's general health status. Patients with diabetes mellitus are more prone to develop

**Table 9.2** Terms used to described changes in skin morphology

| Term | Description |
|---|---|
| Atrophy/atrophic | Fragile, mechanically weak skin, nail or hair, lacking in nutrition |
| Ischaemia/ischaemic | Skin may be white, cyanotic or bright red, cool, very painful |
| Necrosis/necrotic | Skin is black and dry or grey and macerated, with slough and collagen fibres exposed, or a combination of these; painful |
| Hypertrophy/hypertrophic | Increase in bulk or thickening of tissue, e.g. scarring where excess fibroblast activity has caused a thickened patch on the skin |
| Hyperplasia | An increase in the number of cells, e.g. verrucae |
| Anhidrosis/anhidrotic | Dry, often rough skin; fissures around the heel |
| Hyperhidrosis/hyperhidrotic | Overmoist skin |
| Maceration | White, soggy epidermal mass |
| Pruritus | Itchiness |
| Purulent | Presence of pus; may be aseptic or infected |
| Spongiosis | Accumulation of fluid in the stratum spinosum |
| Parakeratosis | Incomplete keratinisation, retention of cell organelles |
| Acanthosis | Increased number of cells in the stratum spinosum |
| Acantholysis | Loss of cohesion between cells in the stratum spinosum |
| Xanthoma | Collection of lipid-filled histiocytic cells in the skin |

bacterial and fungal infections, as are immuno-compromised patients.

# OVERVIEW OF THE ANATOMY, HISTOLOGY, PHYSIOLOGY AND FUNCTION OF SKIN

## ANATOMY AND HISTOLOGY

The skin is composed of two layers (Fig. 9.1); the epidermis (generally 0.06–0.15 mm thick) and the dermis (generally about 2–4 mm thick) which are joined by the dermo-epidermal junction

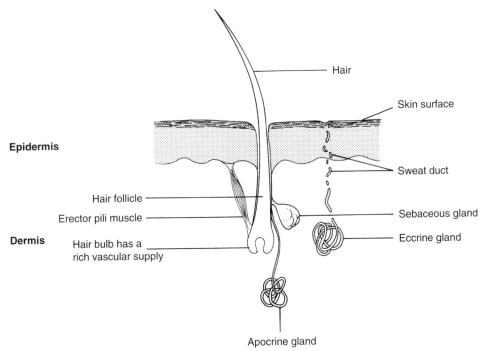

**Figure 9.1** Normal skin (not to scale) showing epidermis and dermis and the skin appendages, excluding nail.

(DEJ), also known as the basement membrane. The skin appendages are hair, nails, sebaceous and sweat glands. Palmar and plantar skin is hairless and has copious eccrine sweat glands. Apocrine sweat glands are present in the axillae.

## Epidermis

The epidermis is a keratinising stratified epithelium which covers the body, changing into a mucosal epithelium at orifices. It does not have a blood supply and obtains its nutrients, via the DEJ, from the papillary blood plexus of the dermis (Fig. 9.2). Undulations between the epidermis and dermis form epidermal rete ridges/pegs and dermal papillae. Other than keratinocytes (corneocytes), the epidermis also contains Merkel cells, which are specialised nerve endings, Langerhans cells, which have an immunological function, and melanocytes, which protect from UV light.

The epidermis has four layers:

### Basal layer (stratum germinativum)

The basal layer is composed of a single layer of columnar epithelial cells which have an oval nucleus and a full complement of cell organelles. There appear to be two different types of basal cell, the serrated stem cells that remain in the basal layer and the smoother daughter cells that migrate to the next layer (Mackenzie 1983). Basal cells abut the DEJ and are linked to this structure via hemidesmosomes and to each other by tight junctions and desmosomes. Each stem cell is surrounded by about six daughter cells which form the epidermal proliferation unit (EPU) (Wright 1983, Millington & Wilkinson 1983).

The dendritic melanocytes present in the basal layer serve about 20 basal cells and secrete melanosomes into them. Melanosomes become arranged superior to the basal cell nucleus. The melanosomes of Caucasians degrade as the cell moves up through the epidermis whereas those of negroid skin do not. Specialised mechanoreceptors, Merkel cells, are situated along the basal layer and free nerve endings may be present in the basal or prickle cell layers.

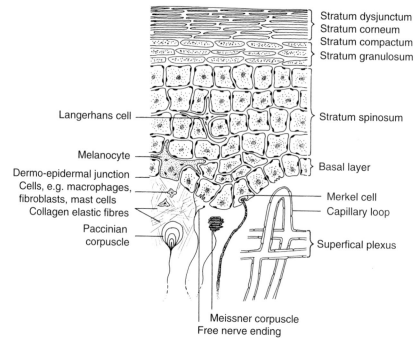

**Figure 9.2** Layers of the epidermis, nerve endings and blood supply to the skin (not to scale).

### Prickle cell layer (stratum spinosum)

The keratinocytes of this layer are still capable of mitosis if required, e.g. during wound healing. The number of layers of cells varies considerably according to site. Skin sites designed to take increased mechanical stress have a thicker prickle cell layer than sites that receive minimal stress. Desmosomes are very noticeable under light microscopy. As the cells from this layer approach the granular layer their cellular contents degrade.

### Granular layer (stratum granulosum)

In this layer there is a drastic change in the appearance of the cells and in cellular content; cells are flatter, have more tonofibrils and contain keratohyalin granules, membrane coating granules (MCGs), hydrolytic and degrading enzymes. The thickness of this layer varies with site; one or two cell layers thick in hairy skin and three to four cell layers in plantar skin (Plates 8 and 9).

### Horny layer (stratum corneum)

This is generally thought to consist of two indistinct sublayers: the deeper stratum compactum (probably the site of what was termed stratum lucidum) and the superficial stratum dysjunctum (Plate 10). The stratum compactum is composed of newly differentiated, tetrakaidecahedral, stacked squames (corneocytes) interposed by lipid lamellae. Intercellular cohesion becomes reduced, allowing cells to shed (desquamate).

## Dermoepidermal junction

The dermoepidermal junction (DEJ) is composed of the lamina lucida and the lamina densa. It supports the hemidesmosomes of the basal layer and is in turn supported by fibrous proteins within the dermis. Epidermal nutrients and products of metabolism must pass through the DEJ to and from the papillary loops and blood plexi.

## Dermis

The dermis is composed of two indistinct layers: papillary and reticular. The papillary dermis is less fibrous than the deeper reticular dermis. The dermis supports vascular structures, nerves, hair follicles and sweat and sebaceous glands (Figs 9.1 and 9.2 and Plates 8 and 9). It consists of interwoven fibres, principally collagen (approximately 80%) but also reticulin and elastic fibres which are contained in a glycosaminoglycans matrix. The main cells of the dermis are fibroblasts; there are smaller numbers of macrophages, lymphocytes, mast cells and Langerhans cells.

The superficial blood plexus is about 2 mm deep from the skin's surface and this supplies papillary loops (capillaries which ascend superficially into the papillae). One ascending arteriole will supply a number of papillary loops creating a candelabra-type structure, which when viewed on the surface appear as a polygon (Ryan 1983). The pattern made by the superficial blood plexus can be seen in livedo reticularis (due to capillary stasis) and erythema ab igne (due to exposure to local heat).

Nerve endings present within the skin are shown in Figure 9.2.

The base of the dermis is bounded by a layer of adipose tissue of irregular contours and the superficial fascia. The thickness of the adipose tissue is greater in women than men.

## PHYSIOLOGY

Keratinocytes go through a process of division, differentiation and desquamation (shedding) to form a protective, pliable outer layer to the body. This process is known as keratinisation (Table 9.3) and was thought to end in cell death. However, the stratum corneum is no longer considered to be an inert structure (McKay & Leigh 1991). The main purpose of the keratinisation process is to form the skin barrier. Normal epidermal turnover time is approximately 30–70 days and the turnover time of cells in the stratum corneum is 14–21 days (Thomas et al 1985). This time is reduced in some hyperproliferative skin disorders, e.g. psoriasis and eczema, and in wound healing. The rate of desquamation should equal the rate of mitosis in the basal and prickle cell layers (Wright 1983). Hair and nail are keratinous structures; their process of formation is similar to that of epidermal keratinisation but

**Table 9.3** Normal keratinisation of human skin (Wertz & Downing 1990)

| Stage | Process |
|---|---|
| Division | The stem cells of the basal layer divide and the daughter cells divide again, amplifying proliferation. The control of epidermal proliferation is complex and much still awaits investigation. Contemporary studies show that biochemical mediators are involved in control of cell growth and differentiation; these include growth factors (interleukins, cytokines and growth factors). Some of these substances stimulate cell division and differentiation, while others appear to inhibit this process. |
| Differentiation | Stratum spinosum, keratohyaline granules appear (thought to be important for the orientation of the keratin fibrils). Some cell division is possible in this layer if required. Granular layer cell contents degrade and the cytoplasm appears to contain granules (keratohyaline granules and membrane coating granules). Membrane coating granules (MCG, also known as Odland bodies or cementasomes) move to the periphery of the cell and disgorge their lamellar contents intercellularly, where they form the lipid lamellae that surround each keratinocyte. |
| Desquamation | Corneocytes at the base of the stratum corneum still have some metabolic activity; if traumatised, cells can release growth factors. Young corneocytes complete the process of keratinisation and desmosomal degradation starts. Old corneocytes in stratum corneum shed in small clumps or singly. |

the resultant protein structure and composition is different (Odland 1983).

The mast cells and macrophages in the dermis can stimulate an inflammatory response, which is then followed by a sequence of cellular and vascular responses so that repair can be initiated and completed. Neuropeptides released by nerve tissue will affect the type and duration of the inflammatory response.

The fibrous components of the dermis are laid down by fibroblasts, and during wound healing myofibroblasts contract the wound margins. Fibroblasts also synthesise the glycosaminoglycans matrix.

The blood vascular system is important in providing nutrients for both the dermis and epidermis, as well as for homoeostasis.

# FUNCTION

Skin is a remarkable viscoelastic organ which allows the body to interact with its environment. It is one of the largest organs of the body and weighs about one eighth of the weight of a normal individual. In its healthy state human skin can contour to contact surfaces without splitting. Skin deforms in response to the application of forces and when these forces are removed its normal configuration is restored. The morphology of macro- and microscopic structures in the skin is convoluted so that each component can take load gradually, thus reducing strain and damage (Ferguson 1980). If the skin's biomechanical behaviour is altered by disease, problems can develop, such as loss of elastic recoil. As a result of the ageing process skin loses its elasticity and wrinkles occur.

Sensory nerve endings allow assessment of the internal and external environment (Fig. 9.2). This permits the body to respond to a variety of stimuli, e.g. moving away from a noxious external stimulus.

The skin blood plexi, their anastomoses (arteriovenous shunts or glomus shunts) and sweat glands are essential in thermoregulation (Ryan 1983). In humans, hair has a vestigial role in thermoregulation. The cutaneous blood plexi are also important in the regulation of blood pressure. Only about 14% of total skin blood flow is required for nutrition purposes. If flow is reduced below this level, e.g. by cold, necrosis may develop.

It is thought that nails have evolved from claws (Finlay 1989). Nails are useful to humans for scratching and also to aid dexterity when trying to pick up tiny objects.

Sweat is slightly acidic; this may help to inhibit pathogen colonisation, particularly yeasts. However, if there is increased activity of the sweat glands this acidity is lost and the pH becomes neutral (pH7). Sebaceous glands duct into hair follicles and secrete sebum. Transepidermal water loss (TEWL) is rate limited by the skin barrier and presence of sebum. Sebum prevents hairy skin from absorbing too much water (bath-time wrinkles) and from dehydrating.

The skin is metabolically active, e.g. it synthesises vitamin D and releases growth factors. The skin also forms a reservoir for drugs and is the site where adverse drug reactions can readily be seen—urticaria, purpura, blisters, maculopapular erythema.

Palmar and plantar skin shows marked skin ridging (dermatoglyphics) which on close inspection appears as a double ridge with sweat duct openings (syringae) in the dent of this double ridge (Fig. 9.3). It is not clear how these striae arise: it is likely to be a combination of the orientation of dermal fibrous proteins, e.g. collagen, undulations of the DEJ and the type of keratin associated with sweat ducts. The striae function like the treads of a car tyre, creating suction with the contact surface, so that objects can be held.

A further, major role of the skin is to form an intact barrier between the body and its environment. This barrier is important for homoeostasis and prevents incursion of pathogens and toxic substances, although some of the latter are capable of penetrating the skin barrier. The site of the primary skin barrier is in the epidermis at the base of the stratum corneum and is formed during the process of keratinisation by the formation of lipid lamellae (bilayers) around the keratinocytes (Wertz & Downing 1990). The water associated with the lipid bilayers and intracellular keratin fibrils permits the stratum corneum to be flexible. 10–20% water content is required for optimal stratum corneum pliability (Blank 1952, Potts 1986). It is not clear to what extent sweat and sebum excretion influence the water content in the skin and control the loss of water (TEWL). The cosmetics industry invests greatly in preparations which hydrate the skin. The lipid bilayers have a further function in that their 'shelf-life' is associated with the ability of cells to desquamate.

The skin may be traumatised if its normal biomechanical behaviour is altered. If the primary barrier of the body is broken and the stratum corneum or deeper viable tissues are traumatised it stimulates the release of growth factors, e.g. EGF, interleukins and/or inflammatory mediators, e.g. serotonin and PGE1.

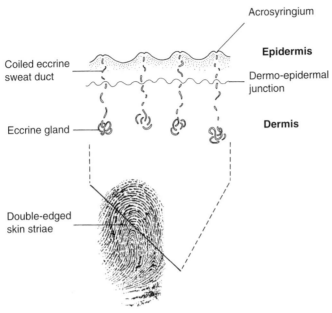

**Figure 9.3**   Thumbprint, showing the dermatoglyphic pattern, and a diagrammatic representation of the skin striae, which consist of a double ridge with sweat ducts opening into the centre of this ridge.

The secondary barrier is provided by the skin-associated cells; Langerhans cells, T-cell sub-populations, keratinocyte-release of interleukins, macrophages and mast cells (Breathnach 1989). In the normal dermis there are large numbers of macrophages, and in the epidermis Langerhans cells; these cells identify 'non-self' and present the antigen to the circulating T-cells. When Langerhans cells move out of the epidermis, in response to exposure to strong sunlight, the mechanism for recognition of 'non-self' is removed and the potential for unrecognised malignant change develops. The mitosing basal cells must then rely entirely upon their supranuclear array of melanosomes for protection from the damaging effects of ultraviolet light.

# THE DERMATOLOGICAL ASSESSMENT

Assessment of the skin and nails involves:

- history taking
- observation
- clinical tests
- special investigations.

Prior to commencing the assessment it is useful to take a brief look at the condition that is causing concern.

## HISTORY TAKING

Tact and sensitivity is required when enquiring about skin conditions, especially if the patient perceives disfigurement or does not understand the purpose of the assessment or why he/she is being asked so many questions. Initially, the patient should be asked about the symptoms and history of the problem (Ch. 3). Patients may be concerned about the appearance of the condition, may be worried that it is infectious and may complain of itching (pruritus), burning, throbbing sensations and pain. The patient may be able to recall having a similar problem in the past.

Skin diseases have psychological effects on sufferers and may cause considerable emotional distress (Burge 1989). When the patient is emotionally stressed some skin conditions worsen, e.g. psoriasis, lichen planus, herpes simplex. The patient may complain of exacerbated symptoms such as pruritus, urticaria, hyperhidrosis. Frequently, it is a great relief to the sufferer to have his/her dermatological problems recognised by the practitioner, even though management options may be limited.

When a history of the condition has been gained patients should be asked about their medical and social history (Ch. 5). Points can be clarified, such as whether the condition is congenital or acquired and whether there is a family history, e.g. of atopic eczema. Questions about occupation and hobbies are also important, especially if a contact dermatitis is suspected.

It is important to ask about diet. Weight-reducing diets where no attention is paid to food values can result in skin conditions such as folliculitis, poor skin tone and skin dryness. If malnutrition is severe, skin changes such as fissures and ulcers develop within a few weeks. It should be noted that gastrointestinal disorders may be responsible for the clinical features of malnutrition.

The patient should be asked about any preparations he/she has been using on the skin. The use of topical steroid creams or ointments may mask the cardinal features of inflammation. Certain preparations can damage or discolour the skin; for example salicylic acid will macerate the skin, leading to tissue breakdown.

Some skin conditions can be obscure, but the patient may suggest a cause (patient's theories), e.g. a resistant mycosis acquired while living in a tropical climate.

## OBSERVATION

The clinical features of skin conditions are many and varied. This is in part due to the dynamic nature of dermatological conditions as they go through a cycle of change from normal to the development of overt clinical features. This sequence may be followed by resolution and eventual clearance or by exacerbation and the condition becoming chronic. In either instance the clinical picture is forever changing; the clinical features of a condition in its acute phase may be very different from those associated with the chronic phase, e.g. eczema.

Observation of skin should be performed under suitable illumination, either colour-corrected light or daylight. A magnifying lens can be used to aid the naked eye. This is particularly helpful when the lesion appearance is complex, e.g. the presence of wart tissue after electrosurgery. Enlarging the structure can allow separation of the macroscopic elements of the lesion to help formation of the diagnosis. Visual assessment should encompass the skin, nails and other skin appendages of the legs, hands, arms and face. Patients should be asked if they have any lesions on parts of their body which are covered, e.g. the trunk.

The following should be noted:

- Presence of primary and secondary skin lesions
- Colour
- Site and distribution
- Size and shape
- Texture
- Smell.

### Primary and secondary skin lesions

Skin lesions can be classified as to whether they are primary or secondary. Primary lesions arise due to the initial effects of a condition; secondary lesions evolve from or as a complication of primary lesions. The distinction between primary and second is not always clear; some lesions can be classed as primary or secondary. The terms commonly used to describe primary and secondary skin lesions are listed in Tables 9.4 and 9.5 respectively. Use of these terms allows comparisons to be made and changes noted from one visit to another (Case history 9.1). They also provide a common language when talking to other practitioners.

### Grading of ulcers

Ulcers affecting the skin can be graded in order that the practitioner can assess the extent of

---

**Case history 9.1**

A patient purchased a pair of walking boots for a walking weekend in the Lake District. He developed severe blisters on the posterior surface of his heels while on the walk. These primary lesions were due to excess frictional stress from ill-fitting footwear. Unfortunately, being far from help, he had to continue walking and the blisters were left untreated. The roof of the blisters became raised and eroded, leaving an area of dermis exposed to further trauma and infection. These lesions developed a secondary bacterial infection which resulted in the development of small, infected ulcers which eventually healed leaving scars—secondary lesions.

---

damage to the skin and the presence of complications. Table 9.6 outlines two grading systems, the Wagner and the Sims. The latter enables the

**Table 9.4** List of primary skin lesions

| Term | Description and example |
|---|---|
| Erythema | Redness, often due to inflammatory response |
| Macule | Flat, differently coloured, e.g. freckles, vitiligo |
| Papule | Palpable, solid bump in skin, e.g. polymorphic light eruption |
| Nodule | Palpable, deeper mass than a papule, e.g. ganglion, rheumatoid nodule |
| Plaque | Elevated, disc-shaped area of skin over 1 cm in diameter, e.g. psoriasis |
| Tumour | Large mass over 2 cm in diameter, e.g. lipoma |
| Cyst | Subdermal, fluid-filled fibrous swelling, loosely attached to deeper structures, e.g. dermal cyst |
| Weal | Large oedematous bump, e.g. insect bite |
| Vesicle | Tiny, pinprick-sized collection of fluid, e.g. mycosis, pompholyx |
| Bulla | Serous fluid/blood-filled intraepidermal or dermoepidermal sac, e.g. bullous pemphigoid |
| Pustule | Vesicle or bulla filled with pus, e.g. acne, pustular psoriasis |
| Burrow | Short, linear mark in skin visible with magnifying lens, e.g. scabies |
| Ecchymosis | Large extravasation of blood into the tissues, i.e. bruising |
| Petechia | Pinhead-sized macule caused by blood seeping into skin |
| Telangiectasiae | Permanently dilated small cutaneous blood vessels |

**Table 9.5** List of secondary skin lesions

| Term | Description and example |
|---|---|
| Scale | Flake of skin, e.g. mycosis, psoriasis |
| Crust | Scab, dried serous exudate, e.g. acute eczema |
| Excoriation | Scratch marks, e.g. pruritus |
| Fissure | Crack in dry or moist skin |
| Necrosis | Non-viable tissue |
| Ulcer | Loss of epidermis; may extend through the dermis to deeper tissue, e.g. venous ulcer |
| Scar | Fibrous tissue production post-healing |
| Keloid | Excessive production of fibrous tissue post-healing |
| Striae | Lines in skin that do not have normal skin tone, e.g. striae tensae in pregnancy, Cushing's disease |
| Purpura | Purplish lesions which do not blanche under pressure, e.g. vitamin C deficiency |
| Urticaria | 'Nettle rash', e.g. drug eruption, allergy, heat |
| Lichenification | Patchy 'toughening' of skin, e.g. chronic eczema |
| Haematoma | Blood-filled blister |
| Sinus | Channel that allows the escape of pus or fluid from tissues. |

early features of ulceration to be assessed in order that preventative measures can be implemented. Neither of these grading systems considers the differential features of ischaemic, venous, neuropathic, trophic/pressure sores or mixed aetiology ulceration; these are discussed in Chapter 17.

*Colour*

It is necessary to establish the normal colour of the patient's skin so that any changes from normal can be identified. Colour changes may affect the whole of the skin, e.g. jaundice, or be localised (Plate 11), e.g. redness associated with eczema, brown/black due to a malignant melanoma. The nail may also show changes in colour in association with disease or disorder (Table 9.11, Plate 12). Colour changes are usually more evident in Caucasian skin than negroid, Asian or oriental skin.

Colour changes commonly seen are:

- redness (erythema, suggestive of inflammation)

**Table 9.6** Classification of skin wounds/ulcers

| Grading | Descriptor |
| --- | --- |
| *Wagner six-level wound/classification system* | |
| Grade 0 | Intact foot, no open lesions |
| Grade I | Full-thickness, superficially located ulcers (including periungual lesions) |
| Grade II | Deep ulcer with penetration through subcutaneous tissue to tendon, ligament, joint capsule or bone |
| Grade III | Deep penetrating ulcer and deep infection (abscess, osteomyelitis, purulent tendinitis or synovitis) |
| Grade IV | A portion of the foot is gangrenous |
| Grade V | The entire foot is gangrenous |
| *Sims et al (1988)/10-grade classification* | |
| Grade 0 | Absent skin lesions |
| Grade 1 | Dense callus lesions but not pre-ulcer or ulcer |
| Grade 2 | Pre-ulcerative changes |
| Grade 3 | Partial-thickness (superficial) ulcer |
| Grade 4 | Full-thickness (deep) ulcer but no involvement of tendon, bone, ligament or joint |
| Grade 5 | Full-thickness (deep) ulcer with involvement of tendon, bone, ligament or joint |
| Grade 6 | Localised infection (abscess or osteomyelitis) |
| Grade 7 | Proximal spread of infection (ascending cellulitis or lymphadenopathy) |
| Grade 8 | Gangrene of forefoot only |
| Grade 9 | Gangrene of majority of foot |

- purple-blue (cyanosis, suggestive of a slow blood flow)
- white (ischaemia, amelanotic)
- black (necrosis, gangrene (Plates 3 and 33))
- yellow (when seen at the base of an ulcer, called slough).

Topical drugs—e.g. silver nitrate, povidone iodine—and shoe dyes may stain the skin, giving it a different hue.

Individual lesions may show colour differences, e.g. the pink and silvery scaled lesions of psoriasis. Haemosiderosis associated with venous hypertension appears as a red-brown discoloration within the skin, often of the anteromedial part of the lower leg (Plate 6). The colour of an ulcer base and the nature of the exudate may be a useful indicator of its cause and progress (Ch. 17). Other colour changes may be seen; for instance, the active margins of tinea pedis are frequently red, scaly and sometimes vesicular, whereas the inner area of the affected skin appears relatively normal, if a little shiny.

White, flat, oval or irregularly shaped patches of non-pigmented skin may occur (vitiligo). A loss of pigmentation in the skin tends to occur with age. In younger people it is associated with hyperthyroidism, diabetes mellitus, pernicious anaemia and Addison's disease. Loss of pigmentation can occur for other reasons, e.g. pityriasis versicolor (mycotic infection). A congenital lack of pigmentation is known as albinism.

### Site and distribution

The site and distribution of lesions can be a diagnostic indicator. For example, lesions that only appear on skin exposed to the sun may be partially or entirely due to sunlight. Note if the distribution is symmetrical, localised or generalised. Symmetrical lesions usually have an endogenous cause whereas asymmetrical lesions tend to have an exogenous cause. On occasions, the cause of a unilateral difference may be obscure, such as a patient who has one white leg and one brown leg due to sunbathing with one leg bandaged. Generalised urticaria implies an aetiology of food or drug allergy, whereas if localised the aetiology is likely to be a contact allergen, such as shoe dye or a topical substance, e.g. perfume, nickel.

The configuration of the lesions should be noted (Fig. 9.4). It should also be noted whether the lesions occur at sites of trauma, e.g. a scratch or skin wound. The presence of a skin condition at the site of trauma is known as Koebner's phenomenon and occurs with psoriasis and lichen planus.

### Size and shape

Ideally the size of the lesion(s) should be measured (see clinical tests). The practitioner should observe whether the lesions are all of a similar size or whether they vary in size. It is important to note the shape of the lesion, in dermatology the following terms are used to describe shape:

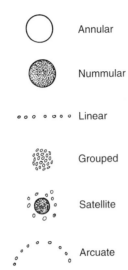

**Figure 9.4** The various configurations of lesion patterns.

- Annular (ring-like)
- Nummular (round, coin-like)
- Discoid (disk-like)
- Retiform or reticulate (net-like)
- Arcuate (curved).

The surface contour of the lesion should also be noted (Fig. 9.5). Observation of the edge/margin of the lesion will show whether it is well or ill-defined.

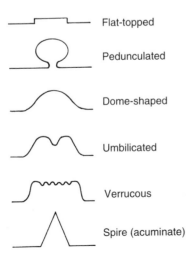

**Figure 9.5** The different surface contours of lesions.

## Texture

It should be noted whether the lesion(s) appears rough, silky, smooth or hard. An anhidrotic skin appears dry, scaly and may display fissures around the ankle (Plate 13). The term 'anhidrosis' implies lack of water; however, it is not clear if the condition is due to a reduction in sweat production by the eccrine glands. Anhidrosis may be a complication of a number of skin conditions, e.g. eczema.

A hyperhidrotic skin appears shiny and moist to the touch and maceration (white tissue) and fissures may be present, especially interdigitally (Plate 14). The condition often starts in adolescence and mostly affects males. The palms and soles are continually moist and can be smelly. Commonly there is no apparent reason for an increase in eccrine gland activity (Manusov & Nadeau 1989). Essential hyperhidrosis needs to be differentiated from pathological hyperhidrosis. Anxiety states may cause localised sweating and hot spicy foods can induce gustatory sweating. Conditions which may cause generalised hyperhidrosis include hyperthyroidism, malaria, pain, pachyonychia congenita and certain abnormalities of the central or peripheral nervous system.

## Smell

While observing the skin the practitioner is also in a position to smell any unusual odours. The smell of wet gangrene (necrotic, infected tissue) is putrid and unmistakable (Ch. 17). Incontinence and poor personal hygiene produce distinctive, acrid smells. Bromhidrosis, the action of bacteria on hyperhidrotic skin, is one of the commonest causes of smelly feet.

Table 9.7 summarises some of the common clinical features observed with skin complaints and gives examples of possible causes.

## CLINICAL TESTS

There are a number of easy to use, relatively economical to perform, clinical tests which can be used to assess the state of the skin. These tests can make a useful adjunct to history taking and observation.

**Table 9.7** Common dermatological clinical features that occur in the lower limb, with examples of the likely causes. This is a guide only and not a definitive list

| Clinical feature | Possible causes |
| --- | --- |
| Raised lesions | Adverse drug reaction<br>Blisters (mechanical, thermal, chemical, disease associated)<br>Chilblains<br>Cysts<br>Dermatofibromas (pink, brownish lesions on legs, commoner in women)<br>Eczema<br>Insect bites<br>Keloid<br>Neurofibroma (von Recklinghausen's disease) |
| Pustules (infection) | Weals (adverse drug reaction, topical substance (e.g. hemlock), associated with an infection)<br>Pustular psoriasis |
| Pruritic lesions | Adverse drug reaction<br>Insect bites, ectoparasites<br>Chilblains<br>Eczema, pompholyx<br>Photosensitivity<br>Psoriasis, especially scalp<br>Tinea pedis<br>Urticaria<br>Bacterial infection may sometimes verge on being itchy rather than painful |
| Skin discolouration | Blue naevus<br>Callus and corns<br>Chilblains and chilling<br>Glomus tumour<br>Hyperpigmentation (haemosiderosis) in venous hypertension<br>Livedo reticularis<br>Melanoma<br>Necrosis/gangrene<br>Purpura<br>Sarcoidosis<br>Telangiectasiae (e.g. spider naevi)<br>Vasculitis (secondary to rheumatoid arthritis, systemic lupus erythematosus, necrotising angiitis, polyarteritis nodosa)<br>White skin (ischaemia, Raynaud's phenomenon, atrophie blanche) |
| Painful lesions | Bacterial infection<br>Bullous disorders<br>Chilblains<br>Eczema (when the dermis is exposed)<br>Erythema nodosum<br>Fissures, dry and moist (may be secondarily infected)<br>Glomus tumour<br>Herpes (not usual in the lower limb)<br>Psoriasis<br>Vasculitis |

**Table 9.7**  (*Cont'd*)

| Clinical feature | Possible causes |
| --- | --- |
| Dry and scaly | Chapping<br>Eczema<br>Ichthyosis<br>Post-acute oedema<br>Psoriasis<br>Tinea pedis |
| Rough | Eczema<br>Psoriasis with hyperkeratosis<br>Seborrhoeic warts<br>Solar keratosis<br>Warts |
| Moist | Erythrasma<br>Hyperhidrosis<br>Maceration<br>Tinea pedis<br>Ulceration |
| 'Tied down' and firm | Fibrous corns<br>Scarring, hypertrophic scarring<br>Systemic sclerosis (scleroderma) |

*Touch*

Epidermal, dermal and subcutaneous tissue changes can be assessed by touch (beware of cross-infection). Palpation of tissues may reveal changes in cutaneous and deeper structures. A light, brushing-type touch should be used to assess surface changes, the assessment of dermal tissue requires a firmer touch with the application of gentle shear to assess tone and the presence of adhesions.

In order to test elasticity a section of skin from the dorsum of the foot can be gently squeezed together between two fingers. On release the time taken for the skin to return to normal should be noted. If it takes more than a couple of seconds this is a sign of loss of elasticity and is a common feature in the skin of the elderly. Tissues can be palpated to help determine whether a swelling is cutaneous, e.g. wart, attached to other structures, e.g. ganglion, or free, e.g. granulation around a cyst or a foreign body. There may be evidence of an unusual skin response to trauma, e.g. hypertrophic scarring, where texturally the skin feels fibrous and non-pliable. Finger- and toenails (Table 9.11) may show evidence of abnormality in texture.

The presence of swelling can be detected through fluctuation. Imagine resting two hands either side of an inflated balloon, apply pressure to the balloon with one hand and feel this effect against the other hand—this is fluctuation.

### Microscope slide

If a microscope slide is pressed against an erythematous area of skin, blanching should occur. This indicates that vascular tissue is associated with the lesion. Non-blanching of skin lesions implies that altered pigmentation has occurred, e.g. post inflammatory hyperpigmentation.

### Microscopy

Microscopy of skin scrapings from an active site can provide immediate confirmation of the presence of fungal infection or parasitic infestation. However, it is more common that these are sent to the pathology laboratory for investigation (Ch. 13).

### Temperature

When the back of the hand is moved from the foot to the leg there may be patches of warmth compared with surrounding skin, suggesting inflammation, e.g. cellulitis, paronychia, chilblain. Skin temperature can be measured using a thermistor, thermometer strip (obtainable from most chemists) or a thermometer with suitable calibration (20–50°C). Normal foot skin temperature has a wide range (24–32°C) and varies according to physiological status and ambient conditions. An increase in skin temperature indicates an inflammatory response.

### Lesion measurement

It is important to record the size of a lesion to aid monitoring of pathological changes and evaluate the effects of treatment. Photographs can be taken to record the progress of the lesion but a measuring scale should be included within the photographic field. Tracings of skin lesions provide a real-size record. Lesionometers are helpful in providing a guide to lesion diameter and a scale rule can be used to measure lesion dimensions. It is not possible to measure topographical features clinically, although skin thickness can be measured with skinfold callipers to give an approximate guide to changes.

## Special investigations

Sometimes it may be necessary to undertake non-routine clinical investigations before a diagnosis can be made. Where possible these should be non-invasive but sometimes it is necessary to use invasive procedures such as biopsy.

### Allergy tests

Allergy tests can be carried out relatively simply. An intracutaneous test involves injecting the allergen into the epidermis. Scratch or prick tests utilise a scratchy instrument to introduce the allergen intraepidermally. An immediate (within 30 min) type 1 or a delayed (24–72 h) type IV hypersensitivity reaction can develop. Patch tests involve applying a number of potential allergens to the patient's back or forearm with a hypoallergenic cover. After 3–4 days the patches are removed and any areas of inflammation are noted. A positive reaction to any or all of the allergens indicates a delayed type IV hypersensitivity reaction.

### Biopsies

Biopsies are useful where the diagnosis is not clear, or if diagnosis is critical, e.g. malignancy. Biopsy· is carried out under a local anaesthetic infiltration (Ch. 13). Many techniques such as monoclonal antibodies and immunocytochemistry are used to investigate the mechanisms of skin abnormality with a view to interrupting or circumventing the pathology. However, traditional techniques such as staining with haematoxylin and eosin dyes (Plate 10) are still useful in visualising tissue and cellular structures.

### Infrared thermography

This provides an expensive but fascinating way of illustrating dynamic temperature changes in skin and deeper tissues. Assessment of temperature gives an indication of the blood supply to the area. Warm spots indicate vasodilation associated with inflammation. Photography with image analysis will provide quantifiable data so that progress can be monitored accurately.

### Skin colour

Colour-sensitive instruments, e.g. erythema meters, are useful for assessing colour changes in a patient. However, they cannot be used to compare the extent of colour changes between patients.

### Skin water content

The water content of skin is difficult to measure non-invasively. Skin conductivity/resistance measurement is a readily available technique but does not always provide valid and reliable results. Resistance-measuring instruments with the required sensitivity tend to be rather expensive. However, data obtained by this method can be useful in monitoring the effect of systemic control of eccrine gland activity and the effects of topical applications, e.g. emollients, and may provide an indirect measure of the quality of the microcirculation.

### Skin imaging

Ultrasound skin imaging (A- or B-scan) instruments are non-invasive and allow measurement of the skin thickness as well as identification of some structures within the skin and deeper tissues (Plate 15). They can be used to locate echogenic foreign bodies prior to excision and may become a method of screening for skin malignancy (Nessi et al 1991, Harland et al 1993). B-scan ultrasound images of ulcers provide data on the depth of the lesion and are very helpful in monitoring change. Magnetic resonance imaging (MRI) provides greater detail but at considerably greater cost.

### Skin blood perfusion

Transcutaneous measurement of the partial pressure of oxygen (TcPO$_2$) was developed as a non-invasive means of monitoring skin perfusion and, therefore, blood supply in neonates (Carter 1993). Laser Doppler flowmetry and laser Doppler Imaging can also be used to measure and monitor cutaneous blood flow.

### Skin biomechanics

Skin biomechanics can be assessed in vivo using extensometry or rheology (the study of flow in a material/tissue) where the tissue response to strain can be measured. Interpretation of data obtained from these instruments requires skill in mechanics, which reduces the popularity of such techniques. Data from these instruments is useful in assessing the effect of different management modalities on a patient's skin or measuring the quality of tissue repair.

## ASSESSMENT OF THE AGEING SKIN

Skin and nails show change with increasing age, especially if exposed to a lot of sunlight (Leveque et al 1984, Helfand 1993). A woman's skin generally remains unchanged until about 40 years of age, a man until 50 years of age, after which there is a slow loss of elastic recoil and the collagen fibres of the dermis realign from a 3D meshwork to a more linear array, parallel to the skin's surface. This means that whilst the tensile strength of the skin is still efficient, it is less resilient to other forces. The effects of ageing on the epidermis are not clear; it is thought that mitotic rate may decrease and there is evidence that the undulations of the DEJ of hairy skin flatten out with increasing age (Smith 1989). There is little change in skin thickness, although skin biomechanical parameters alter with age (see skin function), and so the effects of pressure, shear and torsion are potentially troublesome. Skin lesions such as pressure sores may develop more readily.

In elderly people the nutrition to the skin may change due to the effects of macro- and microvascular disease, poor dietary intake and immobility. The effects of prolonged exposure to sunlight become more pronounced, e.g. solar keratosis, rodent ulcers. Many skin lesions are more common in the elderly; these include telangiectasiae, purpura, skin tags and seborrhoeic warts. Changes to the nail are also more prevalent (Helfand 1993) (Table 9.11).

## ASSESSMENT OF SELF-INFLICTED SKIN LESIONS

The skin and its appendages may also be the site of self-injury (Table 9.8). Many people pick and bite their nails (onychotillomania). Some self-inflicted injuries, e.g. cigarette burns, may indicate a personality disturbance which will need help and counselling by appropriately qualified personnel.

## ASSESSMENT OF CALLUSES AND CORNS

Callus plaques (callosities) are hard, dense, yellowish plaques of hyperkeratotic tissue usually found on the plantar surface of the foot, which may be uncomfortable or painful. Corns appear as darker, harder, invaginated areas of hyperkeratosis present either alone or within a callus plaque. They are frequently painful. Similar clinical features may develop with foreign bodies such as wood or glass splinters. Very new plantar warts often appear similar to tiny plantar corns (0.5–1.0 mm diameter) and have no associated

**Table 9.8**  Skin conditions associated with psychological disorders

| Condition | Description |
| --- | --- |
| Dermatitis artefacta | Cigarette burns on legs |
| Munchausen's syndrome | Repeated fabrication of an illness |
| Parasitophobia | Fear of becoming infested; complaint of itching or crawling sensation on skin |
| Dysmorphobia | Distortions of body image; known as dermatological non-disease as no evidence of disease; skin problem—e.g. baldness or colour of skin—is 'normal' |
| Obsessive–compulsive habits | Plucking out hair and picking skin |
| Onychotillomania | Picking nails |
| Nail biting | Very short nails, uneven appearance |

overlying callus. Wart tissue is moist on excision in comparison with a corn of similar size. Hyperkeratoses of different aetiology, e.g. secondary lesions associated with psoriasis, or Darier's disease, show differential features such as nonusual siting or texture.

Patients with calluses and/or corns complain of a number of symptoms ranging from cosmetic irritation to severe pain. The range of symptoms include a stabbing pain when walking which may persist when resting or subside into a dull, soft tissue ache. They may remark on a corn site feeling as if there was 'something sharp stuck in the skin or shoe' or a callus site as a stinging, burning sensation which is worse just after the start of rest and on resuming weightbearing. An illustrative description of callus being like 'walking on stones' may be given. An erythematous 'halo' may be evident around either lesion type.

Patients may report that they have adopted a different gait to avoid the painful area. These changes in gait may precipitate complications such as knee or lower back pain. So, although calluses and corns are relatively minor conditions, the effects they have may be quite extensive. Public demand for over-the-counter treatments for these conditions is large enough to support a number of pharmaceutical products. This would seem to indicate that corns and calluses interfere noticeably with the everyday life of a large number of people, enough to cause significant expenditure on corn and callus products.

Calluses and corns appear to form in response to over-prolonged and excess mechanical stress from ground reaction forces on the foot and footwear during gait (Springett 1993). The forces exerted on the foot may be in the form of intermittent pressure, shear, friction, torsion, tension or a combination of these. Which combination is influential in the formation of these hyperkeratoses has yet to be identified. However, it is clear that, although vertical force is the greatest, the forces in all three dimensions, as well as torque/torsion (moment), are implicated in the aetiology of callus and corn tissue. Instrumentation capable of providing in-shoe, four-dimensional (vertical, side to side, front to back movement and time) plantar stress analysis is currently being developed and may help to clarify these observations (Cavenagh et al 1992). Footwear may moderate or compound the effects of ground reaction forces. If skin quality is affected by disease or disorder then this biomechanical aetiology becomes more complex.

Corns and callus are always found on areas exposed to mechanical stress and often in a pattern which relates to the biomechanics of foot function (Fig. 9.6). The few surveys undertaken into the incidence of callus and corn lesions on the foot are in general accordance as to their epidemiological features (Gillett 1973, Merriman et al 1986, Whiting 1987, Springett 1993). Diffuse callus over the second, third and fourth metatarsal heads is commonest, followed by callus solely over the second metatarsal head and first and fifth metatarsal heads. Dorsal corns are most common on the fifth toes followed by the fourth, third and second. Interdigital lesions are most common between fourth/fifth toes followed by first/second, third/fourth and finally second/third. The majority of patients have bilateral corns and/or calluses; however, unilateral lesions are a frequent occurrence. Lesion incidence is not associated with a dominant side. Sex incidence ratio is between 1:2 and 1:4 male to female, with mode age of symptomatic onset between 40–70 years. The incidence decreases with reduced weightbearing and shoe wearing.

When tissues are subjected to excess stress for a prolonged period of time it may be assumed the traumatised cells in that area are stimulated to release growth factors and inflammatory mediators (Mackay & Leigh 1991). It is not yet known which substances are released in corn and callus formation nor their influence on the cell cycle and differentiation. However, a sequence of events appears to occur such that callus and corn tissue develops and self-perpetuates (Fig. 9.7). It is not yet known what the mechanism is that stops a callus plaque developing into a corn, but it is feasible the magnitude, duration and direction of force vector are implicated.

Histologically, callus and corn tissues show a number of changes from normal. There is a marked thickening of the stratum corneum, the

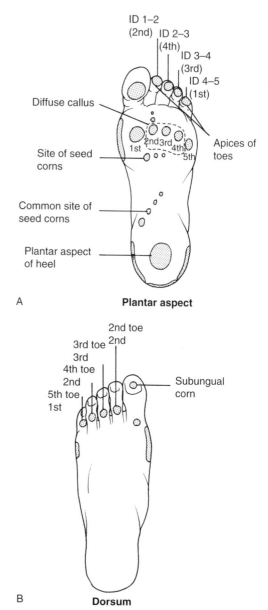

**Figure 9.6** The common sites for corn and callus formation on the feet (Merriman et al 1987).

granular layer thickens and becomes disrupted, and in corns (dorsal and plantar) it disappears completely (Plate 16). The dermal papillae and epidermal rete ridges become elongated and there is slight hyperplasia of basal cells (Thomas et al 1985). Histological evidence suggests that callus tissue is a step along the way to corn for-

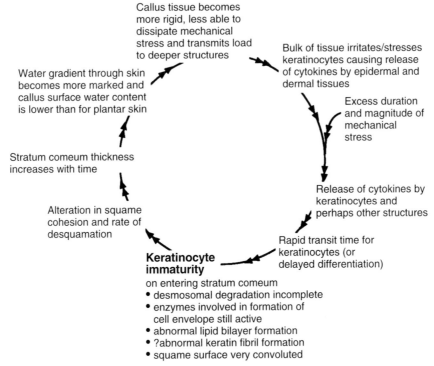

Callus tissue becomes more rigid, less able to dissipate mechanical stress and transmits load to deeper structures

Bulk of tissue irritates/stresses keratinocytes causing release of cytokines by epidermal and dermal tissues

Water gradient through skin becomes more marked and callus surface water content is lower than for plantar skin

Excess duration and magnitude of mechanical stress

Stratum comeum thickness increases with time

Release of cytokines by keratinocytes and perhaps other structures

Alteration in squame cohesion and rate of desquamation

Rapid transit time for keratinocytes (or delayed differentiation)

**Keratinocyte immaturity**
on entering stratum comeum
• desmosomal degradation incomplete
• enzymes involved in formation of cell envelope still active
• abnormal lipid bilayer formation
• ?abnormal keratin fibril formation
• squame surface very convoluted

**Figure 9.7**   A proposed model for callus formation (Springett 1993).

mation (Springett 1993). Corns show additional differences in the ultrastructure of the cells, e.g. in keratin fibril formation, desmosome degradation and cell envelope formation. In the dermis, there may be evidence of capillary angiogenesis (formation of new capillaries in response to demands of new tissue) but generally there is no evidence of an inflammatory process (Thomas et al 1985, Smith & Morrison 1990, Springett 1993). It may therefore be assumed that the skin changes are brought about by local biochemical reactions, probably via growth factors (Mackay & Leigh 1991).

A method of classifying corns and calluses by site and appearance is helpful (Table 9.9). The use of this classification system enables the lesion to be described precisely and allows the progress of the lesion to be monitored and management evaluated. Also, comparison of lesions for research purposes becomes possible. The site of the lesion, an indication of its severity, size, texture (hard and glassy or soft), duration and stimulators/exacerbators, e.g. a particular activity

and/or pair of shoes, should be noted, along with colour differences and lesion contours, bulk, depth and width.

It is assumed that the maceration which appears as a milky yellow region under a callus plaque or corn is due to excess trauma and as a

**Table 9.9**   A classification of callus and corn types and the complications that may arise with these lesions

| Grade | Description |
|---|---|
| 0 | No lesion |
| 1 | No specific callus plaque (callosity), but diffuse or pinch callus tissue present or in narrow bands |
| 2 | Circumscribed, punctate oval or circular, well-defined thickening of keratinised tissue |
| 3 | Corn seed (heloma milliare) or hard corn (heloma durum) with no associated callus tissue |
| 4 | Well-defined callus plaque with definite corn within the lesion |
| 5 | Extravasation, maceration and early breakdown of structures under the callus layer |
| 6 | Complete breakdown of structure of hyperkeratotic tissue, epidermis, extending to superficial dermal involvement |

result water is squeezed from the viable layers of the epidermis into the lower keratinised layers of the stratum corneum. Under greater trauma the contents of the papillary capillaries may be extruded into the epidermis as a brown-black stain (extravasation). The features of maceration and extravasation (Plate 17) may be considered as clinical indicators of marked mechanical stress. Suitable management of these lesions is urgently required to prevent tissue breakdown and ulceration.

## Types of corn

### Seed corns

The aetiology of seed corns (Plate 18) is not clear. The empirically proposed association with tension stress has neither been proved nor disputed. These lesions appear similar in structure and biochemically to other mechanically induced hyperkeratoses. Unpublished work using high-powered liquid chromatography (HPLC) shows that they are not plugs of cholesterol as previously thought but, in common with other hyperkeratoses, have a high cholesterol content compared with normal plantar skin (O'Halloran 1990). Seed corns tend to occur at the margins of weightbearing areas of the plantar aspect of the foot either singly or as disperse clusters.

### Hard corns

A hard corn (Plate 19) appears as a darker patch within the epidermis, often with a callus covering. Texturally it is hard, glassy and dense when touched with a scalpel. When enucleated, a classic corn nucleus appears as a cone, although they may be any shape or multinucleate. Extravasation (Plate 17) may be evident. A corn forming over a bursa may be associated with the formation of a sinus into the bursal sac; infection may result.

### Vascular corns

When the skin is made translucent by application of water, alcohol or oil, clinical signs below the surface of the lesion become apparent. Intrusions of vascularised dermal tissue into the epidermis can be seen in vascular corns and if cut this vascular tissue bleeds profusely. These lesions usually occur at sites of excess mechanical stress, may have a relatively long history and may be painful on direct pressure. These features suggest that the lesion is a vascular corn rather than a foreign body or wart. Some practitioners make a distinction between vascular and neuro-vascular corns; others consider that they are one and the same.

### Soft corns

Soft corns (Plate 20) occur interdigitally and appear as soft, soggy epidermal masses (macerated tissue) which can easily blunt the scalpel blade. Pain is a frequent complaint. The condition appears to be caused by poorly fitting footwear, disease processes affecting the skeleton, e.g. rheumatoid arthritis, or biomechanical anomaly, e.g. excess pronation where the toe tissues are compressed and sheared.

### Fibrous corns

These arise from long-standing corns and involve the presence of fibrous tissue in the dermis below the corn. The affected tissues have an altered biomechanical behaviour: they appear more firmly attached to deeper structures than normal. Shear stresses occur at the tissue interface and, as this tissue is unable to dissipate stress as efficiently as normal tissue, there may be a perpetuation of what appears to be chronic irritation of tissues, causing further fibrosis to develop. The precise aetiology of these lesions is not clear.

### Systemic conditions and hyperkeratoses

Some systemic conditions may lead to hyperkeratosis (Table 9.10). In these instances the hyperkeratosis tends to have a different texture from the mechanically-induced type. For example, in psoriasis the skin may flake off with scalpel use, or chip off and bleed due to malformation of the epidermis (Auspitz's sign). Callus associ-

**Table 9.10**  Causes of non-mechanically-induced hyperkeratosis

| Familial/inherited | Punctate keratoderma |
|---|---|
| | Ichthyosis |
| | Darier's disease |
| | Mal de Meleda |
| | Unna–Thost disease |
| | Disseminated plantar–palmar keratoderma |
| | Papillon–Lefevre syndrome |
| Acquired | Reiter's disease |
| | Keratoderma climacterium |
| | Sezary's syndrome |
| | Chronic contact dermatitis |
| | Hypothyroidism |
| | Lichen planus |
| | Arsenic intoxication |
| | Psoriasis (palmar and plantar) |
| | Syphilis |
| | Tinea of the sole of the foot (tinea rubrum) |

ated with ichthyosis tends to be thick and tough and there is evidence of the condition on other body sites.

## ASSESSMENT OF NAIL PATHOLOGIES

In humans, the purpose of nails is primarily for protection, although they also aid dexterity and allow us to inspect and scratch ourselves and others. Figure 9.8 illustrates the anatomy of the nail. Nails, like the skin, can be used as a cutaneous indicator of disease and disorder; they may also be the site of the primary lesion. Changes in shape, contour, texture and colour should noted. Pain and the appearance of the nail plate are the common presenting problems. Unfortunately, many nail conditions are irreversible, e.g. onychogryphosis.

During the assessment it is worthwhile evaluating how concerned the patient is about the nail condition. Patients may be concerned about the appearance and/or whether it is likely to spread. For example, a patient may be concerned about a fungal infection of a nail (Plate 12) spreading to other nails or members of the family but not about its appearance.

Nails show a number of variations in pathology. The quality and quantity of the nail plate shows the effects of long-term abnormality. Sudden trauma or illness can be identified by the position of Beau's lines (a horizontal indentation across the plate). The expected rate of nail plate growth is about 6 months for a fingernail and 7–12 months for a toenail, but rates vary considerably within individuals. The rate of growth of the nail plate may also be affected by disease, e.g. Raynaud's disease results in a slow-growing nail.

The nail plate may show a characteristic deformity, e.g. club nails (hippocratic nails) due to cardiac or respiratory problems, which will aid diagnosis of the primary aetiology. Table

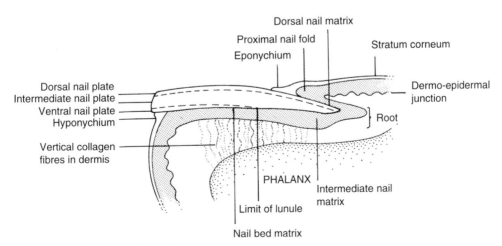

**Figure 9.8**  Structure and anatomy of the nail.

9.11 lists the clinical features associated with local and systemic nail conditions. Table 9.12 gives definitions of common nail conditions.

**Table 9.11**   Clinical features associated with nail conditions

| Clinical feature | Examples of conditions |
| --- | --- |
| *Subungual discoloration* | |
| Brownish | Subungual warts; idiopathic |
| Splinter haemorrhage | Rheumatoid arthritis; naevus; subacute bacterial endocarditis |
| White | Hepatic cirrhosis; anaemia |
| Greenish | *Pseudomonas* infection |
| Yellow | Subungual exostosis; subungual corn; subungual wart; infection |
| Yellowish hyponychium | Psoriasis; Reiter's disease |
| Blue-black | Glomus tumour; subungual haematoma; melanoma |
| *Discolouration of the lunule* | |
| Diffuse red | Congestive cardiac failure; alopecia areata |
| Azure | Hepatolenticular degeneration |
| Brown-black | Haematoma; naevus; melanoma |
| White | Scar from injury |
| *Discolouration of the nail plate* | |
| White | Mycotic infection; maceration; psoriasis; Darier's disease (longitudinal white or dark bands) |
| Yellow | Nicotine stains; yellow nail syndrome associated with lymphoedema; drugs, e.g. tetracyclines |
| Brown | Mycotic or bacterial infection; onychauxis; onychogryphosis; shoe dyes; cosmetics |
| *Deformity of the nail plate* | |
| Atrophied or absent | Ischaemia; systemic sclerosis; epidermolysis bullosa; eczema; pemphigus; occupational; trauma, e.g. onychomadesis; nail–patella syndrome |
| Thickened | Onychauxis; onychogryphosis; onychomycosis; Darier's disease, sarcoidosis; psoriasis; pachyonychia congenita |
| Koilonychia | Iron-deficiency anaemia; nail–patella syndrome; idiopathic |
| Onycholysis | Trauma; psoriasis; dermatitis; thyroid disorders; idiopathic; occupational |
| Clubbing | Cardiac insufficiency; thyrotoxicosis |
| Subungual exostosis | Involuted nails |

**Table 9.11**   *(Cont'd)*

| Clinical feature | Examples of conditions |
| --- | --- |
| *Textural changes* | |
| Brittleness | Idiopathic; topically applied substances; iron-deficiency anaemia |
| Roughness | Psoriasis; Beau's lines; Darier's disease; peripheral vascular disease; alopecia areata; pemphigus |
| Pitting | Psoriasis |
| Splitting | Median nail dystrophy; Beau's lines; occupational effects; trauma; psoriasis; eczema |
| Striations | Variation of normality; lichen planus; Darier's disease; peripheral vascular disease |
| Punched-out areas | Reiter's syndrome |
| *Abnormality of tissues surrounding the nail* | |
| Redness | Paronychia; cosmetic damage; nail and cuticle biting; onychocryptosis; epithelioma |
| Fibroma | Tuberous sclerosis |
| Cysts | Idiopathic |
| Pterygium | Peripheral vascular disease; severe lichen planus; idiopathic |
| Hypergranulation tissue | Ingrown toenail |

Trauma to nails may be mechanical, thermal or chemical and the tissue response may be acute or chronic. Acute trauma to nails is generally defined as being a sudden injury, while chronic trauma usually suggests repeated minor injuries caused by, e.g. poorly fitting footwear (Samman 1986). Fungal infection of the nail plate or bacterial infection of periungual tissue may occur either as a primary lesion or secondary to trauma.

A number of subungual conditions may give rise to pain under or around the nail:

- Subungual exostosis (bony growth on the distal, superior end of the distal phalanx)
- Subungual haematoma (bruising under the nail)
- Subungual heloma durum (hard corn under the nail)
- Subungual ulceration (breakdown of skin under the nail)

**Table 9.12**  Nail conditions and their definitions

| Condition | Definition |
|---|---|
| Onychauxis | Thickened nail, usually due to trauma |
| Onychogryphosis | Thickened nail with deformity (ram's horn) |
| Involution | Transverse plane abnormality of the nail plate, which results in the nail being curved at the edges |
| Onychomycosis | Fungal infection of the nail |
| Onycholysis | Separation of the nail from the nail bed; occurs distal to proximal |
| Onychomadesis | Complete shedding of the nail |
| Onychia | Inflammation of the nail bed |
| Paronychia | Inflammation of the skin surrounding the nail |
| Onychocryptosis | Side of the nail has pierced the skin; results in inflammation and hypergranulation tissue |
| Pterygium | Eponychium grows with the nail plate |
| Beau's lines | Transverse grooves which appear in the nail due to a temporary cessation in growth; may be caused by a systemic illness or malnutrition |
| Hippocratic nails | Clubbing of the nail and distal phalanx due to chronic lung disease and cyanotic heart disease |
| Koilonychia | Spooning and thinning of the nails due to iron deficiency |
| Splinter haemorrhage | Small vertical lines running through nail, usually due to trauma but may be seen with bacterial endocarditis, psoriasis, rheumatoid arthritis |
| Yellow nail syndrome | Nail appears yellow, associated with lymphoedema |

- Glomus tumour (benign growth of the arteriovenous anastomosis under the nail).

The presence of a subungual exostosis may lead to distortion of the nail plate and as a result can be confused with involution. An X-ray is required in order to make a definitive diagnosis. A patient who continues to experience pain some time after a partial or total nail ablation has been performed, for what was thought to be an involuted nail, should receive an X-ray to rule out a possible exostosis. In order to make a diagnosis and effectively treat a subungual haematoma, ulceration or heloma durum it may be necessary to cut back the nail to expose the subungual tissues. This is usually easy to perform as onycholysis occurs with these conditions.

Glomus tumours are composed of a complex of vascular and neural elements. They are pink/purple, painful nodules often found subungually. They can be confused with a subungual corn, subungual naevus or melanoma. The excruciating pain experienced by patients with this problem normally points to the diagnosis. Excision of the lesion and subsequent biopsy usually confirms the clinical diagnosis.

Problems which can arise in the periungual skin include:

- Periungual fibroma (protrusion of fibrous tissue at the side of the nail)
- Periungual warts (verrucae)
- Malignant melanoma
- Paronychia.

The presence of periungual fibromas is associated with tuberous sclerosis. Malignant melanomas can be confused with the clinical features of an ingrown toenail. The presence of periungual problems may distort nail growth, leading to a deformed nail plate.

## ASSESSMENT OF INFECTIONS AND INFESTATIONS

The lower limb, especially the foot, is prone to a range of infections and infestations.

### Viral

The skin may be infected locally with a virus causing lesions to develop, e.g. warts, or there may be a systemic infection where skin abnormalities develop as a secondary complication, e.g. human immunodeficiency disease (HIV). HIV infection may lead to acquired immune disease (AIDS) which gives rise to unusual infections, e.g. histoplasmosis, and recurrent and extensive infections such as candidiasis, tinea and herpes simplex.

#### Verrucae (plantar warts)

Verrucae (Plate 21) are caused by infection of the skin with human papilloma virus (HPV). The virus affects the stratum spinosum and causes hyperplasia and formation of a benign tumour. In the early stages the lesion appears as a small, dark, translucent puncture mark in the skin. More mature lesions show thrombosed capillaries and a 'cauliflower-rough' surface; they are painful when pinched. The patient may complain of increased discomfort on starting to walk after a period of rest, e.g. first thing in the morning. Different types of HPV cause different wart lesions, e.g. flat, genital, plantar (Williams et al 1993). Unless verrucae occur on weightbearing surfaces they protrude above the level of the skin. Those that are found on weightbearing surfaces protrude into the skin and as a result are more painful. Mosaic warts are made up of multiple, small, tightly packed individual warts and may not be painful whereas plantar warts may be single or multiple and are usually painful.

Verrucae can usually be diagnosed from their clinical appearance. They can be confused with corns (particularly neurovascular or fibrous) and foreign bodies. Verrucae can occur on non-weightbearing and weightbearing areas of the foot, unlike corns and most foreign body injuries which occur solely on weightbearing areas. There may be multiple verrucae present, not only on the feet but also on the hands. Pinching the verrucae tends to cause a sharp pain whereas corns and foreign bodies give rise to pain on direct pressure. Verrucae appear encapsulated and the skin striae is broken; corns do not appear encapsulated and the skin striae are not broken but pushed to one side. A biopsy should be undertaken if malignancy is suspected.

### Hand, foot and mouth disease

This is caused by Coxsackievirus and usually affects children. Small, painful vesicles with erythematous halos occur on hands and feet and the buccal mucosa has aphthous-ulcer-type lesions. All lesions and the slight fever usually resolve in 4–8 days. The condition may be confused with pompholyx or herpes simplex. The comparatively short duration of this condition compared to pompholyx is a useful diagnostic indicator. With pompholyx there may be a history of eczema elsewhere and the buccal mucosa is not affected. Herpes simplex gives rise to many of the features of hand, foot and mouth disease and also has a short duration (14 days); however, it does tend to lead to recurrent attacks at the same site.

### Molluscum contagiosum

This is caused by a poxvirus and tends to be more common in children. Clusters of pearly, raised papules 1–2 mm in diameter, often with a depressed centre, appear on the trunk and less frequently on arms and legs. The condition may be confused with verrucae (warts) but the characteristic papules usually enable a clinical diagnosis to be made.

## Fungal

Fungal infection of the skin and nail may be a primary condition, secondary to a bacterial infection or associated with a systemic condition, e.g. diabetes mellitus. The dark, warm, moist environment found in most shod feet is an ideal breeding ground for fungi. The condition can be caused by a dermatophyte infection, e.g. *Trichophyton*, or a yeast infection, e.g. *Candida albicans*, of the keratinised layer of the epidermis.

### Tinea pedis (athlete's foot, fungal infection of the foot)

This condition may manifest on the feet in three ways:

- Interdigital skin may appear macerated (white) and soggy. There may be an unpleasant odour. Moist fissures may be present.
- Patches of skin, or all the skin of the foot, may be affected by recurrent vesicular eruptions. The area affected is itchy and red in colour. The instep is a common site for this type of tinea.
- The soles of the foot may appear dry and scaly. This is usually due to *Trichophyton rubrum*.

When the dermis is exposed the condition is painful and bacterial infection may develop. If the entire plantar surface of the foot is affected, the skin is mechanically weak and sore and fissures can develop. Fungal infections affecting the feet can provoke a secondary pompholyx-like eruption of the hands. Tinea pedis may be confused with dermatitis, psoriasis and erythrasma. A previous history of the complaint, positive laboratory report and resolution of the condition with the use of an appropriate antifungal permit a definite diagnosis to be made. Clinical features may be so obvious that skin scrapings are unnecessary.

### Onychomycosis

Roberts (1992) showed a prevalence of onychomycosis of 1.3% in the 16–34 year age group, 2.4% in the 35–50 age group and 4.7% in those aged 55 years or over. Onychomycosis can be classified into four distinct types:

- *Distal and lateral subungual*: This is the commonest type of dermatophyte onychomycosis. The distal end and side of the nail are affected.
- *Proximal subungual*: This is caused by a yeast infection and arises from the proximal part of the nail. It often occurs secondary to chronic paronychia.
- *Superficial white onychomycosis*: This results in the nail plate appearing white. The nail is affected distal to proximal. The condition is due to *Trichophyton mentagrophytes* and is relatively uncommon.
- *Total dystrophic*: In this type the appearance and texture of the whole nail is affected. It may arise as a consequence of any of the above types.

## Bacterial

Trauma to the foot can result in a break in the skin barrier and put the patient at increased risk of bacterial infection. Corns may become infected due to excessive stresses on the skin leading to tissue breakdown or as a sequel to over-zealous treatment. Those who neglect themselves or are unable to undertake routine footcare are predisposed to infections (Case history 9.2). Systemic conditions that manifest their complications in the foot, e.g. diabetes mellitus, make the foot more prone to infections and ulcerations. Bacterial infection of tissues usually causes an inflammatory response: redness, heat, swelling, pain and the production of pus. Some bacteria cause an acute inflammatory response, e.g. *Streptococcus, Staphylococcus*, while others cause chronic disease, e.g. *Mycobacterium leprae*.

---

**Case history 9.2**

On a home visit an elderly female patient was found to be wearing five layers of clothes. When the layers of stockings and socks had been removed a pair of macerated, acrid-smelling feet were exposed. The skin was deeply pitted, probably due to the keratolytic effects of *Corynebacterium* and/or urea (the patient was incontinent). All nails showed clinical features of paronychia. Beau's lines were present.

History taking revealed that the patient lived alone and had no relatives, friends or neighbours to help her. She had suffered from recurrent chronic infections. It was considered that these had caused the Beau's lines. Results of nail-fold swabs (culture and sensitivity) revealed the presence of *Pseudomonas*; this was likely to be responsible for the pungent odour.

Social services and the district nursing service attempted to improve the patient's living standards and personal hygiene via the home help service, meals on wheels, bath nurse and regular visits from the district nurse.

---

The status of the patient's immune system and general health will influence clinical features and recovery rate (Breathnach 1989). For example, patients on long-term steroids will not show a marked inflammatory response; those who are immunocompromised will not show the normal immunological response to infection. Bacterial infections of the foot should be closely monitored as they may spread and result in cellulitis, osteomyelitis, lymphangitis, lymphadenitis and septicaemia (Ch. 17). A swab should be sent for culture and sensitivity in order that the most appropriate antibiotic may be prescribed (Ch. 13).

## Paronychia

This is frequently due to *Candida albicans* (yeast) and/or *Pseudomonas* (Gram-negative bacillus). The nail bed is painful and inflamed, as are the tissues surrounding the nail. Some exudate may be evident. Paronychia is likely where there is a poor peripheral circulation and in immuno-compromised patients.

## Pitted keratolysis

This condition is due to the growth of organisms that digest keratin, e.g. *Corynebacterium*. It is prevalent in sweaty feet that are shod in occlusive footwear. The soles of the feet are affected by fine punched-out depressions coupled with an unpleasant smell.

## Erythrasma

This condition may arise interdigitally. It is due to diphtheroids, which produce porphyrins that fluoresce coral pink under Wood's light. The condition is usually symptom-free but examination of the toe webs will reveal wrinkled, slightly scaly skin which is either pink, brown or macerated in appearance.

## Erysipelas

This condition is caused by a streptococcal infection which enters a split in the skin, e.g. an interdigital fissure. The area becomes inflamed and has a well-defined advancing edge. Systemic features such as malaise, shivering and fever also occur.

## Necrotising fasciitis

This is a rare but rapidly progressive soft-tissue infection which affects the lower limb. It is due to a mixture of pathogens but usually involves streptococci and anaerobes. Early diagnosis is essential as the condition leads to extensive necrosis of the superficial fascia which can only be effectively treated by amputation.

# Infestations

## Scabies (Sarcoptes scabiei)

Close physical contact is required for transmission. After 4–6 weeks hypersensitivity to mite faeces causes itching to develop, particularly at night. Burrows occur on the sides of fingers and toes, wrists and insteps of the feet. The condition is very itchy; excoriations from scratching can lead to the development of secondary infection. A report of itching in a partner may be relevant to the diagnosis. Diagnosis can usually be reached as a result of the characteristic appearance of the burrows and the presence of the mite or ova, although the condition may be confused with eczema. Microscopy of scrapings of the affected area may demonstrate ova or the mature parasite.

## Fleas

These are parasites which can live on cats, dogs, rabbits and other mammals (human fleas are rare nowadays in the UK). The condition is characterised by pruritic, erythematous papules. Classically, the lesions are clustered, often around ankles as the flea can jump out of the carpet, have a meal, and jump back again. Diagnosis of the condition is via the history of the complaint and observation of the distribution of the lesions and is often aided by the patient's own theories. The clinical features of other insect bites and urticaria may be confused with flea bites.

## Ticks

These animal parasites are common and adhere to their host using a proteinaceous cement around their barbed mouth parts. Once their abdomens are swollen with blood (0.2–0.5 cm diameter or larger) someone with normal sensation and sight will readily see and feel them. Ticks are vectors for Lyme's disease (caused by a spirochaete, *Borrelia burgdorferi*). The symptoms of Lyme's disease include skin soreness, stiff and aching joints and palpitations.

## Insect bites/stings

Many insect bites/stings cause blistering. Usually

the patient is aware of the cause but may be surprised by the vigour of the skin's reaction. Frequently, an urticarial papule develops at the site of a bee sting.

## ASSESSMENT OF CUTANEOUS TUMOURS (BENIGN AND MALIGNANT)

Lumps and bumps on or in the skin need careful diagnosis. Many are benign (do not spread). As the mean age of the population increases, the fashion for a tanned skin continues and the ozone layer depletes, so the prevalence of malignant (spreads to other parts of the body) lesions or those with malignant potential increases. If a malignant lesion is suspected, urgent referral to a dermatologist is essential. Early management of malignancy improves the prognosis considerably. This is particularly important with malignant melanomas, which may metastasise within a short time period (Case history 9.3). Table 9.13 lists the benign and malignant neoplasms that can affect skin.

---

**Case history 9.3**

A mother read about malignancy and moles in a women's magazine and became particularly concerned about the spots on her teenage daughter's back and legs. These spots had developed since being on holiday in Spain. During the holiday the daughter had sunbathed intensively and had suffered from sunburn. The mother wished to consult someone about the likelihood of the moles becoming malignant and what action if any she should take.
This scenario frequently occurs as a result of media coverage of a health issue. With minimum detail and without the affected person being present, the practitioner is in a difficult position. In response to such a query the person should be urged to make an early appointment with their doctor. In this instance the practitioner gave this advice to the mother, discussed the features associated with malignant changes and gave relevant epidemiological information.

---

The skin may also be a marker of an underlying malignancy. A number of conditions are known to herald overt clinical symptoms of malignancy, e.g. acanthosis nigricans, where the

**Table 9.13**  Benign and malignant neoplasms that may affect the lower limb

| Benign | Malignant |
| --- | --- |
| Epidermoid cysts (implantation cysts) | Malignant melanoma |
| Fibroma, e.g. keloid | Bowen's disease |
| Freckles (ephelides, lentigines) | Squamous cell carcinoma |
| Glomus tumour | Kaposi's sarcoma |
| Subungual exostosis | Metastases |
| Melanocytic naevi | |
| Seborrhoeic warts | |
| Viral warts | |
| Lipoma | |
| Pyogenic granuloma | |

palms and soles become rough and thickened. A generalised pruritus can occur in late pregnancy or in old age, but in young people it may be associated with a malignancy such as Hodgkin's disease.

The practitioner should record the size, colour and topography of the lesion (is it flat, raised, warty?) so that changes over time can be evaluated. Photography including a measuring scale is helpful, otherwise size can be recorded by measuring the diameter of the lesion using a lesionometer, or by tracing around it on acetate or sticky tape which is then transferred to the patient's notes. Ultrasound imaging to record the depth of the lesion is useful (Nessi et al 1991, Harland et al 1993). If three or more of the following are noted malignant changes may have occurred:

- Pruritus
- Colour change
- Increase in size
- Irregular shape or surface
- Inflammation
- Ulceration
- Bleeding.

### Squamous cell carcinoma

This involves the epidermis and is usually associated with overexposure to ultraviolet light, topical carcinogens or irritation of chronic skin lesions, e.g. ulcers, warts, scars from lupus erythematosus. The early clinical features are varied (warty lesion, inflammation). Ulceration develops with a palpable infiltrated zone around the lesion. In the lower limb squamous cell carcinoma is likely to arise at the site of an existing lesion, e.g. venous ulcer or subungual ulceration. The practitioner should regularly monitor such lesions and be vigilant for any changes. In cases where there is concern a sample of tissue should be sent for histopathological testing (Ch. 13).

### Kaposi's sarcoma

Associated with acquired immunodeficiency syndrome (AIDS), this usually starts as small purple-brown tumours of proliferating blood vessels and connective tissue on feet or ankles. Oedema may be the first symptom. There is often extravasation and inflammation. The condition can look very similar to purpura. A biopsy should be undertaken to confirm the diagnosis.

### Malignant melanomas

This condition is on the increase. It is more prevalent in Caucasians with blond hair and fair skin who tan poorly. There is a higher incidence in females than males and in Caucasians who live near the equator than those who live in temperate zones. Patients should always be asked about holidays and their sunbathing practices or use of sun beds.

Malignant melanomas can arise from existing moles or spontaneously from apparently normal skin. Metastases form quickly via local infiltration and the lymphatic system, though occasionally it may be years before metastases become evident. Vertical spread as opposed to horizontal spread is of most importance. The prognosis is linked to the depth of the lesion (Breslow thickness). If the Breslow thickness is greater than 3.5 mm the prognosis is poor (40% chance of surviving 5 years).

Changes in the size, depth of pigmentation, extension of the pigmentation or an irregular halo around the lesion should be noted. The dif-

**Table 9.14**  Classification of the different types of malignant melanoma

| Type | Descriptor |
|---|---|
| Superficial spreading | Most common type in Caucasians. Noticeable variation in colour, usually palpable. Increases in diameter. Nodular development indicates dermal invasion. |
| Nodular melanoma | Most rapid growing of the malignant melanomas. Nodular in appearance. |
| Acral lentiginous melanoma | Occurs on palms and soles and in the subungual and periungual tissues. Irregular pigmented macule which becomes nodular when dermal invasion has occurred. Rare in Caucasians; more commonly found in Chinese and Japanese. |
| Lentigo maligna melanoma | Appears on exposed surfaces, usually in the elderly. Grows slowly and has an irregular shape and pigmentation. |

ferent types of malignant melanoma are described in Table 9.14.

The condition should be differentiated from seborrhoeic warts, inflammation in a benign pigmented naevus and subungual haematoma. Excision and biopsy and ultrasound imaging are essential (Nessi et al 1991, Harland et al 1993).

### Bowen's disease

This is an intraepidermal carcinoma and is classed as a carcinoma in situ. In other words it is usually benign but does have the capacity to turn malignant. The lesion is often found on the leg. It is slow-growing, usually singular, with a well-defined border, and may take years to reach a diameter of a few centimetres.

### Metastases (often of lymphosarcoma)

These involve purple-pink nodules within the skin which can occur at any site. Other symptoms include erythroderma and pruritus. Metastasis may be confused with erythema nodosum and naevi. A biopsy should be performed to classify the tumour.

## ASSESSMENT OF THE SKIN'S RESPONSE TO THE EXTERNAL ENVIRONMENT

The skin can be affected by a range of external factors:

- Topically applied chemicals
- Systemically administered chemicals (drugs, food)
- Sunlight
- Cold
- Heat
- Mechanical trauma
- Pathogenic organisms
- Infestations.

The effects of mechanical trauma and infections and infestations have already been discussed. This section will concentrate on the effects of the other external factors listed above.

When describing the skin's reaction to external factors it is important to differentiate between an irritant-type reaction and a hypersensitivity reaction. An irritant reaction occurs when a person is overexposed to a chemical, e.g. solvents or alkalis, or to such factors as powerful sunlight. As a result inflammation occurs. With an irritant reaction everyone exposed is affected although not everyone will react in exactly the same, there may be a range of reactions from severe to relatively mild.

Unlike an irritant reaction not everyone will be affected by a hypersensitivity reaction. Hypersensitivity reactions occur in those who are particularly sensitive to certain external factors (allergens). For example, some people are particularly sensitive to pollens (asthma and hay fever); however, the majority of the population are not. Gell & Coombs (1975) identified four types of hypersensitivity reaction; a fifth type was subsequently added (Table 9.15). These reactions can give rise to localised or systemic effects; the skin is often the primary organ to be affected.

The allergen (antigen) may be a topically applied substance (e.g. perfume, nickel, plant,

**Table 9.15** Types of hypersensitivity reaction

| Type | Reaction |
|---|---|
| I | An immediate reaction due to sensitisation of IgE antibodies, which are bound to mast cells and basophils. Leads to degranulation of mast cells and release of multifunctional lymphokines and cytokines. Response occurs on second or repeated exposure to the sensitising antigen. May cause a general or local response. General anaphylaxis can be fatal. |
| II | Antibodies react with surface antigens on cells resulting in injury to the cell and subsequent complement activation and phagocytosis. May be autoimmune (body no longer recognises self; transplants or due to drug reaction). Presence of skin reaction is dependent upon cells affected. For example, if red blood cells or platelets affected may lead to purpura. |
| III | Caused by reaction of antibody with corresponding soluble antigen, which leads to the deposition of immune complexes. Can result in a general (serum sickness) or a local (Arthus) reaction. Local reactions include vasculitis and rheumatoid nodules as seen in rheumatoid arthritis. |
| IV | Delayed reaction (12–24 h) due to a cell-mediated (T-cell) response to macrophage-bound antigen. Often due to haptens crossing the skin barrier, e.g. contact dermatitis, response to tuberculin bacillus. |
| V | Antibody reacts with a cell surface component such as hormone receptor and 'switches' on the cell, e.g. Graves disease (thyrotoxicosis). |

animal protein) or something systemic, such as food (e.g. nuts, crab) or drugs (e.g. penicillin). The body's reaction to the allergen may be immediate (anaphylaxis) or delayed so that the reaction reaches a maximum after 24–72 hours (delayed hypersensitivity).

The clinical features associated with allergic reactions will vary depending upon the cause and the site of administration of the allergen.

### Photosensitivity

Only skin exposed to sunlight will show a response. UVB (wavelength 280–320 nm) causes sunburn and potentiates malignancy; UVA (320–400 nm) has an adverse effect only on photosensitive skin. Signs and symptoms range from acute erythema, oedema and blistering to chronic changes, e.g. solar keratosis, where early aging of the skin occurs. Photosensitive patients are usually adult and have erythematous papules or urticarial symptoms of varying severity. Some plants, e.g. hemlock, and some drugs, e.g. thiazides and sulphonamides, dyes and perfumes, can photosensitise the skin (increase the skin's reaction to sunlight).

### Contact dermatitis

Contact dermatitis (Plate 22) is due to a cell-mediated (Type IV) hypersensitivity reaction. A range of allergens may be responsible, e.g. nickel, plants, rubber, lanolin, dyes, perfumes, and preservatives in creams and ointments. The skin reacts to the allergen at the site of application; contact dermatitis to shoe adhesives and dyes occurs along the 'slipper-line'. The quality of the skin barrier is important in that if the skin is very moist the percutaneous absorption of substances is enhanced and an allergen can reach responsive tissues more readily (Barry 1989, Walters 1990).

### Juvenile plantar dermatitis

Perpetual or prolonged contact with an allergen may cause chronic contact dermatitis/eczema (Plate 23). Juvenile plantar dermatosis is thought to be a variant of contact dermatitis. It leads to erythema, scaling and sometimes fissuring of the skin (Ead 1992). Differential diagnoses include tinea infection, psoriasis and adverse drug reaction. Patch testing can be used to identify the allergen.

### Drug reactions

Hypersensitivity reactions to drugs may give rise to a range of clinical features:

- Maculopapular rash
- Urticaria and angio-oedema
- Contact dermatitis
- Erythema multiforme
- Toxic epidermal necrolysis
- Fixed drug reaction
- Vasculitis and purpura
- Erythema nodosum.

A maculopapular eruption (exanthematous) is probably the most common response. Urticaria (nettle-rash, hives) is quite common and is characterised by pruritic weals. It may be due to a type I hypersensitivity reaction, in which case the weals arise very rapidly, or to a type III hypersensitivity reaction, in which case it is associated with angio-oedema. Urticaria can occur anywhere on the body but particularly the limbs and trunk. The raised weals may appear white or red according to the stage of formation and may persist for a few minutes to a number of hours (usually resolving within 48 hours).

Vasculitis and purpura occur as a result of a type III hypersensitivity reaction where immune complexes are deposited in blood vessels. Vasculitis leads to painful, palpable purpura. Crops of these lesions appear in particular on the legs and arms.

Erythema multiforme, as the name implies, can present in a number of different ways. Typically, non-scaling macules appear on the palms, soles, arms and legs. Stevens–Johnson syndrome is a severe form of erythema multiforme.

Erythema nodosum is an inflammation of subcutaneous fat (panniculitis). It occurs as a result of an immunological reaction to a variety of stimuli, including drugs. The condition appears as large painful dusky plaques on the shins.

Toxic epidermal necrosis is a very distressing disease where the skin becomes red and intensely painful and then begins to come off in sheets.

## ASSESSMENT OF DISORDERS OF THE EPIDERMIS

Congenital and acquired disorders can affect the epidermis, the following affect the lower limb.

### Ichthyosis

A generalised condition where the skin is dry, scaling and unpliable, often with hyperkeratosis of knees and elbows. There are a number of variants of this condition. Ichthyosis tylosis affects the palms and soles (Plate 24). Clinical features vary according to the severity of the disorder. In severe cases fissures occur due to the limited flexibility of the skin, these extend into the dermis. Differential diagnoses include exfoliative dermatitis and in later life Hodgkin's disease and carcinoma.

## Darier's disease

This is an inherited disorder that causes changes in nails and skin. Wart-like, red-brown papules develop on the dorsum of hands and feet and trunk. Some hyperkeratosis may occur on palmar and plantar skin. White longitudinal bands form on nails. Differential diagnosis includes warts and Reiter's disease. A biopsy should be performed.

## Eczema

Generally the term 'dermatitis' is reserved for conditions where the aetiology is known, while 'eczema' is applied to conditions with an unknown aetiology. Eczema can be classified according to whether it is due to an exogenous or endogenous cause and whether it is acute or chronic (McGibbon 1983). Acute eczema is characterised by a combination of some or all of the following: pruritus, erythema, oedema, papules, vesicles, exudate. Infection is a secondary complication. Chronic eczema is less vesicular and exudative and is characterised by dry, scaly, pigmented skin. Lichenification, dry, thickened skin resembling leather with increased skin markings, secondary to repeated scratching and rubbing, is common.

The clinical features associated with different types of eczema are outlined in Table 9.16.

## Lichen planus

This is a chronic condition of unknown aetiology which occurs most commonly in young to middle-aged people. The clinical features are intensely itchy, flat-topped, shiny, violaceous papules with a white-lace-type surface (Wickham's striae) frequently found on wrists, ankles, forearms, in the lumbar region and at sites of trauma (Koebner phenomenon). On palms and soles the condition may occur as hyperkeratosis. If the nails are involved they show longitudinal ridging. Differ-

**Table 9.16** Types of eczema

| Type | Clinical features |
|---|---|
| Discoid | Affects females more than males. Initially acute but develops into chronic multiple patches of coin-shaped lesions on the trunk and limbs. |
| Seborrhoeic | Most common in adults but can affect infants. Red scaly lesions appear on the scalp, eyebrows, axillae, groin and ear. |
| Gravitational | Occurs as a result of venous insufficiency. Haemosiderosis, telangiectasia, petechiae and atrophie blanche are usually precursors. Very itchy skin may appear scaly or lichenified. May lead to ulceration. |
| Pompholyx | Affects palms and soles. Can be associated with eczema on other parts of the body. Usually an acute form with vesicles and bullae, may extend to digits and dorsum of the foot. |
| Contact dermatitis | Unlike the other types of eczema this is due to exogenous causes. The distribution of the lesions relates to the area that has come into contact with the external agent. Initially acute but on prolonged exposure becomes lichenified. Usually very pruritic. |
| Atopic | Usually appears after three months of age. Familial tendency. Affects flexural surfaces, face, hands, wrists and feet. May also appear on the trunk. Initially shows acute features but eventually becomes lichenified (chronic). May resolve during adolescence or progress into adulthood. Linked with 'atopy' syndrome which involves asthma, hay fever and food allergies. |
| Asteatotic | Dry, atrophic and cracked skin. Very pruritic. Occurs in the elderly especially in winter. |
| Juvenile plantar dermatitis | Cause unclear—probably chronic contact dermatitis. The skin of the soles of the feet, especially weightbearing areas, become dry and shiny and develop fissures. The toes' webs are usually spared. |

ential diagnoses include lichenified eczema, some drug eruptions and guttate psoriasis. Investigations are usually unnecessary as a diagnosis can normally be made through the clinical appearance.

## Psoriasis

Psoriasis is a chronic, non-infectious, inflammatory condition of the skin of unknown aetiology. It is rare under 10 years of age and commonest between 15 and 40 years. It follows an unpredictable course but is usually chronic with exacerbations and remissions. The clinical features associated with different types of psoriasis are summarised in Table 9.17. Koebner's phenomenon and Auspitz's sign are common findings. Psoriatic lesions may be itchy. Of particular interest to the practitioner dealing with the lower limb are psoriatic nails, pustular psoriasis (Plate 25), acral psoriasis and psoriatic arthritis.

Differential diagnosis requires accurate observation of lesion distribution and includes eczema, pityriasis rosea and fungal infection. Hyperkeratotic psoriasis on the soles of the feet may be confused with lichen planus, anhidrotic callus plaques and Reiter's disease. Mycosis fungoides may show pruritic, scaly plaques but should respond to fungicides.

## ASSESSMENT OF BLISTERING DISORDERS

*Vesicles* are fluid-filled sacs less than 0.5 cm in diameter and *bullae* fluid-filled sacs greater than 0.5 cm in diameter. *Blister* is a common term, often used to describe a fluid-filled sac larger than a vesicle but smaller than a bulla. Blisters are classified as to their position in the epidermis.

- *Superficial*: These blisters occur in the stratum corneum and are associated with infections, e.g. tinea pedis
- *Intraepidermal*: These occur in the lower layers of the epidermis, usually the stratum spinosum, and are associated with, for example, acute eczema and viral vesicles
- *Sub epidermal*: These occur at the dermal–epidermal junction and are associated with, for example, epidermolysis bullosa and bullous pemphigoid.

Blisters may occur on the lower limb as a result of a variety of factors (Table 9.18). The soles of the feet are especially prone to developing traumatic blisters. Secondary infection is a common complication.

**Table 9.17** Types of psoriasis

| Type | Description |
| --- | --- |
| Discoid (classic plaque) | Usually affects extensor surfaces with symmetrical distribution. Lesions appear as well demarcated papules/plaques which can be regular or irregular in shape and have a reddish-brown to salmon hue. Scales, silvery white in colour, appear. The condition has periods of remission. The appearance can resemble ringworm. |
| Guttate | Characterised by a crop of evenly distributed pink-red papules which appear on the trunk. It is often preceded by an upper respiratory infection. The lesions may be itchy. After 2–3 weeks can develop into discoid eczema. It usually clears but can become chronic. |
| Flexural | Common in the elderly. Localised to body folds, e.g. beneath the breast. Due to the site, scales are rubbed off, so lesions appear smooth and glazed. |
| Pustular | Usually seen in middle age and more common in women than men. It is usually chronic and intractable. Localised to palms and soles, usually symmetrical. Sterile yellow-white pustules, known as Monro's abscesses, may be seen. |
| Rupoid | Rare type of pustular psoriasis characterised by an extreme thickening of the palms and soles, although it can appear elsewhere. |
| Acral | Very rare form of psoriasis that starts at the fingertips and simulates paronychia in appearance. Digits become progressively involved, leading to disability and discomfort. |
| Nail | Only the nails may be affected or there may be a combination of skin and nails affected. Affects nails in various ways: pitting, onycholysis, onychauxis, discolouration, onychomadesis. |
| Erythrodermic | Localised psoriasis lesions become universal. Skin becomes erythematous and oedematous. The itching and discomfort is considerable. Exfoliation may be negligible or profuse. Causes systemic problems and thermoregulation is affected. |
| Generalised pustular (von Zumbusch's syndrome) | Rare condition that has a dramatic onset. Patient initially suffers from nausea, which develops into a fever. Bright red, burning lesions appear with pustules. |
| Arthritis | Inflammatory polyarthritis seen in approximately 6% of psoriasis sufferers. Affects the terminal IPJs, wrists and the spine. Can be destructive and lead to loss of joint motion. |

**Table 9.18**  Causes of blistering disorders

| Cause | Clinical features |
| --- | --- |
| Adverse drug reaction | Type of blistering depends upon the reaction: urticaria, bullae, vesicles. |
| Bullous pemphigoid | Autoimmune disease that produces subepidermal blisters. Chronic condition, which arises in the elderly. Tense bullae form, especially on flexural surfaces. |
| Epidermolysis bullosa | Genetically determined disorder of which there are at least seven types. Epidermolysis bullosa simplex is the commonest type; large tense bullae appear on the soles and palms in relation to trauma. In its severest form, dystrophic epidermolysis bullosa, large flaccid bullae appear spontaneously. The whole body is affected, including mucous membranes; the condition can be fatal. |
| Friction | Most common reason for blisters to appear on the foot. Blisters of varying size may develop, usually intraepidermal. |
| Hand, foot and mouth disease | Due to viral infection. Produces vesicles on the affected parts. |
| Photosensitivity | Reaction to excessive exposure to ultraviolet light. May produce large bullae. |
| Pompholyx | Vesicles appear around fingers and toes and on the palms and soles. |
| Pustular psoriasis | Sterile yellow-white pustules appear, known as microabscesses of Monro. |
| Tinea pedis | May lead to intensely pruritic crops of vesicles in the arch of the foot or on the dorsum. |
| Dermatitis herpetiformis | Chronic subepidermal blistering disease in which vesicles erupt in groups, as in herpes simplex. Very itchy. Vesicles appear on elbows, knees, buttocks and shoulders. |
| Pemphigus | Autoimmune condition that produces flaccid blisters which initially arise in the mouth. There are various types: pemphigus vulgaris is the most common. |
| Stevens–Johnson syndrome | Rare form of erythema multiforme which involves blister formation. |
| Eczema | Acute forms of eczema will show vesicles which erupt and weep. |

# ASSESSMENT OF CONNECTIVE TISSUE DISORDERS

Many connective tissue disorders are due to autoimmune diseases. They lead to acute and chronic (more common) changes of connective tissue; the skin, joints and other organs may be affected.

## Ehlers–Danlos syndrome

This is an inherited, generalised, connective-tissue defect (Hobson 1994). Signs and symptoms include hyperelasticity of skin, hyper-extensibility of the joints, fragile blood vessels and easy bruising. Differential diagnosis includes Marfan's syndrome and cutis laxa. With Ehlers–Danlos the skin is soft and usually recoils after being pulled; this does not occur in cutis laxa.

## Neurofibromatosis (von Recklinghausen's disease)

This is an inherited disorder which affects 1 in 3000 people. The Schwann cells of cutaneous nerves are affected. Signs and symptoms include oval or round fawn-coloured macules in the skin (café au lait spots), axillary freckling and neuro-fibromas. Neurofibromas may be few or many and some are visible within the skin. The condition is usually benign but may become malignant. Differential diagnoses includes freckles and fibromas. Freckles in the axillae are generally held to be a diagnostic feature.

## Lupus erythematosus (LE)

This condition may affect the skin only (discoid), be associated with some internal problems (disseminated discoid LE) or be a multisystem disorder (systemic lupus erythematosus). It predominantly affects women; the aetiology is unknown. Clinical features include a blotchy, symmetrical butterfly rash across the face, scattered maculopapular lesions, telangiectasia, petechiae (round purple spots caused by capillary haemorrhage), purpura, Raynaud's phenomenon, splinter haemorrhages, vasculitis and urticaria on legs. Systemically it may lead to fever, nephritis, polyarteritis, pericarditis, endocarditis and involvement of the central nervous system. The condition should be differentiated from rheumatoid arthritis, chronic renal disease, adverse drug reaction and chilblains. The history provides important indications. Diagnostic tests involve blood profile and biochemistry.

### Systemic sclerosis (scleroderma)

This condition is characterised by thickening of the connective tissue; it can affect any part of the body. The skin becomes shiny, hard and taut and may be hyperpigmented with telangiectasia and calcinosis. The skin feels as if it is tightly tied to deeper tissues and lacks resilience and recoil. Nails are atrophied and may shed. Raynaud's phenomenon is common as is sclerodactylia (clawing and tapering of the fingers). Small digital ischaemic ulcers may be evident in severe cases. Localised patches of firm, ivory-coloured skin may be called scleroderma, localised scleroderma or morphoea. Facial features are affected: the nose becomes pinched and beak-like and the mouth small and taut; telangiectasia appear on the face. Eventually the lungs, heart and gut are involved. The condition needs to be differentiated from rheumatoid arthritis and ischaemia. The presence of calcinosis may be confused with gouty tophi. Diagnostic tests involve blood profile and biochemistry.

### Sarcoidosis

This chronic condition of unknown aetiology may be systemic or localised to the skin. In those who develop systemic sarcoidosis approximately a third also have skin problems. Dermatological features include brownish-red papules within the skin, erythema nodosum on the anterior shins and chilblains; old scars may show signs of sarcoid papules. Erythema nodosum may be caused by a number of other factors, e.g. streptococcal infection, ulcerative colitis and drug reaction (sulphonamides).

### Erythema multiforme

This may be caused by drugs, infections, preg-nancy or be due to unknown causes. It is often recurrent and in its severe form can be chronic. Initially red macules appear on dorsal and palmar/plantar surfaces, knees, elbows and forearms; these turn into purple 'target' or iris lesions with an erythematous margin. Differential diagnoses include pemphigoid and toxic erythema.

## ASSESSMENT OF SKIN CONDITIONS ASSOCIATED WITH SYSTEMIC DISEASES

A number of systemic disorders may affect the skin and its appendages; the dermatological conditions which develop as a consequence often aid the diagnosis of the primary disorder (Table 9.19). A skin condition secondary to a systemic disorder usually shows generalised effects, e.g. jaundice (yellowish skin) indicative of a liver disorder. However, a systemic disorder may lead

**Table 9.19** Examples of manifestation of systemic diseases in the skin

| Disease/disorder | Conditions |
| --- | --- |
| Diabetes mellitus | Necrobiosis lipoidica, granuloma annulare, Mycotic infections, bacterial infections, xanthoma, neuropathic/ischaemic ulcers, necrosis, dermopathy |
| Chronic liver disease | Pruritus associated with jaundice; spider naevi, white nails, xanthoma, palmar erythema |
| Chronic renal disease | Dry skin, pale and/or shallow yellow colour, half and half nail, pruritus |
| Rheumatoid arthritis | Purpura, vasculitis, fingertip infarcts, periungual erythema, splinter haemorrhage, rheumatoid nodules, ulceration |
| Internal malignancy | Generalised pruritus, acanthosis nigricans, acquired hypertrichosis languinosa |
| Deficiency states: Iron deficiency Vitamin $B_6$ and $B_7$ deficiency Vitamin C deficiency | Dry skin, pruritus Koilonychia Eczema Purpura, ulceration, poor healing |
| Hyperthyroidism | Hyperhidrotic skin, pretibial myxoedema, hair loss, itching and urticaria |
| Hypothyroidism | Sparse hair, dry skin, xanthoma |
| Hyperlipidaemia | Xanthoma |
| Reiter's syndrome | Keratoderma blenhorragica |

to secondary dermatological features which are site-specific, e.g. blistering of the hand in hand, foot and mouth disease and koilonychia in chronic iron deficiency anaemia.

## SUMMARY

There is no point assessing a patient's skin unless the information is to be used to benefit the patient. Usually patients welcome any effort to clear their dermatoses; however, before treatment can be commenced the condition must first be diagnosed. The diagnosis is formulated from all the data gathered from the assessment and the practitioner's knowledge of dermatoses (Case history 9.4).

Epidemiological, information such as age profile and gender may help to reduce the list of likely conditions. Results from observation, clinical tests and special investigations will also help to reduce the list of possible conditions. In most instances, the diagnosis will become obvious, but on occasions it may not be possible to reach a definitive diagnosis. In this case a provisional

---

**Case history 9.4**

A new patient appeared to have psoriatic lesions on the legs and feet. This immediate clinical observation was followed by asking the patient her reason for consultation. The patient complained of a sore lesion on the top of her second toe and recurrent painful toe nails. A brief inspection revealed a slightly red hyperkeratotic dorsal lesion on the IPJ of a hammered second toe. The nails appeared thickened and discoloured.

The purpose of the clinical assessment was explained. Questions were phrased with tact and sensitivity because the patient appeared to be embarrassed about the skin complaint on her legs; she said a lot of people considered her to be 'infectious'.

The patient's general health was assessed as being good and she was not taking any current medication. The systems enquiry did not detect any abnormality. The footwear was ill-fitting; short and narrow in the toe box. Assessment of the locomotor system revealed that there was abnormal pronation during gait which was considered to be due to compensation for a rearfoot varus. It was decided that it was inappropriate to check urine glucose levels as the clinical features and history were not indicative of diabetes mellitus.

From the information obtained it was deduced that the complaint was not a systemic but a local problem. Examination of the complaints (sore toe and nails) showed psoriatic-type lesions with an area of macerated hyperkeratosis. The nails were pitted, discoloured and slightly thickened. The toe lesion had an erythematous periphery; debridement of the superficial callus revealed tissue breakdown (grade 5 lesion). The diameter was measured (US imaging and skin temperature measurement would have been useful if available). Details of the conditions, descriptive and quantitative, were noted.

The skin lesion on the toe could be psoriatic in origin. Psoriasis can give rise to mechanically weak tissue, less able to withstand the stresses imposed on it by abnormal function and tight footwear, hence development of the tissue breakdown. Alternatively, it could be due to tinea pedis, chronic chilling, erythrasma or dermatitis artefacta. The clinical features did not indicate chronic chilling (no scaling of the skin or cyanotic discolouration), dermatitis artefacta (the site could not be easily reached, nor did the patient's demeanour suggest any such problem) or erythrasma (the erythema was not marked and the site was unusual for this condition). There was no evidence of tinea-pedis-type lesions elsewhere; skin scrapings from the lesion might have helped the diagnosis but this would have been a costly exercise when the clinical features suggested the condition was not mycotic in origin.

The peri-lesion erythema was low-grade, which suggested an aseptic tissue breakdown. The patient's general health was good and a marked inflammatory reaction would be expected if infection had been present. Therefore, it was decided that a microbiological swab was also unnecessary. There were numerous psoriatic-type lesions on the leg and elsewhere on the foot and the patient admitted to the condition being a little more severe than normal.

The nail condition may be onychauxis, onychomycosis, psoriatic, hypertrophy associated with eczema or Darier's disease. This last condition could be discarded as there were no other clinical features to support it. The clinical features and history make differential diagnosis between onychauxis, onychomycosis and psoriatic nails difficult. Inspection of the finger nails provided no further clues: these nails appeared normal. As the patient was concerned about the nails, nail scrapings were taken in order to ascertain whether mycelia or yeasts were present. The results of these tests were negative; however, it is possible that this was a false negative. The prognosis for onychauxis and psoriatic hypertrophied nails is poor.

It was then decided the toe lesion was primarily psoriatic in origin. The assessment data suggested that the prognosis for healing of the breakdown was good but might be complicated by psoriasis. A definite diagnosis for the nail condition could not be made: it might be due to trauma (prime cause of onychauxis) or psoriasis.

diagnosis has to be made and the cycle of the disease process must be awaited for further enlightenment. Where a diagnosis is not available the practitioner may decide to treat the symptoms. Occasionally the effect of a treatment can be a diagnostic aid in itself, e.g. a vesicular eruption that resolves with use of an antifungal implies that the aetiology was mycotic. When a condition is diagnosed, the practitioner must decide what action is necessary. The practitioner will use clinical judgement to determine which form of management is required.

## REFERENCES

Barry B W 1989 Percutaneous absorption: transdermal drug delivery systems. In: Marks R, Edwards C, Barton S P (eds) The physical nature of skin. MTP, Lancaster, p 91–100

Blank I 1952 Factors which influence water content of stratum corneum. Journal of Investigative Dermatology 18: 433–408

Breathnach S 1989 Skin as an immunological barrier. In: Marks R, Edwards C, Barton S P (eds) The physical nature of skin. MTP, Lancaster, p 55–60

Burge S M 1989 Darier's disease and other dyskeratoses: response to retinoids. In MacKie R M (ed) Retinoids. Pergamon Press, Oxford

Carter S A 1993 Elective foot surgery in limbs with arterial disease. Clinical Orthopaedics 289: 228–236

Cavenagh P J, Hewitt F G, Perry J E 1992 In-shoe pressure measurement: a review. Foot 2(4): 185–194

Ead R D 1992 Skin disorders in infancy and childhood. Update 1 June: 1009–1022

Ferguson J 1980 Structural and mechanical properties of human stratum corneum. PhD thesis, University of Strathclyde

Finlay A Y 1989 Physical properties and function of nails. In: Marks R, Edwards C, Barton S P (eds) The physical nature of skin. MTP, Lancaster

Finlay A Y 1992 Social aspects of skin disease. Update 15 Jan: 99–101

Gell P, Coombs R, Lachmann (eds) 1975 Clinical aspects of immunology, 3rd edn. Blackwell Scientific, Oxford

Gillet du P 1973 Dorsal digital corns. Chiropodist July

Harland C C, Bamber J C, Gusterson B A, Mortimer P S 1993 High frequency, high resolution B-scan ultrasound in the assessment of skin tumours British Journal of Dermatology 128(5): 525–532

Helfand A E 1993 Onychial disorders in the older patient. In: Helfand A (ed) Clinics in podiatric medicine and surgery, the geriatric patient and considerations of ageing, vol 1. W B Saunders, Philadelphia, PA

Hobson K 1994 Ehlers–Danlos syndrome: a review of the literature with special reference to podiatric implications. British Journal of Podiatric Medicine 49(1): 9–13

Leveque J L, Corcuff P, de Rigal J, Agache P 1984 In vivo studies of the evolution of physical properties of the human skin with age. International Journal of Dermatology 23(5): 322–329

McGibbon D 1983 Dermatology—eczema. Pulse 10: 37–42

McKay I A, Leigh M I 1991 Epidermal cytokines and their roles in cutaneous wound healing. British Journal of Dermatology 124: 216–220

Mackenzie I C 1983 Effects of frictional stimulation of the structure of the stratum corneum. In: Marks R, Plewig G (eds) The stratum corneum. Springer-Verlag, Berlin, p 153–160

Manusov E G and Nadeau M T 1989 Hyperhydrosis: a management dilemma. Journal of Family Practice 28(4): 412–415

Merriman L, Griffiths C, Tollafield D 1986 Plantar lesion patterns. Chiropodist 42: 145–148

Millington P F, Wilkinson R 1983 Biological structure and function: 9. Skin. Cambridge University Press, Cambridge

Nessi R, Blanc M, Bosco M, Dameno S, Venegoni A, Betti R, Bencini P, Crosti C, Uslenghi C 1991 Skin ultrasound in dermatological surgical planning. Jourrnal of Dermatology, Surgery and Oncology 17(1): 38–43

Odland G 1983 Structure of skin. In: Goldsmith L (ed) The biochemistry and physiology of the skin. Oxford University Press, Oxford, p 3–63

O'Halloran N 1990 A biochemical investigation into the cholesterol content of seed corns. BSc dissertation, University of Brighton

Potts R O 1986 Stratum corneum hydration: experimental techniques and interpretation of results. Journal of the Society of Cosmetic Chemists 37: 9–33

Roberts D T 1992 Prevalence of dermatophyte onychomycosis in the United Kingdom: results of an omnibus survey. British Journal of Dermatology 39: 23–27

Ryan T 1983 Cutaneous circulation. In: Goldsmith L (ed) The biochemistry and physiology of the skin. Oxford University Press, Oxford, p 817–876

Samman P D 1986 Nail deformities due to trauma. In: Samman P D, Fenton D A (eds) The nails in disease, 4th edn. William Heinemann Medical Books, London

Sims D S, Cavenagh and Ulbrecht J S 1988 Risk factors in the diabetic foot. Recognition and management. Physical Therapy 68: 1887–1902

Smith L 1989 Histopathologic characteristics and ultrastructre of ageing skin. Cutis 5: 414–424

Smith T J, Morrison D C 1990 Further developments in the use of electrosurgery for the treatment of heloma durum. Chiropodist 45: 67–68

Springett K P 1993 The influence of forces generated during gait on the clinical appearance and physical properties of skin callus. PhD thesis, University of Brighton

Thomas S, Dykes P, Marks R 1985 Plantar hyperkeratoses: a study of callosities and normal plantar skin. Journal of Investigative Dermatology 85: 394–397

Walters K 1990 Penetration enhancers and their use in transdermal therapeutic systems. In: Hadgraft D, Guy R (eds) Transdermal drug delivery systems. Marcel Dekker, New York, p 197–246

Wertz P, Downing D 1990 Hadgraft D, Guy R (eds) Transdermal drug delivery systems. Marcel Dekker, New York, p 1–22

Whiting M F 1987 Survey of patients of large employer in S E England and Dept of Podiatry, University of Brighton. Unpublished, protected data

Williams H C, Pottier A and Strachan D 1993 The descriptive epidemiology of warts in British school children. British Journal of Dermatology 128(5): 504–511

Wright N A 1983 The cell proliferation kinetics of the epidermis. In: Goldsmith L (ed) The biochemistry and physiology of the skin. Oxford University Press, Oxford, p 203–229

## FURTHER READING

Bunney M H, Benton C, Cubie H A 1992 Viral warts: biology and treatment, 2nd edn. Oxford University Press, Oxford

Fry L, Wojnarowska F, Shahrad P 1985 Illustrated encyclopaedia of dermatology, 2nd edn. MTP Press, Lancaster

Graham-Brown R, Burns T 1990 Lecture notes on dermatology, 6th edn. Blackwell Scientific Publications, Oxford

Holdbrook K 1983 Structure of the developing human skin. In: Goldsmith L (ed) The biochemistry and physiology of the skin. Oxford University Press, Oxford

Levene G M, Calnan C D 1974 A colour atlas of dermatology. Wolfe Medical Publications, London

Lovell C R, Maddison P F 1992 Rheumatoid arthritis and the skin. In: Champion R H, Pye R J (eds) Dermatology. Churchill Livingstone, Edinburgh

Marks R, Edwards C, Barton S, 1989 The physical nature of skin. MTP, Lancaster

Roberts D T, Evans E G V, Allen B R 1990 Fungal nail infection. Gower Medical Publishing, London

Vasarinsh P 1982 Clinical dermatology. Butterworths, Boston, MA

Wood E J, Bladon P T 1987 The human skin. Studies in Biology 164. Edward Arnold, London

# 10

# Footwear assessment

*J. R. Hughes*

## INTRODUCTION

Assessment of footwear and hosiery is important as many foot health problems are associated with the foot coverings. Additionally, examination of the footwear can confirm a diagnosis or occasionally suggest a pathology which might not otherwise have been considered.

Effective footwear assessment depends upon the ability to differentiate a suitable from an unsuitable shoe. To do this it is necessary to understand the function of the different parts of a shoe and the properties of the materials used in their construction. This chapter therefore begins with a section about footwear before the methods of assessment are described in detail.

Well-fitting shoes are an essential part of the treatment of foot problems and the ability to assess fit is therefore an important tool. Several methods of measuring fit are described together with some simple observations. The ability to read the pattern of wear on a shoe is a skill that can be used to assess how the foot functions within the shoe. Some of the common patterns are described. It is hoped that this chapter will stimulate the reader to observe footwear and understand its significance.

## Why assess footwear?

Assessment of footwear is essential in the investigation of foot problems for many reasons. Perhaps the most important of these is that shoes give valuable information about how the foot functions during gait. It complements the assessment of the locomotor system (Ch. 8), much of which relies on barefoot observations, by assessing the way the foot functions during daily activity, i.e. wearing shoes. Examination of the wear and crease marks of footwear can be an aid to diagnosis as well as helping to complete the global picture. Another reason for the importance of footwear assessment is that unsuitable footwear can affect the efficacy of treatment or help to prolong a condition which might be alleviated by suitable shoes. In some instances shoes are the cause of the problem and effective treatment will consist simply of suggesting alternative shoes.

Footwear is often neglected by practitioners and its assessment has not always been given the attention it deserves. This type of assessment is more of an art than a science and relies heavily on the experience of the observer. Gaining this experience is complicated by the enormous range of footwear that is available and the many different methods of construction.

Observations of shod and unshod populations in the literature demonstrate that the unshod populations have fewer foot deformities than those who wear shoes. Research has also shown that when members of an unshod population start to wear shoes the incidence of foot problems increases. There is no experimental evidence showing that footwear is the cause but it is clearly implicated.

Simple observation reveals that some feet survive even the most unsuitable footwear. The feet that survive unscathed are probably those with good bone structure and foot function. However, it can be assumed that for some feet inappropriate shoes will certainly cause deformity. Patients with foot deformity often report similar symptoms in relatives but note that they were not present as children.

The shoes most likely to cause problems are those which do not fit well or are in some way unsuitable. Well-fitting, suitable shoes should always be encouraged.

While the basic function of footwear is protection both from hard and rough surfaces and from the cold, the appearance is often more important to the wearer. Patients exhibit strong resistance to change where their footwear is concerned. Many patients, particularly female, choose to ignore advice regarding sensible footwear, believing that what they consider to be an elegant appearance is more important than foot comfort. It is the author's experience that patients are more receptive to footwear advice if the reasons for changing from high-heeled court shoes to lace-ups can be explained. They are also more likely to believe that their shoes are too small when this is demonstrated by a few simple tests. It is important, however, not to be too dogmatic regarding patients' shoes. Advice is more likely to be accepted if it is made clear that smart shoes can still be worn for special occasions.

## THE 'ANATOMY' OF THE SHOE

Figure 10.1A shows the parts that make up an average lace-up shoe. The components can be grouped into those that make up the upper and those which form the sole. They are described individually below. Additionally there are areas which need reinforcement. These are highlighted in Figure 10.1B and described under the area they reinforce.

**Vamp.** The upper is made of two main sections which are together moulded into the shape of the top of the shoe. The front section, which covers the forefoot and toes, is called the vamp. In some shoes the vamp is made of more than one piece, creating a decorative pattern; however, seams other than those joining the main sections are not recommended as they limit stretchability and may rub bony prominences. The vamp is usually reinforced anteriorly by the toe puff, which maintains the shape of this section and protects the toes. In safety shoes this area is reinforced with steel to protect the toes from crushing injury. This reinforcement can be the cause of toe problems if it does not fit well.

**Quarter.** The sides and back of the shoe upper are termed the quarters and their top edge forms the topline of the shoe. The medial and lateral sections often join in a seam at the centre of the heel. In lace-up shoes the eyelets for the laces form the anterior part of this section while the

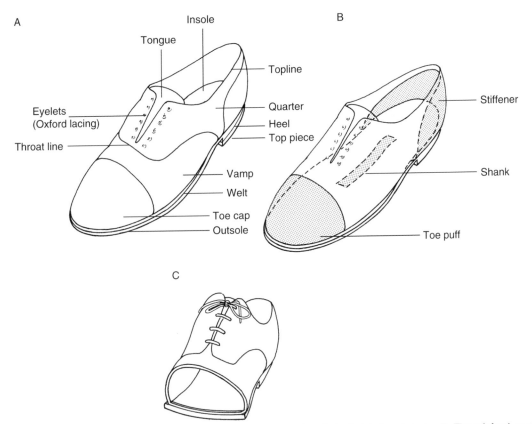

**Figure 10.1** **A.** The 'anatomy' of a lace-up shoe, showing the parts of an Oxford-style laced shoe **B.** The reinforcing within a shoe **C.** Alternative (Gibson) style of lacing.

tongue is attached to the vamp (Oxford style) or forms part of the vamp (Gibson style, Fig. 10.1C). The inside of the quarter is usually reinforced around the heel by the stiffener. This helps to stabilise the hindfoot in the shoe. In some children's shoes and some athletic footwear the stiffener is extended on the medial side to help resist pronation.

**Toecap.** The upper may have a toecap stitched over or replacing the front of the vamp. It is made into a decorative feature in some men's shoes, for example brogues.

**Linings.** Linings (not illustrated) are included in the quarters and vamps of some shoes to increase the comfort and durability. The lining for the bottom of the shoe is called the insock. It may cover the entire length of the shoe, three quarters or just the heel section.

**Throat.** The throat is formed by the seam joining the vamp to the quarter. Its position depends on the style of the shoe. A lower throat line, i.e. a shorter vamp and longer quarters, will give a wider/lower opening. This seam will not stretch and therefore dictates the maximum width of foot for which the shoe can be used.

**Insole.** The insole is the flat inside of the shoe which covers the join between the upper and the sole in most methods of construction.

**Outsole.** The outsole or sole is the under-surface of the shoe.

**Shank.** The shank reinforces the waist of the shoe to prevent it from collapsing or distorting in wear. Shanks may not be needed in shoes with very low heels or in shoes where the sole forms a continuous wedge.

**Heel.** The part of the shoe under the heel of the foot, also called the heel, raises the rear of the shoe above ground level. A shoe without a heel or a midsole wedge may be completely flat or have the heel section lower than the forefoot, in which case it is called a negative heel. The outer covering on the surface of the heel, which can be replaced when worn, is called the top piece.

**Welt.** The welt is a strip of material, usually leather, used to join the upper to the sole in Goodyear-welted construction.

## The 'anatomy' of sports shoes

Since trainers replaced plimsolls sports footwear design has developed considerably, bringing new construction methods and terminology to the footwear industry. The functions of sports shoes are different to those of ordinary shoes as, for example, they may be required to absorb shock or provide some medial to lateral stability. The parts of a sports shoe are shown in Figure 10.2 and the terms illustrated are described below.

**Mudguard.** Reinforcing round the outside of the rim of the toe is called the mudguard.

**Saddle.** The saddle is reinforcing stitched to the outside of the shoe in the area of the arch.

**Collar and heel tab.** The topline of a sports shoe is often padded to form the collar. This may be shaped up around the back of the tendo achilles to form a heel tab. Heel tabs were designed to protect the tendo achilles but sometimes rub sensitive feet and may therefore need to be removed.

**Hindfoot stabiliser.** One of the elements that may be incorporated into a sports shoe to attempt to counter pronation is the hindfoot stabiliser, which consists of a plastic meniscus between the midsole and the stiffener.

## SHOE CONSTRUCTION
### Lasts

The last is the mould on which most shoes are made and its shape and dimensions will dictate the fit and to some extent the durability of the shoe made on it. It is usually hinged around the instep to allow it to be removed from the shoe when construction is completed. Last design and manufacture are skilled occupations involving the use of many measurements, some of which are shown in Figure 10.3. Most of these are volume measurements rather than the traditional length and width measurements associated with shoe fit. The measurements of the last need to be different from the measurements of the foot to allow for movement in walking and the tightness of fit required by the wearer. It is these factors which make it difficult to convert a plaster cast of a foot into a last without considerable modification. Other dimensions are dictated by fashion features and current style. A last for a high-heeled shoe, for example, will need to be much shorter than the foot for which it is being designed to compensate for the shortened equinus position in which the foot is held. Another example is the last for a court shoe, which differs from the last for an equivalent lace-up shoe by

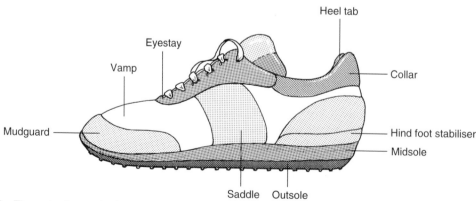

**Figure 10.2** The parts of a sports shoe.

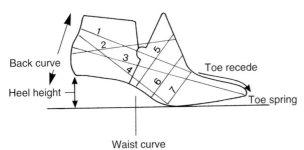

**Figure 10.3**  Some of the measurements used in last design. 1 = throat opening; 2 = heel girth; 3 = length; 4 = heel to ball length; 5 = instep girth; 6 = waist girth; 7 = ball girth (joint).

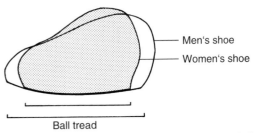

**Figure 10.4**  The different relationship of ball width to ball tread seen in a lady's and a gentleman's shoe. These shoes have identical width fittings.

having an overly curved heel and a shallow toe puff in order to help the shoe stay on the foot. Some features built into the last may affect the fit and are therefore described below.

**Recede.** The recede is the part of the last that projects beyond the tip of the toes and forms the rounded contour of the front of the shoe. A tapering recede, found in some fashion shoes, increases the overall length of the shoe. In a poorly designed last the recede may encroach on to the toes, causing pressure on the tips of the toes in walking.

**Flare.** In the past there used to be no difference between left and right shoes until it was discovered that shoes were more comfortable with a degree of inflare. Now most commercially available shoes are made on lasts with some inflare. Occasionally the flare of the foot does not match that of the shoe, causing characteristic wear marks on the inside of the shoe and pressure lesions on the foot.

**Heel to ball length.** This dimension dictates the position of the hinge and the widest part of the shoe. It is essential that this corresponds to the widest part of the foot, the metatarsophalangeal joint.

**Toe spring.** Toe spring is incorporated into a last to compensate for the stiffness of footwear and is essential for the toe off stage of gait. The more rigid the soling material the greater the toe spring needed.

**Ball tread.** This is the width across the sole under the ball of the foot and it should correspond to the width of the foot at this point. In some ladies' fashion shoes this width is decreased and compensated for with extra girth in order to give the appearance of a thinner, more elegant foot (Fig. 10.4). Thus the shoes will be narrower and deeper than the foot they are designed to fit and when worn the upper will overlap the sole.

## Measurement

The last is designed in a single size and then a set is made in the range of sizes and widths in which the shoes are to be manufactured. Marked sizes will vary slightly from one manufacturer to another.

### Length

Shoes are marked according to one of three different length sizing systems depending on where the shoes were made. Figure 10.5 gives a rough conversion table between the three major systems: United Kingdom, American and Paris Point (Continental). The UK scale starts at 0 for a foot measuring about 102 mm and has 8.4 mm between whole sizes and 4.2 mm between half sizes. After size 13 the scale restarts at size 1 for adult footwear. American shoes are approximately half a size larger than their UK equivalent for all except women's shoes which are one and a half sizes bigger. Paris Point begins at size 0 and increases by 6.5 mm between each size.

### Fittings

Several standard width fittings are available in the UK size system to accommodate differences

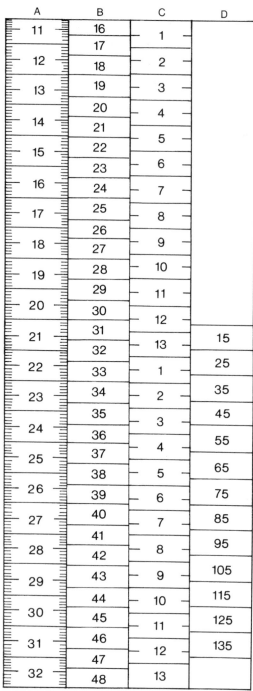

**Figure 10.5** Comparison of measurements of shoe length
**A.** Centimeters   **B.** Paris Point   **C.** English sizing system
**D.** American women's sizes.

in three-dimensional girth. For ladies A is the narrowest and G the widest, for children the range is from A–H and for men it is from 1–8. The girth increase between fittings is normally 6.5 mm. Many lines are only made in one size and this is usually ladies' D or men's 4. The girth around the ball of the foot increases by 5 mm for whole sizes up to children's size $10\frac{1}{2}$ and 6.5 mm for whole sizes above this. In the American system the equivalent to the letter system is two less, for example AAA is equivalent to the UK A. There is no equivalent Continental width fitting system and in general the shoes are narrower than in the UK.

## Methods of construction

Shoes were traditionally made by moulding leather on to a wooden last. Modern technology has brought many new materials to shoe manufacture and has, to some extent, mechanised the construction but it remains a fairly labour-intensive industry.

The first stage in the construction of most shoes is to attach the insole to the undersurface of the last. The remaining construction is split into two main operations, *lasting*, when the upper sections are shaped to the last and attached to the insole, and *bottoming*, when the sole is attached to the upper. There are five main methods of bottoming and the one chosen will influence the price, quality and performance of the final product.

### Stuck-on (cement)

As the name implies, this type of construction involves sticking the sole to the upper (Fig. 10.6A). This method is commonly used for both men's and women's footwear as it produces a lightweight and flexible shoe.

### Goodyear welt

The edge of the sole in a Goodyear-welted shoe is made of two sections. The top section, called the welt, is stitched to the upper and insole rib at the point where it curves under the last (Fig. 10.6B). The outsole is then sewn to the welt

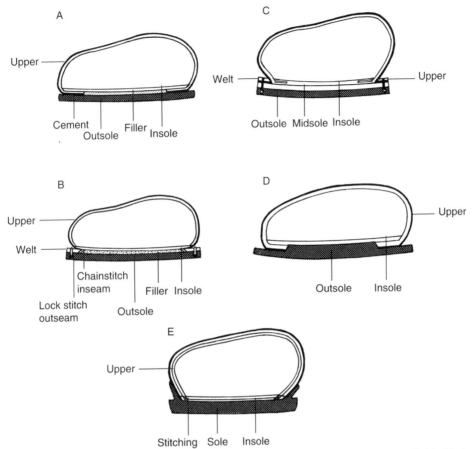

**Figure 10.6** Common methods of shoe construction **A.** Cement **B.** Goodyear **C.** Stitchdown **D.** Moulded **E.** Strobel stitched method.

around the edge. This creates heavier, less flexible footwear and is used for high-quality dress and town shoes.

### Stitchdown

The upper is turned out at the edge of the last instead of being curved under it and attached to a runner (insole) (Fig. 10.6C). The sole is then stitched to the upper and runner. This is a cheaper method of construction. While not as strong as some constructions it produces a lightweight, flexible sole. It is used for children's footwear and some casual shoes.

### Moccasins

In this method the upper is not made in sections and lasted as previously described. A single larger section forms the insole, vamp and quarters, by being moulded upwards from the undersurface of the last. An apron is then stitched to the gathered edges of the vamp and the sole is stitched to the base of the shoe. This method is used for flexible fashion footwear.

### Moulded methods

In these methods the lasted upper is placed in a mould and the sole formed around it by injecting liquid synthetic soling material (Fig. 10.6D). Alternatively, the sole may be vulcanised by converting uncured rubber into a stable compound by heat and pressure. These methods combine the upper permanently into the sole and such shoes cannot therefore be repaired easily. Moulded methods can be used to make most types of footwear.

### Force lasting

There are many variations of this method but the main one, which is increasing in use, is the sewn-in-sock or Strobel-stitched method (Fig. 10.6E). The upper is sewn directly to a sock by means of an overlocking machine (or Strobel stitcher). The upper is then pulled (force lasted) on to a last or moulding foot. Unit soles with raised walls or moulded soles are attached to completely cover the seam. This is a modern method which has evolved from the construction of sports shoes but is increasingly used for casual shoes.

## Materials used in construction

### Leather upper materials

The traditional material for shoe upper manufacture is leather and it still has advantages over synthetic materials. The first of these is its permeability. Permeable materials allow perspiration to escape from the foot, producing a drier environment which is less conducive to fungal growth. The second advantage is that leather stretches with wear and will permanently mould to the shape of the foot. Additionally, leather forms many tiny creases where flexing occurs, giving a smooth contour to the inside of the shoe. It is important to remember that the permeability of leather is likely to be impaired by special coatings, e.g. patent leather.

### Synthetic upper materials

Some synthetic materials (the poromerics) are permeable and allow the shoe to 'breathe' but none have the permanent suppleness found in leather. Most are slightly elastic and will stretch to some extent during wear; however, they will return to their original shape when taken off. For this reason shoes made of these materials

should fit well and will not be as versatile at fitting awkwardly shaped feet as leather. Some synthetic materials may form a single deep crease, which can rub on the foot, instead of the many small creases found in leather. This problem is likely to be more pronounced when the shoes are too big. Many synthetic materials can be produced cheaply and are used to manufacture reasonably priced shoes. Providing they fit well and perspiration is not allowed to build up inside, they can be completely satisfactory.

### Other upper materials

Woven fabrics such as cotton corduroy can be used to make soft uppers. These are classified as breathable fabrics even if made of synthetic fibres; however, they will usually only stretch in one direction. They can make comfortable footwear, but it is essential that these fit well and are well constructed with adequate reinforcement, particularly in the heel area.

### Lining materials

All the materials used for upper construction can also be used for linings; however, the combination of a leather upper with a full lining made of a non-breathable, non-stretch material will have all the disadvantages of the lining materials and none of the advantages of the leather. In practice full linings are rare, but when they are used it is preferable that they be made of thin leather or fabric. Many linings are made of synthetic material but are usually confined to the quarters and the insock, where the loss of permeability and stretchability is not a problem.

### Leather soling materials

The ideal soling material must be waterproof, durable and possess a coefficient of friction high enough to prevent slipping. As for upper construction, leather has been the traditional material for the construction of shoe soles but synthetic materials are much more versatile than leather which, besides being very expensive, has poor gripping qualities.

## Synthetic soling materials

The advantages that man-made soling materials have over leather are that they are more durable, have better resistance to water and have higher coefficients of friction and, therefore, better grip. They can be made of flat material and be stuck or sewn onto the upper like leather, or they can be made in a shaped mould which is either stuck on or moulded directly on to the upper. Extra grip properties can be incorporated in the form of a distinctive sole pattern with well-defined ridges or they can be moulded with cavities to reduce the weight of the sole. These cavities need to be covered with a rigid insole or can be filled with light foam to produce a more flexible sole. Synthetic soling materials have been the subject of a great deal of research, particularly relating to sports shoes, and this has led to new designs and construction methods being used in all types of footwear. For example, two or more materials of different densities can be incorporated into the sole, e.g. to give a hard-wearing outer surface and a softer, more flexible midsole for greater comfort. Many synthetic soling materials possess a degree of shock absorption. Patients can sometimes relieve metatarsalgia by changing from thin soled shoes to shoes with thick soles with good shock absorption properties.

## Shank

The shank can be made of steel, wood or synthetic material and will usually retain a slight degree of flexibility. Shank flexibility can be tested for by pressing down on the inside of the shoe on a flat surface. A suitable shank would be completely rigid or give slightly, but a shank that is too flexible will yield under this pressure and would allow the shoe to twist when weight-bearing.

## Allergy to shoe components

Some components used in shoe construction can cause allergic contact dermatitis. Substances which sometimes cause skin problems are listed below.

**Rubber.** Rubber, used for some soles, can be present even in an all-leather shoe as it is a constituent of many adhesives.

**Chemicals.** The chemicals used in the process which turns animal hide into leather (tanning) and dyes used to colour it can leach out of the leather when the foot sweats.

**Other features.** Materials such as nickel, used in eyelets and shanks, or the fungicides used to protect the leather, can also produce skin irritation.

Diagnosis of these conditions can be made from the localised area affected by the eruption. Treatment involves use of footwear constructed without the causative component. Fortunately these conditions are rare. Help to identify suitable footwear can be obtained in the UK from organisations such as the Disabled Living Foundation and the Shoe and Allied Trades Research Association.

## STYLE

Figure 10.7 shows the seven basic shoe styles, lace-up, moccasin, court, sandal, boot, mule and clog. All shoes are variations on these themes.

## Suitable shoe styles

Only the styles on the left of the illustration, the lace-up, sandal, boot and moccasin styles, fit the definition of a sensible shoe, which must have a mechanism for holding the foot back in the heel of the shoe. Without this fixation the foot is allowed to slip forward into the toe space causing friction on the sole and trauma to the toes. Thus there are two really important parts of an ideal shoe, a band around the instep and corresponding pressure at the heel. These parts, shown in Figure 10.8, should be firm and fit well. The band around the instep prevents the foot from sliding forward. This needs to be well up the instep to be effective. This is counterbalanced by pressure behind the heel to prevent the foot from sliding back.

Support is often listed as being essential in a good shoe, but a normal foot does not need to be supported to function correctly or barefoot walk-

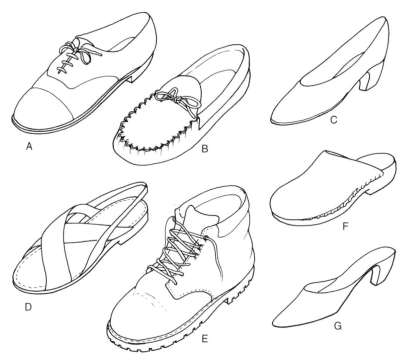

**Figure 10.7** The seven basic shoe styles **A.** Lace-up **B.** Moccasin **C.** Court **D.** Sandal **E.** Boot **F.** Clog **G.** Mule.

ing would be impossible. A good shoe should be firm enough to support itself and provide a solid base from which to push off. Recommending footwear is complicated by the constant changes to styles and models marketed by different manufacturers and the different uses for which shoes are designed. It is better, therefore, to recommend features to be found in a suitable shoe with an explanation of why they are important. To assist this task a list of points to look for in a suitable shoe is included in Table 10.1.

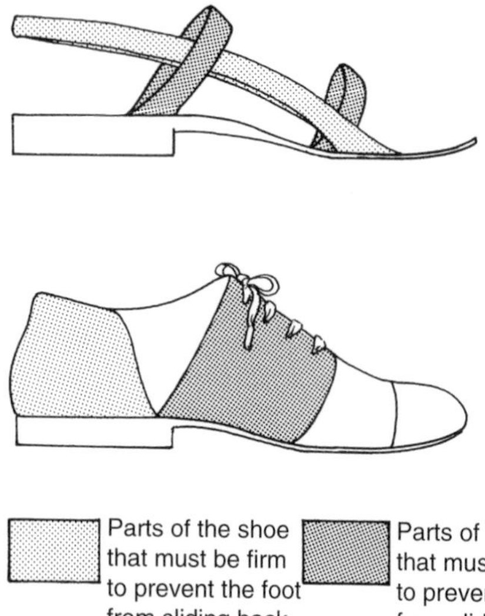

**Table 10.1** Points to look for in an ideal shoe

- Laces with at least three eyelets
- Low, wide heel for good stability
- Good width at the front of the shoe to prevent cramping the toes
- Deep, reinforced toe box
- Firm stiffening round the heel
- Curved back for close fit around the heel
- Shaped topline, high enough up the instep for adequate fixation
- Strong leather upper
- Hard-wearing synthetic sole
- Good fit
- Good condition

Parts of the shoe that must be firm to prevent the foot from sliding back    Parts of the shoe that must fit snugly to prevent the foot from sliding forward

**Figure 10.8** The parts of a shoe needing to fit well to prevent forward or backward movement of the foot.

## Unsuitable styles of footwear

Mules, clogs and court shoes, the styles on the right of Figure 10.7, are unsuitable for regular wear as they have no means of securing the foot. The only way that mules stay on is by being 'gripped' by the toes. This can lead to toe deformity. Slip-on shoes, especially court shoes, are bought too short and inevitably cramp the toes as the only way that they can stay on the foot is by wedging the foot between the curved back of the heel and the toe puff. When tried on in the correct size the foot slips forward into the toe space and the heel lifts out of the shoe on walking, giving the impression that it is too big. Clogs or slip-on shoes that extend right up the instep will limit forward movement to some extent. A properly fitting lace-up is always preferable (Fig. 10.8).

In most shoes, even 'flat' ones, the heel is raised slightly above the level of the ground, so that the foot is in slight equinus. Even a modest height of heel will tend to throw the weight of the foot forward into the toe section unless it is restricted by an adequate fastening. It is therefore even more important for a high-heeled shoe to have a secure fastening. Raised heels are said to have developed as a protection from dirty streets but high heels became associated with fashion and style as early as the 16th century. High heels, defined as those that place the foot in more than slight equinus, are not suitable for everyday wear. In addition to the fact that they are nearly always slip-ons, they alter the normal biomechanics of the lower limb in walking. Habitual wear leads to permanent shortening of the calf muscles, barefoot walking is made uncomfortable and in severe cases the heels may not be able to touch the ground.

## ASSESSMENT OF FOOTWEAR

The assessment of footwear should not be seen as a separate entity to be completed after other aspects of the examination but should be integrated into the global assessment. For example, observation of patients walking in their shoes can often be achieved as they enter the clinic

**Table 10.2** The parts of a simple footwear assessment and the stages at which they can be completed within the global assessment

| Stage of assessment | Test | Brief description |
|---|---|---|
| *In shoes* | | |
| Walking | Observe gait | |
| Standing | Observe stance | |
| | Check length | Palpate end of longest toe |
| | Check heel to ball length | Locate MTPJs in shoe |
| | Check width | Pinch upper over metatarsal heads |
| | Check depth | Palpate toes during flexion |
| *Barefoot* | | |
| Walking | Observe gait | |
| Sitting | History | |
| | Assess suitability of shoes | |
| | Check wear marks | |
| | Examine inside of shoe | |
| Standing | Observe stance | |
| | Note longest toe | |

and there are some checks of fit which should be done before the shoes are removed. This will ensure that the number of times the shoes need to be removed and replaced is kept to a minimum. Table 10.2 lists the tests that should be included in a simple footwear assessment and the stage at which each should be completed. They are described in full below. Performing these checks routinely, as part of a set sequence, will help to ensure that assessment of footwear is completed without undue effort. It should be remembered that hands should be washed between examination of the footwear and the foot. Patients attending for their first appointment should have been warned to bring a selection of their shoes as new or 'best' shoes may not demonstrate the habitual wear pattern found in the shoes worn every day. There may therefore be several pairs of shoes to examine.

### History taking

Background information about the patient's general footwear and purchasing habits is an essential part of the assessment of footwear.

## Financial circumstances

Before suggesting appropriate footwear, it is important to ascertain the financial circumstances of the patient, as this will influence his/her ability to follow the advice given.

## Wardrobe

Questions regarding the number of shoes owned and the number regularly worn may seem irrelevant but can add helpful information. This line of questioning may uncover that special shoes are worn at work and, therefore, need examination in preference to shoes worn only occasionally. There are specialist reinforced shoes for work in dangerous environments, smart shoes may be needed for office work or special shoes may be required for a specific sporting activity.

## Habits

Details of how often shoes are changed and whether long periods are spent wearing slippers or sports shoes can also be important. For example, a lady is unlikely to benefit from having a pair of suitable shoes to go out in once a week when she spends the rest of the week at home in slippers.

## Acquisition of footwear

Information about when, where and how often patients buy their shoes can be useful; for example, do they have their feet measured or visit a self service shop?

## Independence

No assessment of footwear would be complete without noting the patient's ability to put on and take off his/her shoes or to do up and undo the fixation. Many adaptations to footwear and aids to assist independence are available and may form a valuable part of treatment. Sources of information are included in further reading.

# Assessment of shoe fit

Shoe fit is always a compromise as the shape of the foot is changing continually due to many different factors, some of which affect length and some girth. The biggest factor affecting length is weightbearing and measurements of length should, therefore, never be made when the patient is sitting. Girth is affected by body weight but is also highly sensitive to both temperature and swelling. There is thus a tendency for feet to be smaller in the morning than the evening. Measurements taken during the middle of the day will give the most representative results.

Assessment of shoe fit is not an exact science: often observation and common sense are all that is required to decide whether shoes fit correctly. Sometimes a method of measuring fit is useful to demonstrate to the patient that their shoes are inadequate. A well-fitting shoe should fit snugly around the heel and the arch and allow free movement of the toes.

This section includes a comprehensive list of tests for different aspects of fit. It is not intended that all the tests described should be included in each assessment. They are listed partly to demonstrate the range of potential tests, but also to allow selection of an appropriate test to suit the problems experienced by the patient. In most cases the simplest test described will be adequate but occasionally, when more accuracy is required, the more complicated measurements can be useful.

The style of the shoe will to some extent dictate fit: for example, a court or slip-on shoe is likely to be too small in length, width and depth. Additionally, the style of the front of the shoe can have a direct bearing on the fit in this region. Demonstration of poor fit by some of the tests described may help to convert the patient to sensible shoes.

If shoes are really comfortable they are probably a good fit. Strangely, comfort is not as important a factor as might be expected when shoes are being purchased. Colour, style and heel height may compete equally. People, particularly women, seem to be tolerant of minor foot discomfort and it is necessary to explain that ill-fitting footwear may damage feet and that comfort should be paramount when choice of footwear is concerned.

## Length

Correctly-fitting shoes should have a gap between the longest toe and the front of the shoe to allow for elongation of the foot, which takes place when walking. This gap should ideally be about 12 mm. Shoes that are too short will be recognisable as the upper will tend to bulge at heel and toe. There are a number of simple tests with which this observation can be confirmed. They are not all suitable for all types of shoes.

- With the patient standing in his/her shoes palpate the end of the longest toe through the toe puff. This may not be possible if the toe puff is reinforced.
- Sprinkle a little talcum powder into the shoe and ask the patient to walk a few paces. When the shoes are removed an outline of the toes can be seen printed in the powder on the insole from which the gap can be assessed. It may be difficult to see the result of this test in footwear which extends high up the instep (high-waisted).
- Cut a thin strip of card the length of the foot and slide this into the shoe until it touches the tip. This should reveal a gap of about 12 mm between the inside of the heel and the end of the strip of card (Fig. 10.9). This method can be influenced by the shape of the toe puff and is therefore most effective in round-toed shoes. To minimise the error, keep the width of the card narrow and do not slide it right to the end of very pointed-toed shoes.

Shoes that are too short will mould the toes into the shape of the front of the shoe; shoes that are pointed are likely to cause pressure lesions on the toes.

**Length of children's shoes.** Children's shoes need a little more toe space than adults to allow for growth. A gap of 20 mm between the longest toe and the front of the shoe should be present in new shoes, allowing 8–9 mm for growth

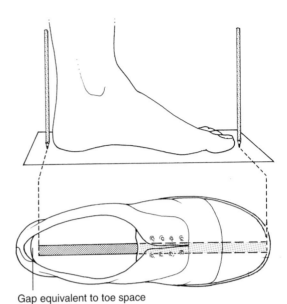

Gap equivalent to toe space

**Figure 10.9** A method of testing a shoe for correct length.

before new shoes are needed. If a child's shoe is worn out it is likely that it is too small, as it is usual for young feet to outgrow the shoe before it is worn out. It is also important to check for sock fit with growing feet as these too can be rapidly outgrown. Hosiery that is too small can cause as much damage as shoes that are too short.

## Heel to ball length

Correctly-fitting heel to ball length will ensure that the hinge of the shoe is correctly aligned with the ball of the foot, and that the widest part of the foot is in the widest part of the shoe. It varies according to the design of the last. Average heel to ball length will be adequate for average feet, and will only need to be assessed if the toes are unusually short or long in relation to the rest of the foot. Heel to ball length will be incorrect if too much room for growth is allowed in children's shoes, when odd-sized feet are not fitted with different-sized shoes or when extra long shoes are bought to fit wide feet. This important measurement should only be assessed once the length of the shoes has been checked and found to be correct. Two techniques for

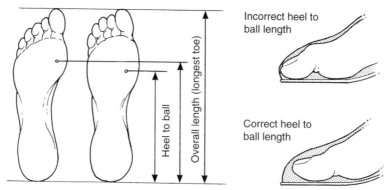

**Figure 10.10**   Illustration of two feet with identical length but different heel to ball length and the result of fitting them both in the same shoe.

measuring heel to ball length, one simple and one more accurate, are described below.

- With the patient standing in his/her shoes feel for the metatarsophalangeal joint. If the bulge of the joint is level with the bulge of the shoe, this measurement is correct.
- Measure the distance from the patient's heel to both the first and fifth metatarsal heads. Flex the ball of the shoe and measure the distance from the heel to the point at which the shoe bends both medially and laterally. The medial and lateral measurements from the foot and the shoe should correspond.

Shoes with a heel to ball length that is too long will put unnecessary pressure and strain on the metatarsophalangeal joints, particularly that of the hallux, as the foot will be trying to flex the shoe where it is still reinforced by the shank. If the heel to ball length is too short, it will cause fewer mechanical problems but will restrict toe room (Fig. 10.10).

### Width

Correct width is also important and should be sufficient to allow the toes to rest flat on the insole without being compressed. Very few fashion shoes are made in width fittings so fashion shoes are often bought either too narrow or a size longer than they should be, to benefit from the corresponding increase in width. In a shoe of inadequate width the upper will overlap the sole. Width can be assessed in a patient's footwear as follows:

- With the patient standing in his/her shoes grasp the upper level with the metatarsal heads and try to pinch the upper material between the finger and thumb. If the upper feels tense and stretched and cannot be pinched, the shoe is not wide enough. If wrinkles appear then the shoe may be too wide.

An additional check on width can be made on shoes with a well-defined throat line. This line governs the maximum width of the shoe as the seam will not stretch. There should ideally be enough space under the throat line to accommodate the tip of a pencil. If this extra space is not available, the throat line can bite into the fleshy dorsal surface of the foot on walking.

Shoes which are too narrow will cause pressure lesions on the first and fifth metatarsophalangeal joints and the interphalangeal joint of the fifth toe. In diabetic patients these pressure lesions can progress rapidly to ulcers.

### Depth

Correct depth is important to prevent pressure being exerted on the tops of the toes. Unlike length and width, there is no increase in depth with an increase in shoe size. The depth of a shoe depends on its last. The degree of recede (Fig. 10.3) incorporated into the last design will also affect the finished depth in the front of the shoe. If the patient is wearing, or needs, an orthosis, or has a toe deformity, then the depth is likely to be a problem. Inadequate depth causes a bulging toe puff. It can be assessed as follows:

- With the patient standing in shoes ask him/her to take a step forward and pause just before toe-off, while still weightbearing equally on both feet. Palpate the upper of the flexed foot above the fourth and fifth toes. If the toes are cramped, then the depth in the toe puff is inadequate.

Shoes which are too shallow will cause pressure lesions on the interphalangeal joints of the toes and can also affect nails.

### Other factors affecting fit

**Shoe flare.** If there is an indication that the flare of the foot does not match that of the shoe, this can be assessed as follows (Fig. 10.11): draw round the standing foot and, on the outline produced, join the centre of the heel to the second toe. Draw an outline of the shoe and join from a point below the heel seam at the back of the shoe

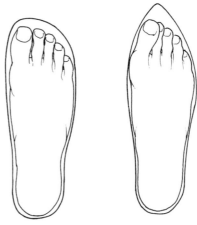

**Figure 10.12** Shoes with a straight and a shaped inside border and the effect on toes.

to a point bisecting the top piece of the heel. Extend the line forward to the tip of the sole. Measure the maximum width of the medial and lateral sections of both outlines, noting which section is the widest. The widest part should be the same in both, and will usually be the medial sections.

**Inside border shape.** Another factor affecting fit is the shape of the front of the shoe and its impact on the inside border (Fig. 10.12). The longest point on the foot is usually the great or second toe, but in shoes, the longest part is traditionally in the centre. Toes can often be painlessly moulded into pointed toe shapes, but this is likely to cause pain and deformity in the long term. A straight inside border is particularly important for patients in whom the longest part of the foot is the hallux or who have a tendency towards hallux valgus. A simple way to demonstrate to a patient that shoes are unsuitable is to ask him/her to stand on an outline of the shoe with the heels aligned. Any overlap of the toes over the edge of the outline indicates that the shoe is incorrectly shaped. Pointed toes are not necessarily unsuitable but the toe shape must start after the toes and the foot must be prevented from slipping forward into the space by a strap or laces.

**Fixation.** The means by which the foot is secured within the shoe will also need to be

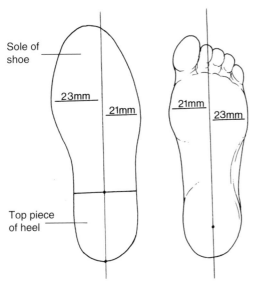

Sole of shoe

23mm

21mm

21mm

23mm

Top piece of heel

**Figure 10.11** The outlines of shoe and foot from an assessment of shoe flare. The medial and lateral measurements are not the same on the two outlines, indicating an inflared shoe but an outflared foot.

checked. Not only should the shoe not be worn too loose or too tight, but some adjustment should always be possible both to tighten or loosen the shoe. In a lace-up this means that there should always be a gap between the rows of eyelets up the front of the shoe. The effectiveness of the fixation can be checked by the following test: with the patient standing with one foot in front of the other grasp the shoe upper and ask the patient to lean forward on to the forward foot. If forward movement can be detected within the shoe, the fixation is inadequate. It is likely to be ineffective if the laces do not come far enough up the instep (three or four eyelet holes will be needed to give adequate fixation and opening) or the patient uses elastic laces or leaves the laces/buckle done up when taking the shoe on and off, making the shoe a slip-on.

**Function.** Most of the aspects considered so far have been static observations. It must be remembered that the shoe is required to function during activity as well as rest. The patient should therefore be observed walking while wearing their shoes and barefoot and any differences between the two noted. If the gait is better barefoot than when shod, there is likely to be some inadequacy of the shoes. Some points to compare when walking in and out of footwear are listed in Table 10.3, together with some possible causes of differences. Additionally, there are some

**Table 10.3**  Points to be observed with the patient walking barefoot and in shoes; any differences between the two sets of observations should be noted

| Observation | Possible causes of differences |
|---|---|
| Step length | High heels will tend to cause a shorter step length |
| Overall stability | This may be affected by sole area |
| Angle of heel | Wear on the inside of a shoe will increase a tendency to valgus in relation to the tibia |
| Heel strike | Some footwear can cause a flat-footed gait |
| Toe-off | Stiff footwear can limit flexion at the metatarsophalangeal joint; incorrect heel to ball length may have the same result |

aspects of shoe fit which can also be assessed when walking: the heel should not lift out of the shoe at each step; the topline should not gape on flexion; there should be no movement of the foot within the shoe.

*Fitting problems*

Anatomical variations mean that some people will have more problems finding shoes that fit than others. An example of this is a combination of a narrow heel and a wide forefoot. A standard shoe bought wide enough for the forefoot will be too loose at the heel. Shoes made on combination lasts used to be available to fit such feet but the best solution is a visit to an experienced shoe fitter who will know what is currently obtainable.

Assessment of the fit of a patient's shoes should be carried out on both feet even if the presenting problem is unilateral. A person's feet are commonly not identical in size and a pair of shoes may fit neither foot adequately. Small differences in size can be managed by shoes which fit the larger foot and adaptation for the shoe of the smaller foot. Differences of two sizes or more will need odd-sized shoes as the discrepancy in heel to ball length will be too great. A list of suppliers of odd-sized pairs can be found by consulting organisations such as the Disabled Living Foundation (DLF) in the United Kingdom. Some adaptations to help overcome the problem are illustrated in leaflets available from the DLF and the books suggested for further reading.

If the assessment shows up any deficiency in fit and the patient is willing and able to buy new shoes, suggest a visit to a shoe shop with a trained shoe fitter and a good stock of different fittings and last styles. Having feet measured may be something many people associate only with buying children's shoes. It is equally important for adults to be measured, particularly those with problem feet. Even specialist shops may have difficulty fitting feet which are bigger, wider or narrower than average. If a patient is having difficulty finding suitable shoes then specialist organisations like the Disabled Living Foundation should be consulted for appropriate manufacturers or stockists.

## Wear marks

Assessment of the pattern of wear on the soles and the uppers of patients' footwear can help to confirm a diagnosis of foot pathology and may also highlight deformity elsewhere, e.g. genu valgum. The patterns are to some extent predictable, given that the shoes enclose the foot and will mould to its shape. Well-defined deformities give classic wear patterns. It is important to be able to recognise the wear expected from a normal foot in order to differentiate that which is abnormal. Abnormal wear presents not only as an unusual pattern, but also as excessive or insufficient wear where some wear should be expected.

Examination of the wear patterns of shoes will also reveal information about foot function. Distortions of the uppers can indicate abnormal frontal plane motion during walking. The wear marks on the heel and sole will reflect the direction of the weightbearing pathway during the gait cycle. Normal wear is the result of a smooth transfer of load from the heel to the forefoot. Some gait analysis equipment (Ch. 12) displays a centre of pressure line and it is logical to assume that normal wear will occur along this path (Fig. 10.13).

The degree as well as the pattern of wear must be assessed, as shoes which are worn out or in

need of repair are unsuitable for regular wear. One check of the degree of wear is to place the shoe on a flat surface and gently touch the back, front and each side. The shoe should be stable and not rock when touched. If rocking is detected than the shoe will provide an unstable base for walking and standing. Checking stance shod and barefoot will confirm these observations.

### Wear on the sole

If the foot is functioning properly and is in a well-fitting shoe the pressure on the sole of the shoe should be even and no one part should wear out excessively. It is normal, however, for signs of wear to occur under the medial central forefoot (Fig. 10.13). It is also normal for there to be a slight curvature of the undersurface of the sole. An element of this is built into the shoe by incorporating toe spring into the last (Fig. 10.3), and this is accentuated by normal toe-off in walking.

Any variation of the above will represent abnormal sole wear. Some examples follow. When the slight curvature on the undersurface of the sole is not apparent, or is not symmetrical or exaggerated, abnormal toe function is indicated. This is often the case in patients with rheumatoid arthritis who may have reduced toe function and a short stride. Insufficient wear on the posterior part of the sole indicates a heel to ball length which is too short and, when combined with excessive wear, at the tip of the sole, means that the whole shoe is not long enough. Wear at the tip of the sole alone may indicate that the shoe has been made on a last designed without enough toe spring, but insufficient wear in this area denotes lack of push-off. Excessive wear to the sole of the shoe may indicate limited dorsiflexion if it is towards the front of the sole, and pes cavus when it is across the tread without extending down the lateral border (Fig. 10.14). An everted forefoot will show excessive wear along the inner aspect and an inverted forefoot will be worn along the outer aspect.

Wear marks indicating a circular contact of the sole with the ground are caused when the

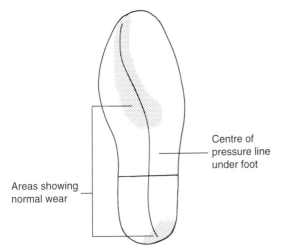

Centre of pressure line under foot

Areas showing normal wear

**Figure 10.13** The 'normal' pattern of wear on the sole and the heel.

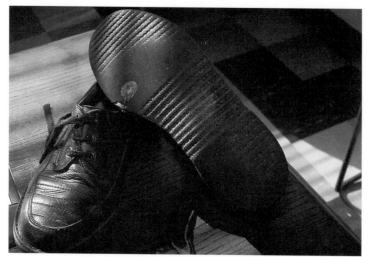

**Figure 10.14**   The pattern of wear seen in the shoe of a patient with pes cavus.

metatarsal area is being used as a pivot, e.g. any condition that makes use of the toes uncomfortable. Examination of the sole will also reveal any areas of abnormally high pressure, e.g. under a single metatarsal head.

### Wear on the heel

The normal wear on a heel, shown in Figure 10.13, spreads along the posterolateral border of the heel. Wear is not central, as might be expected, for several reasons: the entire calcaneus lies towards the lateral side of the inside of the heel of the shoe; the weightbearing tubercle is lateral to the midline of the heel; and the calcaneum is inverted at heel contact.

Excessive wear along the lateral margin of the heel may indicate an inverted hindfoot, but this pattern is also seen in genu varum. Similarly, excessive wear on the inner aspect of the heel may indicate a valgus or everted hindfoot, but is also seen in cases of genu valgum.

### Combined heel and sole wear

A combination of excessive wear on the heel and the ball area of the sole can be seen in pes cavus. Along the medial border of the heel and sole it indicates a valgus or everted foot, and on the outer aspect of the heel and the sole it indicates inversion. This pattern may also be seen in hallux rigidus and severe in-toeing. Wear on the outer side of the heel and the inner side of the sole may be caused by an out-toed gait (external rotation of the hip). Unusual combinations/patterns of wear may simply be the result of a painful area being offloaded; for example, a painful heel may result in insufficient heel wear and abnormal wear in the sole.

### Crease marks in the upper

Normal creasing of the upper due to flexing during walking is slightly oblique and follows the line of the metatarsophalangeal joints. An excessively oblique crease mark is the sign of hallux rigidus in which toe-off occurs on the lateral side of the foot to protect the painful or rigid hallux (Fig. 10.15). The absence of creases in worn shoes indicates absence of toe-off, i.e. a short stride and flat-footed gait.

### Deformation of the upper

Distortions of the shoe's upper are caused by the shoe conforming to common forefoot deformities. Hallux valgus distorts the medial border, bunionette/tailor's bunion the lateral aspect and

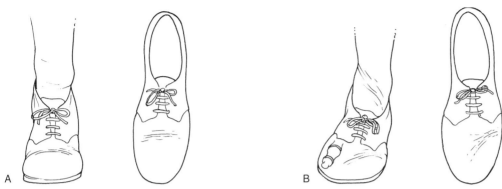

**Figure 10.15**  Crease marks on the upper   **A.** Normal crease marks   **B.** Crease marks with hallux rigidus.

hammer and claw toes create bulges in the top of the toe puff. Additionally, the heel stiffener may be caused to bulge at the back by pump bumps, on the lateral side by a varus or inverted hindfoot, and on the medial side by a valgus or everted hindfoot. Individuals with flat feet may distort the medial border because of the prominence of the talar head (Fig. 10.16). Scuffed toes are seen when there is a foot-drop deformity, as the toes are in ground contact during the swing phase of gait.

### Examination of the inside of the shoe

The assessment of wear should also include an examination of the inside of the shoe. The wear

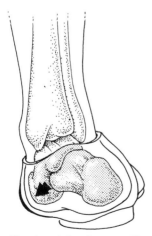

**Figure 10.16**  The shoe deformity caused by medial prominence of the talar head (black arrow) in pes planus.

patterns inside are likely to mirror those found on the heel and sole. Additional features such as creases, seams or rough areas and even nails through the sole may be the cause of localised lesions. The insock will often display a print of the sole of the foot from which the areas taking greatest pressure can be observed.

### Other signs of wear

The shoes of patients with diabetes mellitus may show a characteristic white deposit, sometimes accompanied by deterioration along the inner sides. These signs of wear have been publicised by the Shoe and Allied Trades Research Association (SATRA) who found the white substance to be glucose and the deterioration due to contamination by urine.

## Suitability

Table 10.4 lists the points that should be noted in the examination of shoe suitability, together with the most common observations, divided into good and less good aspects. Such a list could be used as a quick record of the examination by circling the appropriate shoe feature. The suitability/unsuitability would then be shown by the column in which the circles had been made.

A shoe which was originally suitable may become unsuitable through age. Some shoe components deteriorate over time, e.g. the insole, which may become cracked or hollowed. Ad-

**Table 10.4** Points to note in examination of shoe suitability

| Points | | Good | Bad |
|---|---|---|---|
| Style of shoes | | Lace-up, sandal, boot, moccasin | Court, mule, clog |
| Method of fixation | | Lace, buckle and bar, velcro | Elastic, none |
| Heel height | | Flat | High-heeled |
| Upper material | | Leather | Synthetic |
| Sole material | | Synthetic, leather | |
| Condition | | New, scuffed, worn | Worn out |
| Sole wear patterns | | Normal | Abnormal |
| Upper crease pattern | | Normal | Abnormal |
| Fit | Length | Good | Too small/long |
| | Width | Good | Too wide/narrow |
| | Depth | Good | Too shallow/deep |
| | Heel to Ball | Correct | Too long/short |
| | Flare | Good | Bad |
| Construction | | Welted, cemented, moccasin, moulded | |
| Type | | Dress, casual, sports, work | |

ditionally, feet change shape with age and fit may be compromised. A shoe may also be unsuitable if it is inappropriate for the conditions/situation in which it is worn. A common example of this is found in patients with rheumatoid arthritis who, because of the difficulty of finding footwear to fit, wear sandals all year round.

## Everyday shoes

The preceding checks of suitability, fit and wear will only be meaningful if they relate to the patients' everyday shoes. Even if the shoes assessed are representative they may be fairly new or have been recently repaired and there is a great deal of information to be gained from examining more than one pair of shoes. New patients should be routinely asked to bring several pairs of footwear for examination. There are other occasions when it might be helpful to see a selection of footwear, e.g. when assessing a patient for orthoses. Another reason for asking to see additional footwear is to overcome the possibility that the shoes, which apparently conform to the advice given, are being worn only for visits to the clinic.

## Hosiery

Socks and stockings that are too small restrict the circulation to the foot and can do just as much damage to the toes as shoes that do not fit. Hosiery fit should therefore be checked at the same time as shoe fit and this is particularly important in children, where the foot is still growing. Socks and stockings may be outgrown, have shrunk with inappropriate washing or simply have been bought too small. The sizing of stretch socks can lead to confusion as the range of sizes printed on the label indicates the range from unstretched to full stretch. Socks will be more comfortable and cause fewer compression problems if the unstretched size corresponds to the shoe size.

The materials used in the manufacture of hosiery can affect foot health. Socks made of natural fibres may be needed by patients with skin conditions such as eczema, but a mixture of natural fibres and synthetic substances is often an advantage, as the synthetic material can help to keep the foot dry. Natural fibres absorb moisture and remain damp. Synthetic fibres let the moisture pass through to an absorbent surface on the other side, for example a leather upper. This process, known as wicking, keeps the foot dry but will not take place if shoes are made of, or lined with, synthetic material.

## SUMMARY

This chapter has described the factors which should be included in an assessment of footwear. The reader should now be able to judge the suitability of footwear and whether it is contributing to the foot problems experienced by the patient. The ability to use footwear assessment to both the advantage of the patient and the practitioner will come only with experience, but it is hoped that the importance of this often neglected aspect has been clearly demonstrated.

## FURTHER READING

Hughes J R (ed) 1982 Footwear and footcare for children. Disabled Living Foundation, London

Hughes J R 1983 Footcare and footwear for adults. Disabled Living Foundation, London

Hunt G C (ed) 1988 Physical therapy of the foot and ankle. Churchill Livingstone, New York

**Sources of information**

Disabled Living Foundation (DLF) resource on 'Footwear and disability', Section 14 of the DLF Information Service Handbook. DLF, 380–384 Harrow Road, London W9 2HU

Shoe and Allied Trades Research Association (SATRA), Rockingham Road, Kettering, Northants NN16 9JH

# PART 3

# Laboratory and hospital investigations

# 11

# Radiographic assessment

*I. Turbutt*

## INTRODUCTION

The role of the specialist in foot disorders is an expanding one. As the knowledge of foot pathology has increased so has the complexity of referred cases and treatment regimes. Many clinical diagnoses can only be confirmed by the use of one of the imaging modalities. This chapter is designed to give a workable base of information on the ordering and interpretation of X-rays of the foot, and other imaging techniques, together with relevant pathological detail. This knowledge is particularly important for those involved in surgical practice but has great relevance for all progressive practitioners in foot health. The chapter should be seen as a starting point for further reading and development in this fascinating and rewarding field.

The interpretation of X-rays is complex and extremely skilled and it should be borne in mind that it is normal practice within the National Health Service, and good practice in the private sector, for all films taken to be reported by a radiologist. In the light of such a report one may add one's own specific skills and clinical findings to complete the diagnosis.

## GENERATION OF X-RAYS

X-rays are generated by the passage of a high voltage through a heated coiled tungsten wire (the cathode) in a toughened glass tube containing a vacuum, producing free electrons in a process known as thermionic emission. At the other end of the tube is the anode, consisting of a heavy metal disc, normally tungsten, embedded in a copper bar, which rotates to absorb heat. When a high potential difference is applied between the electrodes the electrons from the cathode stream at high velocity towards the anode (cathode rays) and bombard the tungsten target. If a positive nucleus of a target atom is bombarded by fast-moving free negatively-charged electrons from another source a repulsion and braking effect (the *Bremsstrahlung* process) takes place. The electrons decelerate and emit energy in the form of radiation and if the energy levels are high enough the radiation is in the form of X-rays. The bombardment of atoms heavier than sodium, such as tungsten, by free electrons will produce a high energy wave of X-rays in the range $10^{-7}$–$10^{-10}$ cm, as well as other charged particles known as alpha particles, beta particles and gamma rays. The resulting X-rays are focused as required by a light-beam diaphragm—lead shields, visually aligned on the patient with a beam of light.

Radiation is able to penetrate dense objects for a certain distance, dependent upon both the density of the object and the power of the radiation beam. X-rays produced by low voltages, below 50 kV, will not penetrate tissue for any great distance and may be considered 'soft' X-rays. Those produced by higher voltages penetrate for increasing distances and are known as 'hard' X-rays.

When an X-ray beam passes through tissues, such as the foot, and strikes a sensitive film emulsion, it produces a chemical change and forms a negative image of the tissues, which may be viewed once the film has been processed. The most dense tissue, i.e. bone, is shown as white and the less dense tissues are shown as increasing shades of grey and black. In practice it takes quite a large amount of X-radiation to alter the film. In order to reduce the patient dose the film is normally placed in a cassette containing rare earth intensifying screens. These screens fluoresce when struck by relatively small amounts of radiation and it is the fluorescence that changes the film. This reduces the radiation dosage required by up to 90%, depending on the type of screen, and is therefore far safer for the patient and operator. The SI unit of radiation absorbed dose is the gray (Gy).

## The effects of radiation on tissue

All ionising radiations are harmful to living tissue, and must be accorded the greatest respect. It is a firm principle that the advantage to the patient of having a radiographic examination should outweigh the associated radiation hazard. Effects of radiation may be somatic or genetic. Radiation suppresses the ability of cells to reproduce. The sensitivity to radiation is related to oxygen saturation of the cells. Neural tissue is the least sensitive, and blood cells and bone marrow are the most easily damaged, leading to anaemia and leukaemia in severe cases of over-exposure. The thyroid gland and the lens of the eye are also vulnerable. The gonads are radio-sensitive and temporary or permanent sterility, or even genetic mutations, can be caused by the excessive irradiation of the gonads of a person of reproductive age (Swallow et al 1986). However, the low level of dosage received in most properly conducted radiographic examinations, and in particular with the foot, means that there is absolutely minimal risk of any damage.

## ORDERING AN X-RAY

Any practitioner in the United Kingdom who wishes to clinically or physically direct X-radiation must have core knowledge training as stipulated in the Health and Safety Executive Ionising Radiation Regulations (Protection of Persons Undergoing Medical Examination or Treatment) 1988. The course, usually arranged by physicists, will make the practitioner aware of all the safety aspects and the code of practice relating to the direction of radiation. If the patient is referred by the practitioner to an X-ray department the core knowledge training is not necessary as the radiologist is deemed to be clinically directing the examination.

For an investigation to be of maximum use to the practitioner the reason for the referral, any relevant clinical history, the information sought, the views required and whether or not they should be taken weightbearing must be clearly specified to the radiographer and the radiologist. Wasted time, missed diagnoses and unnecessary radiation exposure can result from a poor request.

One of the important questions on any X-ray request form relates to the recent menstrual history of any female patient of childbearing age. This is to protect any early fetus from potential radiation exposure. A female patient of childbearing age should be asked whether or not she might be pregnant. If she cannot be certain the form should be clearly marked accordingly. In fact radiographs of the foot, correctly taken by a radiographer, present no hazard to any fetus, as the dosage is low, the beam is not angled towards the abdomen and gonad protection can be used. It is therefore unlikely that a radiographer will refuse to X-ray the foot of a pregnant woman (National Radiological Protection Board).

It is important that at least two views of any portion of the anatomy are obtained. As an X-ray is a two-dimensional rendition of a three dimensional object pathological changes cannot be properly assessed without more than one perspective. It should also be remembered that an X-ray image will inevitably have some enlargement and distortion of size compared to the actual structures.

In general it may be said that weightbearing views, with the patient standing in normal angle and base of gait, are of most use to the practitioner. It is then legitimate for certain biomechanical features to be deduced as well as pathological features. Otherwise, such deductions are little more than guesswork. However, it should perhaps be noted at this point that the ordering of X-rays for routine biomechanical assessment is not good practice, involving radiation exposure which is generally considered to be unnecessary.

Some of the most commonly requested views, and the reasons for taking them, are shown below. However, it should be borne in mind that there are many variations and other options in favour with various departments of radiology.

## Dorsiplantar view (DP)

This is a general-purpose view, taken either weightbearing (WB) or non-weightbearing (NWB), which will show the majority of the foot from the midtarsal area distally. The X-ray beam is angled at 15° to the naviculocuboid joint as shown in Figure 11.1. Some departments will take both feet simultaneously, and the beam will be directed between the feet at the level of the first metatarsophalangeal joint. The neck of the talus, the distal edge of the calcaneum, the tarsus, metatarsus and digits will be clearly seen (Fig. 11.2). Normally the bodies of the talus and the calcaneum will be occluded by superimposition of the lower ends of the tibia and fibula.

## Lateral view (weightbearing)

This is taken with the beam at right angles to the foot, centred on the styloid process with the medial side of the foot close up against the cassette (Fig. 11.3). The entire lateral view of the foot should be visible (Fig. 11.4). This view will clearly show the tibial and fibular malleoli superimposed over the talus, as well as the calcaneum, the subtalar joint, calcaneocuboid joint and talonavicular joint. The midtarsal complex will be partially obscured by the multiple superimpositions of the cuneiforms and metatar-

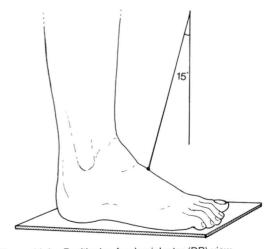

**Figure 11.1**  Positioning for dorsiplantar (DP) view.

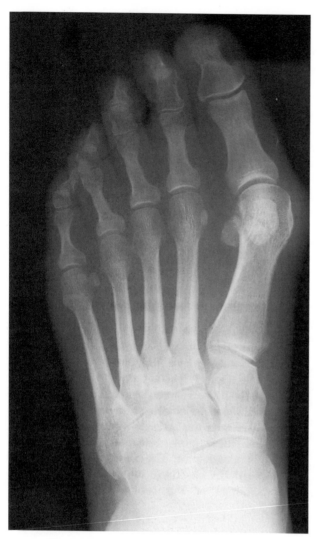

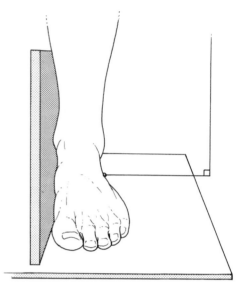

**Figure 11.2** Dorsiplantar view shows a mild hallux abductus deformity. Note also the bipartite medial sesamoid, and additional sesamoids under the second and fifth metatarsal heads.

**Figure 11.3** Positioning for lateral view.

**Figure 11.4** Positioning for lateral view (weightbearing). A typical lateral view, giving a good outline of the talus, calcaneum and medial column. Compare with Figure 11.16.

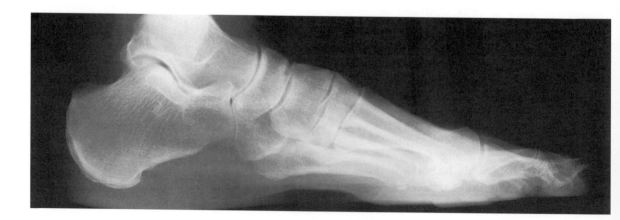

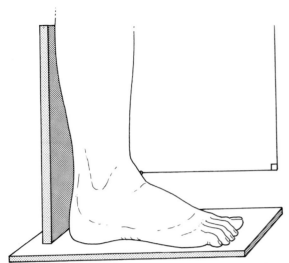

**Figure 11.5**  Positioning for anteroposterior view of ankle (AP ankle).

The lesser metatarsals will be partially super-imposed over each other, although the first metatarsal and hallux, and the structure of the first metatarsophalangeal joint, should be easily distinguishable.

## Anteroposterior ankle (AP ankle)

This is a view taken with the beam directed along the longitudinal axis of the foot towards the ankle (Fig. 11.5). It is particularly ordered when ankle injury is suspected. It will show virtually no detail of the forefoot, due to marked super-imposition, but it is designed to clearly demarcate the trochlear surface of the talus and the articulations with the tibia and fibula (Fig. 11.6). The malleoli are very clearly seen. Avulsion fractures, which occur with inversion and ever-sion injuries, can usually be seen on this view.

This view is sometimes taken as a non-weightbearing *stress radiograph* in which the foot

socuneiform articulations, although the first metatarsocuneiform joint should be well seen.

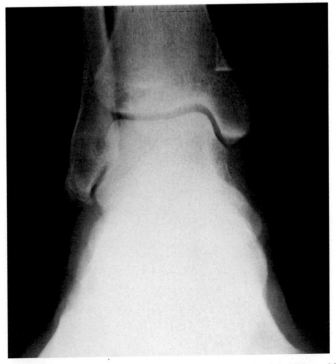

**Figure 11.6**  Anteroposterior view of ankle. This view clearly shows the lower ends of the tibia and fibula and outlines the trochlear surface of the talus. In this case there is a history of an old avulsion fracture of the fibular malleolus and non-union of a small fragment at the apex.

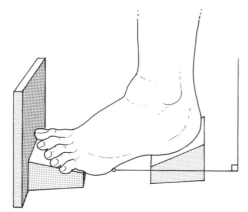

**Figure 11.7**  Positioning for axial view of sesamoids.

is held in inversion or eversion and the amount of ligamentous damage is checked by assessing the degree of tilt of the talus available in the joint. This can naturally be a painful procedure and may require an anaesthetic.

## Axial view of sesamoids

Although not commonly standard this view can be most helpful if degenerative change is suspected in the sesamoids under the first metatarsophalangeal joint. The beam is angled towards the sesamoids with the foot flexed at the metatarsophalangeal joints (Fig. 11.7). A special positioning platform may be used in some departments, but more usually the patient will be asked to retract the toes with the assistance of a loop of bandage. The view will show the ends of the metatarsals, and the sesamoidal relationship with the metatarsal will be clearly demarcated, along with any enlargement or disease (Fig. 11.8).

## Dorsiplantar oblique view

The oblique view is a non-weightbearing view which may be taken in several ways. The most common method is for the patient to sit and incline the foot at approximately 45° to the cassette, with the beam centred on the naviculocuboid joint perpendicular to the dorsum of the foot (Fig. 11.9). This view gives a distorted image of the midtarsal area, but is particularly useful for the open view given of the articular facets in the area (Fig. 11.10). Degenerative changes and pathology such as tarsal coalitions may be readily distinguished.

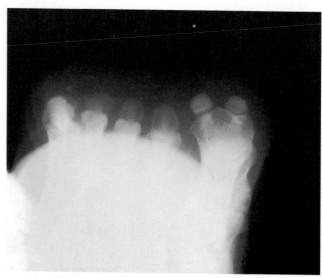

**Figure 11.8**  Axial view of sesamoids. The sesamoids under the head of the first metatarsal are clearly seen, together with the intersesamoidal ridge. In addition there is a sesamoid underlying the fifth metatarsal head.

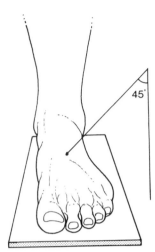

**Figure 11.9**  Positioning for dorsiplantar oblique view (DP oblique).

# BASIC RADIOLOGICAL ASSESSMENT

There is a vast amount of information that may be deduced from the careful study of an X-ray. Increased or decreased bone density, soft tissue abnormalities, age, degenerative change, trauma, metabolic disease, biomechanical abnormalities, foreign bodies and surgical interventions will all be reflected in the film. It takes much practice and knowledge to detect some of the subtler alterations in appearance. For this reason it can help to adopt a system of assessment in order to avoid missing important basic clues to a disorder. A system which has found favour amongst some is known as the ABCS of radiological assessment, where:

A = Alignment and variations
B = Bone density
C = Cartilage
S = Soft tissue.

## Alignment

In order to make judgments about the bio-

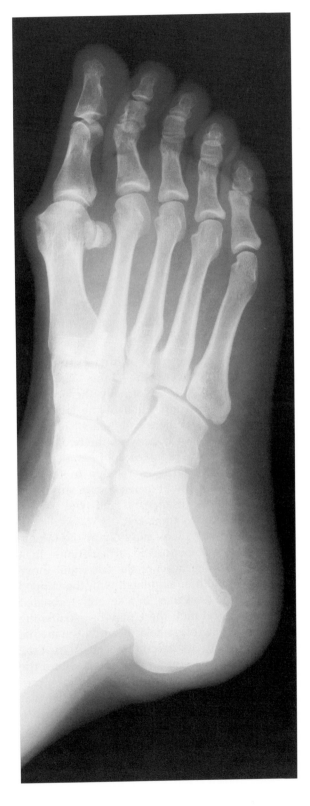

**Figure 11.10**  Dorsiplantar oblique view. In this non-weightbearing view it is possible to see the articular facets of the midtarsal joint complex much more clearly than with a weightbearing DP view. Although distorted, it also gives a useful alternative view of the other joints.

mechanical features of a particular foot as seen on X-ray it is important to decide how the picture was taken. One cannot assess with accuracy any osseous malalignment if the film was not taken weightbearing, and preferably in normal angle and base of gait. Since not many imaging departments actually take films in this way, a cautious approach should be adopted. However, one may certainly make some generalisations about the appearance of a 'normal' foot on weightbearing dorsiplantar and lateral views. It is sometimes useful to draw angles and reference points on acetate sheets overlying the films. Angles quoted below should be considered as broad guidelines only.

In this section the commonly seen anatomical variations, in particular accessory sesamoids, will be discussed.

## Dorsiplantar view (DP)

Commencing at the rearfoot, first examine the relationship between the talus and the calcaneum (Fig. 11.11). Normally there will be considerable superimposition of the talus over the calcaneum, and there will be a small notch, the talocalcaneal notch, between the two at their distal edges. In a pronated foot, as the talus adducts and plantarflexes relative to the calcaneum, this notch will increase. In a supinated foot the notch disappears and the superimposition becomes complete.

Moving distally, look carefully at the talonavicular and calcaneocuboid articulations. In a pronated foot the head of the talus will move progressively out of alignment with the cupped surface of the navicular. In a severely pronated foot of long duration there may be a flattening and remodelling of the talar head on the medial side, with as little as 20% (normal 60–70%) of the articular cartilage surface remaining within the normal confines of the joint. There will be a progressive abduction of the cuboid, the navicular and the three cuneiforms as pronation increases. This *lesser tarsus abduction angle* may be measured against a bisection of the tarsus (Fig. 11.12). The shift of the talus and lesser tarsus are somewhat reversed in a supinated foot structure, although

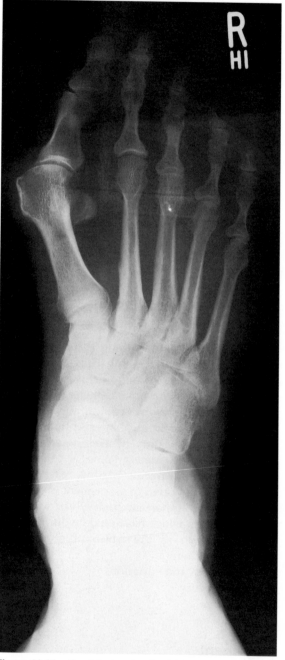

**Figure 11.11**  Dorsiplantar view (weightbearing). A case of a moderate hallux abductovalgus deformity which exhibits mild pronation at the subtalar joint, as evidenced by adduction of the head of the talus and relative abduction of the lesser tarsus. There are increases in the metatarsus primus varus angle and the hallux abductus angle, and the hallux is laterally displaced and slightly rotated into valgus. There is a lateral displacement of the sesamoids into the intermetatarsal space.

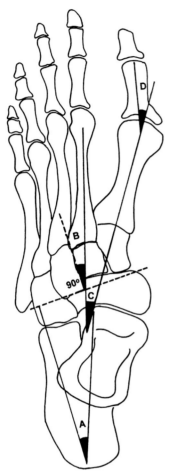

**Figure 11.12** Biomechanical evaluation of a DP view. Diagram to show: lesser tarsus abduction angle (**A**), metatarsus adductus angle (**B**), metatarsus primus adductus angle (**C**) and hallux abductus angle (**D**).

imposed. There is a notch present between the first and second metatarsal bases, the *metatarsocuneiform split*, greater in some cases than others. This may be related to the angle of the distal surface of the medial cuneiform. The base of the first metatarsal appears to have an additional transverse facet. This is in fact a superimposition of the plantar aspect of the metatarsal base, which is cup-shaped.

The lesser four metatarsals are normally parallel and virtually straight, with the fifth metatarsal sometimes exhibiting a lateral bowing, depending on the exact angle of the X-ray beam. A longitudinal bisection may be drawn of the second metatarsal and compared to a bisection of the lesser tarsus. The resulting angle, the *metatarsus adduction angle*, can be of some value in determining whether or not the condition of metatarsus adductus exists (Fig. 11.12). Some authorities believe that a normal range would be 10–20°, with a higher figure indicating that the condition is present. There will be an increase of this angle in a supinated foot and greater superimposition of the metatarsal bases over each other.

Of great importance is the relationship between the first metatarsal and the others. Construction of longitudinal bisections of the first and second metatarsals enables the *metatarsus primus adductus angle* to be measured (Fig. 11.12). Most authorities consider that the norm is 8–10°. Naturally, this angle increases dramatically in cases of metatarsus primus adductus, a component of a hallux abductovalgus deformity, and the intermetatarsal space widens.

The first metatarsal sesamoids normally lie approximately 0.5 cm proximal to the articular surface of the metatarsal head, approximately in the midline, and should appear as two smooth ovoid structures. They may be bipartite or multipartite. This does not necessarily indicate disease or injury, although sesamoids can fracture like any other bone. Since they underlie the metatarsal there is an increased depth of bone for the X-ray to penetrate. As a result they appear more dense than the rest of the metatarsal. In a case of developing hallux abductus, the sesamoids progressively move laterally, with

the talus clearly cannot move very far laterally and there is a denser superimposition of the bones.

The articular surface of the navicular with the three cuneiforms should be clearly visible. It should be possible to see the outlines of the cuneiforms, but it can be difficult to see the facets of all the inter-cuneiform joints due to superimposition. In a case of osteoarthritic degeneration the joints of the whole lesser tarsus can become indistinct.

Further distally the metatarsocuneiform joints, the fifth metatarsocuboid joint and the intermetatarsal joints are visible, although super-

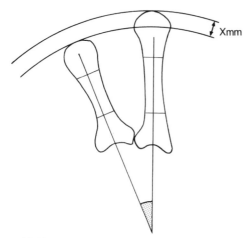

**Figure 11.13**   Measurement of metatarsal protrusion distance. Bisections of the metatarsal shafts are extended proximally, and arcs are drawn to the articular surfaces. The distance between the two arcs is measured.

the lateral sesamoid eventually ending up in the interspace between the first and second metatarsals, the medial sesamoid following closely behind. The *sesamoidal position* can be plotted against the metatarsal bisection if required.

The drawing of arcs from the intersection of the metatarsal bisections allows the relative lengths of the first and second metatarsals to be assessed, the *metatarsal protrusion distance* (Fig. 11.13). This latter measurement is generally considered normal at ± 2 mm.

In the ideal foot the hallux articulates completely with the metatarsal. If a bisection of the shaft is drawn and compared to the metatarsal bisection the *hallux abduction angle* can be measured (Fig. 11.12). The hallux may normally deviate laterally by a small amount, compensating in effect for the normal metatarsus primus adductus angle. Less than 15° is generally considered acceptable. In hallux abductus this angle increases and the articulation becomes progressively less congruous until a partial lateral subluxation occurs, with only a relatively small portion of the cartilaginous surfaces in apposition. The valgus rotation that occurs may be clearly seen in advanced cases, with the plantar condyles of the proximal phalanx becoming progressively more visible. The resultant degenerative changes will be discussed later.

Deviation of the cartilaginous surface of the metatarsal can in some cases be identified and quantified by construction of the *proximal articular set angle* (PASA). This angle has relevance in the planning of surgical procedures for hallux abductovalgus (Fig. 11.14). A deviation in the shaft of the proximal phalanx of the hallux itself can be identified by drawing the distal *articular set angle* (DASA) (Fig. 11.15). This type of deformity is sometimes responsible for the abduction deformity sometimes seen in a hallux when the first metatarsophalangeal joint alignment is normal.

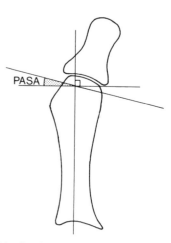

**Figure 11.14**   Proximal articular set angle (PASA). A line representing the limits of the articular cartilage on the metatarsal head is compared to a perpendicular to the bisection of the metatarsal shaft.

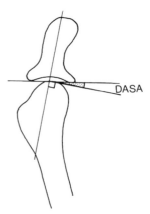

**Figure 11.15**   Distal articular set angle (DASA). A line representing the articular surface of the proximal phalanx is compared to a perpendicular to the bisection of the phalangeal shaft.

Occasionally, a hallux will have an interphalangeal joint abduction deformity which can lead to the distal abduction deformity sometimes referred to as 'terminal valgus'.

The alignment of the digits may vary. Even the most normal toes are not actually straight, but they should sit congruously on to the ends of the metatarsals. However, abduction, adduction, subluxation, dislocation and flexion deformities are exceedingly common. The superimposition of sometimes very small phalanges can sometimes make it difficult to decide on the presence or absence of bony ankyloses or other pathologies.

## Lateral view

A weightbearing lateral view will yield much useful information (Fig. 11.16). The malleoli of the tibia and fibula will be seen superimposed over the trochlear surface of the talus. The malleoli should be smooth in outline, as should the trochlear surface. The talus should be domed. Undue flattening or irregularity may be indicative of degenerative disease.

The facets of the subtalar joint should be clearly demarcated and the sustentaculum tali and sinus tarsi readily apparent. The facets and the sinus tarsi become obscured in a pronated foot and more visible in a supinated one. The calcaneum is inclined to the supporting surface, and the *calcaneal inclination angle* can be easily measured (Fig. 11.17). The normal angle will vary according to the midtarsal joint axes of motion for any particular foot. 0–10° would be considered low, 11–20° medium and 21–30° high. However, the measured angle will vary according to whether or not the foot is abnormally pronated or supinated and clinical

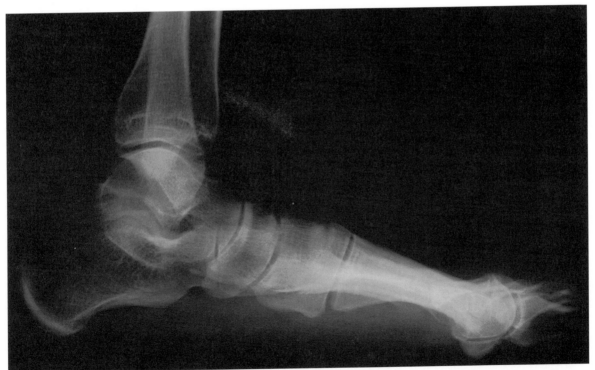

**Figure 11.16** Lateral view (weightbearing). In this pronated foot the talus is displaced medially and plantarly, obscuring the facets of the subtalar joint. The cyma line has a marked anterior break, with the smooth curve being invisible, and a bisection of the talar neck would clearly fall below the level of the first metatarsal shaft. the calcaneal inclination angle is low. Compare this foot to that shown in Figure 11.4.

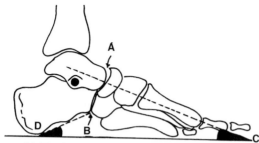

**Figure 11.17** Diagram of lateral view. Note the cyma line (**A–B**), declination of the talus (**C**) and calcaneal inclination angle (**D**).

judgment is important. While looking at the calcaneum one should check for the presence of retrocalcaneal enlargement in the area of the Achilles tendon insertion (Haglund's deformity) or for spur formation on the distal plantar aspect, bearing in mind that many so-called spurs are completely asymptomatic.

A bisection through the sloping body and neck of the talus will demonstrate the *talar declination angle* in relation to the supporting surface (Fig. 11.17). A continuation of this line will normally fall within the confines of the first metatarsal shaft. In a pronated foot the talar declination angle increases and the line falls below the first metatarsal. Conversely it will rise above it in a supinated foot as the talus is relatively adducted and dorsiflexed.

The talonavicular and calcaneocuboid joints together produce a superimposition on a lateral X-ray known as the *cyma line* (Fig. 11.17). These curved joints together form a reverse 'lazy S' as an intact curve in a normal foot. In a pronated foot the 'S' becomes broken as the talonavicular joint moves anterior and plantar to the calcaneocuboid joint, and once again the reverse occurs in a supinated foot.

In a severely pronated foot the talus and navicular plantarflex and exert a downward and retrograde tilting force on the posterior aspect of the medial cuneiform, resulting in a *naviculocuneiform fault*. In such cases the intermediate cuneiform, not normally visible, may be seen protruding above the medial cuneiform.

Less commonly, a *calcaneocuboid fault* may be seen in a high-arched foot. In this situation the cuboid may become partially displaced under the anterior plantar process of the calcaneum.

In a case of restricted subtalar joint motion it is worth carefully assessing the tarsus to eliminate the possibility of a tarsal coalition, although an oblique view is generally more help in this regard.

In the midtarsal region there is considerable superimposition, and it can take some time to distinguish the metatarsal bases from the cuneiforms. Any degenerative changes in the midtarsal region can usually be seen outlined along the dorsal surfaces.

The first and fifth metatarsals are normally easily outlined, with the others being partially superimposed. In a supinated foot one may more clearly see the second, third and fourth metatarsals. In a pronated foot the superimposition becomes more complete, and it may only be possible to clearly distinguish the first metatarsal.

At first metatarsophalangeal joint level one may see the medial and sometimes the lateral sesamoids, appearing as two ovoid structures approximately 1.0 cm diameter that are more dense due to superimposition. Their position and outline, which should normally be smooth, should be ascertained. These sesamoids may be bipartite or multipartite and are as subject to degenerative change as any other osseous structure. Osteoarthritis will produce enlargement and irregularity in the sesamoids. The dorsal aspect of the metatarsophalangeal joint should be assessed for degeneration. The hallux should normally lie in line with the metatarsal, being neither dorsiflexed nor plantarflexed. Similarly, at the interphalangeal joint look for hyperextension, flexion or degeneration. The distal phalanx can be conveniently checked for distal tufting or exostosis formation.

The lesser metatarsophalangeal joints are sometimes visible, and in particular it can be possible to pick out dorsal subluxation or dislocation.

### Anatomical variation

There are many variations of anatomical form, such as the accessory ossicles, which occur fre-

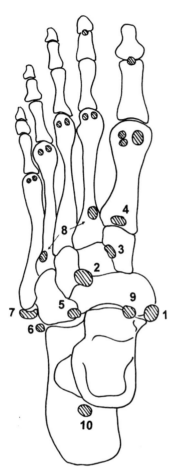

**Figure 11.18**  Accessory ossicle of the foot:  **1.** os tibiale externum;  **2.** processus uncinatus;  **3.** os intercuneiforme;  **4.** parsponea metatarsalia;  **5.** cuboideum secundarium;  **6.** os peroneum;  **7.** os vesalianum;  **8.** os intermetatarseum;  **9.** os naviculare;  **10.** os trigonum.

quently enough to be considered 'normal variants', and others which represent interesting hereditary and congenital malformations of varying degrees of severity. Accessory ossicles occur regularly in association with all the major bones in the foot (Figs 11.18 and 11.19). Most give no cause for concern, but a proportion give rise to symptoms, particularly following trauma or sporting activity, and should certainly be considered in a differential diagnosis.

**Os trigonum** is a secondary epiphysis, found on the posterior aspect of the trochlear surface of the talus, which fails to fuse to the talus in about 8% of the population. It can give rise to symptoms when the foot is regularly plantarflexed, or subject to injury, as in footballers and ballet dancers.

**Os tibiale externum** lies under the insertion of tibialis posterior as it crosses the navicular, and is subject to problems following forced abduction or eversion injuries.

**Os peroneum** lies under peroneus longus in the peroneal groove of the cuboid and is sometimes not noticed except on a lateral or oblique X-ray. Occasionally it can be symptomatic, particularly in a supinated foot.

**Os vesalianum** is a secondary epiphysis at the fifth metatarsal base and must be differentiated from an avulsion fracture. Generally a fracture will have a longitudinal orientation and an irregular outline, compared to the transverse orientation and smooth contour of the ossicle.

**Metatarsophalangeal joint sesamoids and interphalangeal joint sesamoids** occur regularly in varying numbers under any of the joints, and can be symptomatic. In particular, the hallux interphalangeal joint may have a sesamoid which is troublesome, particularly in a hyperextended joint. This sesamoid appears as a small ovoid on a dorsiplantar view, but may have an inverted triangular section on lateral view.

**Polydactyly,** the presence of additional phalanges or complete digits, is common enough to be seen in varying forms. *Brachydactyly*, the partial failure of development of a metatarsal segment or phalanges, is less common and, like polydactyly, has a hereditary predisposition (Fig. 11.20). Cases of *congenital aplasia*, with complete failure of development of a segment, are even more rare.

**Coalitions** may take several forms, and may be fibrous, (syndesmosis), cartilaginous (synchondrosis) or osseous (synostosis). The more common forms are the talonavicular bar, the calcaneonavicular bar and the talocalcaneal bar (Fig. 11.21), all of which will limit subtalar joint motion and are most easily viewed on oblique X-rays. Other coalitions, such as intermetatarsal bars, may also be found. Suspected coalitions need to be confirmed with tomographic scans

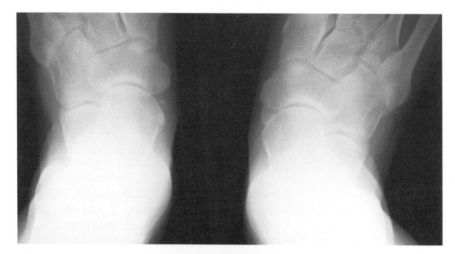

**Figure 11.19** Accessory ossicle—os tibiale externum. In this case os tibiale externum occurs bilaterally in a slightly pronated foot. The ossicle on the right foot is bipartite.

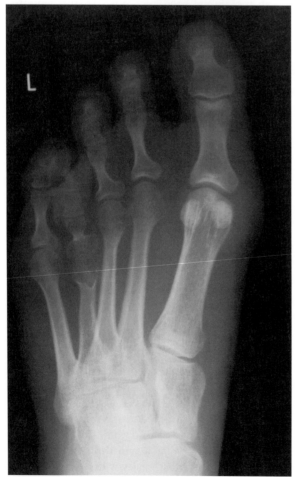

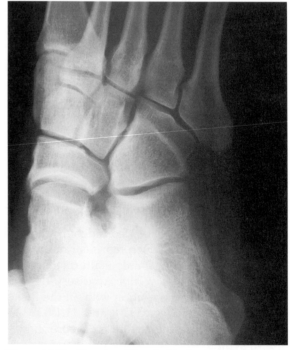

**Figure 11.20** Brachydactyly. There is a marked congenital shortening of the fourth metatarsal and phalanges. The digit is actually dorsally displaced, and in this case the condition was bilateral.

**Figure 11.21** Tarsal coalition. In this dorsiplantar oblique view there is clear evidence of a talocalcaneal coalition. The patient had no subtalar joint motion available and was suffering increasing pain in the rearfoot. The condition was later confirmed with a CT scan which is reproduced later in the chapter.

(CAT) or magnetic resonance imaging (MRI) which can give much more detailed images.

## Bone density

Bone is in a constant state of change, new bone formation by osteoblasts normally being balanced by the resorptive activity of osteoclasts. These activities are governed by the endocrine systems, and are also altered by chemical and vitamin factors in the blood, by diet, by malabsorption from the gut, by disease and repair processes and by physical forces to which the bone is subjected. The growth and maturation processes are beyond the scope of this chapter, but are well described in many standard textbooks, e.g. Parsons 1980, Kumar & Clark 1990.

An area of increased density to X-rays, which will produce a whiter shadow on the film, is known as *increased radiopacity*. Decreased density, which will give a blacker shadow, as *increased radiolucency*. The appearance of increased density of bone on an X-ray is known as *osteosclerosis* or *eburnation*, while decreased density is called *osteopenia*. The term 'osteoporosis' is nowadays reserved for a decrease in bone density due to pathological conditions, and will be dealt with later in the chapter. A sclerotic area will appear whiter on the film, since a greater amount of radiation will have been absorbed by the bone and osteopenic areas will be darker.

Assessment of density by the naked eye is the normal everyday method, but it takes time and much experience before one may be confident of accurate judgment. There are some scientific methods for the evaluation of bone density which may be used by radiologists (National Osteoporosis Society 1993). *Dual energy X-ray absorptiometry* (DEXA) is used on the spine and femoral neck. *Single-photon* or *dual-photon absorptiometry* (SPA or DPA) measures bone density in the forearm. *Quantitative computed tomography* (QCT) is an expensive method used on the spine. Investigations are under way into the effectiveness of *ultrasonic scanning* on the calcaneum. X-rays themselves are of little use for early diagnosis, as bone loss of 30% can occur before radiological changes are apparent.

An adult foot with normal bone density will show several clearly defined features:

- The dense outer cortices will be clearly visible as more sclerotic areas, an average of 1–2 mm thick, around the periphery of the short bones and along the shafts of the long bones, petering out at the metaphyseal areas; in the phalanges, which are considerably narrower, the cortical thickness is still maintained and thus the cortex may appear to account for a relatively larger amount of the shaft.
- The medullary cavities appear as relatively radiolucent areas and the cancellous bone is traversed by fine trabecular patterns which extend into the epiphyses. The trabeculae are lamellae arranged to withstand forces and can be more marked in areas of high stress. The calcaneum often exhibits good examples of trabeculation.
- The proximal and distal articular surfaces of the long bones have a fine sclerotic line around the perimeter, which is normally uninterrupted. This line may increase in thickness if the density of the bone increases when subject to extra stresses, or may disappear in certain disease processes.
- The metatarsals often show a U-shaped sclerotic line at the metaphyseal junction with the epiphysis, which must not be confused with a fracture.

In a juvenile foot the epiphyseal lines will still be visible as radiolucent transverse lines. The appearance of the epiphyses will depend upon the stage of development.

### Osteoporosis

Probably the most well-known cause of osteoporosis is the decrease in hormone production which occurs at the menopause. 30% of postmenopausal women will suffer significant osteoporosis, which is largely preventable with replacement therapy. It is less well known that approximately 5% of men in middle age will also develop osteoporosis (National Osteoporosis Society 1993).

*Hypopituitarism* reduces bone growth and produces short, slender bones with thin cortices. There are delays in epiphyseal fusion.

Hyperactivity of the adrenal glands, or a pituitary adenoma, may cause the generalised osteoporosis of *Cushing's syndrome*. There are around 11 000 sufferers from *Turner's syndrome* in the UK, who have undeveloped ovaries and are likely to have osteoporosis.

*Hyperthyroidism*, which could be due to excessive thyroid hormone replacement therapy, increases the rate of bone remodelling. Faster resorption than new bone formation occurs which may cause thinning of the cortices. Stress fractures can occur in the long bones.

Interference with vitamin D intake or one of several *disorders of vitamin D metabolism* causes rickets in children, i.e. prior to epiphyseal closure, and osteomalacia in adults. Malabsorption due to intestinal disease or gastrectomy may be a factor. Sufferers from anorexia nervosa or bulimia should be considered at-risk patients for osteoporosis, as should ballet dancers and gymnasts who may deliberately starve themselves. In children this leads to characteristic deformities of wrists and legs, with enlargement and irregularities of the epiphyseal plates, and generalised osteoporosis due to failure of the osteoid tissue to mineralise. In the adult there is softening and deformation of the bones, with diminished density. There may be evidence of stress fractures.

*Hyperparathyroidism*, due to hyperplasia of the parathyroid glands (primary type), persistent stimulation due to low serum calcium levels (secondary type) or an adenoma (tertiary type) or carcinoma, will reduce bone density by resorption of calcium salts. Not all cases will show definite osseous changes, but there may be subperiosteal thinning of the long bone cortices, particularly the digits, and distal resorption. 'Brown tumours' may be noted expanding the long bone shafts and there may be calcification of joint cartilages, chondrocalcinosis, in long-standing cases.

Osteoporosis occurs on a local level following a period of disuse of a limb, for example after injury or surgery when immobilisation has been employed. For example, quite marked demineralisation can sometimes be seen, temporarily, following a metatarsal osteotomy, which quickly reverses when stress and function return. Occasionally there is an abnormal response to quite minor injury leading to the condition of *reflex sympathetic dystrophy*. As well as swelling, pain and stiffness which are out of proportion to the injury, there may be radiographic evidence of irregular mottled osteoporosis distal to the injury site. This radiographic appearance is known as Sudeck's atrophy.

Autoimmune disease processes such as rheumatoid arthritis produce specific bone density changes which will be dealt with later.

Finally, it is known that excessive smoking or alcohol intake may play a part in osteoporosis.

## Osteosclerosis

One may also see increased bone density on X-ray. Most commonly it is found in areas of higher stress, where the osteoblastic activity increases to cope with the forces. This will also be observed around healing fracture sites. In these cases the resulting bone will always be sclerotic even after the resorptive osteoclastic activity.

*Hypoparathyroidism*, a deficiency of parathormone, results in blood calcium levels falling and phosphate levels rising. The syndrome can result in short lesser metatarsals, calcification in some ligaments of the spine and in some cases increased sclerosis.

*Hypervitaminosis D* can lead to increased distal metaphyseal calcification and calcium deposits in the skin and periosteum.

*Paget's disease* is a common disorder of unknown origin, although there may be inherited factors. There is speculation and research into a low-grade viral involvement. It is secondary in prevalence to osteoporosis and 0.5–1.0% of 45–54-year-olds and 10–20% of those over 85 will be affected. Males are more commonly affected than females. Symptoms such as paraesthesia and pain are frequently related to nerve compression. The disease causes excessive bone resorption followed by haphazard new bone formation and remodelling. Isolated bones or the entire skeleton may be involved, and severe characteristic thickening and deformity may result. The foot is rarely involved except for the calcaneum. Although the bones are very enlarged and appear dense on X-ray they are of poor quality; microfractures are not uncommon. It should be remembered that Paget's disease predisposes to an increased incidence of osteosarcoma and fibrosarcoma, although less than 1% progress to a malignancy.

*Metastatic bone disease* from primary carcinomata elsewhere, such as the breast, may show sclerotic deposits, although the majority of metastases produce lytic changes. Secondary metastases are uncommon, but not unknown, in the foot. Some primary bone tumours also produce sclerotic changes, and these will be dealt with separately.

*Osteopetrosis* (Albers-Schoenberg disease or marble bone disease) is a rare hereditary disorder causing thickening of the trabeculae in all the bones; in particular there may be dense bands in the vertebrae. Although the bones are dense they are more susceptible to shear forces and may fracture more easily.

*Increased fluorine ingestion* (fluorosis) over many years may result in the laying down of new bone inside the medullary cavity of long bones, leading to a sclerotic appearance. There may also be periosteal outgrowths.

*Epiphyseal, metaphyseal* and *diaphyseal dysplasias*, which form a whole group of hereditary and congenital traits, may lead to many permutations of growth disorders, some of which involve increased bone density.

## Cartilage

Ordinarily one does not see cartilage on X-ray as it is radiolucent. The condition of cartilage really has to be assessed by the relationship of the adjacent bones in a joint. For example a healthy metatarsophalangeal joint will show smoothly outlined joint surfaces evenly separated by 1–2 mm of blackness, which represents the cartilaginous surfaces. Careful examination may reveal the approximate edges of the cartilage surfaces. In a joint which is malaligned or commencing a disease process one of the first signs will be changes in the cartilage space. This can usefully be compared to similar joints elsewhere

in the foot. The space may become narrowed evenly or unevenly, may become calcified and may eventually disappear totally, for example in advanced osteoarthrosis, or may be increased in cases of joint effusion or early rheumatoid disease. These conditions will be dealt with later under the headings of arthritis and rheumatoid disease.

## Soft tissue

On a normal X-ray there will be very little soft tissue evident although the outline of the foot will be delineated. There will be no details elsewhere and any space-occupying lesion would have to be diagnosed purely on bony malalignment in the same way as cartilage damage. For example an intermetatarsal bursa may cause splaying of the adjacent metatarsals and proximal phalanges. It is important in the primary assessment of the film to compare soft-tissue thicknesses and densities with other sections of the feet. With a 'soft' X-ray taken at a lower power there will be progressively more soft tissue visible. If the X-ray has been particularly requested for a suspected soft-tissue lesion this should be clearly stated on the request form. It is sometimes possible to see the shadow of a neoplasm such as a large ganglion (Fig. 11.22), but this cannot be relied on for diagnosis.

Soft tissues can become more visible when involved in disease processes. Long-standing *diabetes* may cause calcification of the small arteries, which appear as small white 'worms', particularly between the first and second metatarsals along the course of the dorsalis pedis artery. Similar changes may be seen in cases of hyperparathyroidism and arteriosclerosis. Other tissues may have calcareous deposits, particularly the muscles and tendons following injury, in which case the condition is known as *myositis ossificans*. All bursae are capable of undergoing degenerative calcification. This is not uncommon at the first metatarsophalangeal joint (Fig. 11.23). Sinus tracts may also calcify.

The skin and subdermal tissues may exhibit the crystalline sodium urate monohydrate deposits of *gout*, usually close to a joint. In

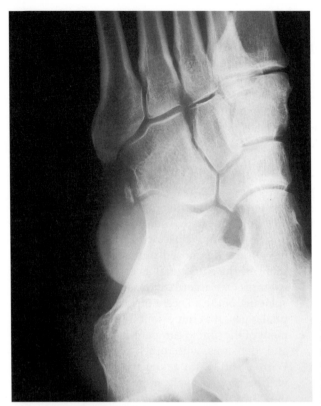

**Figure 11.22** Ganglion. On this dorsiplantar oblique view a large ganglionic cyst is seen arising from the lateral aspect of the tarsus. The X-ray cannot demarcate the origin. Clinically the growth was approximately 4 cm in diameter and very tense. An incidental finding is the presence of an accessory ossicle, os peroneum, on the lateral aspect of the cuboid.

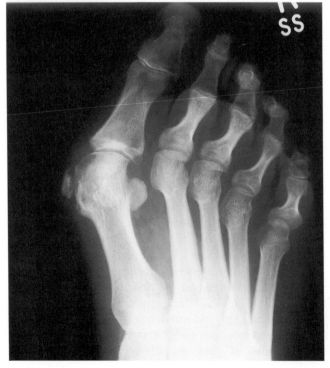

**Figure 11.23** Bursal calcification. This case of hallux abductovalgus had an overlying bursa within which was found an area of calcification. Note also the early manifestations of osteoarthritic degeneration in the joint.

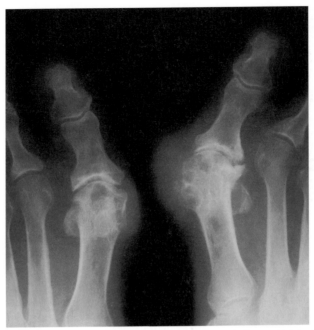

**Figure 11.24** Gout. This radiograph shows gout attacking both first metatarsophalangeal joints. The joints have clearly 'punched-out' erosions associated with gross degenerative changes. There is a large overlying bursa on the right foot.

untreated gout the joint will show degenerative arthritic change with characteristic punched-out erosions near the joint margins (Fig. 11.24). In *pseudogout* there are depositions of pyrophosphate crystals which lead to intracapsular effusion, increased soft tissue density, and increased joint space. Calcium salts may mimic gout in the condition of *calcinosis cutis*, a collagen disease, but the deposits, which are clearly visible, generally occur well away from joint margins.

Normally the periosteum is not visible unless pathological changes are occurring. The periosteum may become elevated and visible due to inflammation, infection or trauma and may in turn become calcified.

The condition of *xanthoma tuberosum multiplex*, believed to be endocrine in origin, can be responsible for large, benign, clearly delineated soft-tissue masses which have a marked increase in density. They can occur in relation to synovial tendon sheaths and bursae in the foot and elsewhere.

## RADIOLOGICAL ASSESSMENT OF SPECIFIC PATHOLOGIES

### Infection

It is important to recognise the development of infection in bone on radiographic evidence as well as by clinical presentation, although radiological changes may not be present in the osseous structures for some time. The first signs are unlikely to appear for 10 days or more. Infection may be blood-borne, or a focus from elsewhere in the body, or secondary to a direct entry wound such as surgery or a compound fracture. Although bone and joint infections can be due to diseases such as tuberculosis (dramatically on the increase worldwide), leprosy, syphilis or viral agents such as smallpox, the most common infections are the acute bacterial infections due to organisms such as *Staphylococcus aureus*, *Staphylococcus pyogenes*, *Salmonella* or *Haemophilus influenzae*. The infection spreads firstly into the medullary bone but will not cross the epiphyseal line. One of the first signs is

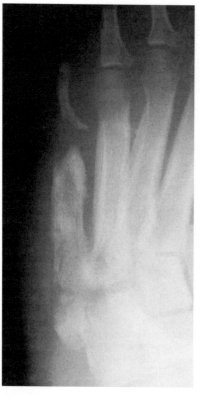

**Figure 11.25** Osteomyelitis. Chronic osteomyelitis in this neuropathic diabetic foot has destroyed much of the fifth metatarsal and phalanges. Note the characteristic fuzzy outline of the elevated periosteum.

increased soft-tissue density and swelling, which should be readily apparent on X-ray. Infection then passes through the cortex and the pus produced elevates and strips the periosteum. The first visible osseous change will often be the subperiosteal reaction, which lifts the periosteum and gives a fuzzy outline to the bone. The bone will lose density and appear hazy. In time a loose body or *sequestrum* may be formed (Figs 11.25 and 11.26). This can be passed to the surface by sinus formation, or it may eventually be reabsorbed or remodelled. In some cases a remodelling of the cortex may produce a sclerotic osseous shell, an *involucrum*, which encapsulates the sequestrum. If treatment is inefficient a chronic walled-off abscess containing debris and sometimes a sequestrum may form and can persist for years. Known as *Brodie's abscess*, this appears as a rarefied ovoid area and may particularly be seen at the metaphyseal areas of long bones.

## Osteoarthritis

The signs and symptoms of degenerative osteoarthritis are well known. On X-ray the earliest signs are irregularity and narrowing of the

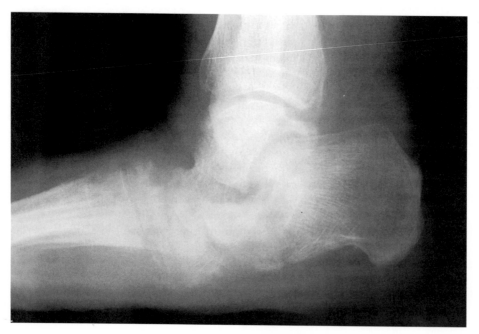

**Figure 11.26** Osteomyelitis. Almost complete destruction of the neck of the talus and all midtarsal bones, due to chronic osteomyelitis.

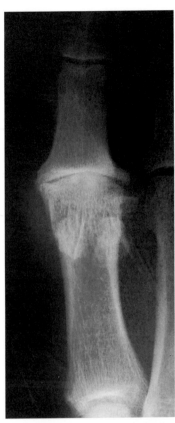

**Figure 11.27**    Osteoarthritis. This case of hallux rigidus shows complete loss of articular cartilage and early osteophytic changes at the joint periphery. There is no deviation in the joint in this case.

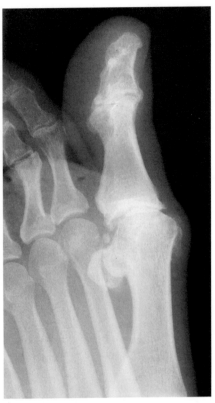

**Figure 11.28**    Osteoarthritis. This oblique view, a more advanced case than that shown in Figure 11.27, shows severe degeneration of the joint margins with obliteration of the joint space. There are multiple osteophytes, some of which have fractured away to become loose bodies within the joint capsule.

cartilaginous space, which may or may not be accompanied by deformity (Fig. 11.27). As the disease progresses the cartilage will degenerate and become calcified (*chondrocalcinosis*) and the joint space slowly disappears. There will be increased sclerosis, and there may be the formation of subchondral cysts. At the periphery of the joint there will be clearly visible spiky outgrowths of bone, *osteophytes*, which tend to grow at right angles to the long bone axis and can attain considerable size. Osteophytes severely limit joint motion and will also cause pain and pressure problems for the patient. In late stages of the disease the joint will become partially or fully ankylosed and the osteophytes may fracture, causing loose bodies within the joint capsule (Fig. 11.28). These osteophytic fractures

and loose bodies are clearly visible on film. While it is relatively easy to diagnose osteoarthritis in the metatarsophalangeal joints, degeneration in the midtarsal area can be masked by superimposition of the bones and may only be seen on lateral or oblique views.

## Autoimmune disease

There are many varieties of autoimmune disease that attack the joints, including rheumatoid arthritis, scleroderma and disseminated lupus erythematosus. Radiographic analysis is only one part of the diagnostic process, but most of the diseases produce similar radiographic features.

Early changes are effusion into the joint capsule as the synovial linings are attacked, with an

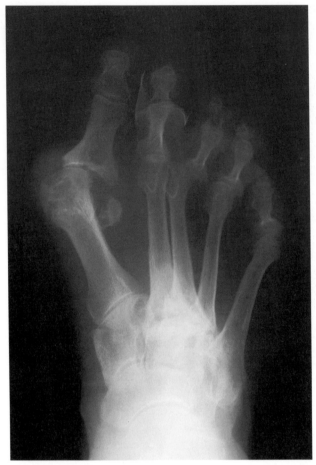

**Figure 11.29** Rheumatoid arthritis. In this long-standing rheumatoid patient one may see gross derangement of all metatarsophalangeal joints, with subluxation in particular of the hallux and third and fourth toes. There is generalised osteoporosis and there are subchondral erosions, particularly seen around the first metatarsophalangeal joint. The midtarsal joints are also affected, with loss of bone density and joint demarcation.

intracapsular increase in density. The joint spaces may increase temporarily. The epiphyses of the long bones become demineralised and as the synovial pannus invades the bone there is a progression towards erosions at the chondral margins, loss of cortex and punched-out peri-articular erosions. There is a progressive loss of normal trabecular patterns and generalised osteoporosis (Fig. 11.29). Articular and bone changes are associated with progressive deformity and characteristic abduction deformities of digits. Gross subluxations and dislocations will be evident in severe cases. There is usually mid-tarsal and rearfoot involvement in long-standing

cases. Radiographic signs of severe pronation may often be seen.

In juvenile disorders such as Still's disease there may be retardation of long bone growth and premature epiphyseal closure, with 'spindling' of the digits.

## Osteochondrosis

This is avascular necrosis of the epiphysis or apophysis, in which there is a well-documented cycle of interference with the vascular supply to an epiphysis, possibly trauma-related but some-times associated with endocrine dysfunction,

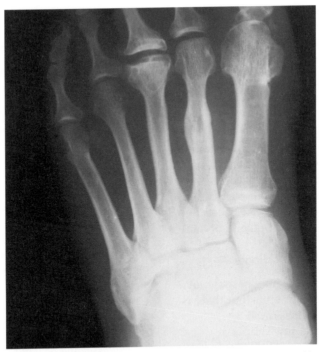

**Figure 11.30**  Freiberg's infraction. The evident flattening and collapse of the third metatarsal head in this middle-aged patient is probably indicative of an old Freiberg's infraction, although this case is unconfirmed. This X-ray also shows: a Keller's arthroplasty, with several loose bodies remaining around the site; an old fracture of the second metatarsal shaft; two sesamoids under the fifth metatarsal head; and a lateral exostectomy of the fifth metatarsal head.

followed by degeneration and later regeneration. It occurs in several sites on the foot, as well as in the femoral epiphysis (*Legg–Calvé–Perthes disease*), vertebral epiphysis (*Schauerman's disease*) and the tibial tubercle (*Osgood–Schlatter's disease*). Over 40 potential sites have been identified. In all the conditions there is a transient increase in sclerosis caused by the failure of the blood supply to remove calcium salts, followed by osteoporosis, crumbling and degeneration of the epiphysis. Revascularisation slowly occurs over a period of months and the epiphysis remodels, sometimes with residual deformity. The conditions are self-limiting and the clinical importance relates to the functional importance of the joint involved. In the foot the common conditions are as follows.

**Freiberg's infraction,** which affects the lesser metatarsal heads, usually the second or third, at the age of about 12–14 years. An increase in the joint space may be noted due to the 'eggshell

crush' degeneration that occurs in the metatarsal head. The finally remodelled head may be flattened or saucer-shaped. In later life it may produce secondary hypertrophic osteoarthritic degeneration (Fig. 11.30).

**Sever's disease** of the calcaneal apophysis usually occurs in the age range 8–12 years. An irregularity and sclerosis may be exhibited along the apophyseal line on the posterior aspect of the calcaneum. However, it should be noted that the apophyseal line is frequently irregular in any case. Some authorities believe that a diagnosis of Sever's disease cannot be made with any certainty on radiographic evidence alone.

**Kohler's disease** of the navicular occurs in youngsters in the age range 2–10 years, with a mean of 3–5 years. 70% of cases are male and there is a familial incidence. The navicular becomes dense initially, followed by porosis and collapse into a disc shape, clearly seen on a lateral view. If untreated the bone may not regain proper form and may remain a lifelong problem.

**Other rarer conditions** are Iselin's disease of the fifth metatarsal base and Bushke's disease of the cuneiforms.

## Trauma

The foot is subject to a wide range of trauma resulting in a variety of pathologies from a hairline stress fracture to major complicated fractures or the presence of foreign bodies. A careful history is required in all cases. At least two radiographic views must be taken of any suspected injury site.

Fractures can be classified as follows:

- *Simple fractures*, where there may or may not be displacement of the bone ends, but there is no penetration through the skin
- *Stress fractures*, extremely fine simple fractures more usually seen on the lesser metatarsals, although the tibia and fibula are also recognised sites, particularly in runners. The fracture may be so fine as to be missed until a later stage when bony callus can be seen around the site. Suspected stress fractures can sometimes only be confirmed using isotope scanning methods
- *Compound fractures*, where the skin has been breached by bone
- *Complicated fractures*, where there is associated trauma or infection involving muscles, tendons and blood vessels
- *Greenstick fractures*, which occur when the bone is bent but only one side of the cortex breaks (frequently seen in children)
- *Comminuted fractures*, in which there is splintering or fragmentation
- *Impacted fractures*, where one bone is driven forcibly into the other
- *Avulsion fractures*, where a chip of bone is ripped away by fibrous attachment such as muscle or ligament. Such fractures can occur in similar sites to accessory ossicles. The fifth metatarsal base is a common site for a fracture and for os vesalianum, and care must be taken to differentiate between them

- *Pathological fractures*, which may occur due to osteoporosis or in cases of primary or secondary neoplastic bone disease.

Certain parts of the foot are prone to specific types of fracture.

- *Pott's fracture* occurs following a forceful direct injury or twist to the ankle and causes a spiral fracture to the fibula approximately 5–8 cm above the malleolus, and also fractures the medial malleolus. There is considerable disruption of the ankle mortise and the articular surfaces between the trochlear surface of the talus and the tibia may be damaged
- *The calcaneum* may suffer from comminuted or stress fractures following a fall from a height or due to disease processes. A comminuted fracture will show as a line of increased density
- *The talar neck* can be fractured in an incident involving forced ankle dorsiflexion
- *Metatarsal and phalangeal fractures* occur very commonly with all forms of injury.

The normal timetable of fracture healing can be found in Table 11.1.

## Foreign bodies

Injuries from foreign body penetration are common in the foot and range from human or animal hairs to metal filings, glass, plastic and wood splinters. Surgical implants are also foreign bodies (Fig. 11.31). Some substances will show as areas of increased density on X-ray, but glass and wood can be difficult to recognise. More than one view is necessary to try and locate a foreign body.

## Neoplasia

The radiological diagnosis of bone tumours requires the expertise of a radiologist. A misdiagnosis could prove fatal to the patient.

A complete classification of tumours with radiological features is beyond the scope of this chapter, but some of the commoner presentations are shown below.

**Table 11.1** Normal timetable for fracture healing

| Time span | Process |
| --- | --- |
| Week 1–2 | Extravasation of blood takes place between the broken ends. X-rays show sharp bone edges with or without displacement and effusion into the soft tissues. |
| Week 2–3 | A fibrosis occurs in the initial blood clot and calcification forms between the broken ends, and may be visualised as a fuzzy plug of tissue. The bone edges will be more blurred. If the fracture is immobilised there will be little or no extra callus formation. A fracture that remains mobile will produce an increased amount of calcified tissue in the area which can be seen clearly on X-ray. |
| Week 3–8 | Calcification in an immobilised fracture should be completed. The fracture line will disappear and remodelling of any excess bone will eventually, over a period of months, restore nearly normal, but slightly thickened contours in the bone (Fig. 11.30). A fracture which has not been immobilised, or in which the bone ends are not apposed, or in a patient with poor circulation or disease processes, may continue to delayed or non-union and exhibit osteoporotic changes with extra bone callus continuing to form; the fracture line will remain evident. |

## Benign bone tumours

**Osteochondroma (osteocartilaginous exostosis).** This may occur as a solitary lesion, developing from the periosteum. It has an equal sex distribution. The tumour shows on X-ray as a mass of trabeculated bone, but it has a cartilaginous cap which is invisible. Many of these growths are asymptomatic, but others may give rise to pain due to pressure on nerves. Practitioners frequently see the pedunculated subungual exostosis on the distal phalanx of the hallux, which may have a traumatic origin (Fig. 11.32). The commonest presentation is in the femur or tibia, and the condition can exist in multiple form as an inherited tendency. Transformation to a malignant chondrosarcoma is rare, but recurrence, the presence of soft tissue shadows or increased cartilaginous thickening should raise suspicion levels.

**Enchondroma.** These benign tumours, which may have a malignant tendency, are caused by the development of embryonic cartilage cells

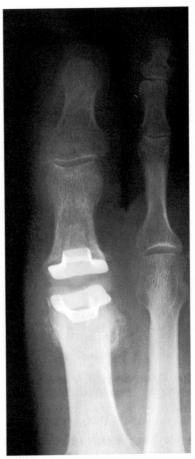

**Figure 11.31** Foreign body—joint replacement. This X-ray shows a Swanson double-stemmed implant in situ following surgery for acute hallux rigidus. The body of the implant can only just be identified between the bone ends, with the stems extending into the medullary canals. The two titanium grommets, through which the stems pass, are clearly seen.

within the shafts of long bones such as metatarsals and phalanges. The tumour is expansile and produces areas of osteoporosis, loss of trabeculation and thin cortices, giving a 'soap bubble' appearance. Pathological fractures can occur. Figure 11.33 shows a multiple enchondromatosis or *Ollier's disease*.

**Solitary (simple) bone cyst.** This is a cyst of unknown origin containing clear or serosanguinous fluid. It generally occurs in the age range 4–15 years and may only be discovered as a result of a pathological fracture. It has a predilection for the humerus and femur, but can

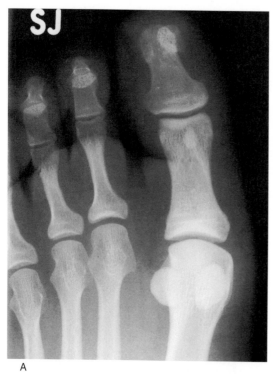
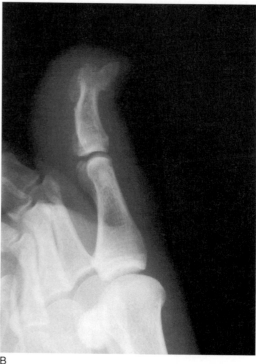

A                                                              B

**Figure 11.32** Osteochondroma. A dorsiplantar view (**A**) and oblique view (**B**) of a subungual exostosis on the hallux, secondary to trauma. These lesions usually have a cartilaginous cap, classifying them as osteochondromata.

occur in the long bones of the foot and the calcaneum. It may cause cortical thinning, with lucent areas in the medulla, but does not always expand the bone.

**Aneurysmal bone cyst.** A sponge-like cyst with blood-filled spaces and fibrous septa, this may arise as the result of a vascular anomaly. It tends to occur in the age range 20–30 years and has equal sex distribution. 50% of the cases are in the long bone metaphyses. There is a rarefied central area with a thin cortical shell and the cyst will rapidly expand and destroy bone tissue.

**Osteoid osteoma.** A most painful lesion which occurs most often in the long bones of the extremities, with over 65% incidence in the femur and tibia. No bones are exempt, including the feet. 75% of cases are in 5–20-year-old patients with a sex ratio of 2:1 male to female. Radiologically it exhibits an ovoid translucent nidus up to 2 cm in diameter surrounded by an area of sclerosis. In fact the sclerosis may be such that it

masks the radiolucent area. The patient may complain of severe pain at night. The differential diagnosis should include Brodie's abscess.

**Synovial chondromatosis.** This condition occurs mainly in young or middle-aged males. Multiple metaplastic cartilaginous bodies form within the synovial membranes around a joint, usually the knee or shoulder but occasionally in the digits. Sometimes they will become true loose bodies within the joint. Radiographic appearance is of multiple small calcified opacities, accompanied by joint effusion and increased soft tissue density.

### Malignant bone tumours

**Osteosarcoma** is the commonest primary malignant bone neoplasm, accounting for 40%. It is not common in the foot, having a 50% incidence in the lower end of the femur and the upper ends of the tibia and humerus. It may

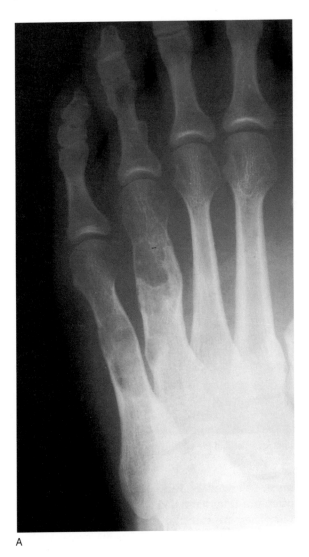

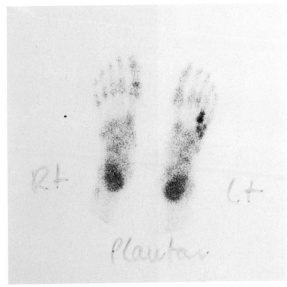

B    Upper

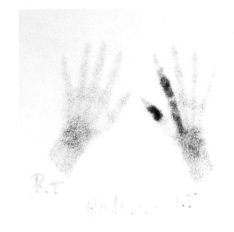

A

B    Lower

**Figure 11.33**   Multiple enchondromatosis. Note the expansile, thin-walled lesions in the fourth and fifth metatarsal shafts (**A**). The patient had similar lesions in the metacarpals of the left hand. The lesions were noted to have increased vascularity on isotope bone scans (**B**).

occur secondarily to Paget's disease. An X-ray may reveal radiating 'sunray' spicules of bone raising the periosteum, although this is not particularly common, and a mixture of lysis or sclerosis within the shaft of the bone. A wedge of ossified tissue can form under the periosteum and is called *Codman's triangle*. Osteosarcoma can occur, but rarely, in soft tissues. Radiologically it shows soft tissue swelling and patchy density.

**Chondrosarcomas** arise from cartilaginous tissue and are second in frequency to osteosarcoma. Primary cases arise within the medulla, mainly in the long bones and ribs, with 10% of cases in the spine. Secondary cases arise from pre-existing cartilaginous pathology. The tumours occur mainly in the age range 50–70 years, with a sex ratio of 2:1 male to female. They are rare in the foot but have been noted in

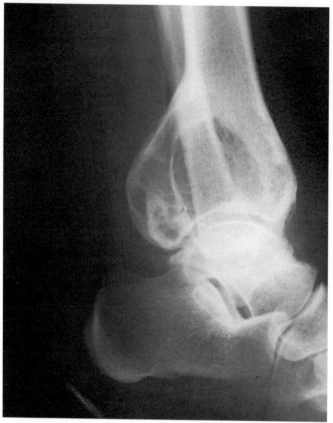

**Figure 11.34** Giant cell tumour: a large vascular tumour affecting the lower end of the tibia.

the calcaneum. Radiologically they can be very varied in appearance, imitating other lesions, but classically they produce expansile 'grape-like' lesions, with a calcified periphery and multiple calcified central foci. Chondrosarcoma can occur in an 'extraosseous form' in soft tissues away from bone.

**Fibrosarcomas** are less common than osteosarcomas and occur primarily in the 40–60 age range. They are highly destructive tumours producing expansile 'motheaten' lesions with slight periosteal reaction in the major long bones and pelvis. 50% of cases occur around the knee joint.

**Giant cell tumours,** of which about 15% are malignant, account for about 4% of histologically identified tumours. They occur primarily in the age range 16–45 years. There is an equal sex distribution. 50% of the growths are around the knee, followed in incidence by the radius and ulna, but they have been observed in hands and feet. They are vascular tumours, which on X-ray present as expanded translucent areas with a thin cortical rim. Sometimes the cortex is breached but there is no active new bone formation present and there may be little periosteal reaction (Fig. 11.34). Differential diagnosis should include the aneurysmal bone cyst.

**Ewing's tumour** is a primary tumour of bone accounting for 5% of primary bone tumours. The age range is generally 5–30 years, with the majority of cases aged 10–20 years. Initially there may only be minor porotic changes visible on X-ray, with early periosteal change and delicate spiculisation being suggestive of osteomyelitis. These later changes cause considerable tissue destruction, with a mottled destructive appearance, cortical penetration and maybe pathological fractures. It has frequently metastasised by the time the patient is first seen.

**Secondary metastases** may occur in bone from malignancies elsewhere, such as the breast, kidney, prostate or bowel.

## OTHER IMAGING MODALITIES

While X-rays provide a considerable amount of information about bone tissue, and are currently the most commonly used imaging modality, there are other methods of obtaining images which are for specific problems and deserve consideration.

## Computed tomography (CT)

In this technique the patient is moved slowly through a circular hole in a gantry containing a mobile X-ray generator and detectors. The X-ray tube rotates completely around the patient in a plane determined by the radiographer. The X-rays generated are picked up by an array of up to 1200 detectors, digitised and fed to a visual display screen via a computer. Hard copy images can also be produced using film. The images produced are in fact slices through the body, and they may be taken at intervals of 2–10 mm. Any portion of the body can be scanned subject to positioning limitations. The images produced give good osseous outline but little detail of the bone substance, even with the enhancement capabilities of the computer. Soft tissues are clearly delineated and a radiologist will be able to differentiate muscle, fat and connective tissues. The CT scan is useful for analysis of suspected coalitions, malformations and trauma in the lower limb. It has a high cost and cannot therefore be used as a routine investigation. It is best used as a secondary test in a case which has already been X-rayed and over which some doubt remains (Fig. 11.35).

## Magnetic resonance imaging (MRI)

At present this is the most expensive imaging technique as the capital cost of the equipment is vast. However it has the ability to produce stunningly accurate images of bone and soft tissues and will prove valuable for the foot as it becomes more readily available. The image is obtained by the application of a pulsed magnetic field, which temporarily realigns the inherent nuclear magnetic field in the atoms of the body tissues. During this realignment energy is emitted in the form of small amounts of very-high-frequency radiowaves. This can be detected and recorded. The images obtained depend on the proton density of the tissue, with hydrogen being the most important nucleus for imaging purposes; this makes the water content very important. Soft tissues that are inflamed contain more water, producing lighter images and very detailed images of soft tissue injuries and pathology can be generated (Fig. 11.36). The images, like those produced by tomography, appear in a sliced format, computer-enhanced.

## Nuclear medicine–isotope scanning

The technique of nuclear labelling is an old one, first used in the 1940s with isotopes such as strontium-87 and fluorine-18. It relies on the fact that an inflamed or pathologically active area of the skeleton has an increased blood flow and bone activity. If a suitable radioisotope is injected intravenously with a phosphate marker it will be taken up by osseous tissue. There is an immediate uptake into the bloodstream and early images, produced by gamma ray emissions, may be taken of the blood flow into the area. Normally the patient will then return 2–4 hours later for assessment of the uptake into the bone. The technique is generally known as a three-phase bone scan (Table 11.2).

**Table 11.2** Isotope scanning: three-phase bone scan

| Phase | Process |
|---|---|
| Phase 1 (flow study) | Images are taken every 5 s for 30 s, giving an indication of blood perfusion into the area |
| Phase 2 (blood pool study) | Images taken when the area is fully perfused |
| Phase 3 (metabolic study) | An image taken 3–4 hours later, giving an indication of the amount of isotope tracer that remains bound to bone |

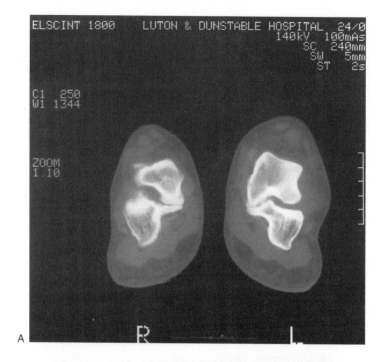

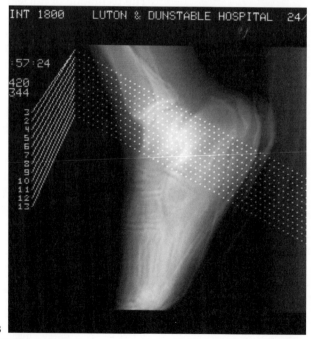

**Figure 11.35** Tarsal coalition. This is the same case as in Figure 11.21 and shows bilateral talocalcaneal bars. The image (**A**) is a single frame from a series of 12 taken as 5-mm 'slices' at right angles to the subtalar joint (**B**) (for orientation purposes the talus is superior to the calcaneum).

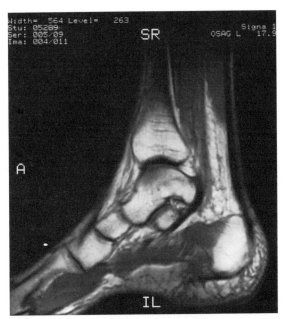

**Figure 11.36** Magnetic resonance imaging. A single frame from a series of slices taken in the sagittal plane.

The most commonly used isotope is technetium-99, derived from molybdenum. It is used because of its short half-life (approximately 8 h). Other isotopes such as gallium are still used, but the trend is towards technetium. The gamma rays emitted are detected by a gamma camera positioned above and close to the patient. The radioactivity is converted into light photons, multiplied and enhanced electronically and displayed on a screen. The image consists of a pattern of dots forming the osseous outline, with the greatest concentration of dots in the area of greatest isotope uptake. Such areas of increased uptake indicate increased activity in the area (Fig. 11.37). This may be due to any inflammatory process such as a primary or secondary neoplasm, injury, stress fracture, or infection. The uptake can be negative in areas of rampant bone infection with destruction. The technique has one great advantage in that it enables detection of bony pathology at a very early stage, unlike other imaging techniques, and it may provide clues in unexplained bone pain. Osteomyelitis and aseptic necrosis may be detected at the earliest stages, and serial scans may be used to track the progress of disease.

## Fluoroscopy

There are certain circumstances, often during operations, where moving images are required,

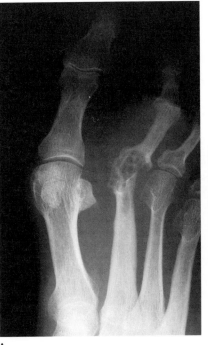

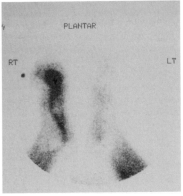

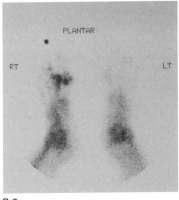

A      B 1      B 2

**Figure 11.37** Large synovial tumour (pigmented villonodular synovitis) which destroyed the 2nd metatarsophalangeal joint. (**A**) X-ray which shows the marked erosions and soft tissue swelling, (**B**) Technetium 99 isotope bone scan which confirmed greatly increased uptake in the blood pool phase, and aided diagnosis.

and the technique of fluoroscopy may be useful. X-rays are produced to cause fluorescence on a screen, most commonly containing caesium iodide. The resultant images are intensified and fed to a display monitor or camera. Modern fluoroscopes can in fact take a series of time-delayed images which, while not a moving picture, are very adequate. This drastically reduces the radiation dosages. In an operating theatre situation the technique is useful for positioning internal or external fixation devices accurately, locating foreign bodies and monitoring procedures.

## SUMMARY

Imaging techniques provide considerable information about many pathologies, but these techniques should only be requested to aid diagnosis and provide effective treatment. Plain X-rays will always have a major role in the diagnosis of foot pathologies. However, the foot specialist must keep abreast of technological developments such as CT scanning, MRI and nuclear isotope scanning which may become more accessible in the future.

## REFERENCES

Kumar P J, Clark M L (eds) 1990 Clinical medicine, 2nd edn. Baillière Tindall, London

National Osteoporosis Society 1993 Menopause and osteoporosis therapy. GP manual. National Osteoporosis Society, London

National Radiological Protection Board 1988 Guidance notes for the protection of persons against ionising radiations arising from medical and dental use. HMSO, London

Parsons V A 1980 Colour atlas of bone disease. Wolfe Medical Publications, London

Swallow R A, Naylor E, Roebuck E J, Whitley A S 1986 Clark's positioning in radiography, 11th edn. Heinemann, London, p 89–107

## FURTHER READING

Aird E G A 1988 Basic physics for medical imaging. Heinemann, London

Berquist T H 1990 Magnetic resonance imaging of the foot and ankle. Seminars in ultrasound, CT and MR 11(4): 327–345

British Institute of Radiology 1992 Pregnancy and work in diagnostic imaging. British Institute of Radiology, London

Gamble F O, Yale I 1975 Clinical foot roentgenology, 2nd edn. Krieger, Basle

McKillop J H, Fogelman I 1991 Benign and malignant bone disease. Clinician's guide to nuclear medicine. Churchill Livingstone, Edinburgh

Murray R O, Jacobson H G, Stoker D J 1990 The radiology of skeletal disorders, 3rd edn. Churchill Livingstone, Edinburgh

Pavlov H 1990 Imaging of the foot and ankle. Radiologic clinics of North America 28: 5: 991–1017

Root M L, Orien W P, Weed J H 1977 Clinical biomechanics, vols 1 and 2. Clinical Biomechanics Corporation, Los Angeles, CA

Taussig M J 1979 Processes in pathology. Blackwell Scientific Publications, Oxford

Warren M J, Jeffree M A, Wilson D J, MacLarnon J C 1990 Computed tomography in suspected tarsal coalition. Acta Orthopaedica Scandinavica 61(6): 554–557

# 12

# Methods of analysing gait

*S. West*

## INTRODUCTION

This chapter presents an overview of the methods employed in modern gait analysis. The advantages and disadvantages of these methods will be highlighted in order to provide practitioners with information that may be of help when assessing patients with gait problems. Information from gait analysis can help identify the cause of a problem and improve the effectiveness of treatment offered to the patient. Technological advances in this field are rapid. New systems are continually being developed. The reader is therefore recommended to review medical and engineering journals to keep abreast of developments.

## What is gait analysis?

Definitions vary. For our purpose gait analysis is defined as the assessment of the way in which people move. In the past there have been differences between practitioners in the terminology used to describe gait. Fortunately, contemporary literature is starting to show a range of common terms.

Gait is divided into a contact phase (stance phase) and a non-contact phase (swing phase). One full gait cycle is the interval of time from heel strike of one foot to heel strike by the same foot at the next step. Practitioners tend to consider gait analysis in terms of evaluating a subject's walking pattern. With the increase in interest in track and field sports, analysis of running gait patterns is becoming an important part of gait analysis.

The objective of gait analysis is to assist in clinical decision making. It forms part of an overall assessment which will normally include detailed history taking and clinical examination. Analysis of a patient's gait will allow the practitioner to formulate ideas about the causes of abnormalities and evaluate the effectiveness of therapeutic intervention. These interventions include the use of orthoses, surgery and physiotherapy. The identification of cause from effect is often difficult because of the highly developed compensatory feedback which operates during the gait cycle and the occurrence of more than one pathology at the same time.

Gross abnormalities, such as a patient with a marked limp or a child who is a toe walker, are relatively easy to identify. Minor variations from the 'normal' cause more difficulty and are harder to spot and describe in a meaningful way. This is not surprising if one considers how fast events occur during walking: it takes only 650 ms to complete one full gait cycle. Practitioners are therefore increasingly looking towards methods of investigating gait in a systematic way, which provides accurate data. In addition, if a system is going to be of any clinical value it must be simple to use, provide repeatable data and be easy and relatively quick to interpret. Fortunately, advances in technology mean that some of these requirements are now being addressed.

## How can gait be analysed?

A variety of methods can be used to provide data. Observation of a patient's gait using the format outlined in Chapter 8 can be assisted by the use of video and treadmills. Simple quantitative measures can be achieved from techniques using paper, pen, tape measure and stop watch. At the other end of the spectrum a comprehensive gait analysis system would include:

- Assessment of high speed videotape recordings
- Cinephotography
- Clinical measurement

- 3D joint kinematics and kinetics
- Electromyographic activity
- Energy expenditure
- Foot loading characteristics
- Foot pressure studies.

Most of the above require expensive equipment and specialist knowledge in the use and interpretation of data. Purpose-designed gait facilities can provide an adjunct to the clinical examination but are often used solely for research purposes.

## Methods used in the observation of gait

These comprise the practitioner's eye, treadmill and video.

### The practitioner's eye

Practitioners frequently undertake gait analysis without the use of equipment. The human eye and brain are more than able to detect and interpret gross changes in gait patterns. The major drawback is that there is no permanent record of the analysis—no opportunity to review the data at a later date or seek a second opinion from a colleague. The analysis is very dependent upon the skill and experience of the observer. All the data is subjective and qualitative. When one observes an individual standing on both feet, it is impossible to predict whether the load (distribution of force) under both feet is equal. This highlights the fundamental drawback of observation of gait: you cannot observe forces and the eye can be easily deceived.

Many practitioners adopt a systematic observation process that allows them to observe gait from key angles, namely the side and front/back. The practitioner will observe several gait cycles, concentrating on specific body or limb segments and identifying key features of gait. These features have already been considered in Chapter 8. Some practitioners find a check list very useful in order to guide their observations and document findings. Even under these circumstances, Krebs et al (1985) found this sort of analysis 'only moderately reliable'.

## Treadmill

One of the most debated areas of gait analysis relates to the length of walkway required in order to achieve 'normal' walking patterns. 4–6 metres is considered appropriate. Many practitioners have heightened the debate by using treadmills rather than long walkways. If a treadmill is used one must ensure that the subject has every opportunity to adapt to treadmill walking prior to analysis being undertaken. This usually requires at least 15 minutes of walking on the treadmill. The more exposure to treadmills, the shorter the time recorded to acclimatise and perform consistently (Tollafield 1990). Clearly, older patients and those with medical conditions are likely to fatigue more quickly.

No matter how sophisticated the system is subjects must feel relaxed and comfortable when being observed. Most authorities now accept that in order to achieve this the subject should be allowed to walk at his/her own cadence rather than being artificially constrained by walking in time to a metronome or some other timing device. A forced gait is of no value to a practitioner attempting to assess walking patterns.

## Video

Observational gait analysis is without question the technique most often used in clinical practice. Qualitative descriptions of gait can be made by observing stability and balance, velocity and control, symmetry of movement of body segments, foot placement and weight transfer.

The practitioner spends a significant proportion of time observing patients walking or running. Human locomotion is a highly complex activity. Many practitioners find it difficult to train their eyes to look for deviations from the normal. This is not surprising, since components of the gait cycle are measured in milliseconds. In order to analyse gait without the need to attach wires to patients or ask them to step on to clearly located force plates and pressure platforms, many practitioners turn to the video camera. Clinically, video analysis is an excellent tool that can be used to supplement the practitioner's eye.

It allows the practitioner more time to review and reflect on information. It provides playback facilities that can be reviewed at a variety of speeds down to single frame analysis. Recent advances in video cameras and playback systems mean that a high-quality unit can be set up economically. This sort of system would give high quality images, 50 frames per second, and play back at different speeds including frame by frame. New video playback recorders have reduced interference patterns and it is possible to split recordings to compare lateral and anterior (or posterior) views on one screen. This type of system is portable and therefore can record activities in a real environment such as an athletics track.

## METHODS OF QUANTITATIVE GAIT ANALYSIS

There are a range of methods which can be used to produce quantitative data on gait (Table 12.1).

### Temporal and spatial parameters

Temporal (time) and spatial (distance) factors include parameters related to stride length, stride time, step length, step time, double support time, mean walking velocity, cadence and the ratios of left to right of these parameters. It also includes toe-out/toe-in angles and width of the walking base. These parameters can be recorded with basic equipment and can provide valuable clinical information (Kippen 1993).

**Step length** is the distance from initial heel strike of one foot to the heel strike of the opposite foot.

**Cadence** is the number of steps taken per unit time, usually per minute. For practical purposes

**Table 12.1** Methods of quantitative gait analysis

- Temporal and spatial parameters
- Kinetics
- Accelerometers
- Kinematics
- Electromyography
- Energy expenditure
- Multisystems

practitioners tend to count the number of steps taken during a period of 10–15 s. When measuring cadence it is important that subjects are told to walk at their normal walking speed and as naturally as possible. The observation count starts once the subject is walking at normal speed. In order to estimate average cadence per minute the following formula should be applied:

Cadence (steps per minute) = steps counted × 60/time(s)

**Stride length** is the distance between two successive placements of the same foot and will therefore consist of two step lengths. This parameter is usually measured in metres.

**The walking base,** also known as **stride width,** is the distance between the feet, usually measured at the midpoint of the heel. This is recorded in millimetres.

**Toe-out and toe-in** are a measure of foot position in relation to the line of forward progression. It has been shown that foot position in relation to the line of forward progression constantly changes during gait. In order to produce an 'average' the position the foot adopts for 10 steps is recorded and the mean is calculated.

**The velocity** of walking is the distance covered by the body in a given time in a particular direction. It is measured in metres per second. The mean velocity can be calculated as the product of cadence and stride length. The cadence is measured in half strides per 60 seconds or full strides per 120 seconds. The velocity can be calculated by the following formula:

Velocity (m/s) = stride length (m) × cadence (steps/min)/120

All of the above data can be collected relatively easily using poster paints or chalk to show footprints on black or white paper. This provides a permanent record of the foot placements during gait and can be used to calculate a variety of parameters, as indicated in Figure 12.1.

Many of the temporal parameters, such as cadence and velocity, can also be measured via simple foot switches attached to the foot and linked into a computer. A foot switch is effectively an on–off button that creates a break in the flow of current between the foot and computer.

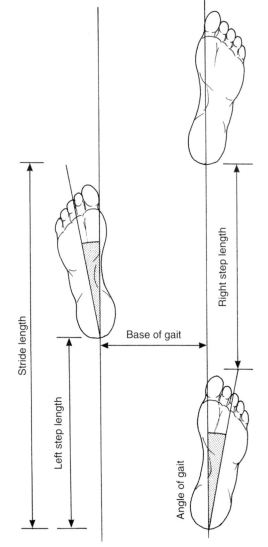

**Figure 12.1** Spatial parameters that can be measured using a simple walkway.

The major disadvantage of such systems is that the foot switch is uncomfortable for some patients and clearly is of little value if subjects do not possess a heel strike and toe-off phase, e.g. patients with cerebral palsy.

To overcome this problem, Crouse et al (1987) described a microcomputer-based system using a resistive grid walkway for recording both spatial and temporal parameters. This system uses a series of circuits designed as a grid. An electrical current passes through the grid. When a load is applied, the resistance varies and can trigger a time display or image of the foot outline. Unfortunately this system has not been used in clinical practice.

Law (1987) published work he had undertaken using a microcomputer-based system which involved attaching a length of perforated computer tape to each foot. As the subject walked the tape streamed through a pair of optical readers which calculated step length, stride time, double support time, walking speed, cadence and maximum velocities. A major disadvantage with the system was that it was attached to the subject and required him/her to walk in a straight line. Optical and electronic systems have also been used to measure these parameters, e.g. video cameras with a date/time generator.

In clinical practice the measurement of temporal and spatial parameters can highlight pathology and changes associated with disease or rehabilitation. Patients such as those with rheumatoid arthritis, Parkinson's disease or paralysis will all show significant deviations from 'normal' parameters, e.g. short stride length, slow or fast cadence. However, it must be recognised that assessment of these parameters on their own is not sufficient for a comprehensive overview of gait. Spatial and temporal parameters vary during walking and from one period of walking to another. In view of this it is important to view the data with caution and to obtain a mean average for any parameter.

## Kinetics of gait

This is the study and measurement of forces and moments exerted on the body that influence movement. Of direct relevance to the practitioner is the recording of forces at the foot/floor interface, measured, for example, via force platforms. Lesion patterns give an indication of the site of excess stresses but quantitative information cannot be gained by observation (Duckworth et al 1985). Consequently, some method of examining the plantar load distribution must be employed.

Many authors use the terms 'force', 'load' and 'pressure' interchangeably. This practice is to be discouraged. It is worth defining these terms and others used in biomechanics (the study of the effect of mechanical laws on the locomotor system) from the outset.

**Force,** as defined by Newton's second law of motion, is mass multiplied by acceleration. This law means that any time a force is applied to an object, the object accelerates. Since acceleration is the change in velocity divided by the change in time, a force applied to an object will produce a change in the object's velocity. Force can therefore be considered as change in momentum divided by change in time. Force is a vector quantity, having both magnitude and direction.

**Pressure** is force divided by area: the larger the area the lower the pressure. This unit has important implications when comparing different measurement systems for measuring pressure under the foot. For example, systems which have large discrete element sizes may not be able to measure the true pressure under a small area of the foot.

At the present time there is considerable interest in the effects of footwear on foot function. Researchers and practitioners are interested in the interaction between the foot and shoe. There are a number of research projects in progress that are attempting to review the effect of footwear and orthoses on foot function. Several studies are comparing the loading characteristics observed in the unshod foot to those in the shod foot. The fundamental questions being asked are:

- Is there a correlation between the loading characteristics of the shod and unshod foot?
- What happens at the foot/shoe interface?
- Is there a correlation between the loading characteristics measured at the shoe/floor interface and those at the foot/floor interface?
- Are the effects of foot orthoses influenced by the type of footwear?

History has seen the development of a variety of systems designed to study the way in which load is distributed over the plantar surface of the foot. These have been extensively reviewed and commented on by Lord (1981), Lord et al (1986) and West (1987). In addition reviews of clinical findings employing particular equipment are continually being published. Many systems described in the literature are designed as part of research projects. These systems have not appeared on the market because of cost, lack of repeatability and technical difficulties that make them difficult to use clinically. The systems currently available to practitioners are:

- Harris & Beath mat
- Pedobarograph
- Kistler force plate
- Musgrave footprint
- In-shoe force measurement.

### Harris & Beath mat

A deformable mat printing technique first employed by Morton in 1935 was modified and adapted for flat-foot studies (Harris & Beath 1947). A three-ridged rubber mat, of 0.002, 0.0025 and 0.0028 inches in height, was designed. The ridged top surface of the mat is spread thinly with soluble printer's ink and then placed on the floor, ridged side up. The mat is covered with a clean sheet of white paper and a static or dynamic footprint is recorded on to it. The differing heights of the ridges produces the effect of increased density of ink in areas of high pressure (Fig. 12.2). An attempt to calibrate the print mat using known size and weight has shown promise but still offers only broad bands of pressure ranges (Silvino et al 1980). This has enabled quantitative data to be collected. Many other authors have adopted the Harris & Beath mat for varying forms of foot analysis (Henry & Waugh 1975, Rose et al 1985, West 1987, Kilmartin & Wallace 1992, Welton 1992). The clinical application of the Harris & Beath mat is far reaching. It can provide data on foot dimensions including foot length, width, arch profile and total foot contact area. In addition, valuable information about loading of the foot can be gathered; high and low loaded areas can be identified.

### Pedobarograph

The pedobarograph was first described by

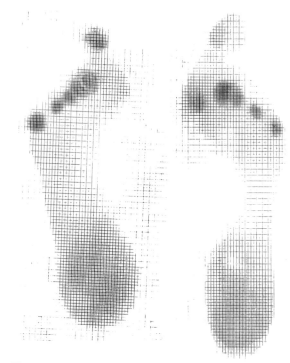

**Figure 12.2** An example of a footprint from the Harris & Beath mat.

Chodera in 1960 and was developed for the investigation of plantar foot pressure measurements. This simple optical system has been used in static and dynamic pressure measurement studies (Betts & Duckworth 1978, Betts et al 1980a). Essentially, the pedobarograph is based on the interruption of a light source by total internal reflection through the highly polished glass edges of a glass plate acting like a lens. An elastic or textured foil is placed between the light-conducting surface and the plantar surface of the foot. Light internally reflecting along the glass is affected by the pressure applied to the foil. The light illuminates the foil which scatters the light back in the area of the pressure. The patterns of the pressure area can be observed and recorded by a camera housed inside the pedobarograph box. Internally, a mirror is angled at 45° to the glass platform which reflects the light image into the lens of the video camera. The pattern observed shows the areas of increased light intensity with pressure. The video output

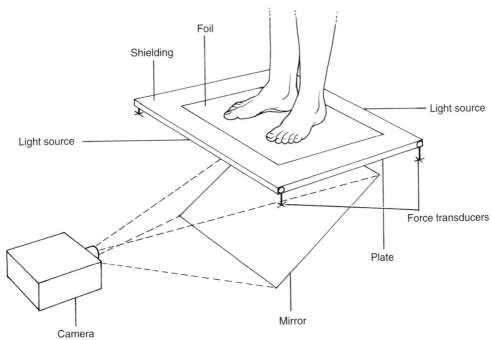

**Figure 12.3**   Cross-section of a pedobarograph.

can be captured via a frame grabber and then manipulated and analysed by software (Fig. 12.3). The pedobarograph is a non-portable system that requires a raised walkway into which it can be placed. The images produced provide high spatial resolution in continuous greyscale or 16 colour zones.

The pedobarograph has been well documented using both dynamic and static data (Betts & Duckworth 1978, Betts et al 1980b, Minns & Craxford 1984, Hughes et al 1990). In most of these studies authors have used computer imaging techniques to zone the greyscale images and enhance them with colour. Several investigations have been undertaken to establish the effects of different foil characteristics on the light intensity emitted. One study by Betts et al (1980b) suggested that photographic paper with a pearl finish would be a suitable foil for calibrated dynamic foot pressure measurements. In their study it was found that the paper showed little viscoelasticity, tackiness or other hysteresis-like effects and no evidence of saturation over the pressure range studied. Hysteresis is the lag

between the release of stress and the cessation of strain in materials subjected to tension or magnetism.

This work highlighted the need for careful interpretation of the data. The systems employed to measure load have within them characteristics that can affect the data. For example, the characteristics of the foil, when measuring static loads, could provide loading data that was too high or too low because of the response time and hysteresis of the material. The recovery time and recovery characteristics of the material, once it has been loaded and unloaded, is especially important when investigating dynamic loading. In the early pedobarograph studies not only was the material slow to recover from loading but it also became tacky and tended to stick to the glass surface even when unloaded. This gave a false loading as a result of the foil characteristics. The pedobarograph system can be calibrated and can measure pressures to $25\,\text{kg/cm}^2$ (2.45 MPa).

Recordings have been made of both static and dynamic loading with feet considered to be normal and abnormal. It has been stated that the distribution of load between the sole of the foot and a supporting surface can reveal information about both the structure and the function of the foot (Lord 1981). As mentioned previously it is desirable to investigate the way in which the plantar surface of the foot bears and transmits loads.

### Kistler force plate

This is a non-portable system, which normally needs to be set in epoxy concrete to prevent interference from vibration, although these vibrations can normally be identified and ignored on gait data. The top surface of the plate can be glass, aluminium or steel. The plates incorporate four quartz rings which exhibit a piezoelectric effect, thus ensuring the system is sensitive to force in three planes: x, y, z. The control unit outputs continuous analogue data via 13 channels, of which eight are normally used. The only limitation of the system is the speed at which data can be received and stored and the analogue-to-digital converter interface which can limit the resolution in time. Each channel can be sampled up to 3000 times per second. The collected data can be displayed on the computer's VDU as digital information or as a series of graphs showing force against time before obtaining a hard copy print. The system provides detailed numerical and graphical data on the forces applied to the foot (Fig. 12.4). The system has poor spatial resolution and does not analyse discrete pressures on the plantar surface of the foot. However, it should be noted that it can be calibrated and has been used to calibrate other force measurement systems.

### Musgrave footprint

The Musgrave footprint is a computer-based system that can be used for the measurement of plantar foot pressures. The footplate is a low-profile plate which uses Interlink force sensitive resistors (FSRs) between an aluminium plate. Each plate has 2032 sensors arranged in a grid pattern. The plates are often used in pairs to

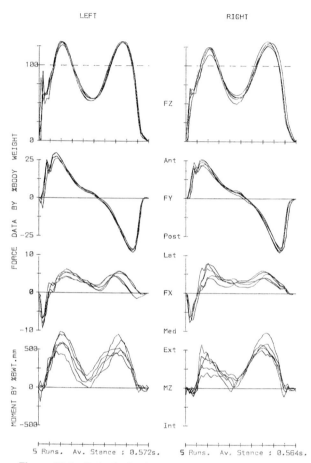

**Figure 12.4** Data display from a Kistler force plate.

provide data of both a temporal and spatial nature. The system is interfaced through a standard PC and is therefore relatively portable.

The Musgrave plate can be calibrated and can record pressures up to 15 kg/cm$^2$ (14.4 MPa). It produces data which can be displayed graphically, numerically or visually. The data presentation is clear and easy to interpret. Little clinical research has been carried out on the system, although several studies are now under way. Young et al (1993) undertook a comparative trial of the system against a pedobarograph and found that the Musgrave plate was unable to measure pressures above 15 kg/cm$^2$. Such pressures have frequently been observed under the metatarsal heads of diabetic patients. The work concluded that in low-pressure areas such as the heel the Musgrave could provide comparable results to the pedobarograph. The Musgrave may be of value in the clinic but possibly not for research, on account of the above points.

The Musgrave footprint tends to illustrate vertical force as pressure values and cannot differentiate high shear force values. Callosity under the foot may not show high values unless the load under the foot has a long duration of contact with the pressure platform.

### In-shoe force measurement

Many methods have been developed for recording foot loading while the foot is shod. Piezoelectric discs have been attached to the plantar surface of the foot to record the different effect of heel height on forefoot loading (Schwartz & Heath 1947). Capacitive pressure transducers have been stuck to the sole of the foot to record peak pressures in predetermined areas during gait in patients affected with Hansen's disease (Bauman & Brand 1963).

Strain gauge transducers have been attached to the forefoot and hindfoot of the sole of the shoe to record the total floor reaction. By this method it was possible to record the heel and sole forces separately (Miyasaki & Iwakura 1978). An insole for recording plantar pressures was developed by Lereim & Serek-Hanssen (1973) in which miniature transducers were accurately positioned against the sole of the foot by the use of X-rays. These were then incorporated into a PVC insole to be worn in the shoe. New insoles had to be made for each subject.

Polchanioff (1983) designed a disposable transducer for the Langer Biomechanics Group using 14 discrete flexible load transducers which could be applied to the plantar surface of the foot. The sensors were designed to provide data on dynamic (vertical) forces occurring under prominent anatomical sites. The device has a waist pack worn by the subject. Information is stored in the waist pack for (up to) seven sensors on each foot. The pack is then downloaded into a PC at a later date. Interpretation of the data is achieved through a computer, using an 'expert system' approach. The system has proved to be fragile. Brand (1988) performed research using discrete transducers working as variable capacitors. The use of discrete sensors has been criticised as it requires assumptions to be made about where peak pressures are likely to be found.

Recently two new insole pressure measurement systems have become commercially available: the German Emed system and the Italian Orthomat. In addition to these a system designed by Tekscan Inc. is now commercially available and is marketed as Fscan.

The Emed system belongs to a class of devices characterised as matrix mats. In these the individual sensors are formed electronically at the intersection of rows and columns of conductive material (Nicol & Henning 1978). The system has been made as a mat and insole unit. The mat has 40 rows and 40 columns, each $1 \times 48$ cm producing a 1600 element mat with $1 \times 1$ cm elements separated by a gap of 2 mm. An electrical component, usually a capacitor or a resistor, varies its properties depending upon the applied load. In the Emed system the active element is a variable capacitor whereas in the Fscan, flexible, pressure sensitive insole, it is a variable resistor.

The Fscan insole system consists of a printed insole approximately 300 mm long, 105 mm wide across the forefoot, 70 mm wide across the heel and 0.02 mm thick. The insole at full size contains 968 sensors, four sensors per square centimetre with a 2 mm inactive area between each sensor. The insole is a multilayer, piezoresistive, screen-printed sensor sandwiched in a moisture-resistant coating. The layers are held together by small glue spots at a repeat distance of 1 cm square. This allows the sensor insole to be cut to fit any size of shoe down to an adult size 4, providing care is taken not to cut through any required silver connecting tracts.

The ink tracts provide multiple sensors of identical characteristics. The sensors relay data (Fig. 12.5) via silver tracts which are banded together to exit the foot on the lateral aspect and insert into a small, lightweight signal processing unit worn by the subject just above the lateral

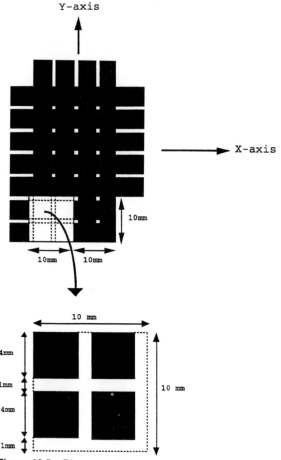

**Figure 12.5** Diagrammatic representation of FSCAN.

pressures. The insoles have a range from 0.57 kg/cm$^2$ (56 kPa) to 8.85 kg/cm$^2$ (868 kPa). The insole unit may be sensitive to temperature and moisture changes. However, well-controlled protocols may be able to reduce this characteristic. Repeatable data collection runs are achievable provided that the sensors are undamaged. Most investigations use each insole unit for a maximum of five data collection runs or approximately 40 gait cycles. The sensor has been shown to exhibit significant decay after this (Rose et al 1992). Unpublished work suggests that the sensor, if laminated with a thin backing material, produces valid and reliable data throughout its working load range for 200 gait cycles. The sensors have shown failure with respect to total breakdown of the silver relay tracks, and loss of individual sensors as a result of marked creasing or cutting. It has also been noted that sensors can be permanently switched on, registering maximum loads. This is thought to be as a result of sensor damage during cutting the insole to fit shoes. Software modifications in the future may allow investigators to delete 'hot' sensors prior to data analysis.

The advantage of the system is that it provides a method for measuring plantar loading of successive steps of each foot while the foot is shod. The foot can be analysed for up to 6 s and the foot-to-shoe or foot-to-orthosis interface can be investigated directly. At the present time the system is being developed to further increase the loading range of the insoles so as to achieve a more acceptable working range to allow analysis of running foot pressures and loads seen in pathological feet.

## Accelerometers

The use of accelerometers in gait analysis has generally been confined to the measurement of impact forces such as those seen at heel strike. Much work has been undertaken by sports footwear manufacturers in the quest for the ideal shock-attenuating insole unit. The 'shock meter' system has been used to investigate shock waves transmitted during gait (Johnson 1990). A few experiments have been undertaken using

malleolus. This processor is then joined via a 10 m thin coaxial cable to an AT-compatible IBM PC. The data is presented to the practitioner via a screen and/or a printer supplying a one-to-one sized printout. The data presentation and collection is achieved via a user-friendly programme using windows and graphic display keys that allows for several alternative data display modes. The sampling rate for the sensor is 0.01 s for 968 cells allowing for display of one frame every 10 ms. Five-bit data acquisition is used with 25 resolvable levels of force giving 32.

The insole sensors do not show a linear relationship between resistance and pressure; algorithms in the software are used to assign levels to pressure. Since this is not linear, different ranges can be achieved for high or low accelerometers mounted on pins and then screwed directly into the bones of volunteers, although this method is clinically unacceptable. Accelerometers have been used to measure acceleration of body parts during motion (Morris 1973). Accelerometers have been used in research but in clinical practice they may not be of much value (Collins & Whittle 1989).

## Kinematics

Kinematics describes angular movement and displacement of joints and the body throughout space. There are a variety of ways in which this data can be measured directly and indirectly.

### Direct method

Direct measurement can be achieved by using goniometers (Chao 1980). These measure joint angle changes. The use of goniometers is becoming increasingly common, especially electro-goniometers and flexible goniometers as supplied by Penny & Giles, Gwent, UK (Fig. 12.6). In addition, potentiometer devices and polarised light goniometers are sometimes used. All these systems are relatively easy to use and provide instant results. They all require careful calibration and setting up in order to achieve valid and reproducible results. Some patients complain of being impeded by the measurement systems. This will affect the results obtained. Another major drawback is the fact that the goniometer can only measure in two dimensions. In practice this means that the goniometer works well when recording sagittal or single-plane motions during activity. Measurement of the small joints within the foot during gait has been more of a challenge and has led to the development and production of small flexible goniometers.

### Indirect methods

Cine photography was the principal technique for gathering kinematic data prior to the introduction of video systems. Muybridge (1955) pioneered the use of cine photography in the study of human and animal locomotion. This

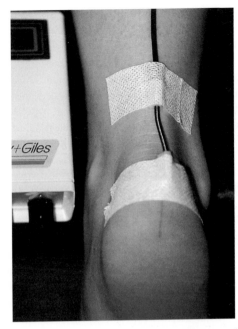

**Figure 12.6**  Electrogoniometer with transducer capable of reading 0.1° of motion (Penny & Giles). The goniometer has been attached to the foot to record subtalar motion.

work was a classic and is still used by scientists and artists today. In the book *Human walking*, Inman et al (1981) demonstrate how the use of cine photography and still pictures can provide valuable information about joint angles and limb placement during locomotion. Data analysis of limb movement became much easier and quicker, although still too slow and time-consuming for routine clinical applications, following digitisation of the images (Sutherland & Hagy 1972).

Modern cine and video recording devices are now available and can be directly interfaced with a computer. Commercially available motion analysis systems use either passive or active discs to track body segments or joint centres in space. The practitioner would require assistance to process and analyse the data. These systems are able to provide both two- and three-dimensional data which is usually reconstructed and displayed as a series of stick figures.

**Passive and active marker systems: Vicon and Selspot.** The Oxford Metrics Vicon system is a good example of how passive infra-red reflective joint markers can be tracked by high-stability television cameras. Although Vicon is described, there are several other systems available that undertake a similar process. Most gait laboratories use three cameras to track the joint markers. The standard camera tracks at 50 frames per second (50 Hz), although high-speed cameras are now available that will track at up to 200 frames per second (200 Hz). The Vicon system is capable of tracking up to 30 markers with accuracy of around 5 mm both horizontally and vertically. Data is presented in movie frames as a 'stick diagram'. One major limitation of the system is that it relies on reflection from the reference discs. This technique may pick up reflections from other sources such as walking aids and jewellery. Selspot is an example of an active marker system. This system uses up to 16 cameras which pick up data from light-emitting diodes (LED) attached to anatomical reference points. Data acquisition is coordinated through a controlling unit and computer and therefore allows the diodes to pulse in sequence, providing automatic identification of markers. The system produces a movie image and 'butterfly diagram' but requires power wires to serve the LED. This is considered to be a major limiting factor of the system since a large number of wires (20 or more) are required to power all diodes attached to the body. Both these systems are commonly employed in research units but they are not routinely used in the clinical setting. This is partly due to the cost and the requirement for a room to be set aside solely for this type of analysis.

**MacReflex.** A new system, MacReflex, has recently been launched. It is used with a Macintosh personal computer and lightweight camera. This piece of technology harnesses the ease of use of the Macintosh computer and one or more CCD cameras. The cameras have an internal light-emitting diode flash for the illumination of reflective discs or tape attached to the body and limbs. The camera automatically reduces its sensitivity so that only markers will be visible on the video image, thus reducing the data considerably and allowing real-time video processing to occur. The data produced by the system provides a series of data coordinates that are fed directly into the serial port of a Macintosh computer. The MacReflex software allows the user to record, sort and track data providing either spreadsheet numerical presentation or simple graphical presentation.

**Digitised video gait analysis.** Some systems are now able to digitise the video image and allow practitioners to identify referenced anatomical points, frame by frame. This allows playback of a digitised image similar to a 'stick diagram'. An example of such a commercially available system is the Salford Gait Station. This uses a frame grabber and computer to generate images similar to 'stick diagrams'. In addition to this feature a time–date generator can provide information that can be used to calculate temporal parameters. Data is presented in a meaningful way via a series of screen windows which are able to show the original video recording, the matchstick figure and the graphical data produced all at the same time. The major drawback is that an element of time is required to achieve manipulation of data. As with any camera system it should be noted that the image is only two-dimensional and many of the movements observed during gait are three-dimensional. It is also important to ensure that camera angles are at 90° to the field to avoid parallax.

# Electromyography (EMG)

The EMG is the electrical signal associated with muscular contraction. EMG analysis can provide information about timing and intensity of muscle contraction. Such information provides data that indicates whether muscles are contracting in the correct order (phasic), at the right time and in an appropriate way. From this phasic muscle activity, tone, continuous and clonic muscle contraction or no muscle activity can be recorded. Data can assist with the assessment and aetiology of movement abnormality or in the review and assessment of physical therapies, rehabilitation or surgical interventions.

Electromyographic data can be collected by using surface or indwelling electrodes. Indwelling electrodes are more definitive than surface electrodes in terms of sampling activity from a particular muscle. These electrodes are also required for analysis of deep muscle activity, e.g. in the deep posterior compartment of the calf. A major problem with this sort of electrode is that they cause intramuscular bleeding and may displace during muscle contraction (Kadaba et al 1985). The use of surface electrodes is clinically more viable as they are non-invasive and less variable than indwelling electrodes. These electrodes are generally used to provide gross information about the activity of muscle groups (Winter 1990) and are therefore less selective. There is also an increased risk of 'cross-talk'—picking up activity from other muscles that are not directly under investigation. The EMG is therefore commonly used to identify gross phasic muscle activity prior to the fitting of orthoses designed to affect muscle activity, or for preoperative planning prior to tendon transfer or lengthening. For routine clinical practice the system is of little value.

## Energy expenditure

Patients who exhibit gross changes in their gait are likely to use more energy than patients with an efficient gait pattern. This is not surprising since the structure and function of the locomotor system is designed to be energy-efficient in terms of its ability both to store and use energy (Ch. 8). The determination of energy expenditure in gait has been undertaken since the 1950s. Many investigations have looked at normal and abnormal gaits in terms of energy cost. Estimation of the energy cost of walking usually involves the measurement of oxygen consumption (Inman et al 1981) or calculation of potential and kinetic energy levels of body segments from their motions and masses (Quanbury et al 1975).

A commercially available device called Caltrac measures the total number of calories used by subjects during walking. An alternative approach is to monitor heart rates as an indication of energy expenditure during activity (Rose et al 1989). In this the 'physiological cost index' (PCI) is calculated as an estimate of energy used. The following formula is used:

PCI = (heart rate walking − heart rate resting)/velocity

The calculation is made using heart rate in beats/min and the velocity in m/min, or beats and velocity in seconds. This is probably more useful in clinical practice than the measurement of oxygen consumption and carbon dioxide production during activity.

The measurement of oxygen consumption requires an analysis of the subject's exhaled air. Normally this requires the use of a 'Douglas Bag' which allows the respiratory quotient to be calculated. Exercise is generally undertaken on a treadmill. Since the equipment required is bulky this sort of assessment is not routinely undertaken in the clinic.

## Multisystems

Several developments are currently under way to provide multiple linked data. These systems may well provide data from energy consumption studies with gait and force plate studies. In some gait laboratories additional information from EMG is also simultaneously presented. The difficulty with these systems is that they tend to cause information overload of the practitioner.

## SUMMARY

Gait analysis is a complex task. Observation of gait can be aided by the collection and analysis of quantitative data. One of the main problems with these methods is the difficulty in establishing what is normal. Gait may alter with every step a person takes; as a result repeatability is a major problem. The practitioner must also be wary of highly technical equipment which will provide complex data that proves difficult to interpret and requires considerable computer power or time.

In the research field, quantitative analysis of gait is making a contribution to our understanding of the complexities of gait. In particular, research into gait is improving our knowledge of its components and is also being used to design and evaluate therapeutic interventions.

## REFERENCES

Bauman J H, Brand P W 1963 Measurement of pressure between foot and shoe. Lancet 3: 629–632

Betts R P, Duckworth T 1978 A device for measuring plantar pressures under the sole of the foot. Engineering in Medicine 7(4): 223–228

Betts R P, Franks C I, Duckworth T, Burke J 1980a Static and dynamic foot pressure measurements in clinical orthopaedics. Journal of Medical and Biological Computing 18: 674–684

Betts R P, Franks C I, Duckworth T 1980b Analysis of pressure and load under the foot. Part 2: Quantitation of the dynamic distribution. Clinical Physical Physiological Measurement 1(2): 113–124

Brand P W Repetative stress in the development of diabetic foot ulcers. In: Levin M E, O'Neal L W (eds) The diabetic foot, 4th edn. C V Mosby, St Louis, MO, p 83–90

Chao E Y S 1980 Justification of triaxial goniometer for the measurement of joint rotation. Journal of Biomechanics 13: 989–1006

Chodera J 1960 Pedobarograph: apparatus for visual display of pressures between contacting surfaces of irregular shape. C25 Patent, 104 514 30d

Collins J J, Whittle M W 1989 Impulsive forces during walking and their clinical implications. Clinical Biomechanics 4: 179–187

Crouse J, Wall J C, Marble A E 1987 Measurement of the temporal and spatial parameters of gait using a microcomputer based system. Journal of Biomedical Engineering 9: 64–68

Duckworth T, Boulton A J M, Betts R P, Franks C I, Ward J D 1985 Plantar pressure measurements and the prevention of ulceration in the diabetic foot. Anatomical Record 59: 481–490

Harris R I, Beath T 1947 Army foot survey. An investigation of foot ailments in Canadian soldiers. Ottawa National Research Council, Canada NRC no. 1574

Henry A P J, Waugh W 1975 The use of footprints in assessing the results of operations for hallux valgus. A comparison of Keller's operation and arthrodesis. Journal of Bone and Joint Surgery 57B(4): 478–481

Hughes J, Clark P, Klenerman L 1990 The importance of toes in walking. Journal of Bone and Joint Surgery 72B(2): 245–251

Inman V T, Ralston H J, Todd F 1981 Human walking. Williams & Wilkins, Baltimore, MD

Johnson G R 1990 Measurement of shock acceleration during walking and running using the shock meter. Clinical Biomechanics 5: 47–50

Kadaba M P, Wootten M E, Gainey J, Cochran G V B 1985 Repeatability of phasic muscle activity: Performance of surface intramuscular wire electrodes in gait analysis. Journal of Orthopaedic Research 3(3): 350–359

Kilmartin T E, Wallace W A 1992 The significance of pes planus in juvenile hallux valgus. Foot and Ankle 13(2): 53–56

Kippen S C 1993 A preliminary assessment of recording the physical dimensions of an inked footprint. Journal of British Podiatric Medicine 48(5): 74–80

Krebs D E, Edlestein J E, Fishman S 1985 Reliability of observational kinematic gait analysis. Physical Therapy 65: 1027–1033

Law H T 1987 Microcomputer-based, low cost method for measurement of spatial and temporal parameters of gait. Journal of Biomedical Engineering 9: 115–120

Lereim P, Serek-Hanssen F 1973 A method of recording plantar pressure distribution under the sole of the foot. Bulletin of Prosthetics Research: 118–125

Lord M, Reynolds D P, Hughes J R 1986 Foot pressure measurement: a review of clinical findings. Journal of Biomedical Engineering 8: 283–294

Lord M 1981 Foot pressure measurement: A review of methodology. Journal of Biomedical Engineering 3(2): 91–99

Minns R J, Craxford A D 1984 Pressure under the forefoot in rheumatoid arthritis; a comparison of static and dynamic methods of assessment. Clinical Orthopaedic and Related Research 187: 235–242

Miyasaki S, Iwakura H 1978 Foot-force measuring device for clinical assessment of pathological gait. Medical Biological Engineering and Computing 16: 429–436

Morris J R W 1973 Accelerometry: a technique for the measurement of human body movements. Journal of Biomechanics 6: 729–736

Morton D J 1935 The human foot. Columbia University Press, New York

Muybridge, Eadweard 1955 The human figure in motion. Dover Publications, New York

Nicol K, Henning E M 1978 Measurement of pressure distribution by means of a flexible large surface mat. In: Asmussen E, Jorgenson K (eds) Biomechanics Vl-A. University Park Press, Baltimore, MD, p 374–380

Polchanioff M 1983 Gait analysis using a portable, micro-processed based segmental foot force measuring system. Proceedings of the IEEE Seventh Annual Symposium on Comput. Applied Medical Care: 897–899

Quanbury A D, Winter D A, Reimer G D 1975 Instantaneous power and power flow in body segments during walking. Journal of Medical Engineering and Technology 7: 273–279

Rose G K 1983 Clinical gait assessment: a personal view. Journal of Medical Engineering and Technology 7: 273–279

Rose G K, Welton E A, Marshall T 1985 The diagnosis of flat foot in the child. Journal of Bone and Joint Surgery 67B: 1

Rose J R, Gamble J G, Medeiros J et al 1989 Energy cost of walking in normal children and those with cerebral palsy: comparison of heart rate and oxygen uptake. Journal of Pediatric Orthopedics 9: 276–279

Rose N E, Feiwell L A, Cracchiolo A 1992 A method for measuring foot pressures using a high resolution, computerized insole sensor: the effect of heel wedges on plantar pressure distribution and centre of force. Foot and Ankle 13(5): 263–270

Schwartz R P, Heath A L 1947 The definition of human locomotion on the basis of measurement. Journal of Bone and Joint Surgery 29(1): 203–214

Silvino N, Evanski P M, Waugh T R 1980 The Harris and Beath mat: diagnostic validity and clinical use. Clinical Orthopaedics and Related Research 151: 265–269

Sutherland D H, Hagy J L 1972 Measurement of gait movements from motion picture film. Journal of Bone and Joint Surgery 54: 787–797

Tollafield D R 1990 A reusable transducer system for measuring foot pressures. A study of reliability in a commercial pressure pad. BSc Thesis, Department of Health Sciences, Coventry Polytechnic

Welton E A 1992 The Harris and Beath footprint: interpretation and clinical value. Foot and Ankle 13(8): 462–468

West P M 1987 The clinical use of the Harris and Beath Footprinting Mat in assessing plantar pressures.

Chiropodist 42(9): 337–348

Winter D A 1990 Biomechanics and motor control of normal human movement, 2nd edn. John Wiley & Sons, New York

Young M J, Murray H J, Veves A, Boulton A J M 1993 A comparison of the Musgrave Footprint and optical pedobarograph systems for measuring dynamic foot pressures in diabetic patients. Foot 3(2): 62–64

# 13

# Laboratory tests

*D. Lodwick*
*D. R. Tollafield*
*J. Cairns*

## INTRODUCTION

This chapter provides an overview of laboratory tests which can be performed on tissue and fluid samples from the lower limb. The tests of most relevance are:

- Urinalysis
- Microbiology
- Blood analysis; haematology, biochemistry and serology
- Histology.

The above play a vital role in enabling the practitioner to understand the nature of local and systemic related pathologies affecting the lower limb. Data from the tests can be used to:

- provide information to aid the diagnostic process
- enable a definitive diagnosis to be made in situations where there may be a number of possible diagnoses
- enable implementation of effective treatment.

Some of the tests can be undertaken in the clinic (near patient testing) but most require the use of laboratory services. On account of the expense and possible inconvenience caused by some of the tests it is important that they are only used where appropriate. Inappropriate use results in wasted resources both for the practitioner and the patient.

# URINALYSIS

## Indications for use

Urinalysis provides a simple, non-invasive method of looking at biochemistry. Examination of urine may reveal:

- the presence of —glucose
                     —protein
                     —ketones
                     —blood
                     —cells/casts
                     —parasites
                     —infection
- changes in    —specific gravity
                     —acidity/alkalinity (pH).

Urinalysis may be used as an aid in the diagnosis of renal and hepatic diseases and diabetes mellitus, all of which can lead to lower limb problems. Diabetes mellitus can have widespread consequences for the lower limb. Kidney (renal) and liver (hepatic) disease may have serious repercussions which complicate diagnosis and affect treatment of lower limb problems.

Urinalysis provides a good method for screening for a range of conditions as it is inexpensive and does not cause undue distress to the patient. Most tests on urine can be undertaken in the clinic (near patient testing). The tests are quick to perform and the results are readily available. In some instances it may be necessary to undertake other more sensitive and/or specific tests. For example, the detection of glucose in the urine alerts the practitioner to the presence of diabetes mellitus. However, blood analysis can provide the practitioner with further information such as the level of glycosylated haemoglobin. This provides a useful indicator of how well the diabetes has been controlled.

## Sampling technique

Patients may bring along a recently produced sample of urine or produce one while at the clinic. The urine should be tested immediately and the data recorded. If it is necessary to send the sample off to a laboratory it should be stored in a clean screw-cap container and labelled with the patient's name and address. If an infection is suspected a midstream sample is usually indicated. In a case of suspected infection the sample must be stored in a sterile container which contains specific chemicals to preserve the sample and prevent invalidation of the lab tests.

## Tests and interpretation of results

Observation, smell and the use of dipsticks are the main methods used to examine urine.

### Observation

Observation of urine should include assessment of colour and turbidity. The colour of urine depends upon the time of collection. The more concentrated the urine, the more yellow the colour. It is likely to be a deeper yellow first thing in the morning. After the ingestion of liquid the urine loses some of its deep yellow colour. Feverish patients may have a dark yellow or brown urine: loss of moisture from sweating increases its concentration. A red tinge, bright red or black colour may be associated with the presence of blood (haematuria); however, blood from menstruation contaminating urine should always be considered. Slight haematuria may cause no discoloration and be detected only by chemical testing or microscopy. Some dietary additives can change the colour, e.g. beetroot (red/pink). Porphyria will cause the urine to fluoresce red. High levels of urochrome produced in the bile will cause the urine to be a deep yellow. In the presence of L-dopa and sometimes in cases of paracetamol poisoning the urine, when left to stand, turns brown.

Urine should be clear and non-turbid (Plate 26). Turbidity can result from the presence of casts. These include various cells such as the epithelial lining of the collecting tubes. The urine of patients with urinary tract infections is often turbid. Blood cells, cells which have become fatty and granular cells that have degenerated may be present. These may reflect the shape of the lumens of the tubules.

## Odour

Normal urine does not have a strong odour but the ammonium salts produced from urea breakdown have an offensive smell. The odour of urine is a useful indicator of metabolic problems. If ketones, such as acetone, are formed as a consequence of low insulin levels a sweet smell is produced. A sweet smell in the presence of a high quantity of ketones suggests diabetes mellitus. The urine of children with undiagnosed phenylketonuria exhibits an unpleasant 'mousy' odour. A pungent and offensive smell might indicate an infection.

## Dip sticks

A variety of dip sticks are available; some are single-test-based (Clinistix), others are multiple-test-based. The Multistix (Plate 27) performs a wide range of tests for protein, glucose, ketones, blood, urobilinogen and pH. The addition of sensitivity to haemolysed blood and specific gravity is helpful in determining kidney disease. Only if one or more of the indicators is abnormal and the patient is unwell or at risk should a sample be sent for culture.

Glycosuria is almost always the result of raised blood glucose associated with diabetes mellitus. However, it can be associated with other factors. Small quantities of glucose in the urine may be due to emotional stress, which results in the mobilisation of glycogen stores from the liver, or temporary alimentary glycosuria. Alimentary glycosuria is associated with an increase in the ingestion of carbohydrate that cannot be metabolised, hence the blood and urine will temporarily show additional levels of glucose. It should also be noted that glycosuria may occur as a result of secondary hyperglycaemia (even if transient) due to thyrotoxicosis, Cushing's disease, steroid use (including the Pill) and acromegaly.

The presence of proteins (proteinuria) is one of the common signs of renal disease. Proteinuria is sometimes seen in joggers and marathon runners and in these cases is due to excessive exercise.

Bilirubin is produced from red cell haemolysis and haemoglobin breakdown. A conjugated form of bilirubin (attached to another compound) is produced in the liver from the unconjugated or the free form. High levels of bilirubin (bilirubinuria) in the urine would suggest liver disease, liver dysfunction or biliary tract obstruction. Bilirubinuria is one of the earliest signs of hepatobiliary disease; it can be easily detected during urinalysis.

The normal pH of urine is between 4.0 and 8.0. Specific gravity should be in the range 1.012–1.030. An abnormally high specific gravity may be due to infection or the presence of large amounts of glucose.

It is not usual to perform other tests unless the patient shows some positive sign of disease. Such tests include culture of pathogens, microscopic examination of cells and centrifugation and tests for the presence of phenylketonuria.

# MICROBIOLOGY

## Indications for use

Routine screening of samples from healthy patients is wasteful in both time and resources and serves little purpose. Skin has a normal and constant functional flora. Unless the skin is broken few problems are likely to exist. Even in situations where the skin is broken pathogens may not always be present. Wounds affecting the foot can yield some potentially significant microbes, yet the extent of pathology is unremarkable. Findings of this nature relate to the patient's ability to provide satisfactory immunity, particularly from bacterial invasion. Beta-haemolytic *Streptococcus* has been found at the first redressing following a nail ablation. The symptoms were not sufficient to warrant antibiotics (Tollafield 1979). *Escherichia coli* is not an unusual finding under atrophic and lytic nail plates and in the toe web space. It is often a sign of poor hygiene.

As with other forms of laboratory testing, microbiological testing should only be considered when it is likely to serve a useful purpose. The circumstances when it is applicable are:

- When the results of testing are likely to influence the choice of treatment and result in more effective treatment for the patient
- If the results will help identify sources of infection that need to be traced (epidemiology).

It is important when treating bacterial infections that the appropriate antibiotic, specific to the causative organism, is used. The repeated use of broad-spectrum antibiotics is costly and can result in certain bacteria becoming resistant to antibiotics. Although initial treatment may be delayed by the time required to undertake microbiological tests when treatment is commenced, with an antibiotic specific to the bacterium, the likelihood of clearing the infection is high.

In the main, with the exception of some of the cutaneous dermatomycoses, bacteria are responsible for most infections occurring in the lower limb. Fungi, yeasts and protozoal organisms are more likely to arise in compromised hosts and from infections associated with tropical regions of the world. In these instances routine tests are not of much use as it is usually difficult to isolate the responsible pathogen. Some of the rare deep fungi such as Madura foot associated with Actinomycetaceae have been excluded from this chapter. In cases of rampant *Candida* in the feet, assessment and tests to detect an underlying disease process such as diabetes mellitus, or inappropriate use of broad-spectrum antibiotics and/or topical steroids may be more effective than skin culture in dealing with the problem.

Verrucae, caused by human papovavirus, can in very rare cases mutate. The clinical signs can be confusing, but rarely would there be a need to perform any virological tests unless there was an association with an occult disease such as HIV.

## Sampling techniques

Certain guidelines should be followed if meaningful results are to be gained from microbiological examination of samples:

- The sample should be taken from the actual site where an infection has been diagnosed or is suspected.
- Skin should not be cleaned with an antiseptic prior to taking the sample.
- Strict aseptic technique must be followed in order to reduce the risk of the sample becoming contaminated by the microbiological flora of either the patient or the person taking the sample.
- Many pathogenic microorganisms are surprisingly delicate. Unless special measures are taken they do not survive for long away from the body. This means it is often vital that specimens are transported to the laboratory without delay.
- If some delay in transporting specimens to the laboratory is anticipated, it is important that steps are taken to prevent significant growth of contaminating normal flora organisms. These organisms grow at room temperature and can swamp the genuine pathogen. Suppression is normally achieved by refrigeration of samples or inclusion of an inhibitor in the transport medium.
- It is important that sufficient sample is supplied so that the laboratory may use different methods for culture and analysis of the sample and thereby maximise their chances of providing meaningful results. Many techniques may not work reliably if insufficient material is provided.
- If at all possible, samples should be taken prior to the commencement of antibiotic therapy. A drug may suppress a pathogen sufficiently to thwart isolation and identification, without actually working well enough to allow the patient to recover.
- It is often desirable for practitioners to wait for the initial results from the laboratory before starting antibiotic therapy. The results will allow practitioners to choose a narrow-spectrum drug which they can be confident will do the job. However, if a life-threatening infection, e.g. meningitis, is suspected a broad-spectrum antibiotic should be prescribed without delay.
- Specimens taken for microbiological analysis

are by their very nature likely to contain pathogenic organisms and therefore should be treated with care. Containers used for transporting specimens should be secure and labelled as potentially hazardous.

- Good documentation is vital to ensure that samples are not mixed up, lost or subjected to inappropriate tests.
- It is vital that there is dialogue between the practitioner taking the sample and the laboratory staff. For more unusual organisms the microbiologist may be able to provide advice about the most appropriate methods of sampling and transportation.
- In order to be effective the laboratory requires good clinical information about the patient. The site of the suspected infection must be stated. The symptoms should be included on the clinical history section. Is there anything in the patient's history or in the clinical features (colour of pus, cellulitis) that might provide a clue as to the type of organism that is causing the problem? It is important to note recent treatment with antibiotics for the reason given above. Without this sort of detailed information, valuable time and resources may be wasted in inappropriate analyses.

### Wounds and mucosal surfaces

If a large quantity of pus is present this may be drained and sent to the laboratory; otherwise a swab should be taken. Great care should be taken to avoid contamination with the normal flora from surrounding healthy tissue. It is important that a sample is taken from the base of the wound. If taken from the superficial edges it could be contaminated by the flora of the adjacent skin. Swabs are placed into tubes containing a semi-solid agar preparation which prevents them from drying out.

### Skin

For mycological (fungal) investigations, nail clippings or skin scrapings from the edge of the lesion, taken with a blunt scalpel, can be placed in either an envelope or a plastic container.

## Tests and interpretation of results

When samples containing suspected bacterial or fungal pathogens are sent to the laboratory, microscopy, culture and sensitivity, or whichever of these is deemed most appropriate to the particular sample, will be undertaken.

### Microscopy

**Bacteria.** Microscopy may be used at different stages in the processing of samples. In general, microscopy of new samples is of little benefit. There may be too few bacteria to see. Even if they are seen, it may be impossible to tell the difference between a normal commensal organism which has contaminated the sample and a pathogen, because many bacteria look very alike under the microscope. Microscopy is normally used on pure cultures of bacteria which have been isolated and grown from the original sample. Living matter does not show up well under the light microscope so smears that have been fixed to a glass slide by heating are stained with dyes. In addition to allowing the bacteria to be seen easily, some react differently to the various stains and this can be used to tell them apart. The most widely used and most useful staining technique is the Gram stain. The majority of bacteria fall into one of two groups (Fig. 13.1): Gram-positive (which stain blue) and Gram-negative (which stain red). The other commonly used stain is the acid-fast stain used for mycobacteria.

The most common occasion when a smear is made directly from the sample is when meningitis is suspected. In this case, speed is of the essence. A presumptive diagnosis of bacterial meningitis can often be made after looking at a Gram-stained smear under the microscope.

**Fungi.** Samples such as skin scrapings can be mounted on slides in a 10% solution of potassium hydroxide, which helps to clear the tissue. Dermatophytes may be stained with lactophenol blue, so that their hyphae and macroconidia can be visualised better. In otherwise healthy patients investigations are seldom considered necessary, but in immunocompromised patients

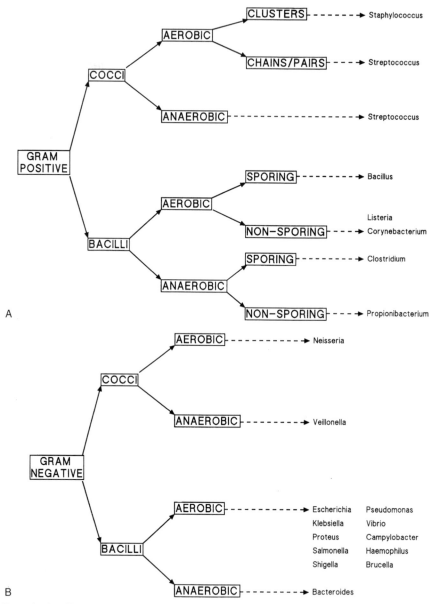

**Figure 13.1** Bacteria classified by staining, shape and use of oxygen   **A.** Gram-positive   **B.** Gram-negative.

fungal infections may be life-threatening. *Cryptococcus neoformans*, which is a cause of meningitis in patients with AIDS, may be demonstrated in cerebrospinal fluid (CSF) by staining with Indian ink prior to microscopy. The pseudohyphae of *Candida albicans*, an opportunistic pathogen and also a significant problem in immunocompromised patients, can often be seen under the microscope.

**Viruses.** Viruses are not large enough to be seen under the light microscope. Although some viruses do differ in shape and they can be seen under the more powerful electron microscope, microscopy is not widely used.

## Isolation and culture

**Bacteria.** A variety of growth media have been designed to promote the growth of different pathogenic bacteria. These are referred to as enrichment media. Bacteria vary considerably in the conditions and nutrients which they require for growth. Some will only grow under aerobic conditions, while others will die unless kept in a strictly anaerobic environment. The most commonly used medium is a nutrient agar to which horse blood has been added. The most fastidious pathogens, such as *Neisseria gonorrhoeae* and *Haemophilus influenzae* (which causes meningitis), require the blood agar to have been heated so that the blood cells burst, releasing nutrients which the bacteria need for growth. The least fussy bacteria such as *Escherichia coli* will grow on almost any medium, so contamination with these members of our normal bacterial flora can pose a problem to microbiologists. Selective media are designed to promote the growth of one type of bacteria whilst discouraging the growth of others.

Not all bacterial pathogens may be easily cultured, e.g. *Treponema pallidum* (the spirochaete which is the cause of syphilis); *Mycobacterium leprae* (the cause of leprosy) can only be cultured in the armadillo.

**Fungi.** Apart from specific fast-growing species such as *Candida albicans*, isolation and culture of fungi is not routinely undertaken. Diagnosis is usually made by clinical means, or after direct examination of the sample under the microscope. Many fungi take a considerable length of time to grow in culture, making isolation of little use. The range of therapies available is limited and the instance of resistance low, so the choice of treatment is usually quite straightforward.

**Viruses.** Viruses are not usually cultured for a variety of reasons. Many cannot practically be grown at all, and others such as HIV are considered too dangerous. In the majority of cases where culture is possible the techniques are expensive and difficult to perform, involving inoculation of fertilised hens eggs, cell cultures or experimental animals. These techniques may take up to 2 weeks to produce a result and are thus of little clinical relevance.

### Identification of bacteria

A wide variety of characteristics may be taken into consideration when attempting to identify an unknown isolate. The microbiologist must decide whether it is Gram-positive or Gram-negative. Determination of shape, production of spores, the ability to thrive as an aerobe or anaerobe (or perhaps both), the medium best supporting growth, the morphology of colonies on an agar plate and types of enzymic production will all feature as questions in arriving at the most likely organism. Once the first question has been answered, the next one follows in a simple and logical sequence. The next question to be asked is dependent on the answer to the previous one. As subsequent questions are answered, the choice of possible species narrows until hopefully only one remains. Table 13.1 lists the types of bacterium found in infections of the lower limb.

**Shape.** There are three basic shapes of bacteria, bacilli (rods), cocci (spheres) or spirals. The spiral-shaped bacteria are quite diverse, ranging from the vibrios, which are comma-shaped, to the spirochaetes, which are like corkscrews. The way in which the individual bacteria are arranged can be quite characteristic of different species or groups. Some streptococci form chains of bacteria where the cells have remained joined together after completing division, whereas *Streptococcus pneumoniae* (a common cause of both pneumonia and meningitis) forms pairs of cells. Staphylococci form bunches of cells.

**Spores.** Some Gram-positive bacilli produce resting forms called endospores, which survive desiccation or exposure to the air. Some species form them in the middle of the bacterium (e.g. *Bacillus anthracis*), others at the ends (e.g. *Clostridium tetani*). If the bacteria are Gram-stained this can be seen under the microscope.

**Oxygen.** Bacteria vary in their need for oxygen. Some like *Mycobacterium tuberculosis* and *Pseudomonas aeruginosa* must have air in

**Table 13.1** Bacterial pathogens found in infections of the lower limb

| Bacteria | Features |
| --- | --- |
| *Staphylococcus aureus* | Gram-positive, aerobic coccus. Most frequent cause of foot infections. Able to form an enzyme which coagulates citrated plasma; therefore the infection tends to remain localised. Responsible for boils, carbuncles, septic toes and osteomyelitis. |
| *Streptococcus pyogenes* | Gram-positive, aerobic or anaerobic coccus. All strains are beta-haemolytic. Produce enzymes which help to break down surrounding connective tissue and thus aid its spread. May lead to cellulitis, lymphangitis and lymphadenitis and may be the prime organism responsible for necrotising fasciitis. |
| *Pseudomonas aeruginosa* | Gram-negative, aerobic bacillus. Gives rise to blue-green pus and produces a pungent odour. May be found in paronychia alongside *Candida albicans*. |
| *Escherichia coli* | Gram-negative, aerobic bacillus usually found in the gut. May be present in mixed infections and also is found alongside *Candida albicans* in paronychia. |
| *Klebsiella* spp. | Gram-negative, aerobic bacillus found in the gut. May be present in mixed wound infections. |
| *Proteus* spp. | Gram-negative, aerobic bacillus found in the gut. May be present in mixed wound infections. |
| *Cornynebacterium minutissimum* | Gram-positive, aerobic bacillus responsible for erythrasma and pitted keratolysis. |
| *Clostridium welchii* | Gram-positive, anaerobic bacillus responsible for gas gangrene. |

order to grow (strict aerobes), whilst others such as *Bacteroides fragilis* are killed by any exposure to oxygen (strict anaerobes). The largest group of medically important species are facultative anaerobes, meaning that they can grow with or without oxygen. Some bacteria, like *Neisseria* spp., use oxygen but grow better if extra $CO_2$ is added to the atmosphere.

**Growth.** The growth of a bacterium on a selective medium may be an important observation. Not only is it important whether the isolate grows or not, but how it grows. Many species produce colonies of a certain morphology, size and colour on different media. For example, *Staphylococcus aureus* produces golden yellow colonies when grown on blood agar. The degree of haemolysis of the blood in a blood agar plate is a useful factor in differentiating between different streptococci. *Streptococcus pneumoniae* colonies are surrounded by a green ring where the haemoglobin in the blood has been altered (alpha-haemolytic) whereas those of *Streptococcus pyogenes* are surrounded by a clear ring where the blood cells have been completely lysed (beta-haemolysis).

**Biochemistry.** Bacteria can perform a wide range of biochemical reactions. Some activities are characteristic of a particular group of species; others can be used to differentiate between two closely related species that otherwise seem to be identical. Staphylococci and streptococci can be separated by performing a test for the enzyme catalase which breaks down hydrogen peroxide. Staphylococci, which are catalase-positive, produce bubbles of oxygen when incubated with hydrogen peroxide. Streptococci, which are catalase-negative, do not. On its own the catalase test is not very helpful, because all bacteria are either catalase-positive or catalase-negative. If a diagnosis of Gram-positive coccus has already been made, suggesting either a staphylococcus or a streptococcus, then it can be of considerable assistance. There are few biochemical tests which are conclusive when taken in isolation, but when the field has been narrowed sufficiently, they can provide vital evidence. The ability to metabolise or ferment different sugars is a widely tested function. Maltose is used to differentiate between *Neisseria meningitides*, which ferments it, and the closely related species *Neisseria gonorrhoea*, which doesn't. One of the most difficult groups of bacteria to separate are the coliform bacteria (Gram-negative bacilli) which includes, among others, the harmless gut bacteria

*Escherichia coli*, *Proteus* and *Klebsiella* spp. and the harmful *Salmonella* and *Shigella* spp., which cause typhoid, food poisoning and dysentery. Several biochemical tests may be necessary to identify the correct organism. Because of the complexity of this process many laboratories now use special testing strips which allow 20 or more tests to be performed simultaneously. Bacterial culture is added to each little plastic chamber, which contains the appropriate substrate plus, if necessary, a dye that will change colour if the test is positive. After a suitable period of incubation the positive reactions can be scored on a scale of 0–5 (0 = negative, 5 = very positive) and a profile of the organism produced. This profile can be checked against a file of standard profiles, allowing the organism to be identified.

**Sensitivity testing.** In many senses the question of which microorganism is responsible for a given set of symptoms is secondary to the question of which treatment will give the best clinical outcome. Obviously knowledge of the type of pathogen will form a large part of the answer, but for bacteria at least, it is often only a part of that answer. The widespread incidence of resistance to antibiotics makes sensitivity testing a crucial part of the microbiologist's role. Resistance to antifungal agents is not particularly common, thus sensitivity testing is rarely undertaken. The limited numbers of antiviral agents available, and the difficulties of testing them, mean testing is not worthwhile in the case of viral pathogens.

*Disk diffusion methods.* A series of small paper disks which have each been impregnated with one of the antibiotics under test are placed on an agar plate on to which has been spread a culture of bacterium. After incubation, for a suitable length of time, the plate is examined. Where a bacterium is resistant to an antibiotic it will grow right up to the edge of the disk, but where it is sensitive to that drug there will be a clear zone surrounding the disk. The radius of this zone of inhibition can be taken as a measure of the degree of sensitivity to that particular drug.

*Minimum inhibitory concentration (MIC).* This assay gives a measure of the minimum dose which is likely to influence the course of an infection. An inoculum of the culture under test is added to each of a series of tubes containing broth, supplemented with increasing concentrations of the drug under test. After incubation, bacterial growth is scored by the turbidity of the culture. The lowest dose of drug which causes the broth to remain clear is termed the MIC. To calculate the minimum bactericidal concentration (MBC) samples from each tube are plated on blood agar plates. The lowest concentration at which no colonies are observed is the MBC. MBC is usually greater than MIC because intermediate doses may inhibit the bacterium without actually killing it. These tests are used where accurate treatment is vital, such as cases of streptococcal myocarditis or in immunosuppression.

**Serology.** Antisera raised against exotoxins or outer-membrane proteins may be used in immunodiffusion tests.

### Identification of fungi

The identification of most fungi is based largely on morphology. For dermatophytes, the structures of their macroconidia (which contain spores) are very individual. For *Candida* spp. pseudomycelium and buds can be observed. On culture some dermatophytes are coloured, e.g. *Trichophyton rubrum* (one of the causes of tinea pedis or athletes foot) which, as its name suggests, produces colonies with a red underside. Table 13.2 lists the types of fungus found in fungal infections affecting the feet.

### Identification of viruses

Most viral infections are diagnosed by the symptoms they cause. In some cases such as suspected HIV or hepatitis, or in transplant patients or other immunocompromised individuals, tests are undertaken. The majority of tests involve either using an antibody-based test for the presence of the virus itself, or screening the patient's serum for antibodies against it (such as the so-called 'AIDS test'). Much of the work going on to develop new diagnostic tests is aimed at finding ways of identifying viral pathogens.

**308** LABORATORY AND HOSPITAL INVESTIGATIONS

**Table 13.2** Fungi responsible for fungal infections of the feet

| Fungus | Features |
|--------|----------|
| *Tricophyton rubrum* | Affects skin and nails. 85% of cases of onychomycosis thought to be due to *T. rubrum*. Can affect skin and hair in a number of ways. Diffuse dry scaling tinea on the soles is usually due to *T. rubrum*. |
| *Tricophyton mentagrophytes* | Affects skin and nails. Can cause a range of skin responses but is especially associated with vesicle eruption. 12% of cases of onychomycosis due to *T. mentagrophytes*. |
| *Epidermophyton floccosum* | Affects skin in a variety of ways but is especially associated with vesicle eruption. Rarely causes onychomycosis. |
| *Scopulariopsis brevicaulis* | Secondary pathogen. Produces a dark green or grey-black discolouration. |
| *Candida* spp. | A yeast of which *Candida albicans* is the most common. Affects skin and nails. In nails it is often responsible for paronychia. |

### New technologies

The need for ever faster and more accurate diagnosis has meant that clinical microbiology must be at the forefront of new technologies. Several recent scientific developments offer major opportunities for faster and more sensitive detection of pathogenic microorganisms, and several systems are already in use. These tests are outside the scope of this chapter and relate to serology (monoclonal antibodies), DNA probing and polymerase chain reaction.

## BLOOD ANALYSIS

## Indications for use

Blood comprises formed elements and chemical substances (Table 13.3). It can be analysed in a variety of ways. Analysis may focus on the cellular content (haematology), blood chemistry (biochemistry) or immunological aspects (serology). Blood tests can aid the diagnosis of the following, all of which are relevant to the practitioner dealing with the lower limb:

- Immunology-related disorders, e.g. seropositive arthritides
- Anaemias, e.g. altered erythrocyte
- Metabolic disorders, e.g. raised serum glucose and ketone levels
- Hormonal disorders, e.g. high level of serum thyroxine
- Systemic inflammation, e.g. raised ESR
- Infections, e.g. raised leucocyte count
- Clotting disorders, e.g. abnormal platelet count
- Leukaemias, e.g. low leucocyte alkaline phosphate.

The use of routine blood screening in patients without symptoms is questionable. The likelihood of detecting an unsuspected abnormality is low, and may be considered insignificant. Routine biochemical screening prior to surgery revealed 0.2%, 0.2% and 1% of abnormality in unsuspected

**Table 13.3** The composition of blood

| Formed elements (45%) | Plasma (55%) |
|-----------------------|--------------|
| Erythrocytes | Proteins—albumin |
| | globulin |
| Leucocytes— neutrophils | fibrinogen |
| eosinophils | |
| basophils | Water |
| lymphocytes | |
| monocytes | Solutes—electrolytes |
| | respiratory gases |
| Thrombocytes (platelets) | enzymes/hormones |
| | nitrogen products |
| | digestion products |

cases (Blery et al 1986, Kaplan et al 1985, McKee & Scott 1987). In cases where abnormality was detected, the results of the tests made no difference to the anaesthetic or surgical management of the patient. Routine haematology screening of GP patients revealed that the older the patient the higher the incidence of abnormality: 1% at age 20 and less than 10% in patients over 70 years.

Blood screening can be useful in detecting sickle-cell anaemia and thalassaemia. Thalassaemia affects 3% of the world's population. 25% of Africans carry the gene related to sickle-cell anaemia. Both conditions can have implications for the management of lower limb problems, especially surgical management. Where surgical intervention is indicated it may be worthwhile to undertake a screening for these conditions in those at particular risk.

In general, patients without clinical signs of disease are unlikely to produce grossly abnormal results. Significant liver disease, for instance, is almost certain to produce jaundice. The appearance of bilirubin in the urine offers a cheap alternative screening test (Jones & Berk 1979). Initial detection of diabetes of any importance can be reliably performed on a urine sample which also has the benefit of revealing proteinuria and unrecognised renal impairment (Payne 1986).

## Sampling technique

An autolet with a disposable needle can be used to produce a small drop of blood from a pinprick. It is usual to prick the distal pulp of the thumb.

For laboratory-based tests a greater quantity of blood than that obtained from a pinprick is required. It is important that the person taking the sample has appropriate and current qualifications. A phlebotomist is a technician who has been trained to take samples of blood. Blood samples are taken from a vein, usually in the forearm. A tourniquet is often used to make the vein visible. A needle is inserted into the vein. This needle is fitted to an evacuated tube which has a double needle at the other end. This allows more than one collection tube to be fitted. As a

result two or more samples of blood can be collected without removal of the needle from the vein.

To ensure appropriate stability of the sample, containers which contain an appropriate additive are used. Many samples must be prevented from clotting. Sodium citrate or ethylenediamine tetra-acetic acid (EDTA) can be used for this purpose. Where an infection is suspected, one type of container is used to collect the blood sample to be tested for the presence of aerobic organisms and another type for anaerobic organisms.

### Guidelines for collecting samples for laboratory investigation

- If appropriately qualified you may take the sample, otherwise the patient will need to be referred to a suitably trained health care worker. Often patients are referred to hospital where a phlebotomist will take the sample.
- Whether you take the sample yourself or refer to a hospital it is essential you provide the laboratory undertaking the tests with relevant information. This will include the patient's personal details, age and sex, current therapy—which may affect the results—and any history that may help point to a diagnosis. The patient's hospital number or laboratory number, if there have been previous tests, will enable current results to be compared with previous test results. Many laboratories produce cumulative results which give an indication of patient progress. Normal ranges vary in pregnancy; for this reason it is vital to provide this information on the request form.
- In the case of some biochemistry tests, the patient must fast before the sample is taken and the time of the last meal recorded. The patient should be fully informed of these requirements.
- If you are taking the sample yourself you must ensure the sample is correctly labelled and that you are aware of the specimen storage conditions for the tests you require. It is important the sample(s) arrives as fresh as

possible. If the sample has not been properly handled, e.g. a sample to be tested for plasma viscosity has been stored in a refrigerator, then the result will be invalidated.

## Tests and interpretation of results

Blood may be tested by two means:

* Clinically via the use of a glucometer for the presence of glucose; this is a form of 'near patient testing'
* By a laboratory when a complete haematological and blood chemistry analysis is required.

### Glucometer

The glucometer uses a small sample of blood to test blood glucose levels (Fig. 13.2). Glucometers vary slightly in design; all come with instructions for use. It is essential that the practitioner follows the manufacturers' guidelines, regularly cleans the equipment and takes care to calibrate the equipment prior to use. The glucometer gives the amount of glucose in the blood, in millimoles per litre, as a digital read out. A normal reading is within the range of 4–8 mmol/l (non-fasting) and 3–5 mmol/l (fasting). Glucometers have been known to give false positive and negative readings. This is usually due to inadequate cleaning, poor calibration or not following the manufacturers' guidelines when carrying out the test.

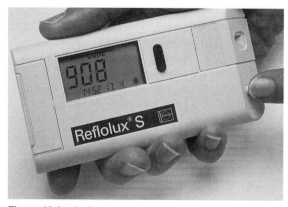

**Figure 13.2** A glucometer.

### Laboratory tests

A range of tests can be undertaken in the laboratory. These can be divided into the following:

* Examination of the relationship between the cellular and plasma content
* Examination of the cellular content
* Chemical tests
* Bacteriological tests
* Serological tests.

The results from a blood test should be compared to the normal value charts (Tables 13.4 and 13.5). Any areas of disparity should be noted and acted upon. Often the laboratory places an asterisk by abnormal results. Some tests, e.g. detection of rheumatoid factor or fasting glucose levels, have to be specifically requested.

The practitioner should be aware of abnormal results from blood tests. Abnormal results may be due to a true positive abnormality or to an error in the collection and/or storage of the specimen. A straightforward example is the reporting of thrombocytopenia (low platelet count). If the collection technique was traumatic then the specimen may have begun to clot in the needle or tube. This will result in a lowered platelet count. This may not be obvious in the laboratory. It is therefore important that the laboratory is informed if the specimen proved difficult to collect. If red blood cells are left in contact with the serum in the tube overnight, serum potassium levels will be high and glucose levels will be erroneously low. Most of these false results can be avoided by adhering to the guidelines for taking blood samples issued by all laboratories.

Tables 13.4 and 13.5 indicate the clinical implications of abnormal readings. Any abnormal finding will be of interest and relevance to the practitioner dealing with lower limb pathologies. The following are of particular interest:

* Erythrocyte sedimentation rate (ESR)
* C-reactive protein
* Rheumatoid factor
* Blood glucose levels
* Glycosylated haemoglobin

**Table 13.4**  Normal values for blood count and coagulation tests and clinical implications of abnormal findings (values vary from source to source)

| Blood count | Measurement | Clinical implication |
| --- | --- | --- |
| Haemoglobin | 14–18 g/dl men<br>12–16 g/dl women | Decrease—anaemia, cirrhosis<br>Increase—polycythaemia |
| Haematocrit (packed cell volume, PCV) | 40–54% men<br>36–47% women | Decrease—anaemia<br>Increase—dehydration |
| Red cell count (RCV) | $4.0\text{–}6.0 \times 10^{12}$/l | Decrease—anaemia |
| Reticulocyte | 0.2–2.0% | Decrease—radiotherapy count<br>Increase—haemolytic anaemia |
| Mean cell volume (MCV) | 80–100 fl | |
| Mean cell diameter | 6.7–7.7 µm | |
| Mean cell haemoglobin (MCH) | 27–32 pg | Decrease—ron deficiency |
| Mean cell haemoglobin concentration (MCHC) | 32–36% | Decrease—iron deficiency |
| Erythrocyte sedimentation rate (ESR) | 3–5 mm/1h men<br>7–12 mm/1h women | Increase—inflammation, infection |
| White cell count (WCC) | $4\text{–}10 \times 10^9$/l | |
| Neutrophils | $2.5\text{–}7.5 \times 10^9$/l | Increase—acute infections |
| Lymphocytes | $1.5\text{–}4.0 \times 10^9$/l | Increase—viral infections |
| Monocytes | $0.2\text{–}0.8 \times 10^9$/l | Increase—chronic infection |
| Basophils | $0.0\text{–}0.1 \times 10^9$/l | Increase—leukaemia |
| Eosinophils | $0.04\text{–}0.44 \times 10^9$/l | Increase—hypersensitivity reaction |
| Platelet count | $150\text{–}400 \times 10^9$/l | Decrease—leukaemia |
| *Coagulation tests* | | |
| Prothrombin time | Within 2 secs of control | |
| Partial thromboplastin time (PTT) | Within 8 secs of control | |
| Bleeding time | Less than 5 min | |
| Plasma fibrinogen | 2.0–4.0 g/l | |

- Uric acid
- Cholesterol and triglycerides
- White blood cell differentials.

**Erythrocyte sedimentation rate.** This is the rate of fall of red cells in a column of blood. ESR increases with age and is higher in females than males. A raised ESR reflects an increase in the plasma concentration of proteins such as fibrinogen and immunoglobulins. It is indicative of diseases associated with malignancy, infections and inflammation. Other measures such as white cell counts may be more sensitive when testing for inflammatory and infectious diseases.

**C-reactive protein.** This measure is replacing the use of ESR. C-reactive protein is synthesised exclusively in the liver. Its presence can be detected in blood within 6 hours of an inflammatory response. It can be detected by using an automated immunoassay.

**Rheumatoid factor.** Conditions associated with unclear causes of joint pain in the foot and lower limb pose a concern for the practitioner, especially where the ankle, subtalar or MTP joints are involved. Seropositive arthritides can be a cause of this type of joint pain. Analysing serum for the presence of rheumatoid factor can

**Table 13.5** Normal biochemistry values of blood and clinical implications of abnormal findings (values vary from source to source)

| Test | Measurement | Clinical implication |
|------|-------------|---------------------|
| Albumin | 27–42 g/l | Decrease—malnutrition |
| Alkaline phosphatase | 100–460 U/l men<br>70–430 U/l women | Increase—Paget's disease, RA |
| Bilirubin | 1–25 mmol/l total | Increase—liver disease |
| Calcium | 2.33–2.6 mmol/l | Decrease—renal disease, osteomalacia |
| Cholesterol | 3.6–6.5 mmol/l | Increase—atheroma |
| High density lipoproteins (HLP) | 0.6–1.6 mmol/l | Increase—atheroma |
| Creatinine | 60–120 µmol/l men<br>50–110 µmol/l women | Increase—renal disease<br>Decrease—muscular dystrophy |
| Glucose | 3.6–5.6 mmol/l fasting | Increase—diabetes mellitus |
| Iron | 14–29 µmol/l | Decrease—anaemia |
| Thyroxine (free) | 11–24 µmol/l | Increase—hyperthyroid<br>Decrease—hypothyroid |
| Urea | 3.5–7.2 mg/dl men<br>2.6–6.0 mg/dl women | Increase—gout? |

be helpful in these instances. Rheumatoid factors are autoantibodies found in the serum, usually of the IgM class, which are directed against human IgG. Their presence can be detected by either the Latex or the Rose Waaler tests. The presence of rheumatoid factors may indicate rheumatoid arthritis (80% of cases), systemic lupus erythematosus (50% of cases), systemic sclerosis (30% of cases), Sjögren's syndrome (90% of cases), polymyositis and dermatomyositis (50% of cases). Occasionally it may be seen in the 'normal' elderly patient, infective endocarditis, primary biliary cirrhosis and autoimmune chronic active hepatitis.

**Blood glucose levels.** Besides the detection of glucose in blood, a fasting glucose tolerance test and the oral glucose tolerance test can be performed. The former is used when there is concern that a high blood glucose level is due to recent carbohydrate intake. The patient is required to fast for a period of time prior to blood glucose levels being assessed. The oral glucose tolerance test is used for borderline cases of diabetes mellitus. The patient is required to fast, the blood is tested for glucose, glucose is

then administered and, after a period of time, the test is repeated.

**Glycosylated haemoglobin.** Under physiological conditions blood sugars bind non-enzymatically to proteins, forming stable covalent linkages. The measurement of glycated derivatives of haemoglobin and plasma proteins has provided a reliable index of long-term blood glucose control in patients with diabetes mellitus and is of proven value. Glycated haemoglobin ($HbA_1$) is the most widely used measure for long-term control of blood glucose level. The level of $HbA_1$ depends on the life-span of red blood cell (RBC) and the prevailing blood glucose concentration. It gives a measure of mean blood sugar level over the preceding 2 months, provided the RBC life-span is normal. It should be remembered that a combination of periods of hyperglycaemia and prolonged hypoglycaemia can result in a normal $HbA_1$ level. Other proteins are glycated and may be useful markers of control. The fructosamine assay has attracted particular interest because it is cheap and rapid to perform. This assay measures glycated serum proteins and so reflects control over a shorter time span (e.g. 2–3 weeks). The total plasma albumin concentration affects all glycated plasma protein methods, making accurate assessment of fructosamine impossible in patients with hypo-albuminaemia.

**Uric acid.** The normal range is 3.5–7.2 mg/dl for males and 2.6–6.0 mg/dl for females. Elevated serum uric acid is not a reliable diagnostic test for gout. However, acute gout never occurs in patients who have a serum uric acid level in the lower half of the normal range. The test can give rise to false negatives and positives. In the first few attacks, when it is often difficult to diagnose, the serum acid level is often below the higher level. Serum uric acid levels can be helpful in monitoring treatment.

**Cholesterol and triglycerides.** Tests for these can now be purchased over the counter in most chemists. They serve as useful indicators of those at risk of severe atheroma formation resulting in peripheral vascular disease. Those with a family history of atheroma and/or diabetics should be tested.

**White blood cell differential count.** As can be seen from Table 13.4 abnormalities in the white blood cell differential count are indicative of a range of infective and immunologically-related disorders that can arise in the lower limb.

## HISTOLOGY

### Indications for use

Histology provides a useful method for clarifying or confirming a diagnosis. Tissue and body fluids (other than blood and urine) can be removed from the lower limb for histological examination.

The indications for histological analysis are as follows:

- When a lesion does not have a clear clinical diagnosis and resists treatment, e.g. neuroma
- When there is no exudate which can be cultured for the presence of pathogens; in this case, a sample of tissue is needed for microbiological purposes and for identification of cellular changes
- Where tissue has an abnormal appearance and malignancy is suspected

- Where the lesion fails to heal, e.g. inclusion cyst, pyogenic granuloma (Plate 28).

## Sampling techniques

Either tissue or fluid can be used for histological examination.

The range of tissues from the lower limb that can be removed for histological analysis can be found in Table 13.6. Various methods can be used to remove tissue or fluid for investigation. The technique used will depend upon the site and the amount that needs to be removed. A wide range of investigations can be performed on tissues taken from the body. Samples should be collected in such a way as to pre-empt the method to be used. The practitioner should therefore decide at the outset what investigations are required. Appropriate collection and storage techniques are vital to preserve the sample.

Most techniques require local anaesthesia. In the case of tissue it is generally advisable to remove a section of surrounding healthy tissue as well as the abnormal tissue; this allows the pathologist to make comparisons between normal and abnormal tissue.

Biopsy is the term used to describe excision of tissue from a living body for microscopic examination in order to make a diagnosis. It consists of removing a piece or the whole of a lesion. Five methods of achieving a biopsy will be considered:

- Excisional
- Incisional
- Endoscopic
- Aspiration
- Amputation.

### Excisional

Excisional biopsy involves the removal of all the abnormal tissue plus a section of the surrounding normal tissue. This procedure permits examination of the abnormal tissue as well as, hopefully, providing treatment at the same time. It is a surgical technique which requires high standards of asepsis. A scalpel is used to incise and

**Table 13.6** Tissues which can be removed from the foot for histological analysis

| | |
|---|---|
| Epithelial | Keratinised stratified epithelial tissue (skin) |
| | Stratified cuboidal epithelium (sweat glands/secretory function) |
| | Multicellular exocrine glands:<br>—coiled tubular eccrine and apocrine (sweat)<br>—branched acinar holocrine (sebaceous) |
| Connective | Mesenchymal found in adult tissue below skin and blood vessels |
| | Loose areolar: subcutaneous layer of skin, blood vessels, nerves associated with fibroblasts, macrophages, mast cells and various fibres |
| | Adipose: under weightbearing surfaces, joints and bone marrow |
| | Dense collagenous: common to fascia, aponeuroses, tendons, ligaments |
| | Elastic and reticular: less abundant in feet |
| | Hyaline and fibrocartilage: chondrocytic cells associated with joints, especially distal metatarsal ends, fibrocartilage submetatarsals, between bones and tendons |
| | Osseous (bone): made of compact (outer), cancellous (inner) and cellular components associated with regeneration |
| Muscle | Skeletal: striated, contractile form attached between bones; mainly intrinsic form in feet in four layers |
| Nerve | Cell body and axons |
| | Neuroglia: found at sites of tumours |
| Synovial membranes | Loose connective tissue: line structures and secrete synovial fluid, tendon lining, bursae, do not contain epithelial cells |
| Tissue repair | Stroma: supporting connective tissue restoration; active repair or scar tissue due to fibroblasts or keloid (overactivity) |
| | Scab/fibrin plug: sealing wound |
| | Granuloma: active repair tissue |

then dissect the abnormal tissue and some surrounding normal tissue from the site. Haemo-stasis should be carefully performed to prevent unnecessary complications. Tissue from skin down to muscle, ligaments and tendon will require careful repair.

Ganglion formation must be removed in total as it has a high recurrence rate. The gelatinous mass is difficult to retrieve. The thin translucent membrane should be included wherever possible. Thicker membranes suggest that they have undergone longer periods of deep trauma.

*Incisional*

An incisional biopsy involves the removal of a small section of abnormal tissue. The procedure is not as extensive as excisional biopsy but is still open to complications such as deep infection. Usually a punch, which consists of a cylinder with a sharp, fine cutting edge, is used. The punch is pushed through epithelial tissue and a small section of epithelial and/or connective tissue is removed. A trephine is a similar instrument to a punch, but much more sturdy. It is used for punching holes in bone. In these cases a larger access hole is necessary. Bone samples should, wherever possible, have clear radiographs attached to assist the determination of the general appearance of the lesion.

The advantage of incisional biopsy lies in the small area of tissue removed. Normal tissue is not usually included. The depth of tissue sampling will depend upon the pressure applied. Incisional biopsy is likely to be used where large areas have been affected and treatment cannot be undertaken at the same time. Unlike excisional biopsy it is purely a diagnostic procedure.

When skin biopsy is performed it is essential to create an unobtrusive scar. In the foot, tissue around digits may require a section of bone to be removed in order to achieve closure. A surgeon specialising in feet should be consulted to reduce the risk of ischaemia.

*Endoscopy*

This is achieved by introducing an endoscope into the body. This procedure is used when it is necessary to remove a piece of tissue from a deep structure, e.g. synovial membrane from a joint.

### Aspiration

Aspiration is the technique used to withdraw fluids from the body, e.g. synovial fluid. Examination of synovial fluid can be very useful when examining for the presence of uric acid crystals (gout), infection or bleeding into a joint space. Where uric acid crystals are suspected the sample of synovial fluid should be placed in absolute alcohol or placed directly on to a slide. Bursae can be aspirated. This usually leads to a temporary relief of symptoms.

### Amputation

Whole parts, such as amputated feet, toes and excised rays, can be sent to the pathology department. Analysis of whole anatomy takes a good deal longer due to the time required to separate and fixate tissues. Bone needs to undergo a decalcification process.

### Transportation and storage

Laboratory personnel will discuss the best mode of collection to ensure that an appropriate sample for testing is achieved. Specimens labelled urgent are unwelcome unless requested during surgery where a quick result is necessary, e.g. in the case of a suspected malignancy, so that appropriate treatment can be performed concomitantly. Even small samples will take 24 hours to fix before the tissue can be usefully analysed.

All specimens should be clearly marked with the patient's name, hospital number, site and the date/time that the sample was taken. A full history of the patient is essential. High risk cases should be identified with a separate 'high risk' label. The specimen should be sealed in a plastic bag, the request form remaining outside.

As with microbiological samples, damage can be sustained by using an incorrect method of transportation. Most tissue samples are placed in a screw-cap container containing buffered formalin solution. Formalin itself constitutes a hazard, especially if spilt on living tissue. Samples for frozen section should be transported dry. They will be damaged if they come into contact with formalin. Frozen sectioning provides rapid results, usually within 5–10 minutes, and is used where results are urgently required.

## Tests and interpretation of results

These fall into several categories depending upon the nature of the lesion and/or suspected pathology. Slides of tissue are produced for microscopy. Often, staining techniques are used in order to show up changes more distinctively.

The main purpose of histological examination is to assess whether the tissue or fluid sample differs from what is normal. Abnormal cellular findings, e.g. changes to the nucleus, may indicate malignant changes. Chronic inflammation may be evident because of the presence of lymphocytes, plasma cells and macrophages. Abnormal findings may relate to the presence of giant cells, a characteristic feature produced by foreign bodies. This is a common feature in the foot.

Scarring and inflammatory changes may tether down tissue which can account for some pain syndromes in both fore and hind parts of the foot. These syndromes are difficult to diagnose accurately other than by exploratory procedures. Nerves fall under this category. They can show marked changes, involving abnormal blood vessels, as in the case of neuromata. Nerve conduction tests may provide evidence of damage prior to surgical investigation in the foot.

## SUMMARY

This chapter has covered the indications for the use of a range of near-patient and laboratory-based tests, appropriate sampling techniques, the principles of testing and interpretation of results. Emphasis has been placed on starting with the most simple tests prior to using more specific and sophisticated tests. The range of tests applicable to the lower limb are summarised in Table 13.7.

The use of laboratory tests can never replace good interview and assessment techniques. Tests

**Table 13.7** Summary of useful tests for diagnosing disease in the lower limb (laboratory sheets adapted from hospital sheet, Cleveland Medical Laboratories, Nuffield Hospital, Leicester)

| *Haematology* | *Biochemistry* |
|---|---|
| Full blood count | Full biochemical screen |
| ESR | Urea electrolytes |
| Viscosity | Liver function |
| Vitamin $B_{12}$/folate | Thyroid function |
| Platelet count | Blood glucose |
| Prothrombin | Serum urate |
| Sickle cell | Acid phosphatase |
| Coagulation screen | Creatinine |
| Glycosylated haemoglobin | Creatinine clearance |
| | Glucose tolerance |
| *Microbiology* | Cholesterol and triglycerides |
| MSU | 24-hour urine |
| Blood culture | |
| Culture and sensitivity (swab) | *Histopathology* |
| Mycology | Nature and site of specimen |
| TB studies | |
| | *Serology* |
| | Rheumatoid factor |
| | C-reactive protein |

should be used economically and wisely, should cause no harm to the patient and above all should be used to support treatment, confirm diagnosis or rule out a suspected malignancy. Results should be acted upon in order to ensure that effective treatment is provided.

REFERENCES

Blery C, Charpak Y, Szatan M et al 1986 Evaluation of a protocol for selective ordering of preoperative tests. Lancet 1: 139–141

Jones E A, Berk P D 1979 Liver function. In: Brown S, Mitchell F L, Young D S (eds) Chemical diagnosis of disease. Elsevier/North Holland Biomedical Press, Amsterdam, p 525–662

Kaplan E B, Sheiner L B, Boeckmann A J et al 1985 The usefulness of preoperative laboratory screening. Journal of the American Medical Association 153: 3576–3581

McKee R F, Scott E M 1987 The value of preoperative investigations. Annals of the Royal College of Surgeons of England 69: 160–162

Payne R B 1986 Creatinine clearance; a redundant clinical investigation. Annals of Clinical Biochemistry 23: 243–250

Tollafield D R 1979 Microbia of the foot and instrument disinfection techniques in chiropody. A two part study. Chiropody Department, Northampton Area Health Authority, Northampton

FURTHER READING

Cano R J, Colome J S 1988 Essentials of microbiology. West
Hoffbrand A V, Pettit J E 1993 Essential haematology. Blackwell Scientific, Oxford
Tortora G J, Anagnostakos N P 1987 Principles of anatomy and physiology. Harper International, New York

Wheater P R, Burkitt H G, Stevens A, Lowe J S 1991 Basic histopathology Churchill Livingstone, Edinburgh
Zatouroff M 1976 A colour atlas of physical signs in general medicine. Wolfe Medical, London

# Specific client groups

# 14

# The paediatric patient

*T. E. Kilmartin*
*D. R. Tollafield*
*P. Nesbitt*

## INTRODUCTION

This chapter is concerned with the assessment of the foot and lower limb of the child. The assessment of a child follows a similar format to that of the adult, except that the practitioner should appreciate that a number of normal developmental changes exists in the first few years. These variations differ from adulthood and may often concern the parent and even confuse the inexperienced practitioner. Such factors must be taken into consideration when examining children from birth to the second decade of life, when skeletal maturity is expected.

It is essential to identify, as early as possible, any problems that might need specialist treatment in order to prevent problems in later life. While the joints, muscles and bones are the major area requiring special scrutiny, it is also important to consider other parts of the primary assessment such as skin and footwear. Common conditions which may arise in the child are listed in Table 14.1.

This chapter considers the normal development process, presents an overview of factors which should be taken into consideration when assessing the child and reviews the assessment findings of specific conditions that arise in the lower limb of children.

## NORMAL DEVELOPMENT

Prior to assessing a child it is important that the practitioner has a good understanding of normal

**Table 14.1** Conditions affecting the lower limbs of children

| | |
|---|---|
| Joints | Congenital dislocation of the hip |
| | Anterior knee pain |
| | Tarsal coalition |
| | Hallux valgus |
| | Digital deformities |
| | Juvenile rheumatoid arthritis |
| Bone | Metatarsus adductus |
| | Talipes equinovarus |
| | Osteochondroses |
| | —Perthes disease |
| | —Köhler's disease |
| | —Freiberg's infraction |
| | Apopyhsitis |
| | —Sever's disease |
| | —Osgood–Schlatter's disease |
| Gait | In-toeing |
| | Genu varum |
| | Genu valgum |
| Neurological | Cerebral palsy |
| | Charcot–Marie–Tooth disease |
| | Friedreich's ataxia |
| Neuromuscular | Duchenne's muscular dystrophy |
| Vascular | Chilblains |
| | Erythrocyanosis |
| | Acrocyanosis |
| Skin | Verruca pedis |
| | Fungal infection |
| | Hyperhidrosis |
| | Bromidrosis |
| | Ingrown toe nail |
| | Epidermolysis bullosa congenita |
| | Traumatic blisters |

**Table 14.2** Prenatal development of the lower limb

| Week | Changes |
|---|---|
| 4 | Limb buds appear |
| 5 | Foot plates appear<br>Nerves to extremities |
| 6 | Limb perpendicular to torso |
| 7 | Lower limbs commence medial rotation towards 90°<br>Feet in equinus and inversion<br>Hallux 50° adducted<br>Digital rays begin to appear with interdigital clefts<br>Muscles appear<br>Ossification points of femur and tibia appear |
| 8 | Distinction between thigh, leg and foot<br>Ossification points of fibular appear |
| 9 | Osseous nuclei of metatarsals and phalanges appear<br>Digits well developed<br>Foot completely inverted |
| 10 | Dorsiflexion of foot begins |
| 12 | Arms and legs move independently of trunk<br>Nails begin to form |
| 16 | Eversion of feet due to valgus torsion of talus and calcaneus commences—it continues until 6 years of age |
| 22 | Toe nails lie in the dorsal position |
| 32–34 | Anterior transverse crease on sole of foot |
| 36–38 | Occasional creases on anterior two-thirds of sole |
| 39–40 | Sole covered with creases |

development and the approximate age by which certain milestones should be met. However, it should be remembered that variations occur even in normal healthy children. Normal prenatal development is summarised in Table 14.2.

## Birth

Apgar scoring is a routine procedure performed at the first and fifth minute after birth. It is used to indicate the cardiovascular, respiratory and neurological status of the neonate.

- A = appearance—colour
- P = pulse—indication of heart rate
- G = grimace—plantar aspect of the foot is stimulated to provoke the child to cry
- A = activity—muscle tone
- R = respiratory effort.

The child's response to each test is rated on a scale of 0–2: 2 is the maximum score. A score of 10 is the maximum and is rarely achieved; a low score below 6 is indicative of problems.

## Early posture

At 6–7 months most babies will sit unassisted and attempt to crawl. They will start to pull themselves up into a standing position and stand holding on to furniture, but they frequently fall backwards into a sitting position. By 12 months the child should be able to stand alone for a few seconds and may possibly walk alone. 97% of children walk between 9 and 16 months; of the remainder only 6% are neurologically compromised (Luder 1988). The child will have a wide base of gait for stability, the arms will be flexed and held high for balance. The base of gait will become narrower as the child gains confidence.

### Determinants of gait

This phrase encompasses the essential developmental milestones, based on six components affecting walking. The various components (Ch. 8) commence at the time the child first starts to walk and continue to the age of 5–6. Learning skills, balance and physiological changes all contribute to the process of maturity, assisting the young child to walk as an adult walks. By the sixth year there is little to differentiate the child's gait from that of the adult (Tollafield 1988). The initial stages of walking involve a 'stomping' gait with the entire limb being lifted, circumducted over the ground and then plunged down again. There is little frontal or sagittal plane movement at the pelvis. The leg is usually maintained in an externally rotated position with little transverse plane motion. The foot neither supinates or pronates and there is little demand on the ankle to either dorsiflex or plantarflex.

Gait is apropulsive, shock absorption minimal and velocity control poor. The child thrusts its head, the heaviest single component of the body, downwards to increase speed and up and backwards to reduce velocity.

## Two years of age

The child's gait will have refined considerably. While the foot is still not capable of supinating at toe off, the pelvis is now beginning to rotate in all three body planes and the leg is showing signs of internal rotation at heel contact. The net result is a much smoother gait. Velocity control is also much improved although the arms still do not swing in coordination with the legs.

## Four years of age

Gait is no longer apropulsive; heel lift and the associated subtalar joint supination are apparent for the first time. Leg and pelvic rotations are now completely developed although arm swing is still not coordinated with leg movement.

## Five to six years of age

Pronation–supination at the contact and propulsive phases of gait will be fully developed, stride length will have increased and foot to ground contact time will be greatly reduced compared to 12 months previously.

## Growth and development

The gradual alteration from specialised chondrocytes to osteocytes creates the ossification process. Knowledge of ossification is important as far as applying effective treatment at the most appropriate time. The lower limb continues to grow in length and girth until the age of 19–20 years in males. Females tend to mature earlier and therefore growth usually ceases around 15–17. The epiphyses at the proximal end of the tibia and fibula are the final bony areas of the lower limb to complete full development and close.

The foot comprises short and long bones.

### Long bones

The matrix of bone starts as a cartilaginous model that develops from mesenchymal tissue; this is apparent from 4 weeks (intra uterine). Metatarsals have a diaphyseal centre and an epiphyseal centre. The phalanges also have two centres of ossification. The epiphyseal centres appear between the second and seventh years for phalanges and around the third and fourth years for metatarsals. The first metatarsal base is the site of the epiphysis whereas the epiphysis of the other metatarsals is located at the metatarsal head. The metatarsals ossify around 14–16 years for females and 16–18 years for males.

Only bone cells with a calcium and phosphate mineral source are readily identified on X-ray film. As the diaphyses are apparent before birth, metatarsals and phalanges can be seen on plain X-ray, albeit as rather poorly defined areas. Ultrasound can be used to study the lower limb in utero and MRI can be useful during childhood.

### Short bones

The calcaneus and talus appear after the first 4 weeks. The subtalar joint is first orientated by the calcaneus, taking a position under the talus at 12 weeks. It is at this point that 'club foot' may occur.

The short bones of the midtarsus are already formed at birth, although the navicular and cuneiforms are rather imprecise (lateral appears first at 3–6 months) and can take another 2–3 years to have a functional calcific appearance. The sesamoids of the first metatarsal appear around 8–10 years of age (Ch. 11).

Most anatomical books will provide a useful table of ossification events and these will therefore not be considered here. When reading X-rays, knowledge of ossification is very important: as some bones may appear differently orientated to those of the adult foot.

# THE ASSESSMENT PROCESS

Assessment can be divided into two areas; history taking and examination.

## Initiating the process

It is usually the parent who draws attention to a foot problem in the child. Parents are often concerned about the manner in which their child is walking or are unhappy about the shape, position or size of the lower limb or foot. The parents' observations or opinions will often be based upon what they, or another family member, consider to be normal. It is the role of the practitioner to identify whether there is an abnormality or, more commonly, to reassure the parents that what appears to them to be abnormal is only part of the normal developmental process. Throughout the developing years there are recognisable features which confirm normal trends.

Information should be taken together with an examination of the whole skeleton, rather than the foot alone. Treatment will only be required if an abnormality is progressive and can be halted. If the condition doesn't warrant treatment then careful monitoring may be desirable to ensure the child develops normally.

It is essential that the practitioner creates a relaxed and conducive environment for the assessment. A casual approach to his/her dress may be desirable. If children have previously undergone medical attention which has involved some form of discomfort, they may associate a white coat with a bad experience. First-name terms may be appropriate. If the child can relate to the practitioner he/she may be more willing to cooperate.

## Interviewing

Interacting with the child, parent or guardian requires interpersonal skills which can elicit important information in a limited period of time. The attention span of a child is generally a lot shorter than that of an adult. It may be easier to interview the parent while the child is playing. Watching the child at play allows evaluation of motor coordination and posture. It may be worthwhile to invest in toys and other amenities to facilitate this informal assessment.

It is important that during any assessment the child is chaperoned. The latter point cannot be ignored these days, when children may misunderstand the nature of examination if left alone with the practitioner. It may be useful to ask parents to dress the child in easy-to-remove clothing so that the process of undressing does not add to the patient's anxiety. Another person who is present—parent, nurse or care assistant—can bear witness to events.

If the child is uncooperative, do not hesitate to temporarily abandon the examination. Arrange a repeat appointment for a time when the child is likely to have rested. Advise the parents to bring along items such as personal toys to create a competitive distraction while being examined.

## HISTORY TAKING

In order to gain a relevant history a structured interview programme is essential. The format of the interview may vary from practitioner to practitioner, but it is essential that a systematic approach is adopted in order to reduce the possibility of omitting relevant details. In addition to the general questions regarding the presenting problem and medical history (Chs 3 and 5), attention should be paid to the following areas:

• Development and birth
• Family history
• Previous consultations.

## Development and birth

It is important to ascertain whether the pregnancy was normal. Did the mother take any medication during her pregnancy? Some drugs, for example phenytoin used to control epilepsy, are known to be teratogenic during the first 3 months of pregnancy. Smoking by the mother has also been reported to retard growth and intellectual development. The practitioner must elicit information without creating anxiety. Some questions may be reserved for cases where visible signs of abnormality are evident. It is important not to alarm the parent as incidental findings are rarely conclusive. The majority of babies encountered are healthy infants.

The mother should be asked about her child's delivery. Incidence of hip dislocation is higher when the foetus is malpositioned in utero or when there are twins. Long deliveries, especially if there was foetal distress, could be significant if there is evidence of poor posture, coordination or motor function. Muscle tone is diminished in premature babies compared to those who reach full term.

## Family history

Family history of problems can provide vital information about the cause and the prognosis of the complaint. Are there other siblings with a similar problem? It is helpful to ascertain any family traits. These can usefully be represented by constructing a pedigree chart (see Fig. 5.1).

## Previous consultations or advice

This should be noted as it may affect the parent's perceptions of the outcome of the child's foot problem. It must be stressed that the majority of paediatric problems are usually normal developmental variations, rarely requir-ing anything more than explanation and reassurance.

## EXAMINATION

Once a clear history has been taken, the child is examined. The younger the child, the more expedient the process needs to be. The examination should consider the following points:

• Footwear
• General walking capability
• Symmetry of body
• Obvious deformity
• Muscle bulk and wasting
• Joint motion
• Vascular and skin quality.

When assessing children, the focus is usually on the locomotor system. In most children a brief vascular, neurological and skin assessment will suffice. Further detailed examination should be performed in cases where the presenting problem, history taking or brief assessment indicates the presence of a significant problem. Tests should only be used in order to clarify an otherwise unclear diagnosis.

Those parts of the examination process which are of particular relevance to the examination of the child are noted below.

## Footwear

Children require their feet to be measured on a regular basis to ensure they have not outgrown their shoes. Often parents present their children to clinic because they are concerned about excessive shoe wear. It is important to determine whether the shoe wear is normal or abnormal. In making this decision it is important to establish how long the shoes are worn each day, the level and type of activity the child engages in and the types of material the shoe is constructed from. Assessment of footwear is considered in detail in Chapter 10.

## Neurological assessment

Neurological assessment implies motor and sensory evaluation. In the UK all neonates are examined by a doctor after delivery; follow-up tests are undertaken by midwives and health visitors during the early years of development. Most neurological abnormalities will be detected during this stage. Reflexes are an important method for determining normal muscle development and innervation in the neonate. Certain involuntary reflexes disappear after the baby reaches specific developmental milestones. Reflexes present during the first year of life are summarised in Table 14.3.

All practitioners should be mindful of skeletal and gait abnormalities which indicate a neuro-

**Table 14.3**   Reflexes associated with development

| Reflex | Descriptor |
| --- | --- |
| Oral reflex | If a finger is placed in a baby's mouth, the baby will automatically suck and swallow. Failure to suck may indicate cerebral problem later leading to motor dysfunction in lower limbs. |
| Moro reflex | This reflex (startle reflex) disappears by 5 months.<br>The infant is raised from a supine position by grasping the hands and is then suddenly released. The normal response is for the baby to spread their arms with hands open and fingers spread apart.<br>The arms are then brought together as if in an embrace. The legs are flexed. Failure to respond suggests weakness. Asymmetry may indicate lower spinal lesion if one leg affected. Hyperactivity suggests CNS infection, reverse Moro, where baby extends limbs with external rotation, basal ganglion disease. |

**Table 14.3**   (Cont'd)

| Reflex | Descriptor |
| --- | --- |
| Grasp reflex | Palmar or plantar response to 9 months. An object is placed in the palm and the fingers automatically flex to grip the object. The foot would be similarly stimulated in the area behind the toes. Failure to respond suggests CNS weakness depending upon symmetry of reflex. |
| Babinski reflex | This is achieved by firmly stroking the lateral sole of the baby's foot and extending the movement across the ball of the foot. A normal response in a child less than 2 years old is dorsiflexion of the hallux and fanning of the lesser toes. There may be an associated withdrawal of the knee and hip. A positive Babinski response after 2 years indicates dysfunction of the upper motor neurones. |
| Placing and walking reflex | If you touch the anterior aspect of either upper or lower limb against the edge of a table (e.g. rest anterior tibia against table) the child will lift the limb to place the foot/hand on to the table top. Alternatively place the dorsum of the foot beneath the table top to attain the same response. This occurs in the newborn up to about 4 weeks of age. If the baby is gently held above a surface with the soles lightly contacting the surface this will elicit walking motion. This response is present until 8 weeks of age. Absence may indicate brain damage. |
| Tonic neck reflex | When the baby is supine and not crying, the head will be turned to one side and the arm on the same side will be extended. The other knee will often be flexed. In normal babies, passive rotation of the head will increase upper body muscle tone on the side to which the head is turned. This reflex is present up to 3 months. |
| Patellar and ankle tendon reflex | Results should be similar to normal adult. |

muscular disorder in later life, e.g. Friedreich's ataxia, Charcot–Marie–Tooth disease and Duchenne's muscular dystrophy. In some cases late walking may be due to neurological dysfunction undetected at birth (Case history 14.1). Neurological tests should be carried out if an abnormality is suspected (Ch. 7).

## Locomotor assessment

This can be subdivided into gait analysis, weight-bearing and non-weightbearing assessment. The examination process outlined in Chapter 8 can be used with children as well as adults, however, the following specific points should be noted.

Walking is perhaps the most sensitive indicator of a child's neuromuscular status. It is an ability that is refined with age and practice, yet many parents are dissatisfied with their child's style of gait—'normal' should be distinguished from 'abnormal'. The developmental milestones such as crawling, sitting, standing and walking may vary from infant to infant. If there is undue delay then pathology such as neuromuscular disease, mental retardation and other physical handicaps must be ruled out.

Parents seek advice less frequently before their children walk. In those cases the complaint usually relates to the shape or the position that the foot or toes are adopting. Once again it is vital to differentiate normal development from true abnormality.

### Gait analysis

It is useful to observe the child's gait when wearing shoes. This can be achieved as the child walks into the clinical area, space permitting. The child should also be observed unshod wear-ing underclothes in order to assess the position of the lower limb, especially the knee. As with all patients it is important to observe the child's gait from head to toe, taking note of any signs of asymmetry of posture. The head should be level in the frontal and transverse planes. The shoulders should be aligned and a child over 6 years should have a symmetrical arm swing. Cerebral palsy affects the appearance of gait quite dramatically (Fig. 14.1).

Asymmetry at the level of the pelvis during walking may indicate pathology associated with a scoliosis or a limb-length discrepancy. Weight-bearing and non-weightbearing examination should be performed on the spine to confirm a tentative diagnosis. Muscle weakness or paralysis associated with hip disorders will cause a distinct lateral lurch in gait as the fulcrum for the muscle is lost.

Equinus may be apparent during gait: in children up to 4 years of age it is not uncommon to observe toe-walking. Abnormal in-toeing (common) or out-toeing should be noted.

### Weightbearing assessment

**Vertebrae**. It is important to check the spine for shape, deformity and movement. Check for normal skin covering and absence of dimpling at the base of the spine over lumbar vertebrae 3/4. If a patient shows signs of dimpling, or a tuft of hair at the base of the spine, it may indicate spina bifida (see Figs 17.2 and 17.3).

The presence of a scoliosis, kyphosis or lordosis should be confirmed and whether it is a functional or fixed deformity. A fixed deformity is usually due to bony abnormality (*structural*) whereas a flexible (*functional*) is due to soft-tissue deformity. Fixed spinal curvatures are retained when sitting and flexing the spine, especially scoliosis. Scoliosis is a frontal plane deformity but can show signs of vertebral rotation causing a kyphotic or humped appearance in the sagittal plane. Progressive thoracolumbar problems can impair pulmonary function and in time cause strain on respiration.

Marked scoliosis in children, especially where epiphyseal growth remains, must be considered

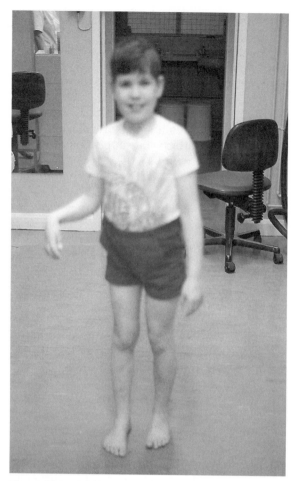

**Figure 14.1**   An 11-year-old boy had suffered cerebral palsy following an infection. Ankle equinus with spasticity has affected the right side of his body.

potentially progressive. These patients should be sent for a specialist opinion. Lordosis is increased forward curvature in the sagittal plane, which commonly affects the lumbar vertebrae.

**Hips**. The Trendelenburg sign may be useful in detecting hip weakness. The Trendelenburg test is a measure of normal muscle action between the pelvis and greater trochanter (gluteus medius). If the mechanism fails, it is deemed positive (Ch. 8).

*Non-weightbearing assessment*

Young children may be best examined on a parent's lap. The lower limb is examined for

pain and swelling, obvious deformity and signs of weakness. Both limbs should appear the same regarding position, muscle bulk and tone. On examination there should be symmetry in ranges of joint motion on each side; the direction of motion should reflect similar values to the opposite limb. Ranges of motion change with development; however, quality of motion should be smooth and unhindered. The temperature of the limb should be warm and the limbs should be examined for dislocations, fractures, soft-tissue lumps and enlargement of bony areas.

**Pelvis and hips**. The gluteal fat folds should appear level. The 'anchor sign' is useful in identifying hip dysplasia in the infant. The altered function of the gluteal muscles change the shape of the buttocks. The central crease forms the central anchor with the two base lines along the buttocks as the bottom of the anchor. If the base lines are altered, this shows as an abnormal anchor sign due to asymmetry. When performing tests on the hips of children, it must be remembered to avoid damaging the blood supply to the femoral head. At birth the head of the femur lies superficially in the acetabulum which gives the appearance that the thigh is externally rotated on the pelvis. As the child develops, the head of the femur goes deeper into the acetabulum, which in turn allows the limb to internally rotate. In a normal neonate there will be little, if any, internal rotation of the hip but up to 60° external rotation. With development, the amount of external rotation reduces as the amount of internal rotation increases, to the point where a normal adult value shows equal internal and external rotation of 45° in each direction.

In the neonate, ligamentous laxity may be present, together with instability of the hip. This is associated with circulating maternal hormones. Care should be taken with the hips to prevent iatrogenic dislocation. Major arteries supply the femoral head by travelling along the femoral neck. Deprivation of blood supply may lead to avascular necrosis of the femoral head. Nerves lying posterior to the hip joint, particularly the sciatic nerve, are subject to trauma in posterior

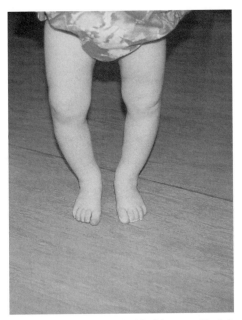

**Figure 14.2** 16-month-old girl with tibia vara of both legs.

hip dislocation. Damage to the nerve may lead to motor and sensory loss.

**Knees**. Newborn babies present with bow legs (genu varum) (Fig. 14.2). The frontal plane angle is formed between a bisection of the tibia and the femur, being on average 16° varus. Within 3 years the knee position will have changed to a mean value of 11° valgus (knock knee); by 9 years of age further developmental change will have reduced it to 6° valgus (Salenius & Vankka 1975).

Bow legs or genu varum reach their optimum value in children of less than 18 months, while maximum knock knee or genu valgum is seen at $3\frac{1}{2}$–4 years. At 4 years of age girls tend to be more knock-kneed than boys (Heath & Staheli 1993). After 4 years the knee gradually straightens.

Knee position should be assessed by pushing the child's knees or ankles together as he/she lies supine with the legs parallel to the examination couch. The distance between knees and ankles can then be measured with a tape measure. At 6 months old the distance between knees should be 2.6 cm; at 3 years of age the genu varum will have reversed and there will now be 3.5 cm between the ankles. At 7 years of

age genu valgum will still be present with a distance of approx 2.1 cm between the ankles.

The child should be observed from the side for genu recurvatum (hyperextension). This deformity occurs in the sagittal plane. In very early childhood, genu recurvatum may be present but should reduce with development as the knee ligaments tighten.

The range of transverse plane motion in the knee should be equal in both directions and be minimal by the age of 4 years. In the newborn 20–30° of total motion may be available (Kilmartin 1988). The amount of rotation of the tibia on the femur should reduce by 10° at 3 years of age and at 6 years of age should show minimal movement.

The tibia and fibula twist with normal development. At birth it will be apparent that the malleoli are on the same level in the frontal plane. As development ensues the distal end of the tibia twists externally (tibial torsion). The lateral malleolus moves to a more posterior position. There is axial rotation of the tibia and fibula as well as twisting within the bone itself. The malleolar position will reach an adult value around 6 years of age with a position of 13–18° external malleolar positioning (Root et al 1977, Spencer 1978, Thomson 1993). This represents a true external tibial torsion of around 18–25°.

*Patellae*. The position of these large sesamoids should be noted. Are they facing forward, inwards or outwards? The patellae may be up to 30° externally rotated at birth. In young children it is considered normal for the patellae to be externally rotated, but by 4 years of age the patellae should face forwards. The position of the patellae is dependent upon normal hip development. The change of DOM and ROM at the hip, femoral torsion and reduction of external position of the femoral head allow the patellae to face anteriorly. These changes may continue until 10 years of age and may give rise to an abnormal foot position.

**Foot**. While a rudimentary examination of the lower limbs is essential, the foot must be carefully examined; each joint should be examined as well as the alignment of the forefoot to the rearfoot. The rearfoot must be examined with the ankle, the forefoot with the midtarsal joint and the toes with the metatarso-phalangeal joints. The overall foot shape is also important.

*Ankle.* In the newborn there is approximately 50° dorsiflexion and 30° plantarflexion at the ankle. The ROM at this joint decreases with development. There should be no deep creasing anterior to the ankle; if present this may indicate a fixed dorsiflexed ankle.

*Rearfoot.* The calcaneus will have a relatively low calcaneal inclination angle in the sagittal plane. In the neonate the neutral position of the calcaneus is 8–10° varus. The talus undergoes valgus rotation up until 6 years. The angle of declination of the talus increases which helps bring the foot from its supinated embryonic position to its more pronated adult position. At birth the forefoot may be slightly inverted, but this will reduce with normal development. The young child has a relatively narrow heel in relation to the breadth of the forefoot. The foot should have a straight lateral border. In a rectus foot a line bisecting the heel to forefoot will demonstrate equal parts medial and lateral to the line. In an adducted foot, the medial side will appear greater and, conversely, in the

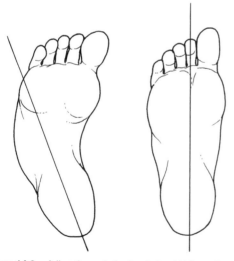

**Figure 14.3** A line through the heel should bisect the forefoot through the second or third toe. The normal foot shape (right) has a straight lateral border and narrow heel, compared to the drawing on the left, which has a marked metatarsus adductus.

abducted foot the lateral side will appear greater (Fig. 14.3).

*Forefoot.* The midtarsus and metatarsus should be examined for frontal plane abnormalities as well as transverse abnormalities. The forefoot in the newborn is 10–15° inverted on the rearfoot (Tax 1980). The latter is easier to identify as it is more obvious. Deformity distal to the metatarsals may be directly related to the metatarsals or may be an isolated deformity.

# CONDITIONS AFFECTING THE LOWER LIMB OF CHILDREN

## CONGENITAL DISLOCATION OF THE HIP (CDH)

This is usually detected shortly after birth, during routine examination of the neonate by the paediatrician. However, it is possible for the condition to be missed and not picked up until later in the child's development. CDH may have serious repercussions leading to osteoarthritis, limb shortening and hip pain.

In a normal hip the quality of motion should be unimpaired when the hip is taken through its range of motion. Various tests are used to establish the presence of CDH, although feeling for displacement of the femoral head may be all that is required. It should be noted that clinical examination may produce false negatives. X-ray and ultrasound imaging can confirm a diagnosis.

**Barlow's test.** The baby is placed supine with hips and knees flexed. Thumb pressure is applied over the lesser trochanter with the middle finger of each hand over the greater trochanter. The femoral head is gently dislocated by moving the pressure on the hand backwards. Consequent release of pressure allows the head to slip back into position. A positive result indicates that the hips are unstable due to ligamentous laxity. The test becomes less useful as the child becomes older (Valmassy 1993).

**Ortolani's manoeuvre.** This is performed by flexing the hips to 90°. The middle fingers are again placed over the greater trochanter and the thigh is lifted and abducted. The hip can be relocated with a palpable (rather than audible) click. This test is reliable in the early months, but clicking can arise from ligaments moving, giving false positives.

**Galleazi's sign.** The infant is observed supine with hips and knees flexed and with the feet placed flat on the couch. In normal limbs the level of the knees should be equal. If one knee is lower than the other this may indicate hip pathology on the low side. This is similar to the skyline test for checking the length of the femur and tibia.

Abducting the hip with the thigh and knee flexed will be resisted on the dislocated side. This is due to contracted muscles such as the adductors. This test is most reliable after 2 months. The anchor sign is abnormal.

## KNEE PAIN IN THE CHILD

Assessment of the painful knee should begin by determining the precise location of the pain. Most commonly it originates from under the medial side of the patella and radiates to the superior and inferior poles of the patella. The severity of the condition should be assessed using the following tests.

**Patella compression test.** With the patient lying supine and the knee extended, the practitioner compresses the patella against the femoral condyles. If this test is performed too vigorously it will cause pain, even in the normal knee. A more sensitive approach of gradually loading the kneecap is preferred and is less distressing for the patient.

**Medial facet tenderness test.** The patella is displaced medially and the practitioner palpates the posterior medial surface. Performing this test also determines whether there is any tightness of the lateral capsule tending to pull the patella laterally, increasing shearing forces on the posterior facets, which may damage the articular cartilage.

**Quadriceps muscle bulk evaluation.** The patient is asked to contract the quadriceps muscle group; the bulk of the vastus medialis muscle is assessed. Loss of muscle bulk can occur with chronic pain or poor mechanical function of the knee.

**Muscle function.** Quadriceps muscle strength and hamstring flexibility should also be assessed. The 90:90 test will determine hamstring tightness which, when present, will tend to flex the knee and increase patellofemoral compression.

**Squatting test.** The patient is asked to stand on both feet and then crouch down. Patients with severe pain will express discomfort; as the knee flexes the posterior surface of the patella is compressed against the femur. The degree to which squatting is restricted will indicate the severity of the condition.

Anterior knee pain is often the young adolescent's first contact with chronic pain. More common in females than males, it is a recalcitrant problem which, in a minority of cases, can be disabling. The pain will be most intense during or after vigorous activity, though kneeling or sitting with a flexed knee for long periods ('*cinema seat*' *sign*) may also incite discomfort.

The aetiology of anterior knee pain is unclear. Biomechanical abnormality, and in particular a high *quadriceps* or '*Q*' *angle* which may alter the normal positioning of the patella in the intratrochanteric fossa, have been suggested as causes. The Q angle is the angle between a line extending from the anterior superior iliac spine to the centre of the patella and a line extending from the tibial tuberosity to the centre of the patella. The angle will increase with internal femoral rotation, external tibial rotation and genu valgum. If present, a full orthopaedic examination of the lower limb is indicated in order to isolate the underlying cause.

**Osgood–Schlatter's disease** may be the cause of a painful knee. It is an apophysitis affecting the tibial tubercle and is associated with patellar tendon strain. It affects males particularly between 10–14 years of age. Pain is anterior and below the knee. It is made worse by strenuous activity. Examination demonstrates the presence of a prominent and tender tibial tubercle. Extending the leg against resistance exacerbates the symptoms. Radiographs may show fragmentation of the tibial prominence at the tendon insertion.

# ABNORMAL KNEE POSITION

Parental concern about knock knees or bow legs is a common presenting complaint (Case history 14.2), already highlighted earlier in this chapter.

---

**Case history 14.2**

The parents of a 3-year-old boy were concerned about his knock knees. Non-weightbearing examination indicated marked genu valgum with a gap of 6 cm between the ankles when the medial condyles of the knee were placed together.

The parents had two other sons, aged 9 and 7, who similarly had severe knock knee appearance around the age of 3. On non-weightbearing examination the older siblings were found to have straight legs with no gap between the malleoli or the femoral condyles when the legs were placed together.

Because the older siblings were now normal, the parents were reassured that no treatment was necessary. It was decided to monitor the leg position on a regular basis. Annual review followed until the child was discharged, aged 6, with straight legs and a normal distance between the malleoli and femoral condyles.

**Conclusion**: Genu valgum may not require treatment. Monitoring is a valuable method to ensure that early intervention can be considered if required.

---

## Genu varum

If a child presents with bow legs at 3–4 years of age, further investigation and treatment may be necessary. A distance of more than 5 cm between the knees, at any age, is cause for concern and necessitates further investigation (Sharrard 1976). Rickets and Blount's disease are two conditions predisposing to genu vara with tibial vara.

### Rickets

Rickets will present as genu varum as well as anterior bowing at the junction of the middle and lower one-third of the tibia. Swelling of the wrists and ankles and bossing of the cranium is also seen in rickets. Radiological investigation will show the epiphyses to be widened and irregular, while the metaphyses, the region just adjacent to the growth plate, will appear 'cupped'.

Biochemical tests are performed to determine levels of vitamin D, calcium and phosphate which may be reduced due to dietary deficiency, malabsorption, renal disease or hypophosphotasia. If biochemical tests prove normal, Blount's disease may be suspected.

### Blount's disease

This is a condition affecting the growth of the medial upper tibial epiphysis. Cessation of the growth plate causes the tibia to develop a lateral varus tilt. This condition has an estimated incidence of 0.05 per 1000 live births and is due to the lateral side of the growth plate expanding faster than the medial side. Blount's disease is thought to be a combination of obesity and marked physiological bowing. This will have the effect of compressing the medial side of the growth plate which causes further bowing of the tibia. The lateral epiphysis continues to expand as pressure is released. The medial epiphysis will appear fragmented on X-ray. Blount's disease may appear at any time between the ages of 18 months and 4 years. Referral for treatment should be initiated as the condition will invariably progress without treatment. In the infant, Blount's disease is often severe with both knees affected. Arrest of the medial growth plate may also affect older children, aged between 6 and 13, in whom the deformity is usually unilateral and less severe than the infantile variety, though no less certain to progress without treatment. Unilateral tibia vara can contribute to limb-length discrepancy.

## Genu valgum

If the distance between the malleoli is greater than 10 cm in children aged between three to four years, genu valgum (genu valga) is suspected. This condition is often known as knock knees. In severe unremitting cases radiological examination should be used to rule out developmental or metabolic abnormalities of the epiphyses. Surgical correction may have to be considered, although this is rare. Unilateral knock knee should be investigated as it is almost always a pathological defect of the epiphysis associated with either trauma, osteomyelitis, tumour or developmental bone disturbance.

Excessive subtalar joint pronation of the foot has been associated with genu valgum, as it throws body weight medial to the central axis of the foot and hence tends to force the foot into pronation. Conversely, excessive varus deformity of the forefoot may create frontal plane movement of the knee, in order to bring the entire forefoot into ground contact. Genu valgum will result.

## IN-TOEING PROBLEMS

In-toeing is often a cause for considerable parental or grandparental concern. Many families fear that the condition will lead to long-term disabilities. It is important to establish exactly what the family's worries are because resolving those fears provides an important goal of treatment. It is also helpful to establish and agree with the parents exactly what the problem is. Many will complain that the foot is turned in or out when really their concern is that the foot is pronating.

30% of children in-toe at the age of 4, but the condition persists in only 4% of adults (Svenningsen et al 1990). It was once thought to cause osteoarthrosis of the hip and poor sporting ability (Alvik 1960), but it has subsequently been shown to be unimportant in osteoarthrosis of the hip (Hubbard et al 1988), while the sporting performance of women with internal femoral position has been found to be equivalent to normal controls (Staheli et al 1977).

Resolution of the in-toeing gait usually occurs between the ages of 4 and 11 (Fabry et al 1973, Svenningsen et al 1990). In a significant proportion of in-toeing children there is no obvious structural abnormality of the foot or leg. In the absence of abnormality, it is difficult for the practitioner to know at which level to apply treatment. Reassurance is probably most appropriate, the parents simply being advised that the child is adopting an in-toeing habit and is quite capable of walking straight if reminded to do so.

Whether or not treatment is necessary, management of in-toeing depends upon the level at which the abnormality originates as well as the possibility of harmful compensations occurring at another joint. In-toeing is also significant when it causes the child to trip constantly. In cases of tripping, bruising and even broken bones may be reported.

Assessment commences with gait analysis; even in the very early walker this can be achieved with the parents supporting the child's upper body. The key to accurate diagnosis is the position of the patella. In the in-toeing child, the patella will either point in the direction of progression or it will be internally rotated or 'squinting'. A squinting patella indicates that the cause of the gait defect is proximal to the knee joint. Severely adducted feet in the presence of a forward-looking patella occur in cases of metatarsus adductus (forefoot), internal genicular position (knee) and internal tibial torsion (leg) (Fig. 14.4).

Following gait analysis, the ranges of motion at the hip and knee joint and the position of the transmalleolar axis and forefoot should be assessed. The range of hip rotation is assessed with the knee and hip extended, the leg is brought to the neutral position where the patella is facing directly upwards, in other words lying parallel with the frontal plane. While viewing the patella, the leg is internally and then externally rotated and the degree of rotation estimated. In children of less than 4 years, an excessive internal range of hip motion is considered abnormal and will often explain an in-toeing style of gait. In children older than 4, asymmetry of motion may be significant.

A common finding on hip examination of the in-toeing child is 40–60° internal range of hip motion but just 20° external range of motion. In such cases there is obviously sufficient range of external motion to allow normal walking; however, the child continues to walk in-toed because it is easier to do so. The parents should be told that the child is simply walking along the line of least tension. Most children who present with internal femoral position grow out of the condition. In a study of 1522 hips the development of a larger range of external hip motion was found not to be the cause (Fabry et al 1973).

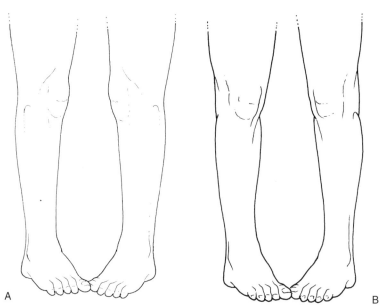

**Figure 14.4**   Squinting patellae indicate that the cause of intoeing is likely to be above the knee joint (**A**). Adducted feet in the presence of forward looking patellae indicate that the cause of intoeing originates from below the knee joint (**B**).

While internal rotation falls from about 60° at age 4 to under 40° in the adult, decreasing 2–3° per year (Staheli 1993), external rotation remains at a constant 40° from 4 years of age to adulthood. The net result is loss of total rotation with age and less internal bias to gait.

## Hamstring shortening

Hamstring, and more specifically medial hamstring, shortening is a common cause of asymmetrical hip motion and subsequent in-toeing. Diagnosis is made by flexing the hip to 90° and then attempting to extend the knee using the 90:90 test (Fig. 14.5). In children under 10 years, less than 70% extension is unsatisfactory. Quality of motion is also evaluated while performing the 90:90 test. If the final 30° of motion is resisted by the hamstrings it is usual for the child to experience discomfort, which indicates an abnormal tightness. The medial hamstring tension can be tested by internally rotating the flexed upper thigh while gradually extending the knee. If, with internal rotation of the thigh, knee extension is limited and uncomfortable, then the medial hamstring is the principal cause

of the complaint.

On standing, children with tight hamstrings will often assume a normal angle and base of stance, the feet being abducted 20–30°. It is only on walking, as the knee extends just prior to heel contact, that the tight medial hamstring will abruptly rotate the leg internally. Such cases will also demonstrate a windmilling style of running, the lower leg being circumducted during the late swing phase of running in order to 'short-cut' around the extended knee position. Growing pains are common in such in-toers. Hamstrings should therefore be tested in any child complaining of persistent nocturnal leg pains.

## Tibial torsion and internal genicular position

Clinical diagnosis of internal tibial torsion is made by measuring the transmalleolar axis which is formed between the midpoints of the medial and lateral malleoli and the frontal plane. The transmalleolar axis increases during the first few years of life from 2–4° at birth to 10–20° in the adult. Many complex methods have been described for measuring tibial torsion

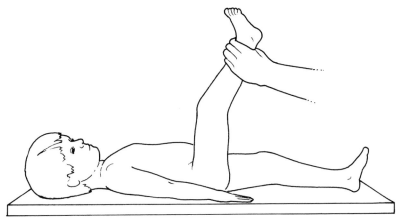

**Figure 14.5**    To determine hamstring tightness, lay the child supine, flex the hip to 90° and attempt to extend the knee to 90°.

(Reikeras & Hoiseth 1989). A quick clinical estimation is made by placing the thumb of each hand anterior to the malleoli; the medial malleoli should be one thumb's thickness anterior to the lateral malleoli (Fig. 14.6).

The incidence of internal tibial torsion has been reported to range from 1–40% (Hutter & Scott 1949, Michele & Nielsen 1976). In some cases the transmalleolar axis will appear normal though it is apparent on gait analysis that the

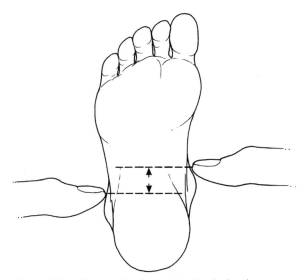

**Figure 14.6**    Check malleolar position by placing the thumbs on the anterior surface of the malleoli. There should be one thumb's thickness difference between the medial and lateral malleoli.

whole tibia is internally rotated on the knee. This condition is called *internal tibial position* or *internal genicular position*. An internal genicular position is an important cause of in-toeing and is so similar to tibial torsion that it is quite likely to be misdiagnosed as such.

Internal genicular position only becomes a cause for concern for the parents when the child starts to walk. Examination will reveal a normal transmalleolar axis but an abnormally high internal range of motion at the knee. This is estimated by stabilising the thigh initially and then grasping the foot to produce a long lever arm on the knee joint, rotating the tibia internally and then externally (Fig. 14.7). Normally a small but symmetrical range of motion of 10–20° will be evident. In cases of internal genicular position, 45° or more of internal rotation may be present. External rotation usually remains no more than 10–20°, although in some cases it is completely absent.

The prognosis without treatment for internal genicular position and internal tibial torsion is good. It tends to resolve spontaneously around 5–6 years of age. Its significance lies in the fact that it can cause frequent tripping. There is also some evidence to suggest that it could be an important factor in the development of osteoarthrosis of the knee joint. One study of 1200 knee clinic patients with arthritis found 64% showed signs of internal tibial torsion (Turner & Smillie 1981). For that reason it is worthwhile

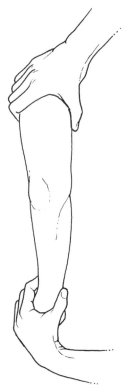

**Figure 14.7** Internal tibial position is estimated by internally and externally rotating the tibia on the knee joint.

monitoring the child to ensure that resolution does occur. The patient should be seen every 6 months, gait analysis performed and the range of motion at the knee and the transmalleolar axis measured. If tripping and clumsiness is severe, treatment may be considered.

## Metatarsus adductus

Internal tibial torsion and abnormal knee position may also occur in combination with metatarsus adductus. This is a common cause of abnormal foot shape and hence of in-toeing. Metatarsus adductus is a deformity of the tarso-metatarsal or Lis Franc's joint. The condition was first recognised in 1864 by Henke, who considered it a contracture of the metatarsus. Although he labelled the condition metatarsus adductus, a number of other names, including skewfoot, metatarsus varus, Z foot, serpentine foot, one-third of a clubfoot and hookfoot, have subsequently been used. Some of these terms have proved useful when describing more complex variants of the basic condition. The hallmark of the deformity is a C-shaped curvature of the lateral border of the foot (Fig. 14.8). Other less significant signs can help confirm the

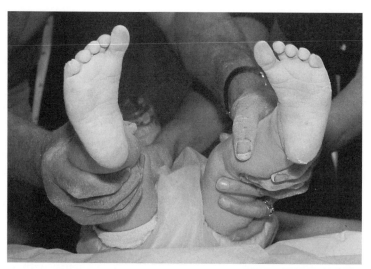

**Figure 14.8** A C-shaped curvature of the lateral border of the foot is the hallmark of metatarsus adductus. This 2-year-old boy responded poorly to treatment as the deformity was quite rigid. The early management of metatarsus adductus is desirable.

diagnosis; they include wrinkling of the skin in the medial longitudinal arch as a consequence of bunching of the metatarsal bases, a dorsal plantar crease medial to the first metatarsal cuneiform joint, a high arch profile created by adduction of the forefoot on the rearfoot and, if the child is walking, a marked tendency to lateral weightbearing.

The cause of metatarsus adductus is unknown. A number of theories have been proposed, although intrauterine moulding remains the most popular. Wedging of the lateral side of the foot against the wall of the uterus is thought to push the forefoot into adductus. If this is the case it would seem logical to expect that most metatarsus adductus children would be born to young primigravida mothers. Rushforth (1978) tested this logic by assessing the maternal age and history in 130 cases of 'hooked forefoot'. Although the age ranged from 15–36, the mean age was 27 and half the children were second-born.

Cessation of fetal development has been associated with transient or permanent loss of amniotic fluid, which is the dialysate of maternal serum, blood and fetal urine in which the foetus 'floats' (Melincoff & Davis 1978). DeMyer & Baird (1969) aspirated amniotic fluid from a study group of pregnant rats to reduce the fluid volume. Compared to controls, foetuses subjected to amniotic fluid aspiration were born with a higher incidence of clubfoot. The authors considered that this finding might have been a consequence of a reduction in fluid leading to a relative immobilisation of the foetus.

Loss of amniotic fluid due to premature 'breaking of the waters' has also been found to be significant in cases of human clubfoot (Blane et al 1971). Rupture of the amniotic membrane often results from a fetal limb being thrust through it. Strands of amnion have been reported to entwine around the limb and cause a variety of limb defects. In 400 cases of constricting amniotic bands reviewed by Torpin (1968), 131 had clubfoot deformity.

The foetal environment, then, is clearly very important, but the intrauterine moulding theory does appear to be somewhat flawed, not least because from the 17th week of foetal life the mother is aware that the fetus is moving, pushing up against and away from the highly elastic uterine wall. The direct deforming influence of constricting amniotic bands, as well as foetal immobility caused by loss of amniotic fluid has, however, been shown by controlled experiment to be associated with clubfoot. Metatarsus adductus, 'one-third of a clubfoot', may well have similar origins.

Metatarsus adductus is thought to resolve spontaneously in more than 90% of cases (Staheli 1993). Ponsetti & Becker (1966) found that only 11.6% of their patients required treatment while Rushforth (1978), in an 11-year follow-up of 83 children, found that 86% demonstrated complete resolution of the deformity. Both studies concluded that feet which could be passively corrected did not require treatment.

Personal observation indicates that metatarsus adductus is rare among geriatrics. Until it can be proved that metatarsus adductus is definitely associated with specific foot pathologies, a case for treatment can only really be made for those moderately or severely deformed feet that provide resistance to manipulation. Eversion of the heel, medial bulging of the talonavicular joint and 'humping' of the dorsolateral midfoot also indicate that spontaneous correction is unlikely.

Metatarsus adductus represents a spectrum of mild, moderate and severe deformity. Assessment of the foot's flexibility is the practitioner's primary objective. The child's heel should be cupped in one hand while the other hand attempts to push the foot straight (Fig. 14.9). If the foot can easily be corrected and the adductus position is mild, the prognosis for spontaneous resolution is excellent. As the deformity becomes more marked it is quite likely that there will be a corresponding increase in rigidity. Uncompensated metatarsus adductus appears as a high-arched supinated foot; symptoms are usually minimal and, in the author's experience, limited to skin lesions under the fifth metatarsophalangeal joint. Accordingly, prognosis is less favourable and treatment should be instigated as soon as possible. Another significant finding on assessment is the presence of a vertical crease

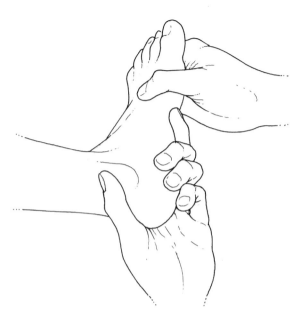

**Figure 14.9** Assessing flexibility of the metatarsus adductus foot by cupping the heel in inversion while pushing the forefoot straight.

overlying the medial cuneiform. The vertical cuneiform crease presents only in the more severely affected feet.

Radiographic examination can assist the evaluation of metatarsus adductus, especially if there is rearfoot involvement as is the case with the skew or Z foot. In this complex variant of metatarsus adductus, the rearfoot is everted and the talus plantarflexed and adducted. Several charting techniques have been developed to measure metatarsus adductus and its variants (Berg 1986). The value of radiography is, however, somewhat limited by the fact that the bones involved at the level of the deformity will not ossify until the patient is 3–4 years old; moreover, in the non-weightbearing patient the plate will simply show the position the foot was held in for X-ray.

Only rarely in metatarsus adductus does the original parental complaint concern the shape of the foot. It is far more likely to result from dissatisfaction with the patient's adducted style of gait. To ensure consistent and reliable diagnosis, all other causes of adducted gait, including internal femoral rotation, internal tibial torsion, genicular position and hallux varus, must be ruled out. In conclusion the 'level of deformity' may be quite different. It is also important to note any element of these conditions which may be superimposed upon the metatarsus adductus, as management of more than one condition may be necessary.

# CONGENITAL CLUBFOOT (TALIPES EQUINOVARUS)

In congenital talipes equinovarus, the adductus of the forefoot occurs not at the tarsometatarsal joint but at the midtarsal joint. There are four components to the deformity: equinus, inversion of the rearfoot, adductus and pronation of the forefoot. The most severe deformities, however, occur in the rearfoot. The talus is abducted and the calcaneus is in equinus. The calcaneus is also inverted while the navicular is displaced medial to the head of the talus. The posterior and medial soft tissues, including tibialis posterior, flexor digitorum longus and triceps surae, are also shortened and atrophied, forming a 'pipe stem' shape to the leg.

Congenital clubfoot is difficult to correct and there is a known tendency for recurrence in children and adolescents, especially if first attempts at correction are not entirely successful. It is well documented that it is easier to correct a clubfoot deformity in the first few days of life than after even a few weeks (Ponsetti 1992).

Assessment of the clubfoot should address the relative severity of each of the four components of the condition. The plantarflexed first metatarsal component is critical but usually yields well to manipulative correction. The equinus and inversion components of the rearfoot and the adduction of the forefoot at the talonavicular joint are more resistant to correction. Internal tibial torsion may also occur with clubfoot and must be also be corrected.

No matter how effective initial treatment, clubfoot will always result in shortening of the foot, reduced calf muscle circumference and reduced ankle and subtalar joint motion. Medial displacement of the navicular and abduction of the talus on the calcaneus may also persist. In less well corrected clubfeet, poor gait and abnormal forefoot loading results in plantar callus and shoe-fitting difficulties.

## FLAT FEET

Following a survey of London school children, Morley (1957) suggested that children under 5 years of age appeared to have flat feet because the medial longitudinal arch was filled with fat. Radiological studies of toddlers' feet have subsequently proved Morley wrong. All children under 5 years have a depressed medial longitudinal arch because of the low calcaneal inclination angle. It is only with external torsion of the tibia, in the first 5 years of life, that the calcaneus begins to assume its normal 20° angle of inclination and the medial longitudinal arch becomes apparent. However, in the neonate, fat deposits are retained for a short period and tend to be quite marked on the dorsum of the foot. This fat distribution does contribute to an immature foot shape, which disappears quite rapidly after the first 12 months.

'Flat foot' is a common term used by health care professionals and lay people alike. 'Excessive pronation of the foot' is a more accurate term because, as well as a lowered medial longitudinal arch, the flat foot may also present the following clinical signs (Fig. 14.10):

- Eversion of the heel
- Bulging of the talus as it adducts out of the talonavicular joint
- Abduction of the forefoot.

Eversion of the heel, or Helbing's sign, can be recognised as a bowing of the tendo achillis as it inserts into the calcaneus. Helbing's sign is not always reliable. This is so when the foot maximally pronates from a supinated position associated with rearfoot varus. Pronation can occur using the available range of subtalar joint motion, but the calcaneus may still remain in a relatively inverted position. This is commonly referred to as 'partially compensated rearfoot varus'. Marked eversion of the calcaneus will inevitably lower the medial longitudinal arch. With calcaneal eversion there will also be abduction of the distal end of the calcaneus, allowing the talus to assume a more adducted and plantarflexed position which can be seen clinically as medial bulging in the area of the talonavicular joint. As the talus adducts, the forefoot will assume an abducted position relative to the rearfoot. This abnormality will manifest clinically as the 'too

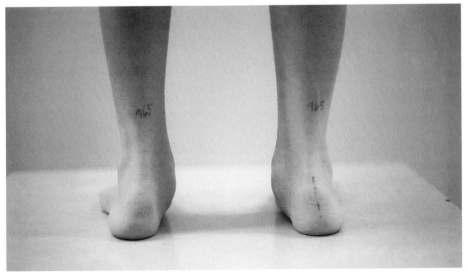

**Figure 14.10**   10-year-old boy with moderate pronation. Calcaneal eversion, medial talonavicular bulging and forefoot abduction characterise excessive subtalar joint pronation associated with forefoot varus of both feet.

many toes sign'. When a normal foot is observed from the rear, it is possible to see the fifth and sometimes the fourth toe. In a pronated foot the third toe may be seen as well. The lateral border of the foot will be C-shaped with the concavity of the 'C' overlying the calcaneocuboid joint.

The aforementioned clinical signs associated with excessive pronation will occur with varying degrees of severity. In some cases the only abnormality will be a lowering of the medial longitudinal arch: all other signs will be absent. Such feet are not a cause for concern; indeed, a study of 295 Israeli army recruits undergoing basic training found that the incidence of stress fractures was reduced in individuals with low-arched feet (Giladi et al 1985).

Objective assessment of the pronated (flat) foot is vital in order to measure how the patient's foot is changing with the passage of time or indeed how it is responding to treatment. Staheli et al (1987) performed a footprint examination of 441 normal individuals aged between 1 and 80 years. The area of the medial longitudinal arch in contact with the ground was then determined by measuring the narrowest point of the arch and the widest point of the heel. The arch width was divided by the heel width to give an arch index value. The mean arch index values were then used to generate a table of normal values for 21 different age groups (Fig. 14.11). Staheli recommended that his graph of normal values should be used to determine which children were abnormal and required treatment. However, in practice Staheli's normal limits have proved to be very wide. Moreover the height of the arch alone is not a reliable indicator of excessive pronation of the foot as the arch is not flat in every pronated foot. Some patients will present with calcaneal eversion and talonavicular bulging, but the medial longitudinal arch may still be apparent.

Rose's valgus index takes into account the eversion of the foot relative to the leg and can be used in conjunction with Staheli's index to obtain more valid information about the degree of pronation (Fig. 14.12) (Rose et al 1985). Rose's technique measures the displacement of the medial malleolus relative to the weightbearing

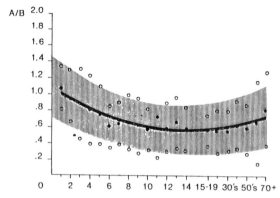

**Figure 14.11**   Staheli's table of normal arch index values. The mean values for the arch index and two standard deviations for each of the twenty-one age-groups. The solid line shows the mean changes with age; the shaded area shows the normal ranges. The actual values for each age-group are represented by solid circles for the mean and open circles for two standard deviations. (Reproduced by kind permission of the *Journal of Bone and Joint Surgery.*)

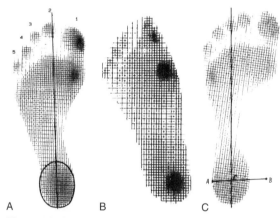

**Figure 14.12**   Rose's valgus index. Footprints to show diagnostic features. **A**—The orientation of the heel oval, in this case pointing towards the second toe. **B**—The medial pressure pattern which is commonly found in flat foot. **C**—To show the measurements for calculation of the valgus index, which equals

$$\frac{1}{2}AB - AC \times \frac{100}{AB},$$

where *A* and *B* are vertically beneath each malleolus and *C* is the centre of the heel print. (Reproduced by kind permission of the *Journal of Bone and Joint Surgery.*)

surface of the heel. The more the foot pronates, the greater the medial displacement of the malleoli. Valgus index values for 257 children and 100 adults with no foot pain or abnormalities were calculated using the formula (Fig. 14.12). Values greater than 24 were considered beyond normal limits.

The Rose and Staheli indexes should be used to determine objectively foot position and arch height. Footprints should be repeated once yearly in an attempt to identify change. The footprint indices should not be used alone to determine which children require treatment and which do not; that decision should be made only after obtaining information on family history and assessing the magnitude of symptoms.

Medial bulging indicates talonavicular subluxation. The other clinical sign, forefoot abduction, is largely a secondary effect of talonavicular bulging. The forefoot assumes an abducted position relative to the adducted rearfoot. Once congruency is lost at the talonavicular joint, progressive subluxation of the joint follows.

The patient with excessive pronation may suffer from chronic low-grade discomfort in the medial longitudinal arch or talonavicular area of the foot, or pain in the muscles of the leg, or even all three. The tibialis anterior muscle is particularly prone to causing discomfort where the foot is excessively pronated. This could arise because the excessive pronation movement of the foot causes the muscle to work aphasically. In many cases, such leg pain may be written off as untreatable 'growing pains'. The condition is, however, very responsive to conservative orthotic treatment.

While the young patient's foot may be severely pronated, it usually remains quite flexible, as demonstrated by the hallux dorsiflexion (Jack's test) and tiptoe-standing tests. This invokes the windlass mechanism associated with the plantar aponeurosis, affording a rise in arch height where the foot is flexible. This test is negative for rigid flat feet. In a rigid pronated foot the arch will not rise upon dorsiflexion of the hallux, neither will the rearfoot invert when the individual stands on tiptoes.

## Rigid flat feet

A rigid pronated foot is a rare but significant finding, usually indicative of tarsal coalition and peroneal spastic flat foot. Tarsal coalition is a fibrous, cartilaginous, or osseous union of two or more tarsal bones and is congenital in origin (Mosier & Asher 1984). Coalition between the calcaneus and the navicular and the middle facet of the subtalar joint is the most common presentation and is conclusively linked with the syndrome of peroneal spastic flat foot, which is a painful rigid pronation of the foot with tonic spasm of the peroneal muscles.

Tarsal coalitions usually become painful during the second decade of life when the coalition starts to ossify, and may be associated in the rearfoot with a sudden injury. The child will present with mild deep pain in the subtalar joint and limitation of subtalar joint movement. Generally the more severe the limitation of movement, the more severe the pain. Talocalcaneal coalition tends to produce the most severe pronation of the foot.

If the tarsal coalition has ossified, its presence can be confirmed by radiographic examination of the foot. The calcaneonavicular coalition is best demonstrated by a medial oblique radiograph. In non-ossified calcaneonavicular coalition the proximity of the two bones and flattening of the navicular as it approaches the calcaneus should arouse suspicion. The talocalcaneal joint most commonly shows a coalition in the middle facet which is best seen on a Harris–Beath or ski-jumper's view of the rearfoot. Recently tomography and bone scans have been shown to be useful in identifying both cartilaginous and osseous coalitions of the talonavicular joint.

The peroneal muscle spasm, which may be occasional or continuous, is probably the response of the peroneal muscles to effusion into the subtalar joint. It has been demonstrated that the posterior subtalar joint intra-articular pressure is less in eversion than in inversion (Kyne & Mankin 1965). The peroneal spasm can be reduced by a local anaesthetic block of the common peroneal nerve as it passes around the neck of the fibular (Harris 1965). The spasm, a protective mechanism, can be induced by forceful inversion of the foot.

# DIGITAL DEFORMITIES

## Hallux valgus

While not a common condition, juvenile hallux valgus is a very significant foot problem. Although it begins as an isolated abnormality of the first metatarsophalangeal joint, as the condition progresses it affects the entire forefoot. Advanced hallux valgus is known to be associated with hammer second toe and crowding of the other lesser digits, widening of the forefoot leading to footwear-fitting problems, and plantar callosity and metatarsalgia.

A survey of 6000 9-year-olds determined a 2% incidence of hallux valgus (Kilmartin et al 1991). Although it is possible to detect hallux valgus in children younger than 9 years, the changes are often very subtle. On the other hand, in adolescents the condition may have already progressed to the point where it is involving the other lesser digits. Therefore 9 years is probably the optimum age for assessment and treatment.

The condition is known to be inherited (Johnston 1959), so children with the complaint are often presented by parents who are only too familiar with the long-term effects of 'bunions'. Diagnosis may be confirmed using the following three criteria:

- A first metatarsophalangeal joint angle in excess of 15°. This may be measured clinically with a digital goniometer or on a dorso-plantar weightbearing X-ray. If radiographs are taken, the first–second intermetatarsal angle should also be measured. An angle in excess of the normal 9° is known to be the forerunner of clinically apparent hallux valgus (Kilmartin et al 1994).
- Osteophytic thickening of the first metatarsophalangeal joint. Visible thickening of the joint indicates hypertrophy of the metatarsal head caused by loss of congruency of the joint and subsequent early degeneration of the joint surface.
- A strong family history of the complaint. A family history of hallux valgus, while not confirming diagnosis, must arouse suspicion.

When hallux valgus is present in the child, family history may also indicate the likely prognosis for the child. A history of severe deformity affecting siblings, parents and grandparents is very significant.

Pain is not usually a feature of hallux valgus until the deformity is more advanced. Pain can be associated with footwear irritation of the skin overlying the medial eminence or, more significantly, a dull ache within the joint which can rarely be produced clinically, but occurs on activity or is induced by damp, cold weather or ill-fitting footwear. Pain deep within the joint is caused by degenerative joint changes.

Because of the progressive nature of hallux valgus, once the diagnosis is made, assessment and review is likely to be a long-term commitment for both patient and practitioner. Dorso-plantar weightbearing radiographs will allow accurate assessment of the following:

- First metatarsophalangeal joint space
- Hallux valgus angle
- First–second intermetatarsal angle
- Medial eminence
- Osteophytic development
- Sesamoid position.

Radiographic changes are likely to be very subtle in the short term. Three yearly X-ray reviews are therefore indicated. Objective clinical assessment can be made by taking a digital goniometer measurement of the first metatarsophalangeal joint angle. This value should be recorded after drawing around the weightbearing foot on a blank sheet of paper. When stored in the patient's records, this can provide a visual indication of the effectiveness of treatment. Because hallux valgus is usually a bilateral condition, both feet can be assessed in this manner even if at first only one foot is affected.

## Lesser digit deformity

The following lesser digit deformities are common cause for parental concern:

- Adductovarus third, fourth, fifth toes
- Dorsiflexed second toe

- Overriding fifth toe
- Underriding third and fourth toes.

Although the abnormal position is often real enough, the condition may be quite benign. It is essential that the practitioner applies the following criteria to determine which lesser digit problems require treatment.

1. Is weightbearing on the apex of the toe rather than the soft plantar pulp? Apical weightbearing may lead to the development of painful corns and callus.
2. Is the malposition of one digit likely to influence the position of an adjacent, otherwise normal digit? For example, a dorsiflexed second toe will lead to loss of buttress effect on the hallux which will predispose to hallux valgus.
3. Is the malpositioned digit likely to be irritated by footwear or cause footwear-fitting problems?
4. Is the type of digital deformity likely to respond to conservative or surgical treatment? Transverse and frontal plane deformities are resistant to conservative treatment, while sagittal plane deformities and even the sagittal plane component of complex digital deformities respond more favourably to conservative treatment. In children older than 9, conservative treatment becomes progressively less effective. In infants younger than 2, corrective devices are poorly tolerated and technically difficult to make because of the size of the digits.

If treatment is indicated, conservative treatment should always be attempted first. Response to treatment should be measured using a Harris & Beath mat. The child should be asked to step on and then off the mat. Digital purchase will be recorded by the mat. Apical weightbearing by the digits will be recorded as a very small area of digital contact, while adductovarus will often appear as the lateral side of the digit in contact with the mat. In overriding digits, toe purchase with the ground will be absent. Following treatment, the foot printing procedure should be repeated.

Drawing around the toes on blank paper, photocopying the undersurface of the foot while supporting the child's weight, or photographing the digits will also facilitate objective assessment of treatment success.

## CONDITIONS ASSOCIATED WITH PAIN

The painful foot in the child is a problem creating considerable concern. Evaluation must be carried out with care and sympathy. Sources of such pain may be visible or hidden. It may indicate inflammation and infection. Chapter 16 considers the painful foot, but to complete the paediatric examination, the practitioner should be aware of common entities likely to be associated with pain.

### Tumours

These are rare but if expansile cause discomfort and pain. Malignant bone tumours are rare but do occur more commonly in children than in adults. Subungual exostosis is a common benign *osteochondroma* lying on the dorsal tip of the distal phalanx. The nail is deformed centrally or along one edge, causing the nail to be humped up.

Small naevi should not be painful, with the exception of *angioleiomyoma*, which is found in association with blood vessels as a dark, well-defined but tender lesion.

Cysts affect soft tissue as well as bone; bone cysts may occur within the calcaneus. Pain associated with a bone cyst usually responds to paracetamol but may require operation.

### Osteochondroses

This group of disorders is associated with trauma and altered vascular supply to bone, usually at critical stages in development.

#### Legg–Calvé–Perthes disease

This is considered to be an avascular necrosis of the femoral head. It usually presents in children over 3 years old. Clinical signs may be detected as a reduced range of motion, especially internal rotation and abduction, and muscle wasting of the buttocks on the affected side. The patient may present with a positive Trendelenburg sign. If both hips are affected the patient may walk with a waddling or swaying gait. A limp may be present. Pain may be detected over the anterior or lateral hip and there is general hip joint tenderness. In some cases the pain is referred to the knee. It can lead to osteoarthrosis of the hip in the young adult.

### Köhler's disease

Pain in the midfoot is associated with Köhler's osteochondrosis of the navicular. Köhler's disease is rare but may be a cause of limping in the young child. It will present as tenderness and swelling over the dorsal midfoot region. Boys are more commonly affected than girls; the peak incidence in both sexes is around 4–5 years of age. There is no apparent family tendency. It is usually unilateral and one-third of cases have a history of associated trauma.

The diagnosis of Köhler's disease is made on the basis of clinical and radiographic findings. Waugh (1958) described two distinct radiographic presentations. The more common presentation is the flattened, irregularly shaped and sclerotic appearance of the navicular. Alternatively the navicular may be normal in shape and contour but uniformly increased in density, as in a 'silver sixpence'.

Köhler's disease is self-limiting. The navicular returns to regular size, shape and density within 2–4 years, suggesting that the condition may be nothing more than an alternative sequence of tarsal ossification. Another suggested cause of Köhler's disease is compression of the bone's vascular supply due to repeated microtrauma which creates avascular necrosis.

Other osteochondroses of the tarsus have been recorded and include *Buschke's disease* of the cuneiforms and *Iselin's disease* of the fifth metatarsal. The latter may not, however, be a true osteochondrosis but rather a traction apophysitis.

### Sever's disease of the heel

This, like Osgood–Schlatter's disease, is a traction apophysitis and an extremely common complaint among young adolescents, especially boys aged 8–12. Heel pain related to Sever's disease will be most noticeable before and after sport. The pain originates from the posterior apophysis of the calcaneus. This is because the tendo achilles is inserted at this point and leads to pulling against the bone. Strong shearing and tensile forces may result in inflammation of the weakest point of the calcaneus, the superior centre of ossification of the posterior apophysis. Radiological assessment of suspected Sever's disease may be misleading. Tachdjian (1985) found that irregularity of ossification and sclerosis of the apophysis was a normal finding. A normal calcaneal apophysis may be bipartite, tripartite or divided even further. While a lateral X-ray of the calcaneus may assist differential diagnosis, Sever's disease is a straightforward clinical diagnosis based upon patient age, subcalcaneal pain on activity and tenderness on applying pressure to the medial and lateral sides of the calcaneus. Sever's disease is a self-limiting condition: the pain will resolve once calcaneal ossification is complete and the apophysis fused.

### Freiberg's disease

Freiberg's disease, osteochondrosis of the lesser metatarsal heads, carries the worst prognosis of all the osteochondroses affecting the foot. The condition may be defined as a degenerative aseptic necrosis of the secondary ossification centre in the lesser metatarsal head which leads to disorganised regeneration and predisposes to premature osteoarthrosis of the metatarsophalangeal joint. The condition was first described by Freiberg in 1914, although Köhler in Germany had given a more detailed account earlier. While the second metatarsal head is affected in 68% of cases, the third metatarsal head is involved in 27% of cases and the fourth in 5%. It is extremely rare for the fifth metatarsal to be involved (Gauthier & Elbaz 1979).

Osteochondrosis of the lesser metatarsal heads is often, but not always, associated with a single incidence of trauma. Repeated low-grade trauma has also been implicated as a cause of the impaired metatarsal head vascular supply. It usually affects children in their early teens. Girls are affected three times more than boys. The involved metatarsophalangeal joint will present as hard, swollen and tender on movement. While this is a relatively late stage according to Smillie (1969), acute tenderness may be present without such changes if the patient is referred early in the pathology. Dorsiflexion and plantarflexion of the digit will cause moderate to severe pain and demonstrate considerable limitation if the problem persists. Activities that require metatarsophalangeal joint extension, such as hill walking, climbing stairs or wearing high-heeled shoes, will likewise provoke pain from the joint. Radiological assessment is indicated, although in the early stages there may be no changes other than slight sclerosis of the metatarsal head.

Pain from the acute stage may subside in time, although pain is likely to recur in the mid-teens to early 20s when poor mechanical function of the joint leads to early degeneration of the joint surface. At this stage the joint will appear thickened on palpation, digital dorsiflexion will be limited and dorsoplantar and medial oblique radiological views will show a flattened metatarsal head and, occasionally, loose bodies within the joint (Case history 14.3).

## Infections

Skin infections should be relatively obvious. Verrucae are endemic in children, particularly between 6 years of age and the late teens. The source of the viral infection is often hard to identify and advice will depend upon duration, symptoms, activities and attitude toward the problem. The presence of tinea pedis is diagnosed from skin scrapings; teenage boys are particularly susceptible to fungal infections associated with hyperhidrosis.

## Juvenile plantar dermatitis

Another seasonal condition is forefoot eczema or juvenile plantar dermatosis. The aetiology is uncertain but it is not thought to be a chronic contact dermatitis. A rash appears on the weightbearing area of the foot. A pink, shiny or glazed appearance is noted with scaling. The skin thins and is inflexible, with resultant fissures forming. Differential diagnosis includes tinea.

## Vasospastic disorders

These used to be very common in children because of poor economic and housing conditions. Their incidence has declined in recent decades. However, chilblains still occur in children who are exposed to extremes of temperature due to inadequate footwear and hosiery in winter or poor home conditions. They appear as red, blotchy, intensely itchy areas. Broken chilblains may become infected.

Dark mauve swellings around calf muscles, thighs and buttocks indicate erythrocyanosis. This affects overweight females in particular. Acrocyanosis, reddening of the hands and feet, may also occur in children. Both erythrocyanosis

---

**Case history 14.3**

A 14-year-old boy presented with a painful second metatarsophalangeal joint. The boy reported that the joint was most painful during and after competing in cross-country running events.

The foot had previously been investigated radiologically after the subject had dropped a dumbbell on his foot while partaking in weightlifting exercise. At the time, the foot had swelled, caused pain and made walking difficult. The radiograph, however, showed no bony abnormality.

On examination the second metatarsophalangeal joint was palpably enlarged. Dorsiflexion of the digit was restricted and the boy complained of pain on the dorsal surface of the metatarsal head with forced dorsiflexion. Freiberg's disease was suspected and, although the parents were adamant that osteochondrosis had been ruled out by the previous X-ray, repeat dorsoplantar and medial oblique views showed a flattened second metatarsal head and increased joint space consistent with osteochondrosis of the second metatarsal head.

**Conclusion**: Single X-rays taken early in the course of a pathology should not be relied on, as a false negative result can be drawn. Inadequate follow-up can lead to this type of misdiagnosis.

and acrocyanosis are indicative of poor blood supply and response to cold.

## SUMMARY

Although the assessment process is similar, the skills required to assess the child do differ from those used to assess an adult.

Assessment of the child requires sufficient knowledge of normal development and the ability to differentiate between self-limiting developmental conditions and significant, persistent abnormalities, and those that warrant further evaluation. The practitioner must appreciate normal developmental milestones in order to undertake a thorough assessment.

This chapter has primarily concentrated on common orthopaedic conditions associated with the lower limb. Brief discussion has considered pertinent vascular, dermatological conditions that lead to patients seeking advice. The practitioner must identify the cause of any pain and be vigilant for signs of neuromuscular deficit. In a well-resourced country such as the UK, most severe problems associated with the foot and lower limb are detected at birth. However, all practitioners should be aware of problems that may have missed detection or which are relatively mild, but may still lead to functional problems in later life.

## REFERENCES

Alvik L 1960 Increased anteversion of the femoral neck as a sole sign of dysplasia coxae. Acta Orthopaedica Scandinavica 29: 301–306

Berg E E 1986 A reappraisal of metatarsus adductus and skewfoot. Journal of Bone and Joint Surgery 68-A: 1185–1196

Blane W A, Mattison D R, Kane R 1971 LDS intrauterine amputations and amniotic band syndrome. Lancet 2: 158

DeMyer W, Baird I 1969 Mortality and skeletal malformations from amniocentesis and oligohydramniosis in rats. Teratology 2: 33–40

Fabry G, McEwan G D, Shands A R 1973 Torsion of the femur (a follow up study in normal and abnormal conditions). Journal of Bone and Joint Surgery 55A: 1726–1738

Gauthier G, Elbaz R 1979 Freiberg's infraction: a subchondral bone fatigue fracture. A new surgical treatment. Clinical Orthopaedics and Related Research 142: 93–95

Giladi M, Milgrom C, Stein M et al 1985 The low arch, a protective factor in stress fractures. Orthopaedic Review 14: 709–712

Harris R I 1965 Peroneal spastic flat foot (rigid valgus foot). Journal of Bone and Joint Surgery 47-A: 1657–1667

Heath C H, Staheli, L T 1993 Normal limits of knee angle in white children—genu varum and genu valgum. Journal of Paediatric Orthopaedics 13: 259–262

Hubbard D D, Staheli L T, Chew D E 1988 Medial femoral torsion and osteoarthrosis. Journal of Paediatric Orthopaedics 8: 540–542

Hutter C G, Scott W 1949 Tibial torsion. Journal of Bone and Joint Surgery 31-A: 511–518

Johnston O 1959 Further studies of the inheritance of hand and foot anomalies. Clinical Orthopaedics 8: 146–159

Kilmartin T E 1988 Medial genicular rotation: aetiology and management. Chiropodist 43: 181–184

Kilmartin T E, Barrington R L, Wallace W A 1991 Metatarsus primus varus. Journal of Bone and Joint Surgery 73B: 937–940

Kilmartin T E, Barrington R L, Wallace W A 1994 A controlled prospective trial of a foot orthosis in the treatment of juvenile hallux valgus. Journal of Bone and Joint Surgery 76B: 210–214

Kyne P J, Mankin H J 1965 Changes in intrarticular pressure with subtalar joint motion with special reference to the etiology of peroneal spastic flat foot. Bulletin of the Hospital for Joint Diseases 26: 181–186

Luder J 1988 Early recognition of cerebral palsy. Update 15 March: 1955–1963

Melincoff R H, Davis M H 1978 The development of lower extremity deformity. Journal of the American Podiatry Association 60: 631–635

Michele A A, Nielsen P M 1976 Tibiotalar torsion: bioengineering paradigm. Orthopedic Clinics of North America 7: 929–947

Morley A J M 1957 Knock knees in children. British Medical Journal 2: 976–979

Mosier K M, Asher M 1984 Tarsal coalitions and peroneal spastic flat foot. Journal of Bone and Joint Surgery 66-A: 976–984

Ponsetti I V 1992 Current concepts review. Treatment of congenital clubfoot. Journal of Bone and Joint Surgery 74-A: 448–454

Ponsetti I V, Becker J R 1966 Congenital metatarsus adductus, the results of treatment. Journal of Bone and Joint Surgery 74-A: 702–711

Reikeras O, Hoiseth A 1989 Torsion of the leg determined by computerized tomography. Acta Orthopaedica Scandinavica 60: 330–333

Root M L, Orien W P, Weed J H 1977 Normal and abnormal function of the foot, vol II. Clinical Biomechanics Corporation, Los Angeles, CA

Rose G K, Welton E A, Marshall T 1985 The diagnosis of flat foot in the child. Journal of Bone and Joint Surgery 67-B: 71–78

Rushforth G F 1978 The natural history of hooked forefoot. Journal of Bone and Joint Surgery 60-B: 530–532

Salenius P, Vankka E 1975 The development of the tibio-femoral angle in children. Journal of Bone and Joint Surgery 57: 259–261

Sharrard W J W 1976 Intoeing and flat feet. British Medical Journal 1: 888–889

Smillie I S 1969 Treatment of Freiberg's infraction. Proc. R. Soc. Med. 60: 29–31

Spencer A M 1978 Practical podiatric orthopaedic procedures. Ohio College of Podiatric Medicine, OH

Staheli L T, Lippert F, Denotter P 1977 Femoral anteversion and physical performance in adolescent and adult life. Clinical Orthopaedics 129: 213–216

Staheli L T, Chew D E, Corbett M 1987 The longitudinal arch. Journal of Bone and Joint Surgery 69-A: 426–428

Staheli L T 1993 Rotational problems in childhood. Journal of Bone and Joint Surgery 75-A: 939–949

Svenningsen S, Tierjesen T, Auflem M 1990 Hip rotation and intoeing gait. Clinical Orthopaedics and Related Research 251: 177–182

Tachdjian M O 1985 The child's foot. W B Saunders, Philadelphia, PA

Tax H 1980 Podopaediatrics. Williams & Wilkins, Baltimore, MD, p 68–85

Thomson P (ed) 1993 Introduction to podopaediatrics. W B Saunders, London

Tollafield D R 1988 The child's gait (video presentation). Northampton Health Authority video services/Nene College, Northampton

Torpin R 1968 Fetal malformations caused by amniotic rupture during gestation. Charles C Thomas, Springfield, IL

Turner M S, Smillie I S 1981 The effect of tibial torsion on the pathology of the knee. Journal of Bone and Joint Surgery 63-B: 396–398

Valmassy R L 1993 In: Thomson P (ed) 1993 Introduction to podopaediatrics. W B Saunders , London, p 29–31

Waugh W 1958 The ossification and vascularisation of the tarsal navicular and their relation to Köhler's disease. Journal of Bone and Joint Surgery 403-B: 765–768

## FURTHER REFERENCES

Illingworth R S 1990 The development of the infant and the young child. Churchill Livingstone, Edinburgh

Berkow R (ed) 1987 The Merck manual, 15th edn. Merck Sharp & Dohme Research Laboratories

McCrea J D 1985 Pediatric orthopaedics of the lower extremity. Futura, New York

Sheridan M D 1975 Children's development progress. NFER Publishing Co

# 15

# The sports patient

*W. Turner*
*S. J. Avil*

## INTRODUCTION

More and more people are participating in exercise in order to keep fit. Unfortunately, sports injuries are a by-product of this health 'craze', often occurring as a result of people being ill-prepared for their sport, being unfit or placing too much stress on their musculoskeletal system.

Injury commonly arises as a result of:

1. 'Normal' physical structure and function but inadequate preparation for sport and excessive demands placed on tissues
2. 'Abnormal' physical structure and function coupled with a demand over and above everyday stresses on tissues.

This chapter confines itself to building on previous chapters that have already covered a wide range of assessment activities. Patients with a particular interest in sports activities should be carefully evaluated. The locomotor system examination (Ch. 8) covers techniques for evaluating joints, muscles and skeletal deformity. It is not intended, therefore, to repeat the process of full locomotor system analysis in this chapter, although the discussion is pertinent to some of the activities, such as gait analysis. Chapter 16 provides examples of common foot problems associated with stress exercise.

The practitioner will need to consider an examination scheme. In order that previous chapters are placed in perspective, a summary is included in Table 15.1.

**Table 15.1** Examination scheme for sports injuries

- Personal details
- Complaint (symptoms)
- Psychological profile
- Sporting history
- Footwear
- Relevant medical history
- Current health status
- Medication currently used
- Locomotor assessment
- Vascular
- Neurological
- Dermatological

The assessment of an athlete is dependent upon the practitioner's preferred approach, which might include working with other professionals as a team in a health centre, within the framework of a larger organisation such as a football club or on one's own.

The chapter is confined to sports psychology and related physical examination. The main features of the sports assessment are considered in Figure 15.1.

## The basis for sports injury consultations

The World Health Organization has recently suggested that the damaging effect of not taking

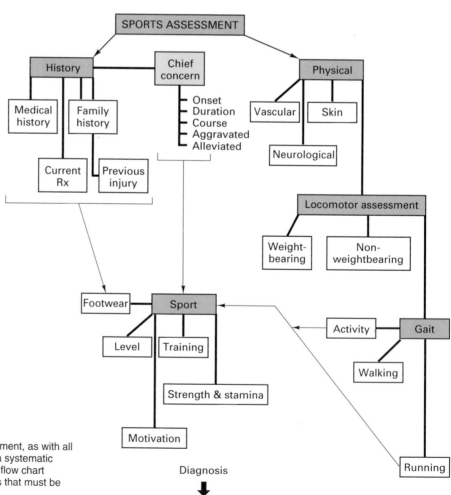

**Figure 15.1** Sports assessment, as with all patient categories, requires a systematic approach to the patient. The flow chart provides a summary of areas that must be included.

**Table 15.2** Incidence of sport-related injury (n = 1600). Source: Glasgow Royal Infirmary 1984

| Site | Incidence |
| --- | --- |
| Head and neck | 17.7 |
| Upper limb | 30.7 |
| Trunk | 6.4 |
| Thigh and pelvis | 2.2 |
| Knee | 10.4 |
| Leg, foot and ankle | 32.6 |

exercise is equivalent to smoking 20 cigarettes a day. Publicity has encouraged people to take part in sporting activities.

Sports medicine is a young subspecialty of medicine in the UK. The novice practitioner has to deal with two problems: the patient and the system. Fortunately there has been much advancement in knowledge of sport pathology, but in the UK not all hospitals have the expertise to deal with sports problems let alone those associated with the lower limb. In this respect the private sector, where multidisciplinary teams cooperate, has expanded considerably.

### Defining the problem

Assessment of the patient with sports injuries is becoming an important part of clinical practice. The increase in the number of people engaged in sports has lead to an inevitable rise in the number of injuries sustained as a result of sporting activity. Most forms of sport and exercise are weightbearing and therefore place stress on the lower extremity. Stresses through the lower limbs can increase by up to five times as a result of such exercise. It is not surprising therefore to find that about 45% of all sports injuries occur below the hip (Table 15.2).

### Making a case for dealing with sportspeople differently

Practitioners involved in treating sports injuries make the common mistake of assessing the patient in terms of structural and functional assessment only. This type of assessment will be insufficient for the majority of sports patients. It is necessary to combine physical assessment with a knowledge of the sport and a thorough understanding of the patient and the patient's approach to sport.

The practitioner starting out in practice can find sports medicine daunting. Sports podiatry concerns itself with only a part of sports medicine, although knowledge should not be restricted to the foot alone. A number of professional groups do overlap and this is where collaboration can be an advantage. Many newly qualified practitioners shy away from sports medicine as a specialty for several reasons:

- Requirement by health service managers to concentrate on other client groups (e.g. the elderly, children, etc)
- Inadequate provision of support services essential to the sports medicine practitioner (e.g. X-ray facilities, orthotic and gait analysis services)
- Inadequate undergraduate or postgraduate training in sports medicine
- Fear of litigation
- Lack of adequate career structure and remuneration.

Practitioners who opt to specialise in sports medicine and who overcome associated problems can expect a wide and varied caseload.

### Patient compliance

A common problem of treating the sportsperson can be the patient's unwillingness to accept assessment or treatment. The problem of compliance is common amongst sportspeople. Often the patient's anxiety to return to training and exercise as soon as possible results in him/her placing unrealistic demands on the sports practitioner. These patients often demand spot diagnoses and expect treatment to take effect immediately. Practitioners will find that this presents two problems. The first is getting the patient to allow sufficient time for appropriate investigations in order that a diagnosis can be made. Secondly, patients who have started a treatment plan may lose interest in it if it does not show immediate results. All too often such patients return to sport too soon, only to find that their injuries still give them problems, or to sustain new injuries.

Occasionally, sports patients will readily accept a clinical diagnosis but may find it difficult to accept the treatment plan. This is a particular problem if the treatment plan includes a period of abstinence from sport, or if the patient is requested to modify his/her training programme. Case history 15.1 shows how this can be a particular problem for the sports practitioner.

## Sports patients

The types of person engaged in sport vary

---

**Case history 15.1**

A 22-year-old male patient attended the clinic following a running injury. His primary sport was long-distance running and secondary sports were swimming and weight-training. He complained of severe, disabling pain in his right shin that was exacerbated by running. He ran for around 3 hours a day and represented his county at national competitions. His coach was preparing him for international trials. Examination revealed a tender region along the anterior right tibia, consistent with the origin of tibialis anterior.

**Diagnosis**: A diagnosis of anterior tibial shin splints was made. The patient had a forefoot varus deformity, with plantarflexed first rays.

**Discussion**: The treatment plan consisted of shock-absorbing insoles with anti-pronatory control. The patient was advised to rest the limb for 2 weeks except for swimming. The patient returned 2 weeks later. He had not worn the insoles because they took up too much room in his running shoes, nor had he rested the area. The patient complained that inappropriate treatment had been prescribed and discharged himself from the care of the attending podiatrist. He failed to make the England squad.

**Conclusion**: This case highlights the problem of non-compliance which may be detected in advance of devising the treatment plan. It is important to use this knowledge to ensure that the patient understands the principles of the assessment and treatment and accepts their role in the overall management of the problem. However, it is equally important to avoid making uncertain diagnoses or overestimating the potential success of treatment as this may affect the patient's willingness to comply in the long term and may cause him/her to lose confidence in the practitioner's assessment skills.

---

widely in terms of physical shape and psychological approach to sport. The desire for a healthier lifestyle has resulted in many unfit and overweight people taking up exercise. At the opposite end of the spectrum are accomplished athletes, for whom athletic activity is essential for self-fulfilment, achievement and satisfaction. Prior to any discussion regarding physical examination it is worthwhile considering the types of patient who could present to a clinic for preliminary examination.

### Children and sports injuries

Certain injuries are more common in certain age groups. Children, in particular, present an interesting assessment problem. Most schoolchildren participate in organised sport and exercise in physical education classes. Children may compete individually or for a team. Children of the same age often develop physically at different rates. Variations in development and morphological characteristics can lead to some children being more at risk on exercising.

Peer group pressure amongst children should not be underestimated as a causative factor for sports injuries. Often children are encouraged to take part in exercise by their friends and form strong competitive tendencies which can cause a child to push him/herself over the threshold for injury.

Highly competitive children, like adults, can develop an obsessive desire to improve their performance time and become addicted to sport. Injury is sustained by the child placing excessive demands on his/her body during key developmental stages and can result in lifelong problems. Obsessive physical education teachers and parents can make the situation worse by putting pressure on the child to improve performance and take part in competition.

Motivation to do sport can be difficult to assess in children. Hopefully, children are motivated as a result of performing well at a particular sport, or from the enjoyment derived from exercise. However, there are occasions when children do not perform well, are not selected for team sports by their peers and derive little enjoyment from exercise. These children are at risk from injury as a result of losing soft-tissue tone, joint stability and possibly becoming overweight.

### Age and sex distributions

The type of injury sustained by adults may be related to natural 'wear and tear' factors. Injury in the sportsperson over 50 years of age is often related to general degenerative changes, for example, osteoarthrosis. Painful joints in the older sportsperson may exclude him/her from weightbearing sports.

Adults in the second and third decades commonly present with overuse injuries. These occur as a result of either placing too great a demand on normal structures or increasing the demand on abnormal structures, causing increased compensation.

The distribution of injuries among adults may show a pattern according to the age and sex of the sportsperson identified in a recent report from Denmark. Before the age of 30, males develop considerably more injuries than females. However, females over 40 years of age have a higher incidence of foot sprains; 62% of which occurred outdoors. By the age of 70, the sexes are equal again (Holmer et al 1994).

More women are participating in sport in efforts to become fit and lead a healthier life. The uptake of aerobic dance classes and fitness videos in recent years is largely among women in the third and fourth decades. In addition to this involvement in exercise, the number of women competing in sport and taking part in team sports is increasing. Injuries amongst women taking part in sport may be due to any of the factors already discussed: excessive demands on normal or abnormal structure and function, and lack of preparation for sport.

## HISTORY

A significant part of the interview will be taken up by listening to the patient and asking questions. Examination is important, but more

can be learned by looking and listening. The general overview involves:

- Personal details
- Complaint
- Psychological profile
- Sporting history
- Current health status
- Medical history
- Medication
- Diet.

## Personal details

Personal details are essential. Names and addresses of contacts such as team coaches might be helpful. When managing children, the name of the school and the name of the physical education teacher is useful. Sometimes this part of the assessment may reveal common patterns associated with injury in particular schools. It is important to recognise these patterns and to communicate with the school, the teacher and the children in order to prevent further injuries.

## Presenting complaint

It is essential to find out what the presenting complaint or concern is. Why has the patient asked for a consultation? It is valuable to obtain a perspective from the patient of how they view the problem. Often the patient will complain of a number of pathologies that he/she feels are related to lower limb function or associated with injury. It is important to encourage the patient to rank them in order from pathologies of least concern to pathologies of greater concern. The following should be covered:

- When did the symptoms start?
- Is the pain constant or intermittent?
- When is the pain a problem?
- What makes the pain worse?
- What alleviates the pain?
- How long is the pain present (all the time, occasional, only on exercise, at rest only)?

It is also useful to ask the patient's opinion about the cause of the problem. It is important that the patient's perception of the pathology is identified and either confirmed or denied as a result of clinical examination.

Previous sporting injuries and treatment should be recorded. All too often the sports practitioner will find that the same factors that have been responsible for causing previous injury are likely causes of current injury. This line of questioning will help to identify cases where recurrent injury is due to non-compliance or previous treatment which has been ineffective.

## Motivation to do sport

It is also useful to determine factors which motivate a patient to participate in sport. Motivation is an extremely important aspect of the assessment of the sports patient. Common examples of motivating factors are desires to:

- attain or maintain fitness
- lose weight
- feel part of a team
- occupy spare time
- win competitions
- escape from day-to-day life
- stimulate endorphins ('runner's high')
- achieve
- conform to the expectations of others.

Knowing what motivates someone to take part in sport will help to form an overall assessment profile and help significantly with treatment planning. Motivating factors, together with what 'phase' the sportsperson falls into, can help the practitioner determine the level of compliance that can be expected from the patient.

Practical assessment of motivation is sometimes difficult to carry out. It is important to determine what motivating factors exist for every sport the patient participates in. This will also help in identification of the patient's primary, secondary and accessory sporting activities.

It is also important to identify what motivates the patient to seek help for injury. Examples of motivating factors include the desire to:

- return to sporting activity quickly
- be free from pain
- improve performance
- improve health overall
- prevent further injury
- learn improved training techniques.

The practitioner should also be aware that some patients may be addicted to their sport. Various researchers have investigated the psychological effects of sport on the body. Kostrubala (1976) described the 'runner's high' as a mild euphoria. It became clear that runners return to running to repeatedly experience this 'high'.

Research into the runner's high seems to demonstrate that the elation takes place in the second half of the run. It has been suggested that autohypnosis is a factor in rhythmic running. The runner's high has also been linked to raised levels of noradrenaline, beta-endorphins and serotonin. The exact neurophysiological nature of the runner's high is not fully understood. It seems likely that both psychological and physiological factors contribute.

## Psychological profiling

Subotnick (1989) describes four 'phases' of runner (although these phases could be applied to any sport) from the point of view of the range of injuries presenting for assessment.

### Phase I

Phase I sportspeople are people who have just begun taking exercise. Very often they have returned to sporting activity after a long period of rest or relative inactivity. Typically, these people are in their third or fourth decade and have not taken part in formal sporting activity since leaving school. As a result of this long period of inactivity, these people have a tendency towards being overweight and unfit. The prime motivation is the desire to get fit and have a healthier lifestyle. A gradual, controlled return to sport is likely to be beneficial. The person will notice a gradual improvement in performance, feeling less out of breath and being able to sustain activity for longer or at an increased intensity as time goes by. This improved performance is a result of cardiovascular changes and a consequence of aerobic exercise.

It is important, in the case of injury, to assess the patient's approach to sport. There is a danger that the return to exercise may have been too demanding, resulting in the person becoming exhausted, suffering muscular aches and pains and becoming liable to injury. Apart from the physical effects of this overexertion, the person's motivation to continue with sport may suffer adversely. This is extremely common amongst people who join formalised exercise (aerobics) classes to find that the exercise routines are too demanding, leaving them feeling exhausted and in pain.

Phase I people who sensibly manage their return to exercise will soon experience the beneficial health effects of exercise. Physically, a loss of weight and improved cardiovascular function will lead to improved fitness and reduce the chances of cardiovascular disease. Psychologically, these people often find that as a result of exercise, they are able to accomplish more in everyday life, feeling more at ease than they did before they started exercising.

## Phase II

These people have moved a stage further, occasionally taking part in sport competitively. It is important to assess the patient's competitive attitude toward the sport. Often they are motivated to do sport for the prospect of winning. This win can be either winning as part of a team, or beating another individual. Sometimes a win can simply mean beating a 'personal best'.

Phase II sportspeople enjoy the benefits of aerobic exercise, experience the beneficial psychological and cardiovascular effects. They sometimes use exercise to achieve stress reduction, although this can sometimes be a difficult factor to assess. Exercise is undertaken between two and five times a week, with periods when exercise is relaxed.

## Phase III

This type of sportsperson becomes obsessive and compulsive; they are physically and psychologically dependent upon their sport. Sport is used as a safety valve for stress, to escape from the everyday stresses of life. Exercise is undertaken seven days a week with feelings of guilt if they are unable to exercise every day. Their obsession with sport often means that their work, social and personal lives suffer.

Phase III people often believe that they are immune from injury and have a cavalier attitude to training. Often the warm-up and stretching routines are omitted in order to spend the maximum time at sport.

When injury does occur, they are keen to blame anyone or anything for their injury other than themselves. Rarely do they accept responsibility for their injury. For instance, blame is often placed on their coach, doctor or family or they may say that the weather, the surface or their footwear is responsible.

Phase III sportspeople are difficult to assess. They often demand spot diagnoses and are sometimes reluctant to seek assessment. Frequently they only attend for assessment after they have unsuccessfully tried to treat themselves. They may have rigid ideas about the cause of their injuries and place unrealistic demands on the practitioner, often wanting an immediate diagnosis and results of treatment.

Such patients may become impatient and are generally not compliant. From the point of view of assessment, it is important to identify the phase III person as soon as possible, as the underlying reason for the injury often stems from the patient's attitude to sport.

## Phase IV

This group has usually passed through phase III but has 'mellowed out'. They tend to be much more sensible about their sport. They have come to realise that their injury and poor performance occur as a result of overexertion and to accept more responsibility for their injuries. Phase IV people are much more compliant and have developed a good background knowledge of their sport and factors responsible for causing injury.

## Drawing conclusions from profiles

Assessment of the category or 'phase' which a particular sports patient fits into can be a useful adjunct to physical examination and injury history. The practitioner can assess patient compliance by forming an opinion about his/her sport type. Subotnick's phases give an overall picture of the wide range of people taking part in sport and exercise.

Often, injury arises as a result of components from both of the above. To illustrate this concept further, two case histories (Case histories 15.2 and 15.3) are illustrated to show how this relationship can help to explain the cause of sports injury.

---

**Case history 15.2**

An overweight, 35-year-old male sales representative decided to get fit. He had not participated in sporting activity since he was at school. He decided to enter a local fun run and raise some money for his favourite charity at the same time. Pressure at work prevented him from training for the event and he soon found that the date of the fun run had arrived. Because he had obtained many sponsors and raised £60 he felt compelled to complete the run. He turned up on the morning; the weather was cold and wet. The run took place on roads and involved hill work. He commenced without stretching or warming up his joints or muscles. After a few minutes he became breathless and perspired heavily. He continued to run, attempting to keep up with his neighbour who had also entered, but who had some training prior to the run. 2 miles into the run he was stopped suddenly by an agonising pain in the posterior right thigh.

**Diagnosis**: A hamstring tear was diagnosed at the hospital accident department.

**Conclusion**: This was a patient with normal physical structure and function who placed excessive demands on an ill-prepared body resulting in damage to tissue.

---

## Sporting history

It is essential for the complete assessment of the sports patient to include thorough details of the

---

**Case history 15.3**

An 18-year-old female played in three basketball matches over consecutive weekends. She decided to train four times a week in order to achieve the required standard. Training consisted of warming-up on a cycle ergometer followed by gentle stretching exercises. This was followed by team activity and short games of basketball. Towards the middle of the second week of training, she noticed a dull ache in the anterior left shin which gradually deteriorated over the following week. She was prevented from playing basketball on the final weekend because the pain in her shin prevented her from running.

**Diagnosis**: Anterior tibial shin splints due to tibia vara compensated by subtalar joint pronation with resultant overuse of tibialis anterior.

**Conclusion**: Injury can occur in a relatively well-prepared athlete as a result of abnormal physical structure and function (tibia vara). It is important to recognise that abnormal structure and function does not necessarily result in injury. Injury will occur when the demands placed upon this abnormal structure exceed an individual threshold. Injury occurred as a result of imposing extra demands on an abnormal structure, pushing the patient's system over the threshold for injury.

---

patient's sport and training programme. Sporting history assessment should include details of:

- type and level of sport
- motivation to do sport
- training and stretch routines.

### Type and level of sport

It is important to obtain details concerning all sports and activities that the patient is involved in. This should include the patient's occupation and level of occupational activity. Details of the patient's main or primary sport should be taken. The primary sport is usually the sport or activity which the patient takes most seriously. Frequently the primary sport is one in which the patient competes. In phase I patients who do not compete but participate in sport purely to improve fitness, the primary sport will be the sport they spend most time on.

Secondary or complementary sports should also be discussed with the patient. Often phase II and III patients who compete in a primary sport, supplement their training programme by a secondary activity. This activity is often designed by the sportsperson to complement their primary sport. For example, a patient who runs competitively may supplement this activity with a sport such as weight-training in order to improve lower limb muscle strength.

Sometimes the primary and secondary sports require similar attributes, as in the case of racket sports. A particularly interesting combination of sports may be carried out by a patient in order to enter a specific competition, for instance triathlon or pentathlon. These sports are extremely demanding, testing strength and stamina and placing stress on both upper and lower body musculature.

Information about activities used for recreation and enjoyment should be recorded. For example, a person whose primary sport is running and who has weight-training as a secondary sport may enjoy a game of golf as a recreational activity.

Information about the type and level of sport should be recorded and should include:

- Frequency of participation (number of times sport is carried out per week/month)
- Duration of each session and distance run
- Frequency and level of competition
- If team sport, what position is played.

### Negative addiction

The runner's 'high' is a rewarding and stimulating experience and ensures the runner's continuance of the sport. However, this can result in an uncontrollable need to train, letting nothing prevent it. Occasionally sportspeople will miss holidays, work and other appointments in order to train. This syndrome has been described as *negative addiction* and is comparable to other forms of *negative addiction* such as alcohol, drugs and smoking. Negative addiction can be just as difficult to overcome as drug addiction.

Negative addiction to sport can be recognised if the patient requires daily exercise to cope with the stresses of life or to escape from reality. These people often suffer from the effects of withdrawal if exercise ceases, demonstrating some or all of the following features:

- Restlessness
- Unpredictable mood swings
- Fatigue and malaise
- Lethargy
- Insomnia
- Irritability
- Dysphoria
- Upper/lower gastrointestinal symptoms.

Patients who become negatively addicted to their sport are often phase III people who have become physically and psychologically dependent on it. The symptoms described are not dissimilar to those associated with stress. Eventually the patient's work and personal life suffers from the effects of withdrawal. Most negatively-addicted athletes will continue exercising even when exercise is medically, vocationally and socially contraindicated (Morgan 1979).

Patients who are negatively addicted to their sport present a particular problem to the practitioner. They may offer poor compliance with treatment plans that involve abstinence from sport. The patient may undergo a process similar to bereavement and suffer withdrawal symptoms.

Assessment of the negatively-addicted sportsperson may be further complicated by the fact that these patients often hide their injuries or report dramatic improvements, when in fact there have been none, in order to resume training. If the sportsperson is a professional competitor, it may be the trainer or coach who refers the patient for assessment. The patient him/herself may resent medical intervention and continue with his/her training schedule, ignoring advice. Often the patient's prime goal is to return to the usual sporting activity as soon as possible, and he/she can often mislead coaches and health care staff in order to do this.

### Training and stretch routines

The patient's training routine should include activities to prevent injury and build strength. For effective, safe sporting activity, it is important for the sportsperson to be adequately prepared. Preparation prior to sport usually consists of a routine of stretching exercises, the aim of which is to increase the range of motion at joints and also to reduce the risk of injury. Training routines are also used to bring the sportsperson up to a level of strength and fitness necessary for their chosen sport.

Sports assessment should aim to determine the level of training and details of the training programme carried out by the sports patient and include details of pre-sport and post-sport stretching programmes.

Assessment of the athlete's training programme (or lack of one) may provide the clinician with the key to the problem. For example, patients who spend three or four consecutive days doing demanding 'workouts' will undoubtedly cause strain and fatigue of muscles and predispose to soft-tissue injury. Training should include knowledge of the benefits brought about by warming up before any exercise. Joints and surrounding connective tissue will respond to greater stresses when warmed through gentle movements. Joints should be moved to improve the dynamic properties of synovial fluid and tendons, muscle fibres and ligaments stretched to reduce tensile resistance and yet retain strength within biomechanical tolerances.

### Aerobic activities

Physical activities produce aerobic effects. Aerobic exercise is defined as any activity which causes the following physiological effects:

- Heart rate increased to 70% of maximum heart rate (MHR)
- Increased heart rate sustained for minimum of 12–15 minutes.

Aerobics was made popular in 1968 by Kenneth Cooper in his book *Aerobics*, which described techniques to overload the cardiovascular system. This overload has the effect of improving physical fitness and cardiovascular function.

Initially, aerobics focused on running as the exercise of choice, but it now includes many other forms of sporting and recreational activity including dance, vigorous swimming, circuit training, football and netball, to mention but a few.

Much has been stated about how often and for how long a person should train to obtain an aerobic (or training) effect. It is now generally accepted that three to five sessions of aerobic exercise per week will improve cardiovascular condition and physical fitness. Six days a week is the upper limit of activity to reduce the risk of injury.

The intensity of the workout is just as important as the frequency in order to achieve maximum fitness. The aim is to achieve 70–80% MHR and maintain this for 12–15 minutes. Initially, workouts will achieve this level of MHR very quickly, so workouts should be correspondingly short. It is not uncommon, therefore for a person beginning an aerobic exercise regime to spend no more than 20 minutes per session achieving a training effect. This time would include warm up, preliminary stretches and warm down.

As the sportsperson begins to benefit physiologically from the effects of aerobic exercise, the amount of activity necessary to bring about a rise in MHR will increase. It may be necessary for the sportsperson to work out harder and for longer to bring about the rise in MHR necessary for a training effect.

Professional athletes usually have coaches or trainers to advise them on their aerobic programmes. Their exercise routines are gradually increased to the optimum level required for maintenance of the physical condition necessary for their sport. The level will depend upon the athlete's cardiovascular fitness and stamina.

The amateur sportsperson will not generally have the benefit of professional exercise planning. Injury is likely where the sportsperson rapidly increases the intensity or duration of the aerobic workout, or trains too often, not enabling the body to adapt to demands.

The FITT principle can be applied to assessment of aerobic training, and information should be gained regarding each of the elements of FITT assessment:

- F: Frequency of training
- I: Intensity of workout
- T: Time taken for workout
- T: Technique adopted for workout.

In a similar way that the cardiovascular system has to be overloaded to achieve a training effect, muscle needs to be overloaded to improve strength and muscle bulk. Many sporting injuries occur as a result of this overload on muscle being too great. Overload of muscle may result from functional abnormality, or from excessive demands being placed on the muscle structure. Overdemand with overload from forces resulting in injury usually occurs as a result of excessive factors associated with the FITT assessment process. FITT assessment of muscle strength training will help to identify the cause of injury. Careful locomotor assessment will help to identify muscle overuse injury as a result of excessive mechanical forces.

### Anaerobic activity

Many sports and activities will also involve a substantial amount of anaerobic energy demand. Anaerobic energy pathways provide much ATP to meet the demands of exercising muscles. This process involves the breakdown of glucose or glycogen to pyruvic acid (in the process of glycolysis). Pyruvic acid is then converted to lactic acid. Through an 11-step process there is an overall gain in ATP produced. This ATP is then available to provide energy for muscle contraction.

Many athletes have an anaerobic training programme in addition to aerobic training programmes. Assessment of the sportsperson's anaerobic training regime is important for assessment of sports injury. Anaerobic exercise requires a higher intensity than aerobic exercise. The duration of the workouts is often shorter and the workouts are often less frequent. Often, anaerobic exercise is the predominant feature of the sportsperson's secondary sport, as in weight-training.

The FITT assessment principle can also be applied to the anaerobic training regime. A very effective way to train the anaerobic energy system is 'interval training'. This involves a series of highly intense activities followed by periods of rest. An example of interval training is the bicycle ergometer interval training technique, in which the sportsperson cycles extremely hard against resistance for a set period of time. When the time elapses, the person stops exercising and rests for the same amount of time. This process is repeated for a predetermined number of times. By adjusting the frequency, intensity, time and technique it is possible for the sportsperson to alter the anaerobic training effect achieved.

Most sportspeople combine both aerobic and anaerobic exercise in training programmes. This combination ensures that both stamina and strength are improved, which in turn will improve the athlete's performance in sport. Muscle function will be improved, partly as a result of increased energy availability resulting from anaerobic training, and partly due to increased muscle tone and strength due to muscle overload.

## Footwear assessment

Sports footwear shows signs of wear more rapidly than walking shoes. Wear patterns may be characteristic of functional foot pathology and should be noted.

Specific sports and exercises place particular demands on footwear. The sports shoe should always be chosen with the sport in mind. The qualities of a sports shoe include:

- light weight
- provision of shock absorption
- good fastening
- overall comfort
- rearfoot stability.

Certain sports may require additional qualities, for example footwear used by the sprinter may necessitate firm ground-grip and usually has a spiked sole. Field sports often require studded-soled shoes to give a firm grip on a muddy surface. Road and track sports often require shoes with a flexible but shock-absorbing sole. Cycling requires shoes that clip on to the pedal, restricting foot and ankle movements in the transverse and frontal planes.

The shoe acts as an interface between the patient's foot and the ground. Through its presenting wear patterns, the practitioner may interpret the way in which the foot reacts to these ground reaction stresses.

The basic details of age, size, shape and type of shoe are important to take into consideration. An old, worn-out shoe will offer little protection to the wearer during sporting activity. If the size and shape is wrong for the foot, injury may be more likely. Excessive lateral heel wear will sustain an undesirable inversion position at heel strike. A crushed heel counter will result in inadequate rearfoot control and therefore affect heel stability. Worn-out soling that has perished will affect the physical properties, e.g. water resistance, shock attenuation, stiffness. A toe box loses its strength and protection if it is crushed in storage. Shoes that fall into disrepair offer a lower level of safety for the wearer. The practitioner must make the message clear to any athlete: poor footwear leads to reduced performance and safety.

There have been many developments in the design and manufacture of shoes in proportion to the growth of sport and exercise amongst the general population. There are now hundreds of different styles and types of shoe for various sports and for people of all ages. This in itself may present problems for the patient. Many sports shoes are marketed as multipurpose and many include particular gimmicks and features. Common among these are devices that purport to aid shock attenuation, devices that allow the first ray to plantarflex and additions to 'control' or influence subtalar joint motion. Other devices are marketed through their special fastening systems or air-filled insoles. Such shoes are not necessarily designed with the sportsperson in mind, but have been launched on a fashion-conscious market. As a result of the demand for high-fashion sports shoes, the sports footwear industry is now a multi-million-pound operation. This is reflected in the high prices attached to certain shoes. As a general rule the higher the price the more likely the addition of frills and gimmicks. High heel counters were introduced in the 1980s with tags to pull shoes on. Such modifications may result in skin lesions over the tendo achilles and may have to be trimmed before use.

The best sports shoe, particularly for running, is not always the most expensive. Indeed, some of the more expensive running shoes, with their anti-pronatory devices and shock-absorbing modifications, may cause problems for the wearer. The basic requirements of the running shoe are minimal, but it is essential for it to have a shock-absorbing sole. Ethyl vinyl acetate (EVA) is an excellent shock absorber and is used for the soles of the cheapest running shoes. One problem with EVA is its tendency to deform and 'bottom out' after about 500 miles. Regular replacement of cheaper shoes may be desirable, and may prove cheaper than expensive footwear with various modifications that may not be helpful to all sportspeople. Careful examination by a professional is advised wherever the foot type suggests a complicated biomechanical problem.

Sports shoes must always be correctly fitted. Assessment of the patient's foot size and the size of the shoes is an important part of the footwear appraisal. A shoe which is too small for the foot is likely to lead to forefoot pathology and damage to the nail structure. Shoes that are too tight may interfere with the normal elongation of the foot that takes place on pronation, and therefore affect shock absorption. Conversely, a shoe that is too big for the foot is likely to cause blistering and may become detached from the foot during exercise, causing the patient to fall and sustain injury.

The mode of fastening of the shoe is an important consideration. Sports shoes should be adequately fastened (preferably with laces) to avoid the foot slipping forward and causing digital impaction within the toe-box. On the other hand, laces should not be so tight as to cause trauma to the dorsum of the foot. It is sometimes useful to examine the foot for tell-tale pressure points from shoes that have been fastened too tightly or that are too small.

## Sole and upper wear marks

In order for this part of the footwear assessment to be useful, it is important to determine the age and duration of wear of the shoes. All shoes at some time or other will show some degree of wear. The important indicators are the pattern of wear and the speed at which wear occurred. Heavy heel wear may be indicative of a particularly heavy heel strike, or excessive subtalar joint pronation. Uneven forefoot wear may indicate a plantarflexed metatarsal, compensatory forefoot shear or limitation of metatarsophalangeal joint motion. Examination of the shoe uppers is just as important as examination of the sole; medial bulging of the upper might be indicative of excessive subtalar pronation. A hole, or wear of the upper, around the hallux may indicate a hyperextended hallux or overuse of extensor hallucis longus, with risk of deformation to the nail plate (Ch. 10).

## Medical history

So far the likely extrinsic and psychological intrinsic causes associated with the patient's complaint have been discussed. In this section comment is directed to the place of medical history taking. The medical history has been comprehensively considered in Chapter 5 and should be applied to all patients. Medical assessment of the sports patient is regarded as essential in determining their suitability to participate in sporting activities. The medical history may also result in an increased susceptibility to injury.

Particular attention should be paid to the patient's current health status, i.e. any current illnesses, injuries or diseases and the remaining effects of previous pathology. When questioning the patient about medical history it is valuable to determine when the medical condition started to be a problem, what symptoms were present, when treatment was first sought, who was consulted and where treatment was carried out. It is also a good idea to obtain the name, department and hospital or clinic address of any specialist with whom the patient still maintains regular contact.

Details of medication should include prescription and non-prescription systemic and topical medication. It is important to include details of recent drug therapy, especially medication stopped within the last few months. This is especially important in the case of drugs which have a latent effect or a long half-life, or are indicative of particular intermittent disease processes as in depression. Details of any previous adverse drug reactions should be included. Non-steroidal anti-inflammatory drugs are popular for the management of sports injuries, but these drugs are contraindicated for patients with peptic or duodenal ulceration and should be used with caution in asthmatics.

Determining someone's fitness for sport is often a difficult assessment to make. However, injury is likely if a patient participates in unaccustomed strenuous activity with little preparation. Similarly, an unfit person is more likely to suffer from sporting injury than a well-prepared sportsperson with good cardiovascular fitness and muscle strength. Often these patients raise their mean heart rate (MHR) to 80% very quickly, and maintain it for longer than necessary. The result can lead to the patient experiencing exhaustion and severe muscle pain following such exercise.

Various tests of the patient's fitness may be carried out. The aim of fitness tests are to determine whether the patient achieves 70–80% MHR and to monitor speed of recovery of heart rate to resting heart rate following cessation of exercise. A very simple test which may be carried out by the sports practitioner using a treadmill or cycle ergometer is the 'talk test'. The patient is instructed to run or cycle for a period of time associated with their usual exercise. If at the end of the exercise test (whilst still exercising) the patient can talk to the practitioner, then it is likely that the patient's MHR does not exceed 70–80%. However, if the patient becomes breathless and cannot hold a conversation, then it is likely that the MHR has exceeded 80% and the exercise regime has been too intense or has lasted too long. This indicates that the patient's aerobic schedule is too rigorous.

Warning—never carry out a talk test or other test of fitness using motorised treadmills or ergometers on patients with suspected cardio-vascular or peripheral vascular disease. If in doubt about a patient's fitness to undergo exercise stress tests, liaison with the general practitioner is essential.

Fitness for sport also includes assessment of the patient's overall physical condition. Assessment of the patient's height and weight should be carried out. Percentage body fat measurements can be carried out using calibrated callipers. Patients who are assessed as overweight may be unsuitable for particular high impact sports, as excess weight would place excessive stresses and predispose lower limb structures to injury. Obviously these sportspeople tend to lose weight as a result of controlled aerobic exercise and may increase the intensity or type of activity they participate in as their overall fitness and condition improves.

### Nutritional needs

Assessment of the patient's diet is often worthwhile. Professional athletes in particular pay special attention to their diet. Generally, a balanced diet is essential for health and performance. Assessment of the patient's diet will occasionally be necessary in cases of suspected malnutrition, vitamin deficiency syndromes or rapid weight change.

The main functions of foodstuffs are:

* Provision of energy
* Growth and repair of body tissues
* Regulation of body processes.

Provision of energy is satisfied by carbohydrates, fats and to some degree proteins. Growth and repair of body tissues is satisfied by proteins, vitamins and minerals. Regulation of body processes is satisfied by minerals, fibre and water.

By selecting foodstuffs from all of the above groups, an individual should obtain enough essential nutrients to satisfy their needs. If the sports practitioner suspects that diet and nutrition are unsatisfactory, referral to a dietician might be considered.

### Specific medical conditions

Patients with diabetes mellitus participating in exercise programmes may suffer complications. Unaccustomed exercise in patients with diabetes can cause a sudden rise in glucose demand and a correspondingly sharp decline in blood glucose levels. If the patient is receiving regular injections of insulin, this can result in exercise triggering a hypoglycaemic coma. Most diabetic patients will realise when their blood sugar level is decreasing and, if exercising, will carry oral glucose solution or tablets to deal with hypoglycaemia. Diabetic patients should be encouraged to take part in exercise, but may need to adjust insulin levels, decrease the number of units of insulin injected prior to their activity and be prepared with glucose during or shortly after sporting activity.

Patients with peripheral vascular disease also present a particular problem. It is unlikely that someone with advanced peripheral vascular disease with symptoms of intermittent claudication, nocturnal or rest pain will be participating in sport. However, patients with mild ischaemia and peripheral venous disorders may take part in sporting activity and may suffer unusual complications or injury. Exercise invariably causes a rise in temperature of musculature and skin and therefore increases the metabolic rate of tissues. This increased metabolic rate places a demand on the vascular system to supply blood and nutrients to the active tissue and to drain metabolites away into the systemic circulation. If there is mild arterial occlusion or vasospastic disorders such as Raynaud's phenomenon then arterial supply may be unable to meet these demands, resulting in local tissue hypoxia. Clinical features of ischaemia include coldness, pallor, pulselessness and cramping pain. This may affect the whole of the lower limb, e.g. calf, medial arch, or even a single digit. Ischaemic pain may only be apparent on exercise and exertion, and is an important differential diagnosis for many other conditions, e.g. shin splints, metatarsalgia, plantar fasciitis.

Patients with joint disease also require careful assessment. There appears to be an increasing tendency for exercise to be advocated for the management and rehabilitation of patients with joint disease. Much of this rehabilitation will be supervised by physiotherapists who have particular skills in this area. Radiographs may prove useful in the assessment of patients with joint pain, to ascertain the extent of degeneration to articular surfaces. Degenerative joint pathology may occur secondary to functional biomechanical pathology or impact injury, and it is important for the assessment to highlight functional or traumatic arthropathies. Unilateral arthropathies may result in an antalgic (avoiding pain) gait and running style, which may ultimately contribute to injury on the unaffected limb.

Patients with neurological lesions may also require assessment for sporting injury. Upper or lower motor neurone disease should be identified if clinical features are present (Ch. 7). Neurological lesions can result in a cavoid foot type, which produces inefficient contact-phase shock absorption. During normal walking activity this deficient shock absorption may not be a problem. However, if the patient places additional stress through the lower limb, such as that arising from running, then absorption of shock may become a problem.

The patient's medical status is important in order to help prevent injury. The patient is placed at risk from injury or complications when suffering from obesity, joint disease, diabetes and other metabolic problems affecting the skeleton or endocrine system. Predisposing factors like diabetes or joint disease cannot be eliminated, but safe continuance of athletic activity is to be encouraged providing such exercise does not increase the risk of injury, ischaemia or avoidable collapse. The goal of good assessment and management must determine the optimum conditions for both sporting and recreational activities. Discussion with the patient about such risk factors and the appropriateness of their chosen sport can often go some way to preventing injury and complications of existing disease processes.

Medical history taking should never be rushed or overlooked; to do so could mean time wasted in unnecessary assessment or inappropriate treatment. At worse, a poor medical history could result in the patient suffering recurrence of injury, permanent injury or adverse reaction to treatment.

## LOCOMOTOR ASSESSMENT

The structure of the body and foot need to be assessed to determine whether injury has occurred or is likely to occur as a result of compensatory or overuse syndromes (Ch. 8). It is necessary to consider whether an individual's structure is a causative or predisposing factor to injury. Biomechanical abnormalities may be present, but their relevance to injury needs to be determined.

The aim of the orthopaedic assessment is to gain an overall understanding of mechanical function by assessing joint position and range, direction, quality and symmetry of joint motion. From the locomotor assessment it is then possible for the practitioner to form a clear idea of the role of the patient's anatomical and biomechanical structure in relation to function and factors responsible for injury.

Locomotor assessment should consist of observation, active and passive movement, movement against resistance and palpation; this will include the manoeuvres look, feel and move. Initially, it is useful to view the patient walking or running to avoid any preconceived ideas about joint problems, limb-length discrepancies or skin lesions on the foot.

### Assessment of gait

A major component of the assessment of the sports patient is analysis of gait. Several options for gait analysis exist:

- Walking gait analysis
- Treadmill running analysis
- In-activity analysis.

The objective of gait analysis is to gain an appreciation of how the patient's foot functions during gait. This includes an appreciation of biomechanical compensatory mechanisms and muscle activity.

The walking gait analysis is a good starting point. The patient is asked to walk up and down a corridor, or on a treadmill. It is probably more effective to allow the patient time to acclimatise to the new walking environment before analysis begins. Examination is aided by video-recording a number of gait cycles. A good quality video camera with high-speed shutter and a video recorder capable of quality slow motion and freeze frame is desirable. The patient may initially feel embarrassed or uncomfortable by being filmed in this way. The practitioner needs to be mindful of the patient's self-consciousness and should appreciate the effect this may have on the normal gait pattern.

Running gait analysis is particularly useful. This is rather more important than recording slower velocity movement as the patient's pathology may be more easily identified following a period of time at a constant velocity. In cases such as this it is important to gain an estimate of either time or distance into the run at which pain first becomes noticeable. For accurate analysis of running it is essential to use a treadmill. Video recording is an essential part of assessment as the human eye cannot assimilate information fast enough beyond simple walking. The patient is then left to run on the treadmill for a period of time close to that which would result in pain. A video recording is made which includes film of the beginning, middle and end of the run. Some treadmills simulate uphill activity by raising the front of the treadmill to a preset gradient. This is useful for analysis of pain that is noticeably worsened by uphill runs.

Analysis of the patient's gait may also be undertaken by observing the patient participating in his/her usual sporting activity. This can be done in a variety of ways. Firstly, it is possible for the practitioner to directly observe patients taking part in their sports by attending runs, sports meetings or games. Direct observation is then possible, with or without video camera recording. The advantage of this technique is that it enables the practitioner to gain direct knowledge of how the patient functions during sport. Analysis is interactive in the sense that the practitioner can change position to observe the patient from different angles. If injury is present, or pain becomes evident during the sporting activity, then the practitioner will have seen the events leading up to pain. The main disadvantage of this method of analysis is that it is extremely time-consuming.

An alternative technique for the examination of a patient's gait during sport is to ask the patient to provide an amateur video recording of his/her activity and performance. Most people, if asked, will be able to arrange for loan of a camcorder and persuade a friend or preferably a fellow sportsman to video them taking part in sport. The video cassette can then be viewed on equipment with slow motion and freeze frame facilities to help with gait analysis. The obvious advantage of this technique is that the practitioner does not have to attend the event and can view the video recording during a clinical session.

Whichever technique is used, the practitioner should aim to observe the following:

- Posture of torso/shoulders during sporting activity
- Any shoulder or spinal positional abnormalities
- Any restrictions of motion at pelvis, hip or knee
- Transverse plane motion of the leg (knee)
- Shock absorption including signs of heavy heel strike
- Early or delayed heel lift
- Excessive subtalar joint pronation with medial bulging of the navicular
- Midtarsal joint hypermobility, shape of lateral border
- Action of the toes, including signs of hyperextension (when barefoot or distortion of uppers)
- Forefoot motion, including abductory twist
- Function of the first ray and hallux, including any sign of medial roll-off
- Muscle activity, including signs of overactivity of tibialis anterior/posterior

### Referred pain

Pain syndromes are covered in Chapter 16.

Referred pain is an important cause of pain in the foot. Findings may suggest pain referred from the sacral or lumbar plexus. Muscle weakness may occur as a result of lower-motor neurone damage. Examination of the back must not be ignored; any relevant injuries associated with the vertebral column should be identified.

## Non-weightbearing examination

Following a short warm-up period, the patient is laid supine on a flat examination couch. Once in this position, systematic examination of the patient from waist to toe may be performed.

An appreciation of quality of motion (QOM), symmetry of motion (SOM), direction of motion (DOM) and range of motion (ROM) of the joints should be obtained. While taking joints through their ranges of motion, the practitioner may assess muscular strength by asking the patient to resist passive motion.

A structured approach to examination of the lower limbs is important and may highlight areas for further, more detailed, investigation. The examination should include hips, knees, tibiae, ankles, rearfoot to leg, forefoot to rearfoot, first rays and toes.

By aligning the legs with the torso, a leg-length discrepancy may be diagnosed by observing the level of the knee joints and the malleoli. If a difference in leg length is suspected, a tape measure can be used to measure from the anterior superior iliac spine to the medial malleolus or xiphisternum or umbilicus to the medial malleolus (Ch. 8). Small values of difference have a greater effect on the human frame at higher velocities than when standing or walking. This is based on the simple equation: force is proportional to mass and acceleration, according to Newton's second law of motion.

With the patient in the supine position, it is possible to appreciate any frontal plane deformities, e.g. coxa vara or valga, or genu varum or valgum. Internal and external rotation at the hip may be assessed and any limitation of motion investigated.

Knee joint assessment is particularly important: around 10% of all sports injuries affect the knee (Table 15.2). Medial and lateral stability of the knee should be assessed for medial or lateral collateral ligament strength and capsular integrity. Anterior and posterior cruciate ligaments should also be assessed, as should the knee menisci. Abnormal patella position or tracking should be examined and noted. Compression of the patella, with or without active quadriceps contraction, may help to detect symptoms associated with maltracking or retropatellar damage. With the patella in a neutral position—neither internally or externally positioned—the tibiae may be examined to identify frontal plane deformity, i.e. tibial varum or valgum. An increase in the curvature of the lower third of the tibiae (tibia vara) will cause the foot to be presented to the ground in an inverted position. Compensation for this position will usually take place by subtalar joint pronation, which enables the medial border of the foot to ground contact.

General assessment of joint ligamentous stability is also important. A joint which has lax ligaments, or where ligamentous injury has taken place, may have a large or abnormal range or direction of motion.

The ankle (talocrural) joint should be examined and any limitation of dorsiflexion or plantarflexion noted. A limitation of dorsiflexion may result in an early heel-off and affect the foot's stability during the contact phase. This joint is essential for multidirectional sports and should be examined to ensure all anatomical sites are normal. Anterior–posterior drawer test, lateral stress ·test and special attention to the talar plafond and posterior Stieda process should be considered where pain is present. The use of arthroscopy is becoming popular as a investigation for painful syndromes associated with the ankle.

The relationship of the rearfoot to the leg can be assessed by bisecting the lower third of the tibia and the posterior surface of the calcaneus. When the subtalar joint is placed in its neutral position with the midtarsal joint maximally pronated, it is possible to see whether the calcaneus is inverted or everted in relation to the leg. In addition, an appreciation of the range of motion of the subtalar joint will help to identify any functional deformity.

The forefoot to rearfoot relationship is also an important factor as a forefoot varus or valgus may result in compensatory subtalar pronation with resultant lower-limb pathology. Similarly, the sagittal position of the first ray and the quality of its motion can help to identify functional abnormality and compensatory motion.

It is important to remember that assessment of the lower limb should involve soft-tissue assessment. Observation for any swelling or redness may indicate sites of inflammation or acute injury. Swelling with no apparent redness might indicate chronic injury. Assessment of muscle bulk is important. Muscle bulk, particularly of the thigh and calf, should be examined and any asymmetry of mass noted.

## Weightbearing examination

**Head and torso:** Starting at the head, the position at which the head is held may yield information relating to abnormal curvature of the cervical spine. The shoulders and spine may be considered together. Imbalance in shoulder height (shoulder drop) should be noted, and might indicate either spinal scoliosis, hemiplegic paralysis or severe limb-length discrepancy. The spine may be assessed by asking the patient to touch his/her toes. From the back, obvious spinal deformity may be apparent and this may be accentuated by observing the shape of the spine as the patient moves upright from this flexed position. Observation of any muscle spasm in the back may be relevant to further assessment findings.

**Pelvis:** Observation of the pelvis in the relaxed calcaneal stance position may show abnormalities of position. Palpation of the anterior superior iliac spines may show whether there is a right- or left-sided frontal plane tilt to the pelvis. Often this is a result of a spinal scoliosis, or secondary to a limb-length discrepancy. Any excessive transverse plane rotation of the pelvis may occur as a result of spinal kyphosis and may lead to further compensatory changes in the lower-limb, e.g. genu recurvatum attempting to gain greater extension of the knee.

**Hip and lower limb overview:** Looking at the thighs, the muscle appearance and bulk should be compared. The knees are observed for any positional abnormalities, e.g. hyperextension or relaxed flexed position. The patella may serve as a useful indicator of transverse plane position, i.e. is the knee internally rotated or externally rotated? An assessment of the Q angle may also be made at this point (Ch. 8). This is a measurement which represents the pull of the quadriceps muscles on the patella and its influence on patella tracking and alignment. The Q angle is formed from the anterior superior spine of the pelvis to a vertical line through the midpoint of the patella and a line from the centre of the patella to the centre of the tibial tubercle. It should be measured in the weightbearing position. A large Q angle is seen in patients with genu valgum and coxa vara. The shape of the pelvic girdle is associated with a larger Q angle in females than males. The Q angle can also be increased by subtalar pronation bringing about closed kinetic chain internal rotation of the tibia. An abnormal Q angle can lead to patellar malalignment syndrome and pain in the anterior knee and peripatellar pain. The relaxed calcaneal position can also be useful to determine if the legs and knees show any frontal plane positional abnormalities. Knock knees (genu valgum), bowed knees (genu varum) or bowing of the tibia (tibia vara) may be seen in the relaxed position and may exert an influence on overall lower limb function and result in compensation.

**Feet and ankles:** The angle and base of gait should be observed and excessive abduction or adduction of the feet noted. An abducted angle of gait may show a lowering of the medial longitudinal arch and a medial 'roll-off' when walking. An adducted foot might lead to excessive pressure on the lateral aspect of the foot during the propulsive phase of gait, or may lead to compensatory subtalar joint pronation. The position of the subtalar joint may be determined in the relaxed calcaneal stance position from the front, rear and sides. A pronated subtalar joint will be detected by eversion of the calcaneus. A flattening of the medial longitudinal arches, visible from the sides, supports the observation of subtalar joint pronation, as does medial bulging of the navicular.

**Forefoot:** Abnormalities of midtarsal joint and forefoot position may also be detected in the relaxed calcaneal stance position, particularly the transverse plane position of the forefoot. An adducted or abducted forefoot might indicate congenital deformity or midtarsal joint compensatory motion. Determination of rigid or flexible flat foot is essential. *Jack's test*, discussed in Chapter 14, offers a guide to presence of a flexible flat foot. Dorsiflexion of the great toe will invoke the windlass mechanism and the arch will rise. This will not happen when the foot is rigid. The dorsal humping of the metatarsal cuneiform bones across the midfoot can give rise to footwear problems, especially if the patient has an existing bursa overlying a bony exostosis. Position of the toes in the relaxed calcaneal stance position should be noted, as should any hyperextended digital positions or flexion deformities, and may be indicative of abnormal intrinsic muscle function or excessive pronation.

## VASCULAR, NEUROLOGICAL AND DERMATOLOGICAL ASSESSMENT

The other key systems—skin, nerve and blood supply—should be considered. The importance of examination has been covered in detail in the respective chapters. Differential diagnosis is essential and may well point to a systemic condition if trauma is not involved.

### Dermatology

Dermatological assessment may reveal skin and nail conditions which may themselves serve as clues to the underlying functional foot pathology. Hyperkeratosis in particular, and the exact location of lesions, can suggest a particular functional foot type. Plantar callus overlying the first and fifth metatarsal heads suggests a cavus or high arched foot type. The features of heavy callus can be associated with poor shock absorption. Trauma from sports footwear may leave

characteristic changes to the nail plate. Footballers and rugby players with tight boots often present with thickened toenails and sometimes with subungual haematoma. Similarly, long-distance runners may present complaining of accelerated wear of the toe-box of training shoes and discomfort of both hallux nails. This pattern is seen in patients who have plantarflexed first rays and a hyperextended hallux and can lead to onychauxis (thickened toenail) or subungual haematoma. The presence of mycotic infection such as tinea pedis or onychomycosis may suggest occlusive footwear, poor foot hygiene, or fatigue leading to hyperhidrosis.

Blistering of the skin is a common finding in sportspeople. Traumatic blisters occur where there is excessive shear placed upon the skin, leading to damage to the skin and creating local inflammatory changes. Occasionally, blisters may be filled with inflammatory exudate or blood, indicating deeper levels of damage. Blisters provide a useful indication of foot function and footwear suitability. The exact nature and site of blisters should always be noted.

## SUMMARY

The importance of a structured approach to the assessment of the sports patient should not be underestimated. Each practitioner should develop an assessment scheme which will ensure that all aspects of the patient's personal, medical, physical and sporting details are taken into consideration for diagnosis and subsequent treatment planning. Emphasis should be placed upon patient psychology. The time spent with the sportsperson can vary and may depend not only on the type of problem but the type of person.

Dealing with foot problems associated with sporting activities demands that the practitioner has some knowledge of the requirements of particular sports. It may not be surprising to learn that subsport specialties exist at highly competitive levels. It would be perfectly appropriate for practitioners to refer to colleagues who specialise in a particular area of sporting activity. In this latter respect many texts have been produced dealing with interests such as dancing and running. The easy availability of detailed knowledge about a range of sports means that sports enthusiasts are highly educated in their area of interest. This point is worth bearing in mind, as many patients will expect a special approach.

The practitioner should never underestimate the importance of the patient's role in the assessment process. The patient should be encouraged to understand the pathological processes and injury as well as the factors that have been responsible for the injury. In this way it is possible to educate the patient about how to avoid future injury.

REFERENCES

Cooper K 1968 Aerobics. Bantam Books, New York
Glasgow Royal Infirmary 1989 Incidence of sports injuries (personal communication)
Holmer P, Sondergaard L, Konradsen L, Nielsen P T, Jorgensen 1994 Epidemiology of sprains in the lateral ankle and foot. Foot and Ankle 15(2): 72–74

Kostrubula T 1976 Joy of running. J B Lippincott, New York
Morgan W P 1979 Negative addiction in runners. Physician Sports Medicine 7(2): 57
Subotnick S 1989 Sports medicine of the lower extremity. Churchill Livingstone, Edinburgh

# 16

# The painful foot

*P. Laing*

## INTRODUCTION

The painful adult foot may present from a rich diversity of sources. A painful foot is one which causes loss of normal function. Dysfunction may range from the occasional to constant manifestation and individuals will be affected differently. The variability from one person to another may often be described as the individuals having different pain thresholds. Patients often seek help after the problem has reached an inconvenient level of discomfort.

Pain may arise locally and be obvious; the pain from a hammer toe is unlikely to be confusing. Equally, pain may be diffuse, or perhaps referred from elsewhere. Pain described by the patient as being around the ankle joint but arising from the subtalar joint, a common trap in rheumatoid arthritis, or perhaps from a trapped nerve root in the back, is a challenge. To circumvent nature's attempts to confuse us we need a logical, systematic approach to each patient, remembering that the foot is an appendage which should not be considered in isolation.

The first step is to listen to the patient's own story (Chs 2 and 3). Let the patient show you where he/she feels the pain and where it is maximal. Patients have a poor understanding of anatomy and it is helpful if they indicate where pain in the 'ankle', 'foot', etc really is. This may localise the pain from, say, a fibular impingement syndrome, rather than taking the ankle as the global assumption. Patience in letting the patient explain the symptoms may stop you jumping to an erroneous diagnosis, asking only those questions which confirm your premature conclusion. The essential questions which will lead on to further questioning and examination prior to ordering specific tests, if needed, are:

- What was the patient doing? (injury)
- How long has this been present?
- Define the type of pain (e.g. sharp, dull, aching, intermittent or continuous)
- When does it arise? (time, activity, related to other source)
- What makes it worse or better?
- Recent treatments?
- Recent medical problems?

Some general information should be sought, such as occupation and whether the problem is related to an accident, either at work or elsewhere, for which there is any outstanding medicolegal claim. Regrettably, such patients may not recover fully until the claim is settled and you should be aware of this. Any previous operations on the foot are clearly relevant, but equally so are any spinal operations which potentially may have affected nerve roots causing sensory or motor loss in the lower limb. Similarly, a history of vascular surgery will cause you to carefully examine the circulation to the lower limb. The patient's general health, past and present, is relevant; for instance, rheumatoid arthritis and diabetes cause foot problems. Heart disease may cause bilateral ankle swelling in the patient with cardiac failure; unilateral swelling is more likely to be due to a local cause. Skin diseases such as psoriasis may be associated with arthritis in the foot, although the stigmata may be apparent elsewhere.

In all of these instances the history is guiding you towards a correct diagnosis, usually giving clues but sometimes trawling brightly coloured herrings to confuse and deceive. A thorough examination is essential to expose any such creatures.

## EXAMINATION

Your first observation should be to look at the patient, not the foot. It is useful to highlight those traits that have been discussed under medical history (Ch. 5) as the source of pain can be explained by general disease processes. These are listed below. Assess the patient's attitude. This may reveal psychological variations from normal and may influence the outcome in terms of treatment. General pointers concerning health include:

- Does the patient look well?
- Is the patient well nourished (obese or thin and wasted)?
- Colour (pale and anaemic, jaundiced)?
- Look at the hands (rheumatoid arthritis).

The physical examination may reveal findings that should bring about caution. For example, a manual worker who has thick calluses on his hands, yet says he cannot work because of the pain in his foot, may be less than fully honest.

Examination of the foot begins with watching the patient walk. While this has been mentioned in Chapter 8, the appearance of pain as an antalgic limp, when the patient will spend only a short time on the painful foot, is a clear positive sign. The limp may be linked with other problems associated with proximal joints or the back; these have to be excluded. Look at shoe wear on the sole. This may indicate an abnormal gait pattern. Are the toes severely clawed, suggesting a neurological problem?

The rest of the examination should follow the pattern of look, feel, move (Ch. 8). It is important to note any callosities, both dorsally and on the sole, as these indicate areas of high pressure and friction. Similarly, one must remember all the structures running under any area of tenderness.

The sources of pain are numerous (Table 16.1) and can be subdivided for convenience into problems affecting different tissues, generalised disorders and referred pain. The table provides an overview of typical problems associated with the painful foot. In many cases the origins are not clear and assessment and investigations are necessary to isolate the cause.

## ARTICULAR AND BONE CONDITIONS
## Osteoarthritis (OA)

Degenerative arthritis may affect any of the joints

**Table 16.1** Sources of pain classified under tissue types. The table provides an overview of typical problems associated with the painful foot. In many cases the origins are not clear and assessment and investigations are necessary to isolate the cause

| Condition | Aetiology |
|---|---|
| *Articular and bone* | |
| Osteoarthritis | General degeneration |
| Footballer's ankle | Chronic injury |
| Osteochondritis dissecans | Chronic injury |
| Hallux rigidus | General degeneration |
| Toe deformities | Congenital and acquired |
| Accessory ossicles | Congenital/injury |
| Stress fractures | Repetitive injury |
| Subungual exostosis | Repetitive injury |
| Exostoses | Injury/dislocation/ biomechanical |
| Tarsal coalition | Congenital |
| Metatarsalgia | General degeneration/referred/ multifactorial/rheumatoid |
| Sesamoiditis | Repetitive injury/degenerative |
| Bony or cartilaginous tumours | Neoplastic metastasis, primary or secondary |
| Periosteal/joint | Infective/neoplastic metabolic/ autoimmune reactive |
| *Soft tissue* | |
| Tendonitis Subluxing peroneal tendons Chronic ankle sprain Compartment syndrome | Most of these are associated with injury |
| Sinus tarsi | Degenerative/trauma or rheumatoid manifestation |
| Nodules | Dermatological/rheumatoid Ganglia/cysts |
| *Nerves* | |
| Tarsal tunnel | Degenerative/biomechanical |
| Peripheral neuropathies | Metabolic/endocrine/proximal entrapment or trauma |
| Interdigital neuromata | Repetitive injury and (Morton's) degenerative |
| Hereditary and motor sensory neuropathies (HMSN) | Congenital with hereditary predisposition |
| Radicular pain | Lumbar referred pain |
| *Vascular* | |
| Peripheral vascular disease | Socioenvironmental/endocrine and metabolic |
| Acute embolism | Secondary to other factors, e.g. atherosclerosis |
| Buerger's disease | Ethnic and social factors predispose to manifestation |

**Table 16.1**  (*Cont'd*)

| Condition | Aetiology |
|---|---|
| *Skin and subcutaneous* | |
| Retrocalcaneal bursitis | Repetitive injury/mechanical rheumatoid |
| Heel pad | Obesity/occupational referred from back |
| Plantar fasciitis | Repetitive injury, biomechanical |
| Onychocryptosis | Iatrogenic/congenital |
| Plantar warts | Infective |
| Callosity/corns | Biomechanical/deformity/ endocrine/footwear design |
| Ulcers | Vascular/infective/traumatic/ dermatological/neoplastic |

of the foot and ankle. The joints most commonly affected are the ankle, subtalar, calcaneocuboid, talonavicular, first tarsometatarsal and first metatarsophalangeal joint (MTPJ). The first MTPJ will be considered separately under the heading of hallux rigidus.

### Aetiology

This may be primary with no known cause but, while such arthritis is common in the hip and knee, it is rare in the ankle. Far more commonly OA is secondary to some insult to the joint and may follow major injury, such as a fracture extending into the joint, a dislocation or repeated minor trauma. Fractures of the neck of the talus may also lead to OA of the ankle.

Other causes can include:

- *Infection in the joint.* Septic arthritis, unless diagnosed and treated early, will lead to lysis of cartilage and secondary OA
- *Inflammatory arthropathies* such as rheumatoid arthritis and the seronegative arthritides, e.g. psoriatic arthritis, Reiter's disease and ankylosing spondylitis
- *Metabolic disorders* such as gout and pseudogout
- *Systemic diseases* such as diabetes mellitus, which can lead to Charcot foot or ankle; the ankle is affected in about 10% of Charcot foot cases

- *Proximal malalignment*, e.g. following a malunited fractured tibia, has frequently been stated to lead to arthritis by imposing abnormal stresses on distal joints. While some authors have allowed up to 10° in the sagittal or frontal plane (Nicoll 1964), others have felt that even a few degrees of angulation may lead to significant problems (Johnson 1987). Merchant disputed this in a long-term follow-up study when he could find no correlation between the degree of malunion and the occurrence of OA (Merchant & Dietz 1989)
- *Other miscellaneous conditions* such as haemophilia or avascular necrosis (Freiberg's disease affecting second metatarsal head).

### Presenting symptoms

Generally these will be pain and stiffness in the area of the affected joint. Symptoms may start as aching after exercise and progress to pain after walking a distance. With time and progression of the arthritis the distance the patient can walk without pain gradually reduces. Pain may become constant and also present at night, disturbing sleep. How much pain the patient is experiencing is important to know but quantifying pain is difficult, because individual patients will have different tolerances to pain and different attitudes to the degree of their disability. While one can ask the patient to quantify their pain on a visual analogue scale of, say, 1–10, it is function which probably influences us most when it comes to determining treatment. While one must beware the stoic who pushes him/herself on regardless of the pain (and vice versa), how much a patient can do is often a good indicator of how severe the symptoms are. Stiffness may initially occur after the joint has been rested for a while, but with time the range of movement in the affected joint will decrease. Dorsiflexion is usually the first movement to be lost and shoes with a slight heel raise may therefore be more comfortable. In severe OA the joint may completely lose movement and become virtually ankylosed. Patients may also complain of a limp, swelling or joint deformity.

### Signs

The joint may appear swollen or deformed or be held in an abnormal position. The joint may feel warm if the underlying cause is infection or an inflammatory arthropathy, but otherwise not. An effusion may be present in ankle OA but is not usually clinically detectable in OA of other foot joints. Osteophytes may be felt in superficial joints as hard bony swellings and represent new bone formation around the periphery of affected joints. Localised tenderness may also be found. The range of movement of the joint will be reduced, the degree depending on how advanced the arthritis is, and movement will be painful, more so at extremes. Often movement may feel 'dry', rather than smooth and easy. In advanced OA grating or crunching may be felt by the examiner as the joint is moved.

### Investigations

Plain X-rays, generally standing anteroposterior (AP for ankle, DP for foot) and lateral, are essential (Ch. 11). The cardinal signs of OA are reduced joint space, sclerosis, cysts and osteophytes (Fig. 11.27). Standing films are helpful as they may demonstrate deformity under load and the true loss of joint space due to cartilage erosion. Special views may be helpful to show the subtalar joint; Anthonsen's view shows the medial and posterior subtalar facets. If infection is suspected then any open wounds can be swabbed. Aspiration of the joint to obtain bacteriology may be helpful. Results from blood tests will be normal and are unhelpful unless the OA is secondary to a systemic disease, infection or metabolic cause such as gout (Ch. 13). Further to the discussion on pain it should be noted that the degree of X-ray change does not always correlate in a linear fashion with the patient's symptoms or disability. It is always important to treat the patient and not the X-ray.

### Differential diagnosis

In early OA, when X-rays are normal, a presumptive diagnosis may be made solely on information from the history, symptoms and signs. Other periarticular causes should be considered however. In established OA, with X-ray changes, the differential will usually lie in determining the underlying cause.

## Footballer's ankle

### Aetiology

This condition was well described by McMurray in 1950 and occurs in soccer players as a result of repeated kicking of the ball with the foot held in equinus (McMurray 1950). In this position the anterior capsule largely takes the strain, as the extensor tendons are mechanically disadvantaged, and bony traction spurs develop.

### Presenting symptoms

These will be pain, often on kicking a stationary ball, but also on dorsiflexion of the ankle. The patient may complain of some restriction of dorsiflexion.

### Signs

Local tenderness over the neck of the talus and anterior tibial margin; pain on dorsiflexion of the ankle and perhaps some restriction of this movement.

### Investigations

Plain X-rays will demonstrate a dorsal talar spur and also a spur on the anterior lip of the tibia. The spur on the anterior lip of the tibia can be subtle, appearing as a convex margin rather than the normal concave one (Fig. 16.1). Both these spurs are intracapsular although this may be difficult to appreciate on a plain X-ray.

### Differential diagnosis

This is mainly associated with early OA of the ankle. It should be noted, though, that in a true footballer's ankle the articular surfaces are normal

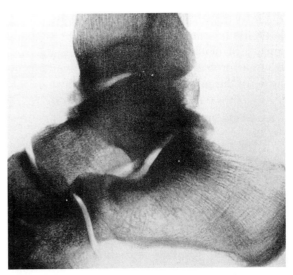

**Figure 16.1** X-ray showing footballer's ankle with an anterior tibial spur—lateral view.

when these bony spurs are removed surgically (Case history 16.1).

---

**Case history 16.1**

**Patient:** 24-year-old professional footballer.
**Presenting symptoms:** 1 year history of pain over dorsum of the right ankle. This had gradually increased and was painful especially when running. There was no history of instability. 3 months previously the patient had undergone removal of 'bony spur' by the club doctor, but symptoms had persisted and he was currently unable to play football.
**Signs:** Some discomfort on full dorsiflexion but no discernible loss of movement.
**Investigations:** Plain X-rays showed osteophytic lip to anterior margin of right tibia, with evidence of previous removal of talar spur.
**Diagnosis:** Partially treated footballer's ankle.
**Operative findings:** Arthroscopy showed synovitis of ankle and confirmed osteophytic anterior tibial margin. This was resected.
Postoperatively the patient made a good recovery and returned to the first team.

---

## Osteochondritis dissecans (ankle/talocrural joint)

### Aetiology

This is an interesting condition in which an osteochondral fragment becomes separated from the talar dome, usually posteromedially or mid-laterally. It is now thought that all of the lateral and most of the medial lesions originate from trauma, probably associated with inversion injuries of the ankle (De Smet et al 1990).

### Presenting symptoms

Because of the aetiology the diagnosis may be missed acutely and the patient treated for a simple sprain or malleolar fracture. If, however, symptoms persist after adequate treatment of the recognised injury, an osteochondral fracture should be suspected. Acute symptoms will be those of a sprained ankle, the patient complaining of pain, swelling and difficulty walking. Chronic symptoms are more general, with patients complaining of discomfort, pain and perhaps stiffness during or after exercise. If an osteochondral fragment has become detached from the talar dome then there may be locking and giving way in the ankle, suggestive of a loose body.

### Signs

Acute signs will include swelling and tenderness over the lateral ligament complex with pain on inversion of the ankle. It may be possible to locate tenderness over the talar dome mid-laterally or behind the medial malleolus.

### Investigations

AP, lateral and oblique (10° of medial rotation) plain X-rays of the ankle should initially be requested. Lateral lesions classically are shallow, horizontal and often detached or elevated. Medial lesions are frequently cup-shaped and deeper (Canale & Belding 1980), shown by line drawing in Figure 16.2. In the acute stage X-rays may appear normal, especially if the lesion is stage 1, i.e. only the articular cartilage is damaged (Berndt & Harty 1959). Even in a chronic lesion it may be difficult to detect any changes on plain X-ray. A bone scan is extremely useful as it will usually be positive. Magnetic resonance imaging (MRI) is the most sensitive, as well as the most expensive way of demonstrating the osteo-

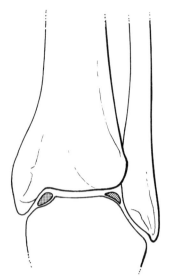

**Figure 16.2** Osteochondritis dissecans: line drawing of anterior view of the ankle mortice. Lateral lesions tend to be horizontal and shallow, medial ones tend to be deeper and cup-shaped.

chondral fractures. Blood tests are of no value in the investigation of this condition.

### Differential diagnosis

Acutely this will be the co-existent trauma. Chronically it will be other conditions around the ankle such as anterolateral impingement syndrome, tendinitis of any of the tendons crossing the ankle joint and early OA.

## Hallux rigidus

### Aetiology

Hallux rigidus is a condition in which dorsiflexion of the MTPJ of the hallux is restricted and painful on movement. Plantarflexion may also be limited but dorsiflexion is the functional movement affected by the pathology. It may occur secondary to an osteochondritis dissecans of the first metatarsal head in adolescents, usually females. In adults males tend to predominate and it can be secondary to a systemic disease such as RA or gout, but most commonly is primarily due to a local arthritic degeneration. Various theories have been advanced for the primary cause, such as a long first metatarsal and hallux and repeated minor trauma; patients tend to have pronated, narrow, long feet with a flat longitudinal arch. Hallux plexus was a term originally used to describe hallux rigidus. It is now used in connotation with a severe form where the proximal phalanx becomes flexed at the MTPJ and the first metatarsal becomes secondarily elevated.

### Presenting symptoms

Intermittent pain in adolescents, who may experience episodes of acute pain made worse by walking. Adults present with pain on walking, stiffness and pain over the dorsal exostosis in more advanced cases, although lateral joint pain may be observed as well.

### Signs

The hallux is commonly straight and a dorsal bony prominence, with perhaps a bunion (soft bursa swelling), may be found. Locally there may be some tenderness over the exostosis and around the first MTPJ. The range of movement should be assessed with the foot in a plantigrade position but also in a plantarflexed position. A grind test, in which the hallux is compressed longitudinally with rotation, may be painful where the joint is not stiff. In advanced cases compensatory secondary hyperextension of the interphalangeal joint (IPJ) may be found and commonly there is a callosity on the medial plantar aspect of the head of the proximal phalanx or base of the distal phalanx.

### Investigations

Plain X-rays of the first MTPJ may be normal or show a dorsal exostosis with a normal-looking joint (Figs 11.27 and 11.28). In more advanced cases degenerative changes will be apparent with progressive OA. If hallux rigidus is due to gout or RA then periarticular erosions may be present with osteoporosis. Blood tests are only indicated if a systemic disease is suspected.

### Differential diagnosis

In flexor hallucis longus tenosynovitis, dorsiflexion of the hallux may be restricted and painful. Resisted plantarflexion of the hallux will be painful and local tenderness may be felt posterior to the medial malleolus.

## Accessory ossicles

### Aetiology

There are at least 15 accessory ossicles around the foot and ankle (Romanowski & Barrington 1991). Most are anatomical variants in origin (Fig. 11.18). Only two are rarely likely to cause symptoms. Around the hindfoot there is the *os trigonum*, on the posterior aspect of the talus close to the lateral tubercle, and the *accessory navicular* (Figs 16.3 and 11.19). The type II accessory navicular is roughly 1 cm in size and united to the main body of the navicular by a synchondrosis of about 12 mm (Romanowski & Barrington 1991).

### Presenting symptoms

The os trigonum causes symptoms with activities in repeated plantar flexion, affecting football

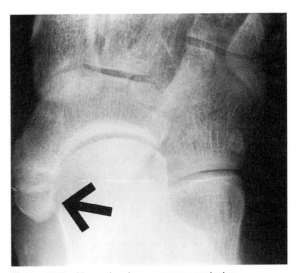

**Figure 16.3**   X-ray showing accessory navicular—dorsiplantar view

players and dancers standing 'en pointe'. Patients complain of posterolateral ankle pain when the ankle is plantarflexed and impingement occurs. An accessory navicular may cause rubbing in a shoe, because of local pressure, or may become symptomatic following a twisting injury to the foot.

### Signs

With a symptomatic os trigonum tenderness may be felt behind the lateral malleolus and peroneal tendons and forced passive plantarflexion of the ankle will be painful. When an accessory navicular is present there will be local tenderness in association with a prominent navicular and perhaps pain on resisted inversion.

### Investigations

Plain X-rays will demonstrate the presence of accessory ossicles but their presence is not proof of their guilt. A bone scan may help to demonstrate a symptomatic os trigonum.

### Differential diagnosis

A symptomatic os trigonum may be mistaken for peroneal tendinitis, flexor hallucis longus tendinitis or a fracture of the lateral process of the posterior talar tubercle. A symptomatic accessory navicular is usually obvious because of local tenderness but should not be confused with tibialis posterior tendinitis.

## Stress fractures

### Aetiology

Stress fractures occur due to overuse in unadapted feet or when surgery in the foot leads to high stresses elsewhere. Fractures have been reported in groups such as runners, army recruits and dancers. They may also occur, though rarely, after first ray surgery, e.g. Keller's excisional arthroplasty operation, which increases stresses on the lesser metatarsals. From whatever cause the most common site is a metatarsal shaft. Stress fractures have also been reported in

the calcaneus, navicular, cuboid and proximal phalanx of the hallux.

### Presenting symptoms

Pain occurs in relation to activity. Initially it may be vague and difficult to localise but settles on rest. With time the patient may complain of a limp.

### Signs

In the early stages there may be little to find on clinical examination but if activity continues then local tenderness and swelling will develop. A limp may be present.

### Investigations

Plain X-rays may often be normal in the early stages and it can be 2–3 weeks before changes become apparent for metatarsal stress fractures and up to 5 weeks for calcaneal ones. In the metatarsal shafts early changes may be a fine line of bone resorption followed either by sclerosis or periosteal callus, depending on whether the cortex has been breached. In the calcaneum the fractures tend to occur in the posterior part and appear as endosteal callus with an intact cortex on X-ray. Because of the delay in plain radiographs a bone scan may be helpful if there is doubt about the diagnosis. CT or MRI scans may be helpful to show stress fractures which are difficult to depict on plain X-ray.

### Differential diagnosis

The clinical picture, relation to activity and local tenderness should point towards the correct diagnosis. One should beware metatarsal 'stress fractures' in the diabetic as they may be the precursor of a Charcot foot.

## Subungual exostosis

### Aetiology

This is a bony spur usually arising from the dorsomedial aspect of the distal phalanx of the hallux. Rarely it may arise from the lesser toes. It is generally a benign osteochondroma, congenital in origin, and may be noticed from adolescence up to early middle age. There is some suggestion that those occurring in young adult athletes may be the result of repetitive minor trauma inside the shoe.

### Presenting symptoms

Patients may notice a swelling under the nail or may complain of pain on walking or running with shoes on.

### Signs

The nail may be elevated and there may be a darkish discoloration, resembling a haematoma, apparent under the nail. The distal nail edge may be elevated, suggesting an enlarged distal tuft.

### Investigations

Plain X-rays will show the exostosis. Medial oblique views are most helpful but DP and lateral may be required to establish the extent of the projection. As cartilage is not radio-opaque, the practitioner should not be lulled into thinking that the swelling is small (Fig. 11.32).

### Differential diagnosis

A subungual exostosis may be confused with other conditions, such as a glomus tumour or subungual wart.

## Tarsal coalition

### Aetiology

This is a congenital condition, inherited as an autosomal dominant trait in which adjacent tarsal bones have a fibrous, cartilage or bone connection or bridge which progressively restricts normal movement. This may be termed syndesmosis, synchondrosis or synostosis respectively and occurs in less than 1% of the population (Mosier & Asher 1984). Generally, it begins as a fibrous union in infancy and progresses to cartilaginous

and then bony union; however, it may remain fibrous. The most common coalition is probably talocalcaneal, followed by calcaneonavicular (Stormont & Peterson 1983). Although rare, most other possible combinations have been described.

### Presenting symptoms

Although these coalitions usually ossify between 8 and 16, symptoms may not develop until late childhood or into adulthood. Sometimes patients never develop symptoms and the diagnosis is made incidentally. When they do present, patients may complain of stiffness and ankle pain when playing sport. They may also complain of recurrent ankle sprains.

### Signs

Stiffness in the subtalar or midtarsal joint movements is usually the predominant sign. They may also have a valgus flatfoot with subtalar irritability, characterised by pain on forced plantarflexion of the ankle joint and some peroneal spasm. In childhood presentation like this is known as peroneal spastic flat foot.

### Investigations

Appropriate plain X-rays may demonstrate a coalition; DP, lateral and medial oblique films should be taken. Medial oblique views show the calcaneonavicular coalition (Fig. 16.4). A Harris axial view may show a talocalcaneal coalition. Dorsal beaking on the head of the talus is a secondary change to abnormal movement also suggesting this type of pathology (Case history 16.2). A long anterior calcaneal process may indicate a calcaneonavicular coalition although this coalition is usually well demonstrated on plain films (Fig. 11.35). If X-rays are not diagnostic then a CT scan in the frontal plane may confirm the diagnosis.

### Differential diagnosis

Other conditions leading to stiff subtalar or midtarsal joints, such as degenerative or inflammatory arthritis.

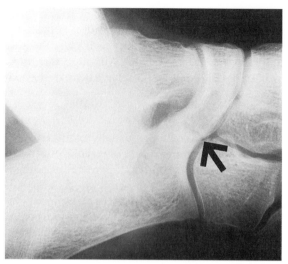

**Figure 16.4** X-ray illustrating calcaneonavicular coalition—medial oblique view.

---

**Case history 16.2**

**Patient:** 25-year-old female.
  **Presenting symptoms:** The patient had a history of bilateral flat feet since childhood. She was now getting pain on walking after half a mile which was interfering with normal living.
  **Signs:** There was a normal range of movement in both ankle joints but both subtalar joints were rigid; there was slight decreased range of movement in the midtarsal joints bilaterally.
  **Investigations:** Plain X-rays showed talar beaking bilaterally. A CT scan showed bony left talocalcaneal fusion. On the right there was virtual talocalcaneal apposition but bony fusion could not be demonstrated and a fibrous union was surmised.
  **Diagnosis:** Bilateral talocalcaneal tarsal coalition with secondary arthritic changes in the midtarsal joints.
  **Operation:** Planned staged triple arthrodeses to give the patient plantigrade pain-free feet for walking.

---

# Metatarsalgia

## Aetiology

Metatarsalgia is characterised by pain felt under one or more metatarsal heads when weight-bearing. It may be due to a number of causes:

- *Atrophy of the plantar fat pad with age.* This results in a generalised metatarsalgia because of loss of the cushioning effect of the fat pad

- *Increased pressure under the lesser metatarsals* following first MTPJ surgery, e.g. for hallux valgus or Keller's operation
- *Metatarsophalangeal joint problems.* Subluxation or dislocation of the proximal phalanx may lead to a pistoning effect which depresses the metatarsal head, increasing its load. This may occur in inflammatory arthropathies or in a cavus foot with claw toes. Claw toes that dorsiflex on the metatarsal head pull the fat pad forward, exposing the metatarsal head to greater loading during stance. Case history 16.3 illustrates the effect of hallux valgus on the forefoot
- *A prominent fibular (lateral) condyle on a metatarsal head* may cause a very local plantar callosity with pain on weightbearing
- *Proximal stiffness or malalignment*, e.g. a pes cavus foot, may lead to excessive loading on one side of the foot.

---

**Case history 16.3**

**Patient:** 58-year-old garage mechanic.
  **Presenting symptoms:** The patient presented with a large bunion on his left foot and discomfort under the centre of the ball of his foot on walking.
  **Signs:** A gross hallux valgus was present, along with pronation of the hallux. There was some callosity formation under the second and third metatarsal heads and discomfort on direct palpation of the heads. The rest of the foot was normal.
  **Investigations:** Plain X-rays showed a hallux valgus of 55° with lateral subluxation of the proximal phalanx at the first MTPJ. Some minor degenerative changes were present in this joint.
  **Diagnosis:** Gross hallux valgus with secondary transfer metatarsalgia due to unloading of the first ray.
  **Operation:** Arthrodesis of the first MTPJ to correct the hallux valgus and allow better weightbearing through the first ray, thus relieving the transfer metatarsalgia. Usually a secondary reduction in the intermetatarsal angle also occurs. Correcting gross hallux valgus is difficult with realignment (osteotomy) operations. Postoperatively the patient's symptoms were relieved.

---

## Presenting symptoms

Patients complain of pain under the ball of the foot on walking, made worse by walking barefoot. Well-padded shoes such as trainers can reduce symptoms effectively. Patients may also complain of hard skin continually building up under the foot which adds to the general discomfort.

### Signs

The main sign is tenderness under the metatarsal heads on palpation; callosities may be present under the symptomatic heads indicating the increased load. With a prominent fibular condyle the callosity is small and well-defined and has a central keratotic core. This may be described as a localised intractable plantar keratoma. The other type of callosity observed will be a diffuse lesion without a central keratotic core. Prominent metatarsal heads may be palpated and their degree of rigidity should be assessed, as should the mobility of the toes. It is important to assess the mobility of the proximal joints to ensure they are supple.

### Investigations

Plain X-rays will demonstrate evidence of any inflammatory arthropathy and any changes in a metatarsophalangeal joint. If available, dynamic pressure studies will show the distribution of pressure under the metatarsal heads. The plain X-ray view has not been shown to provide an objective measurement of metatarsal plantarflexion in the case of lesser metatarsals.

### Differential diagnosis

This lies between the various causes of metatarsalgia. A wart may cause a plantar callosity but does not normally occur under a metatarsal head. A Morton's neuroma is commonly referred to as Morton's metatarsalgia, although the pain and tenderness is actually between metatarsals, radiating into toes (digital neuritis).

## Sesamoiditis

### Aetiology

Flexor hallucis brevis inserts into the base of the proximal phalanx of the hallux and within its tendons two sesamoid bones lie under the first metatarsal head. These may give rise to pain if they become arthritic. This can occur secondary to hallux rigidus or inflammatory arthropathies such as rheumatoid arthritis. Chondromalacia-type changes have also been reported. Rarely, sesamoids may fracture following trauma and stress fractures have been reported. Hypertrophy of a sesamoid can lead to a painful plantar callosity.

### Presenting symptoms

Pain under the first metatarsal head on weight-bearing is the main symptom; patients may notice this particularly on toe-off.

### Signs

Tenderness may be localised to one or both sesamoids. Extension at the first MTPJ may be limited and painful and a plantar callosity may be present.

### Investigations

A standing DP and lateral X-rays should be taken and also a skyline view of the sesamoids. If X-rays are normal a bone scan may be helpful.

### Differential diagnosis

Other causes of pain around the first MTPJ, such as hallux rigidus. The high incidence of bipartite sesamoids (figures vary from 10–30%) may lead to a false diagnosis of a fracture (Hubay 1949).

## Tumours

### Aetiology

Bony or cartilaginous tumours are fortunately rare in the foot. Nevertheless a number have been reported, both benign and malignant. Among the most common benign ones are *osteoid osteoma*, *enchondroma* and *osteochondroma*. Osteoid osteomas may occur in the tarsus in the foot, enchondromas in metatarsals or phalanges

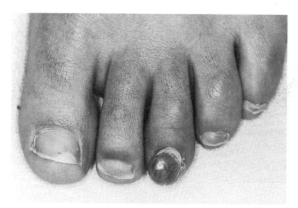

**Figure 16.5** Subungual exostosis on dorsum of third toe with gross nail displacement.

and osteochondromas normally only occur as subungual exostoses (Fig. 16.5). Malignant tumours reported include *osteosarcoma, chondrosarcoma* and *Ewing's tumour*. Osteosarcomas and chondrosarcomas have been reported in the tarsus and metatarsals, Ewing's in the tarsus. Although a secondary deposit is the most common bony tumour in the body as a whole, secondaries are rare in the foot but may occur. If they do the most likely primary is a bronchial carcinoma.

### Presenting symptoms

This will depend on the individual tumour. Osteoid osteomas tend to occur in young adults and classically give rise to night pain relieved by aspirin. Enchondromas may cause cortical thinning of a metatarsal and therefore present with acute pain from a pathological fracture. Malignant tumours may present with pain and/or swelling.

### Signs

These depend on the diagnosis and may vary from nil to tenderness and swelling from a pathological fracture.

### Investigations

Plain X-rays will demonstrate most of these lesions, showing areas of bone destruction, ex-

pansion or new bone formation. An osteoid osteoma may be seen as a central nidus with surrounding sclerosis, but can be very difficult to see and a bone scan may help by showing it as a concentrated hot spot. MRI is extremely helpful both in diagnosis and delineating the extent of a malignant tumour. Before any definitive treatment is planned a biopsy of the tumour is usually necessary. As well as imaging bony tumours, a full blood screen will usually be performed, along with a chest X-ray and bone scan, unless the tumour is simple and benign.

### Differential diagnosis

The first consideration with any lesion suspected of being a tumour is whether it is benign or malignant. Infection should always be considered as it may sometimes be difficult to differentiate. Although it should not cause any confusion in diagnosis, an old fracture may sometimes look suspicious to the untutored eye.

## SOFT TISSUE, TENDONS AND LIGAMENTS

## Tendinitis

### Aetiology

Peritendinitis may affect any of the tendons crossing the ankle into the foot but most commonly involves the tendo achilles and tibialis posterior. Achilles tendinitis occurs usually in young adults who are joggers or athletes. Tibialis posterior tenosynovitis (inflammation of its tendon sheath) normally occurs in late middle age. Less commonly, tenosynovitis of a peroneal tendon may occur and in dancers tenosynovitis of the flexor hallucis longus tendon can occur where it passes in a groove behind the talus.

### Presenting symptoms

Patients with peritendinitis will present with pain on exercise, usually along the course of the tendon; they may also notice some swelling. It is worth enquiring whether they have recently changed running shoes.

### Signs

In Achilles tendinitis the tendon will be painful to palpation about 5 cm proximal to its distal insertion; with time swelling and crepitus may be found. In tibialis posterior tenosynovitis there will be tenderness behind the medial malleolus with pain on resisted inversion and perhaps passive eversion. It is important to rule out ruptured tibialis posterior tendon. In this case the patient may present with vague pain on the medial aspect and a spontaneous flat foot. The hindfoot will be in valgus and the heel will not invert if the patient stands on tiptoe. When looked at from behind, the forefoot is abducted, producing the 'too many toes sign' (Johnson 1983).

For the peroneal tendons tenderness will be felt distal to the lateral malleolus, along the course of the tendons, with pain on inversion and plantar flexion. Differentiating between brevis and longus may be difficult; tenderness on the sole of the foot between the cuboid and base of the first metatarsal will suggest problems with peroneus longus. Evert the hindfoot actively against resistance to clarify such involvement.

In tenosynovitis of flexor hallucis longus there will be tenderness posterior to the medial malleolus with pain on passive extension of the hallux. Occasionally tenderness can be found at the level of the sesamoids and may cause limitation of movement at the first MTPJ.

### Investigations

Peritendinitis is largely a clinical diagnosis; if doubt exists then MRI may be helpful in showing fluid in the tendon sheath. Abolition of the patient's symptoms by injection of local anaesthetic may also be diagnostic.

### Differential diagnosis

In Achilles tendinitis it is important not to miss a rupture. Up to 25% of acute ruptures are missed (Lutter 1991). Similarly, with tibialis posterior, tenosynovitis rupture should be looked for. Tenderness at the insertion may be due to an accessory navicular.

## Subluxing peroneal tendons

### Aetiology

The peroneal tendons are held behind the lateral malleolus by the retinaculum and this may be ruptured in an acute injury. Following that the tendons are free to sublux.

### Presenting symptoms

The patient may complain of a painful snapping sensation at the ankle on certain movements.

### Signs

There will be tenderness along the peroneal tendons behind the lateral malleolus and the tendons may sublux anteriorly with resisted eversion and dorsiflexion.

### Investigations

Again, this is mainly a clinical diagnosis but if doubt exists then a peroneal tenogram may show dye leakage, indicating a torn retinaculum.

### Differential diagnosis

Acutely with a sprained ankle and more chronically with peroneal tenosynovitis.

## Chronic ankle sprain

### Aetiology

Chronic lateral pain following an acute inversion injury of the ankle is common, being reported in up to 50% of some patient groups (Ferkel et al 1991). This may be due to residual instability, causing recurrent sprains, but most commonly is due to soft tissue impingement in the lateral gutter. The initial sprain leads to inflammation, synovitis and then scar tissue and fibrosis.

### Presenting symptoms

Patients complain of pain over the anterolateral aspect of the ankle on walking, and often weakness and a feeling of giving way.

### Signs

Tenderness is present over the anterolateral gutter of the ankle. Ankle and subtalar joint movement is usually normal. Instability should be carefully looked for. Clinically this is done by comparing inversion between the two ankles and doing an anterior drawer test. In this test the patient lies supine with the knee flexed and the examiner sits on the patient's foot to stabilise it. The tibia is then pushed back on the talus. Instability is shown by excessive movement by comparison to the other ankle. A clunking sensation may be elicited sometimes. This may be a difficult test to do without the patient fully relaxed under a general anaesthetic.

### Investigations

Plain X-rays are usually normal but may show small bony spurs or calcification. Stress X-rays for instability will be normal. A bone scan may show mildly increased uptake and is only useful in excluding other causes of pain. MRI is the only tool which can show increased soft tissue in the lateral gutter.

### Differential diagnosis

Other local causes of pain should be excluded such as an osteochondral fracture, peroneal tendon problems and arthritis of the ankle joint.

## Sinus tarsi syndrome

### Aetiology

This condition was first described in 1958 by O'Connor, but has remained somewhat nebulous

(O'Connor 1958). It follows a sprained ankle which does not resolve in the normal time and may be due to degeneration of the fatty soft tissue in the sinus tarsi. Although such changes have been shown, in O'Connor's original series of 14 patients treated operatively histology of excised tissue was normal. Some consider that the condition represents a mild form of subtalar instability.

### Presenting symptoms

The patient will complain of chronic pain, situated laterally, following a sprained ankle.

### Signs

Apart from tenderness over the sinus tarsi there is little to find.

### Investigations

Plain X-rays will be normal. An injection of local anaesthetic into the sinus tarsi should provide some temporary relief of symptoms and is diagnostically useful.

### Differential diagnosis

Other causes of continued pain following a sprained ankle.

## Compartment syndrome

### Aetiology

The muscles and nerves in the leg are contained within four compartments each of which has fascial or fascial and osseous boundaries. The foot also has four compartments. A compartment syndrome results from ischaemia to muscles, and may involve nerves, secondary to raised pressure within that compartment. It may occur acutely following a fracture or soft-tissue trauma or chronically with symptoms after a certain level of exercise. Mild compartment syndromes are not infrequently missed following a fractured tibia and present with residual sequelae such as claw toes. Chronic compartment syndromes only will be discussed.

### Presenting symptoms

Chronic compartment syndromes of the leg will present with pain in the involved compartment after a degree of exercise, usually running. The pain settles on rest but symptoms may become worse with time. If the anterior compartment is involved then pain and paraesthesia may radiate into the dorsum of the foot and ankle from involvement of the superficial peroneal nerve. If the deep posterior compartment is involved then pain and paraesthesia over the sole of the foot, in the distribution of the posterior tibial nerve, may be felt.

### Signs

At rest physical examination may be normal, although there may be some tenderness over the distal tibia. This may become more marked if the patient exercises on a treadmill to produce symptoms.

### Investigations

Plain X-rays should be taken to exclude a stress fracture or other osseous causes of leg pain. Measuring compartment pressures with a catheter introduced under local anaesthetic is the most useful way to confirm the diagnosis.

Pressures are measured before and after exercise. There is some debate as to the correct abnormal compartment pressures. Generally, intracompartmental pressures at rest should be less than 15 mmHg and 5–10 minutes following exercise should have returned to 15 mmHg or less (Pedowitz et al 1990).

### Differential diagnosis

Shin splints or stress fractures of the tibia will be the main differential diagnosis for leg pains. For neurological symptoms in the foot an entrapment neuropathy should be excluded.

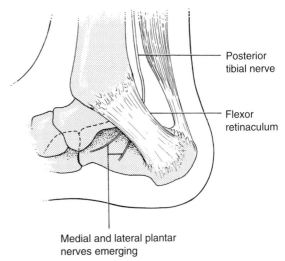

**Figure 16.6** Line drawing to show gross anatomy of the tarsal tunnel—lateral view.

Posterior tibial nerve

Flexor retinaculum

Medial and lateral plantar nerves emerging

## NERVES

A number of nerves may be compressed at sites around the ankle and foot, resulting in entrapment neuropathies.

## Tarsal tunnel syndrome

### Aetiology

The posterior tibial nerve, a branch of the sciatic nerve, may become compressed as it passes under the flexor retinaculum behind the medial malleolus (Fig. 16.6). Interestingly, tarsal tunnel syndrome is a relatively new diagnosis, having only been properly first described in 1962 (Keck 1962, Lam 1962) The condition is analogous to carpal tunnel syndrome in the wrist but nowhere near as common. The compression may cause direct pressure, leading to motor and sensory symptoms, or may compress the vascular supply, the vasa nervorum, causing sensory symptoms only. Aetiology of tarsal tunnel syndrome is idiopathic, trauma or associated with bony alignment (Cimino 1990). Other cases may be related to problems such as rheumatoid arthritis or compression within the tunnel associated with a ganglion, lipoma or venous varicosities.

*Presenting symptoms*

The patient is likely to complain of a diffuse, burning type of pain on the sole of the foot. With time symptoms may become more localised. Often pain is worse on activity and better at rest. A proportion of patients get night-time pain and some 30% have proximal radiation of pain to the midcalf region, known as the Valleix phenomenon (Mann 1993).

*Signs*

Sensory or motor weakness is rare to find but should be carefully looked for. Most useful is a positive Tinel sign, obtained by starting proximally and percussing along the course of the nerve. At the site of entrapment percussion will cause radiation of pain along the course of the nerve.

*Investigations*

Plain X-rays may demonstrate any post-traumatic bony spurs causing compression but do not in themselves make a diagnosis. Electrodiagnostic tests are necessary for this: nerve conduction studies looking at sensory conduction velocities and the amplitude and duration of motor evoked potentials (Ch. 7). Tests should be performed bilaterally and a peripheral neuropathy should be excluded. If an extrinsic compression in the tunnel is suspected then an MRI may be helpful.

*Differential diagnosis*

Because of the diffuse nature of the symptoms the differential diagnosis is quite wide, but two possibilities should be particularly looked for. A peripheral neuropathy, e.g. from diabetes, may cause burning pains in the foot, but is usually bilateral. Sciatica with nerve root irritation causing distal pain also needs to be excluded. Straight leg raising will be restricted and painful.

## Other entrapments

*Aetiology*

Other entrapments which have been described include the deep peroneal nerve under the inferior extensor retinaculum and the superficial peroneal nerve as it exits the deep fascia about 11.5 cm above the lateral malleolus, the medial plantar nerve at the master knot of Henry and the first branch of the lateral plantar nerve between abductor hallucis and quadratus plantae muscles. Most of these entrapments occur in runners or athletes.

*Symptoms and signs*

**Deep peroneal nerve:** Patients complain of pain over the dorsum of the foot and sometimes numbness and paraesthesia in the first web space. There may be altered sensation in the first web space and a positive Tinel sign.

**Superficial peroneal nerve:** Symptoms include pain over the dorsum of the foot and ankle and inferior lateral border of the calf. As a sensory nerve there are no motor signs but there may be a positive Tinel sign. A fascial defect or muscle herniation where the nerve exits the deep fascia should be looked for.

**Medial plantar nerve:** Patients complain of an aching pain over the medial aspect of the arch, often radiating into the medial three toes, becoming worse on running. Again a positive Tinel sign may be found and also tenderness under the medial arch (Case history 16.4).

**First branch of lateral plantar nerve:** Patients complain of chronic pain, often increased on running but sometimes present on waking. On examination there will be tenderness over the nerve deep to abductor hallucis and pressure reproduces the patient's symptoms.

*Investigations*

Nerve conduction studies may help with the diagnosis of deep peroneal nerve entrapment, but are less useful in diagnosing the others. More recently abnormalities of nerve conduction and electromyography have demonstrated plantar nerve abnormalities (Schon et al 1993). Injection of local anaesthetic at the site of entrapment may act as a diagnostic test if it abolishes symptoms.

---

**Case history 16.4**

**Patient:** 48-year-old keen runner; squash and badminton player.

**Presenting symptoms:** 18-month history of bilateral paraesthesia affecting the medial aspect of the soles of both feet, in the distribution of the medial plantar nerve, when running. Symptoms initially settled after exercise but over the next 6 months the patient developed shooting pains without any pattern of onset with increasing numbness in both feet.

**Signs:** A positive Tinel sign above both medial malleoli. Some loss of sharp and blunt sensory discrimination on the medial aspect of the sole was identified.

**Investigations:** Nerve conduction studies showed conduction blocks bilaterally at the level of the tarsal tunnel. Medial plantar responses were absent on the right and delayed on the left.

**Diagnosis:** Bilateral tarsal tunnel syndrome.

**Operative findings:** On both sides there was a high division of the posterior tibial nerve into medial and lateral plantar branches. A sharp edge to abductor hallucis was found to be compressing the medial plantar nerve bilaterally. In addition there was a large vascular pedicle crossing the medial plantar nerve and compressing it more proximally. Pain settled following surgery.

---

*Differential diagnosis*

As for tarsal tunnel syndrome.

## Peripheral neuropathy

*Aetiology*

Peripheral neuropathies may be due to a variety of causes. In the West the leading cause is diabetes and in the Third World it is leprosy. Other causes include spina bifida, pernicious anaemia, drugs and alcoholism. The different patterns of peripheral neuropathy may vary but in diabetics the most common is a symmetrical distal polyneuropathy, encompassing motor, sensory and autonomic components.

*Presenting symptoms*

Patients may notice no symptoms at all if the neuropathy presents as a painless one. The first inkling of a problem may be when a patient presents with a complication such as ulceration or infection. In a diabetic who normally has a painless foot with no sensation the presence of pain is important and may indicate deep infection, such as an abscess or osteomyelitis. If the presentation is of a painful neuropathy the patient may complain of a burning sensation in the legs and feet, commonly worse at night.

*Signs*

In a diabetic the foot may adopt a cavus appearance with clawed toes. In the absence of vascular disease the foot will feel warm and there may be distended veins. Sensation to light touch and pinprick will be reduced and joint position sense may be impaired. The toes may be clawed with wasting of the intrinsic foot muscles and the ankle jerk absent. Callosities may be present under the metatarsal heads and heel.

*Investigations*

In evaluating a peripheral neuropathy it is important to look for an underlying cause. The urine should be tested for sugar and a random blood glucose test performed to look for the most common cause. A careful history and examination should uncover evidence of other causes. Nerve conduction studies may be helpful to rule out an entrapment neuropathy.

## Morton's metatarsalgia (neuroma)

*Aetiology*

This condition is a type of entrapment neuropathy affecting a plantar digital nerve. It most commonly affects the common digital nerve to the 3/4 interspace, but may also occur in the 2/3 interspace. The diagnosis probably does not exist in the 1st or 4th webspaces, although there has been much debate about this. The incidence of a second neuroma in the same foot is 4% (Thompson & Deland 1993). Women are affected at least four times more often than men and the condition can affect adults of any age. The nerve develops a fusiform swelling, just proximal to its bifurcation, at the level of the intermetatarsal

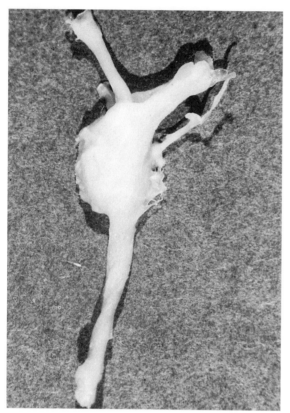

**Figure 16.7** Resected Morton's neuroma showing terminal digital branches following operation.

bursa (Fig. 16.7). Although frequently termed a neuroma, technically it is not as the histology shows a degenerative process rather than a proliferative one.

### Presenting symptoms

The patient complains of a burning pain on the sole of the foot, at the level of the metatarsal heads and commonly radiating into one or two toes. It may feel to the patient like walking on a sharp pebble. Occasionally pain will radiate proximally. Pain is often worse on walking and may be particularly exacerbated by tight-fitting shoes, as these will compress the metatarsal heads together, thus 'trapping' the nerve. Resting or removing tight shoes may settle the pain. Less than half the patients complain of numbness in the toes.

### Signs

On palpation of the relevant interspace the patient's pain will be reproduced, sometimes with radiation into a toe. However it may be difficult to elicit conclusive evidence on examination. If pressure is maintained in the interspace with one hand, while the other alternately squeezes the forefoot from side to side to compress the metatarsal heads together, then a painful click may be obtained. This is known as Mulder's click and is only helpful if it reproduces pain (Mulder 1951). It is important to ensure that any tenderness is not over the metatarsal heads, rather than intermetatarsal, although in rare cases nerves may become entrapped under a metatarsal head. Sensation in the toes is usually normal, but may vary.

### Investigations

Plain X-rays should be taken to rule out other pathology. Although ultrasound and MRI have been used to look for the swelling in the nerve they have not generally proved reliable enough to be used as diagnostic tools. Ultrasound has been reported as useful if the neuroma is 5 mm in diameter (Pollak et al 1992). Nerve conduction studies are not helpful. A diagnostic injection of local anaesthetic may be helpful if it abolishes the patient's pain.

### Differential diagnosis

Problems affecting the metatarsal head, such as synovitis, intermetatarsal bursa and Freiberg's disease should be considered. It is important to be careful about whether the tenderness is under a metatarsal head or intermetatarsal. Pain from a neurological cause, such as tarsal tunnel syndrome, peripheral neuropathy or referred pain from the back should be excluded.

## SKIN AND SUBCUTANEOUS TISSUES

## Retrocalcaneal bursitis

### Aetiology

There are two bursae at the heel; one is deep to

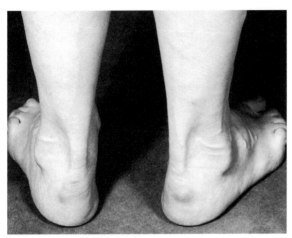

**Figure 16.8**    Bilateral heel bumps with superolateral prominence on the heel, also known as Haglund's deformity.

the tendo achilles and the other lies superficial to its insertion. The deep bursa is infrequently affected but, as it has a synovial lining, symptoms may be early indicators of an inflammatory arthropathy such as rheumatoid arthritis. Men are affected more often than women. Symptoms in the subcutaneous bursa affect adolescent females most frequently.

### Presenting symptoms

For the subcutaneous bursa the symptoms are well described by some of the eponyms for the condition, such as 'pump or heel bumps'. The patient complains of a tender prominence at the heel when wearing shoes (Fig. 16.8).

### Signs

Inflammation of the deep bursa will produce tenderness deep to the tendo achilles. In heel bumps there is variable tenderness over a thickened bursa situated just lateral to the tendo achillis attachment.

### Investigations

A plain lateral X-ray should be taken. With deep bursitis calcaneal erosions should be looked for.

In heel bumps the X-ray is usually normal with no evidence of any posterosuperior prominence to the calcaneus.

### Differential diagnosis

This is mainly with other causes of heel pain and with Achilles tendonitis.

## Heel pad syndrome

### Aetiology

This is a chronic inflammatory process within the heel fat pad. The heel is subject to repetitive impact loading on walking which can exceed body weight; with running these forces can rise to 3–8 times body weight (Riegler 1987). Predisposing symptoms may be running on hard surfaces, e.g. roads, obesity and increasing age.

### Presenting symptoms

Patients complain of heel pain, worse in the early morning and on weightbearing. They may have a limp.

### Signs

There is localised central tenderness under the heel.

### Investigations

This is essentially a clinical diagnosis. X-rays or ultrasonography are not helpful.

### Differential diagnosis

This will include plantar fasciitis and entrapment neuropathies, particularly of the nerve to abductor digiti quinti.

## Plantar fasciitis

### Aetiology

This is a chronic inflammation at the site of the attachment of the plantar fascia to the medial tubercle of the calcaneum. It possibly represents a traction periostitis and may be precipitated by overuse and occurs in middle-aged people and with a male predominance.

### Presenting symptoms

Patients complain of pain under the heel on weightbearing; this may be particularly acute on getting up in the morning.

### Signs

There is tenderness along the anteromedial border of the calcaneum which may be increased by passive dorsiflexion of the toes.

### Investigations

The diagnosis is clinical although a bone scan may show increased uptake locally. Plain X-rays may show a spur on the inferior border of the calcaneum but this is equally found in asymptomatic people.

### Differential diagnosis

As in heel pad syndrome.

## Soft tissue masses or tumours

### Aetiology

Some benign soft-tissue masses, such as *ganglions*, are common in the foot. A ganglion is a mucoid cyst which usually arises from an underlying joint. In the foot they most commonly occur over the dorsum of the ankle (Fig. 16.9). *Plantar fibromatosis* is analogous to Dupuytren's contracture in the hand and is a proliferation of the plantar aponeurosis to form discrete nodules, usually in the instep. A *glomus tumour* is a benign bright red vascular tumour, the size of a small pea, and usually located subungually or in a web space.

### Presenting symptoms

A ganglion presents as a painful lump inside footwear. Plantar fibromatosis may present with

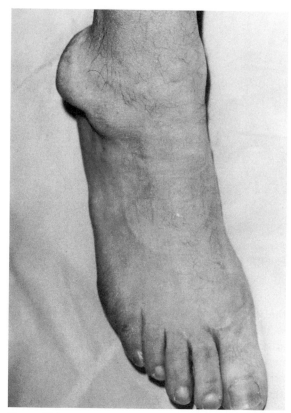

**Figure 16.9**  Large ganglion on lateral aspect of the ankle.

painful nodules, although often the patient only notices some mild discomfort or simply a swelling. A glomus tumour, however, may present with marked pain.

### Signs

A ganglion will appear as a mobile subcutaneous lump of variable size. Small ones may appear quite firm whereas larger ones often have a more spongy feel. The nodules of plantar fibromatosis are felt as firm, fairly immobile nodules, often along the edge of the plantar fascia and under the instep. A glomus tumour will appear as a subungual mass or may be palpated as a small nodule in a web space.

### Investigations

Plain X-rays may distinguish a glomus tumour

from a subungual exostosis. Otherwise the diagnosis is made from clinical information.

### Differential diagnosis

Multiple ganglions around the extensor tendons on the dorsum of the ankle should arouse suspicion of rheumatoid arthritis. A lipoma may be mistaken for a ganglion and is commonly located on the dorsolateral aspect of the ankle.

## GENERAL

## Crystal arthritis

### Aetiology

Arthritic changes may be caused by the deposition of crystals within a joint. This may be sodium urate crystals in *gout* or calcium pyrophosphate dihydrate crystals in *pseudogout*. Gout is a disease characterised by a disorder of purine metabolism and is associated with hyperuricaemia. It may be primary with a strong hereditary factor or be secondary to other problems such as renal failure. Pseudogout is sometimes associated with other metabolic conditions, such as hyperparathyroidism, but otherwise it is idiopathic.

### Presenting symptoms

Up to 75% of initial attacks of gout affect the big toe (Jacoby & Dixon 1991). The patient complains of acute onset of a swollen, very painful first MTPJ. Pseudogout may present with gout-like attacks but these are usually less severe. About 50% of patients, however, will present with progressive degeneration of joints. In the foot the ankle, subtalar and talonavicular joints are most commonly affected.

### Signs

In the acute stage of gout the great toe will be swollen, inflamed and very tender (Fig. 16.10). In chronic cases the signs of osteoarthritis will be present. Gouty tophi (deposits of sodium urate) may be found in the cartilages of the ears and in bursae, tendons and soft tissues generally.

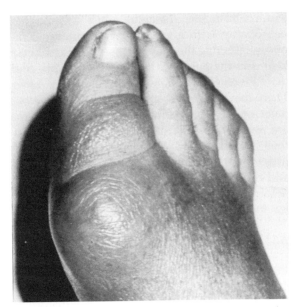

**Figure 16.10**  Acute gout in the first metatarsophalangeal joint.

### Investigations

Acutely the serum uric acid may be raised but acute attacks can occur with a normal uric acid level. Aspiration of joint fluid and examination under polarising lens will show brightly birefringent needle-like crystals in gout and more pleomorphic rectangular crystals in pseudogout. Chronically X-rays will show degenerative changes in joints affected. Gout gives a characteristic appearance of sharp, punched-out juxta-articular lesions, with little reactive sclerosis and no general osteoporosis.

### Differential diagnosis

Acutely this will be with acute infection and septic arthritis. Chronic forms will be associated with other causes of degenerative joint disease.

## Hereditary and motor sensory neuropathy

### Aetiology

This condition is also known as *peroneal muscular atrophy* and was first described by Charcot, Marie and Tooth in 1886. Essentially it is an inherited neuropathy with a predominantly motor component affecting the lower limbs. Motor weakness begins in the peronei, then the dorsiflexors, and may involve all the muscles below the knee. There may also be sensory changes and involvement of the upper limb. The initial symptoms are usually in childhood but the neuropathy then slowly progresses. The adult may then present with a cavus foot, claw toes and pain and callosities over the metatarsal heads. Fixed deformities may develop with equinus of the forefoot and varus of the hindfoot (Mann 1983).

### Presenting symptoms

This will depend on how far the disease has progressed. Initially, the patient may present with just a clumsy gait and perhaps a history of recurrent ankle sprains. With time the weakness and changes in the shape of the foot become more apparent. The patient may then complain of footwear problems and pain along the lateral border of the foot because of the varus heel.

### Signs

In the established case there will be a cavus foot with a high arch, a plantarflexed first ray, clawing of the toes and peroneal and intrinsic muscle weakness. Weakness of other muscle groups should be looked for and the hands examined. Sensory changes, if present, are usually mild.

### Investigations

A careful clinical examination is important because of the differential diagnosis. Plain X-rays, standing AP and lateral, will show the cavus and demonstrate any degenerative changes when fixed deformities are present. Nerve conduction studies and electromyography are important for accurate diagnosis and to rule out other causes of pes cavus.

### Differential diagnosis

This is from other causes of pes cavus, which will include idiopathic, muscular diseases such as muscular dystrophy, neurological problems such as cerebral palsy, Friedreich's ataxia, poliomyelitis and spinal cord problems. In addition, pes cavus may be due to residual club foot or compartment syndrome.

## Infection

### Aetiology

Infection may occur in the soft tissues, as osteomyelitis in the bone or as septic arthritis in a joint. The cause may be direct inoculation following an open wound, either traumatic or surgically created, or via haematogenous spread.

Traumatic or surgical infection may occur at any time but septic arthritis is more likely to occur in the very young or the elderly or immunocompromised. Bony infections are most commonly due to *Staphylococcus aureus* but streptococci may also be associated with soft-tissue infections.

### Presenting symptoms

These will vary according to the tissue involved and degree of infection. Cellulitis will present with pain, swelling and erythema of the involved area. Because the bones are very superficial in the foot, osteomyelitis should always be suspected under any area of cellulitis. Septic arthritis is likely to present with exquisite pain on moving a joint, usually the ankle, and with overlying swelling and erythema. However, in the elderly or immunocompromised, symptoms may be strikingly muted, reducing suspicion of an underlying joint infection. In acute septic arthritis or osteomyelitis the patient is likely to have systemic signs of being unwell.

### Signs

Swelling, tenderness and erythema of the soft tissues will be noted. In septic arthritis there is likely to be marked pain on very limited movement of the joint. If marked local tenderness is elicited over a bony area this should alert you to the possibility of underlying osteomyelitis. If infection spreads to a tendon sheath, causing a tenosynovitis, then passive movement of the tendon will be limited and very painful and tenderness may be present along the length of the tendon.

*Investigations*

Plain X-rays are necessary to exclude or demonstrate osteomyelitis. However, it may take 10 days to show any changes. A bone scan will be positive well before plain X-rays and may help. In septic arthritis a diminution in joint space or adjacent osteomyelitis may be seen. Aspiration of fluid from a joint and Gram stain and culture can provide a diagnosis. Blood cultures should also be done: a full blood count will show a raised white cell count and the ESR or C-reactive protein will be high. Obviously, if there is an open discharge with pus then swabs should be taken.

*Differential diagnosis*

Infection is a clinical diagnosis. Usually the question to be decided is whether there is underlying bony or joint infection.

## Reflex sympathetic dystrophy (RSD)

*Aetiology*

This is an interesting condition which is poorly understood but results from a dysfunction of the sympathetic nervous system. It can follow trauma, sometimes minor in nature, after a fracture or following surgery. Pain can become so unremitting that the patient wishes amputation and may also develop depression and personality changes.

*Presenting symptoms*

Patients complain of a burning pain, often out of proportion to the injury. Initially, this will be due to the trauma or surgery but, instead of settling, the pain increases and becomes the dominant complaint. Pain can occur at rest, with movement and may well trouble the patient at night. The weight of blankets on the bed, or even a sheet, may be intolerable. As well as affecting the injured area the patient may experience pain over the whole foot in a global distribution.

*Signs*

These may vary according to the stage of the condition. The limb may be swollen and may have a shiny dry appearance. There may be hair and nail changes, joint stiffness and sudomotor changes, with dry skin or excessive sweating. The affected area may become very sensitive and even light touch may evoke considerable and prolonged pain. Because of muscular spasm patients may develop fixed equinus at the ankle or claw toes.

*Investigations*

Plain X-rays may show osteopenia within a few weeks and subperiosteal bone resorption. A bone scan is very helpful as it will show generalised increased uptake in the affected area. Patients have a characteristic delayed bone scan pattern of diffuse increased tracer throughout the foot, with juxta-articular uptake accentuation (Holder et al 1992). Temporary pain relief from a lumbar sympathetic block is also a useful test, although a negative test does not exclude RSD. Case history 16.5 belies some of the problems of treating and diagnosing this pain syndrome early. Both psychological and organic problems can arise, making the problem intractable.

*Differential diagnosis*

It can be difficult sometimes to decide if mild RSD is present or if the patient simply has a very painful injury, or one is missing a component of that injury.

## Referred pain

*Aetiology*

Referred pain has been mentioned in connection with compartment syndrome involving the deep

Case history 16.5

**Patient:** A 13-year-old schoolgirl presented following a nail surgery (phenolisation) with positive subungual exostosis over the left hallux. This was confirmed by X-ray. Following an exostectomy to remove the bone, intractable pain developed in a pattern unusual for postoperative events.

**Presenting symptoms:** Pain following two operations at 6 weeks. Stabbing and crushing pain was described, with extreme sensitivity over the foot.

**Signs:** The foot was swollen and blue. Analgesics were of minimal help. The patient had a tendency to hysterical fits. Over an 18-month period the contralateral side became affected.

**Investigations:** Infection was excluded. Surgery was performed on two further occasions by different surgeons in case an exostosis was still present. Amytriptyline 10 mg at night provided minimal help in reducing vasomotor activity. A lumbar sympathectomy (guanethidine) only gave temporary relief. Psychiatric assessment was considered.

**Diagnosis:** Reflex sympathetic dystrophy with hysteria.

**Conclusion:** This case history highlights the ease with which inappropriate management and additional physical insult can elevate the patient's problem. RSD is a difficult problem to manage and non-invasive techniques should be emphasised, with total pain-blocking control and maintenance of mobility if the pain syndrome is diagnosed (Tollafield 1991).

peroneal and posterior tibial nerves. The main source of referred pain, however, is sciatica due to nerve root compression in the back. Most commonly this is due to a prolapsed intervertebral disc and over 90% of these occur at the L4/5 or L5/S1 levels.

### Presenting symptoms

Patients will usually complain of low back pain radiating into a buttock and down the leg. They may have little back pain and mainly leg pain. A careful history may indicate the nerve root involved. Pain radiating down the back of the leg into the sole of the foot is generally S1 in origin

and down the lateral border of the leg and into the hallux is generally L5 in origin.

### Signs

In an acute disc prolapse the patient experiences considerable pain and is unable to move easily. He/she may have a scoliotic tilt to the spine when viewed from behind, paraspinal muscle spasm and tenderness in the buttock. Straight leg raising will be restricted and causes pain in the distribution of the nerve root. Sensory changes and muscle weakness appropriate to that nerve root may be found but not invariably. Reflexes may be diminished; the knee jerk is L3/4 and the ankle jerk is L5/S1.

### Investigations

Plain X-rays should be taken of the lumbosacral spine. If surgery is contemplated, or the diagnosis is unclear, then an MRI scan or CT scan is necessary.

### Differential diagnosis

The symptomatology is usually clear but back pain is very common and a more distal problem co-existing with long-standing back pain and sciatica should always be considered.

## SUMMARY

The causes of foot pain are numerous. Not all are listed here as several conditions are covered in other chapters. A careful history, examination and relevant investigations are necessary to make a correct diagnosis. Despite such attention there will occasionally be patients who fail to fall neatly into the right category. With such patients local anaesthetic injections can be very useful in determining which structures are giving rise to the symptoms.

## REFERENCES

Berndt A L, Harty M 1959 Transchondral fractures (osteochondritis dissecans) of the talus. Journal of Bone and Joint Surgery 41-A: 988–1020

Canale S T, Belding R H 1980 Osteochondral lesions of the talus. Journal of Bone and Joint Surgery 60-A: 97–102

Cimino W R 1990 Tarsal tunnel syndrome: a review of the literature. Foot and Ankle 11: 47–52

De Smet A A, Fisher D R, Burnstein M I et al 1990 Value of MR imaging in staging osteochondral lesions of the talus (osteochondritis dissecans). American Journal of Roentgenology 154: 555–558

Ferkel R D, Karzel R P, Del Pizzo W et al 1991 Arthroscopic treatment of anterolateral impingement of the ankle. American Journal of Sports Medicine 19: 440–446

Holder L E, Cole L A, Myerson M S 1992 Reflex sympathetic dystrophy in the foot: clinical and scintigraphic criteria. Radiology 184(2): 531–535

Hubay C A 1949 Sesamoid bones of the hands and feet. American Journal of Roentgenology 61: 493–505

Jacoby R K, Dixon A StJ 1991 The painful foot in systemic disorders. In: Klenerman L. (ed) The foot and its disorders, 3rd edn. Blackwell Scientific Publications, Oxford

Johnson K A 1983 Tibialis posterior tendon rupture. Clinical Orthopaedics and Related Research 177: 140–147

Johnson K D 1987 Management of malunion and nonunion of the tibia. Orthopaedic Clinics of North America 18: 157–172

Keck C 1962 The tarsal tunnel syndrome. Journal of Bone and Joint Surgery 44-A: 180–182

Lam S J S 1962 The tarsal tunnel syndrome. Lancet 2: 1354–1355

Lutter L D 1991 Achilles tendon rupture. AAOS fourth annual comprehensive foot and ankle course

McMurray T P 1950 Footballer's ankle. Journal of Bone and Joint Surgery 32-B: 68–69

Mann R A 1993 Diseases of the nerves. In: Mann R A, Coughlin R J (ed) Surgery of the foot and ankle, 6th edn.

C V Mosby, St Louis, MO

Mann R A, Missirian J 1983 Pathophysiology of Charcot–Marie–Tooth disease. Orthopaedic Transactions 7: 167

Merchant T C, Dietz F R 1989 Long term follow-up after fractures of the tibial and fibular shafts. Journal of Bone and Joint Surgery 71-A: 599–606

Mosier K M, Asher M 1984 Tarsal coalitions and peroneal spastic flat foot. A review. Journal of Bone and Joint Surgery 66-A: 976–984

Mulder J D 1951 The causative mechanism in Morton's. Journal of Bone and Joint Surgery 33-B: 94–95

Nicoll E A 1964 Fractures of the tibial shaft. A survey of 705 cases. Journal of Bone and Joint Surgery 46-B: 373–387

O'Connor D 1958 Sinus tarsi syndrome. A clinical entity. Journal of Bone and Joint Surgery 40-A: 720

Pedowitz R A, Hargens A R, Mubarak S J et al 1990 Modified criteria for the objective diagnosis of chronic compartment syndrome of the leg. American Journal of Sports Medicine 18: 35–40

Pollak R A, Bellacosa R A, Dornbluth N C et al 1992 Sonographic analysis of Morton's neuroma. Journal of Foot Surgery 31(6): 534–537

Riegler H E 1987 Orthotic devices for the foot. Orthopaedic Revue 16: 27–37

Romanowski C A J, Barrington N A 1991 The accessory ossicles of the foot. Foot 2: 61–70

Schon L C, Glennon T P, Baxter D E 1993 Heel pain syndrome: electrodiagnostic support for nerve entrapment. Foot and Ankle 14: 129–135

Stormont D M, Peterson H A 1983 The relative incidence of tarsal coalition. Clinical Orthopaedics and Related Research 181: 28–36

Thompson F M, Deland J T 1993 Occurrence of two interdigital neuromas in one foot. Foot and Ankle 14: 15–17

Tollafield D R 1991 Reflex sympathetic dystrophy in day case foot surgery. British Journal of Podiatric Medicine and Surgery 3(1): 2–6

# Assessment of the 'at risk' foot

*J. Mooney*
*L. Merriman*

## INTRODUCTION

An 'at risk' foot is one which is more likely than the 'normal' foot to develop:

- ulceration
- infection
- necrosis/gangrene
- deformity.

The first part of this chapter examines why it is important to identify the 'at risk' foot and discusses the factors which may cause a foot to be labelled thus. This is followed by a discussion on how to identify the 'at risk' foot, the complications which may arise in such a foot and the factors which may affect its prognosis. The chapter concludes by looking at the assessment findings of a range of conditions associated with the 'at risk' foot.

### Why is it important to identify the 'at risk' foot?

Problems which arise in the 'at risk' foot can affect both the quality and quantity of life. Amputation may be the last resort in the management of these problems, with all the ensuing physical and psychosocial effects from this radical procedure. It is, therefore, important that the practitioner identifies those patients who are at risk in order that:

- preventative action can be taken
- a base line can be established for monitoring any changes.

# What causes an 'at risk' limb?

One or more of the following factors may lead to a foot being classed as 'at risk':

- Poor arterial blood supply to the foot or poor venous drainage from the foot and leg
- Sensory neuropathy
- A compromised immune system
- Excessive weightbearing on a part of the foot.

The causes and the effects of reduced blood supply to and return from the foot and leg are discussed in detail in Chapter 6. Whether the problem is arterial, venous or lymphatic or a combination of these the nutrition of foot tissues will be compromised. The tissues will become prone to ulceration and necrosis. Infection is also more likely if the skin barrier is broken or there is a reduction in the number of phagocytic and T cells that can reach the site.

The causes and effects of sensory neuropathy are discussed in detail in Chapter 7. Sensory neuropathy can affect one or more of the sensory modalities. Unconscious trauma leads to breaks in the skin integrity and ulceration.

Patients with a compromised immune system are not able to mount the body's normal response to pathogenic microorganisms. The factors which may lead to a compromised immune system are outlined in Table 17.1. Immunocompromised patients are at an even greater risk of infection if there is a break in their skin.

Excessive weightbearing on a part of the foot results in the tissues at that part being subjected to high levels of stress, causing tissue breakdown. This problem is compounded if the patient has peripheral vascular disease or sensory neuropathy. Many conditions can lead to deformity of the foot and hence affect the normal weightbearing pattern of the foot (Table 17.2).

## ASSESSMENT OF THE 'AT RISK' FOOT

Assessment involves identification of:
- whether the foot can be classed as 'at risk'
- any complications that may have occurred
- any factors that may affect the prognosis.

**Table 17.1** Factors which may lead to a compromised immune system (*more common causes in italics*)

| | |
|---|---|
| Congenital | DiGeorge syndrome<br>Chronic granulomatous disease |
| Infections | Human immunodeficiency virus<br>Cytomegalovirus<br>*Infectious mononucleosis*<br>Acute bacterial disease<br>Severe mycobacterial or fungal disease |
| Endocrine/metabolic | *Diabetes mellitus*<br>Malnutrition |
| Immunosuppressive agents | *Long-term steroid use*<br>Immunosuppressive drugs<br>Radiation |
| Haematological disorders | Leukaemia<br>Hodgkin's disease<br>Lymphoma<br>Sarcoidosis |
| Miscellaneous | Burns<br>*Ageing*<br>Cirrhosis<br>Lupus erythematosus |

**Table 17.2** Some causes of foot deformities that may result in abnormal stresses on a part of the foot

| | |
|---|---|
| Congenital | Spina bifida<br>Talipes equinovarus<br>Talipes calcaneovalgus<br>Vertical talus |
| Acquired | Diabetes mellitus<br>Charcot's joints<br>Upper motor neurone lesions, e.g. CVA, cerebral palsy<br>Lower motor neurone lesions, e.g. polio, trauma<br>Leprosy (Hansen's disease)<br>Abnormal pronation<br>Pes cavus foot type<br>Rheumatoid arthritis<br>Osteoarthrosis |

## IDENTIFICATION OF THE 'AT RISK' FOOT

An assessment of a patient's risk status can be made from the medical and social history (Ch. 5) and by meticulous observation and examination. This will include an assessment of the vascular (Ch. 6), neurological (Ch. 7) and locomotor

(Ch. 8) systems as well as an assessment of the skin and its appendages (Ch. 9) and footwear (Ch. 10). In particular, changes of temperature, discoloration, absent pulses and altered sensation should be noted. Identification of gait and biomechanical abnormalities is essential, as these can lead to areas of the foot being subjected to increased mechanical forces. Clinical and laboratory analysis of urine and blood should be undertaken as necessary (Ch. 13). X-rays may be used to help diagnose certain conditions (Ch. 11).

The information from the above assessments should be systematically recorded. The presenting signs and symptoms should be reviewed at every visit and any improvement or deterioration noted. Action should be taken to prevent complications from arising in those assessed to be 'at risk'.

## IDENTIFICATION OF COMPLICATIONS

As highlighted in the introduction an 'at risk' foot may develop ulceration, infection, necrosis/gangrene and/or deformity. It is important that the practitioner identifies these complications which occur and the extent of any pathological changes.

## Ulceration

An ulcer is a loss of full skin thickness with exposure of dermal and, potentially, subdermal tissue. The term 'ulcer' is used to denote loss of skin due to an internal cause, e.g. ischaemic ulcer, whereas 'wound' is used to denote loss of skin due to an external cause, e.g. gunshot. Ulcers are associated with a loss of normal tissue viability. The prime pathological process is ischaemia (lack of blood). Ischaemia may occur as a result of one or more of the following: arterial disease, venous disease, blood disease, trauma, infection, deformity and reduced joint mobility, neurological disorders, endocrine disorders, connective tissue disorders. These factors lead to ischaemia in one or more of the following ways:

- By reducing or inhibiting completely the flow of blood to the area through
  - restriction of the lumen of the arteries, e.g. atheroma vasospacticity
  - complete restriction of blood flow due to, e.g.
    infection (blood flow restricted because of mass of white blood cells in the area)
    blood clot (thrombus)
    embolus (fragment of thrombus which lodges in a small vessel)
    tourniquet
    sickle cell disease
- By reducing the oxygen-carrying capacity of the blood (anaemia)
- By stagnation of blood and accumulation of metabolites and waste products (poor venous or lymphatic drainage).

Although the pathological process is primarily ischaemia, ulcers are classified as to their cause. Six types of ulcer are found in the leg/foot:

- Ischaemic
- Neuropathic
- Venous
- Pressure (decubitus)
- Mixed (ischaemic/neuropathic), sometimes known as diabetic
- Neoplastic.

The most common type of ulceration is venous (80% of ulcers); the least common are those ulcers associated with neoplasia. The practitioner should be able to distinguish between the various types.

### Ischaemic ulcers

These result from inadequate blood supply (Ch. 6). Common sites affected are the apices of toes, medial and lateral border of the foot and the heel. They are usually painful and small with a 'punched-out' appearance (Plate 2). The base is often laden with tough, adherent, yellowish necrotic tissue, lacking in granulation tissue. They are very difficult to heal unless the blood supply to the area can be improved. They are more likely to develop in winter, and may

**Table 17.3** Causes of neuropathic ulceration

- Diabetes mellitus
- Poliomyelitis
- Spina bifida
- Neurosyphilis (tabes dorsalis)
- Leprosy (tuberculoid and lepromatous)
- Syringomyelia
- Trauma or tumour of spinal cord or peripheral nerves
- Pernicious anaemia

heal during the summer if the initial cause can be treated or prevented. Patients with ischaemic ulcers present with the following clinical features:

- Pain
- Absent or faint pulses
- Dry, shiny, hairless skin (Plate 1)
- Crumbly, thickened nails
- Pale, cool limb and foot
- Paraesthesia (Ch. 6).

The ankle brachial index is less than 0.6 unless the arteries are calcified. Infection may be present but the signs of inflammation may be inhibited because of the inadequate blood supply. A swab should be taken if in doubt (Ch. 13).

### Neuropathic ulcers

These result from damage to one or more parts of the nervous system; sensory, motor or autonomic. The sensory part of the nervous system is always involved (Table 17.3). Sometimes a neuropathic ulcer is due to lack of awareness of a harmful stimulus, e.g. a stone in the shoe, or putting a foot into very hot water. However, damage to the motor system and autonomic nervous system can compound the problems associated with sensory neuropathy and result in a greater risk of ulceration. Motor damage can lead to deformity and abnormal weightbearing, e.g. wasting of the intrinsic muscles of the foot results in clawed toes and plantarflexed metatarsals which in turn leads to excessive weightbearing on the metatarsal heads. An impaired autonomic nervous system may affect the blood supply to the skin and as a result impair the

skin's normal resilience to stress.

In the presence of neuropathy these ulcers may be painless and patients may present with advanced ulceration, infection or gangrene. The typical neuropathic ulcer is found on the weight-bearing plantar surface of the foot, the digits. These ulcers present with hyperkeratotic (callused) borders and are often very deep, extending down to tendon and bone (Plate 29). Sometimes the practitioner may expose a neuropathic ulcer after debriding an area of callus or the site of ulceration may be preceded by the development of bullae and an area of necrosis.

The ulcer base may be dry or moist and show granulation tissue or be sloughy (Plate 29). These ulcers can perforate, penetrating deep into the tissues, exposing tendons, joints and bone, leading to osteomyelitis or eventual arthritis (Plate 30). Sequestra, pieces of dead bone which separate from healthy bone, may be found. As with all ulcers there may be secondary infection leading to cellulitis which may track to other parts of the foot.

### Venous ulcers

These are associated with chronic venous insufficiency (Ch. 6). Gravitational eczema, deposits of haemosiderin, oedema and atrophie blanche are likely to be present. These ulcers commonly occur around the malleoli, especially the medial malleolus (great saphenous vein). Venous ulcers are small initially but gradually increase in size, so that they may encircle the ankle (Plate 7). They may be shallow or deep with sharply demarcated borders. This type of ulcer may cause pain, but is not normally as painful as an ischaemic ulcer. There is usually a copious exudate, and often a secondary infection may occur. Such ulcers are often indolent (fail to heal) and in some cases a squamous cell carcinoma may develop at the site.

### Mixed ulcers

These occur where there is a combination of ischaemia and sensory neuropathy (Plate 31) and are typical of diabetes mellitus.

## Pressure ulcers

These occur as a result of prolonged compression and shear stress to tissues that exceeds capillary pressure (normally 20–30 mmHg). The magnitude of the stress is not as important as the duration of force application. Patients with a poor peripheral blood supply, whose healing potential is reduced through disease or malnutrition and who spend a long time in one position (chair or bed bound) are particularly prone to developing this form of ulceration. The initial sign of this type of ulcer is an area of blanching erythema over a bony prominence such as the sacrum, femoral trochanters and condyles, malleoli, heel, base of the fifth metatarsal and heads of the first and fifth metatarsals. Eventually the area becomes non-blanching. A blister may form prior to ulceration. The patient usually complains of pain. The ulcer may extend to involve subcutaneous tissues.

## Neoplasia

The excessive cell division that occurs with neoplasia, especially when malignant, is accompanied by angiogenesis (development of blood vessels). When the neoplasia outgrows its blood supply the area ulcerates. This type of ulcer tends to have rolled edges and an unusual appearance, e.g. malignant melanoma.

Table 17.4 compares the three most common types of ulcer found in the lower limb: venous, neuropathic and ischaemic.

# Infection

There are two reasons why an 'at risk' patient is more prone to develop an infection:

- Loss of the skin barrier
- Impaired immunity.

In many cases where there the immune system is compromised, there is also an increased risk of ulceration. The infection may originate as contamination of a break in the skin, by tracking or spread of infection from a primary source or by blood-borne spread, e.g. from a dental abscess. For example, diabetics are prone to ischaemic, neuropathic and mixed ulcers but at the same time are also more at risk of *Candida* and bacterial infections because of the effects of diabetes on the immune system. Rheumatoid arthritis may be treated with long-term steroids. These medications increase skin fragility, and increase the likelihood of ulceration in response to 'relatively normal stresses'. Steroids also interfere with the immune system and depress the inflammatory response, so the signs of infection are less.

Local infection may spread to adjacent tissues and become disseminated. *Cellulitis* is the term

**Table 17.4** Comparison of neuropathic, ischaemic and venous ulcers

| Neuropathic | Ischaemic | Venous |
|---|---|---|
| Pain-free | Excessively painful | May be painful |
| Hyperkeratotic edges | May be slight hyperkeratosis | No hyperkeratosis |
| May be macerated | Usually dry unless infected | Area oedematous |
| Occur on areas of pressure and shear | Occur at extremities | Occur around the malleoli, especially the medial malleoli |
| Medium to large | Initially small | Large and shallow |
| Undermined walls | Vertical walls (punched-out) | Sloping walls |
| Yellow purulent slough | Thick adherent slough | Thin, watery slough |
| Copious discharge (may be bloody) | Seropurulent discharge | Seropurulent discharge |
| General/local neuropathy | Associated signs of ischaemia | Signs of venous stasis |

used to describe the spread of infection to adjacent connective tissue (Plate 32). *Osteomyelitis* is infection of bone, usually due to staphylococci. *Lymphangitis*, inflammation of the lymph vessels and *lymphadenitis*, inflammation of the lymph nodes, usually result from streptococcal infection (Ch. 13). Red lines extending from the site of the infection up the leg indicate lymphangitis which may lead to lymphadenitis (swelling of the inguinal nodes). *Bacteraemia* refers to the presence of bacteria in the blood and, if the organisms go on to multiply, in the blood, *septicaemia. Toxaemia* is even more serious and implies that the host is poisoned by bacterial products and damaged tissues.

Some 'at risk' patients may develop an infection without an underlying ulcer. Patients with acquired immune deficiency syndrome (AIDS) develop unusual infections, e.g. *Pneumocystis carinii*. Patients with T cell deficiencies are predisposed to a range of infections, particularly verrucae.

An increasing problem is the development of antibiotic-resistant bacteria, 'super-bugs'. Of particular concern is *Staphylococcus aureus*, which accounts for one in five of the infections acquired by patients during treatment. Naturally-occurring strains of *Staphylococcus aureus* have developed a resistance to all antibiotics except vancomycin. These strains have occurred as a result of the overuse and misuse of antibiotics. Other bacteria have also developed resistant strains, e.g. *Streptococcus pneumoniae* and *Mycobacterium tuberculosis*.

## Necrosis and gangrene

Where there is severe ischaemia, necrosis (localised death of tissue) will result and may progress to gangrene. Gangrene denotes the digestion of dead tissues by saprophytic bacteria, which are incapable of invading and multiplying in living tissues. Gangrene can be classified as primary or secondary, depending on the cause of the tissue necrosis. Primary gangrene, e.g. gas gangrene, is brought about by toxins of bacteria that invade the tissues and cause necrosis whereas secondary gangrene occurs in tissues that are already necrotic. Various bacteria lead to the breakdown of tissue proteins, carbohydrates and fats, the end products of which give off a characteristic foul odour. Secondary gangrene may be classed as *dry* or *wet*.

### Dry gangrene (Plate 3)

The affected tissues gradually undergo mummification, shrink and become clearly demarcated from the surrounding healthier tissues, with only minimal peripheral inflammation. The skin becomes dark in colour as a result of the breakdown of haemoglobin. Saprophytic organisms are usually present in relatively small numbers except at the junction between viable and nonviable tissue, which is the site of slow putrefaction. Amputation may be necessary to prevent infection and relieve intractable, severe pain.

### Wet gangrene (Plate 33)

Purulent necrosis arises as the result of a combination of local ischaemia due to infective vasculitis and bacterial toxins (Delbridge et al 1985). There is no clear line of demarcation between viable and non-viable tissue as in dry gangrene. Wet gangrene is likely to occur in a leg which is oedematous due to congestive heart failure or chronic venous insufficiency. If the underlying blood supply is reasonable healing may be promoted by thorough surgical debridement and parenteral antibiotics. However, there is always a high risk of amputation.

Gangrene can also arise as a severe complication of other conditions, such as sickle cell anaemia and frostbite. Erythrocytes in small blood vessels clump when tissue oxygen tension is low, leading to capillary and arteriolar thrombosis. Thus digital tourniquets should never be used in subjects with sickle cell anaemia. The disease also causes the superficial tissues to be poorly perfused, resulting in oedema and extensive skin ulceration, particularly around the malleoli.

## Deformity

A range of conditions, particularly those which

affect the nervous system, may result in lower limb deformities. For example, a cerebral vascular accident (CVA) can lead to an inverted foot with a circumducted gait; spina bifida can lead to marked foot deformity. Rheumatoid arthritis, an autoimmune disease affecting joints and other connective tissue, can lead to severe forefoot and rearfoot deformities. Osteoporosis of the spine can lead to spinal deformity and nerve entrapment, causing pain in the lower limb and altered gait and lower limb alignment.

These deformities, whatever their cause, affect the pattern of weightbearing. This often results in the build-up of pressure on particular parts of the foot, e.g. under one of the metatarsal heads (Mueller et al 1990). Pathological changes occur in the skin in response to these stresses, leading to hyperkeratosis (corn and callus formation) and in turn aseptic breakdown.

Of particular interest to practitioners dealing with the lower limb is the development of Charcot joints (Plate 34). Charcot joints (neuropathic arthropathy) occur as the result of autonomic neuropathy and resultant loss of vasomotor control of bone perfusion. Bone becomes increasingly fragile, and fractures occur spontaneously. Neuropathic patients are unaware of the local damage, and may present with an area of inflammation and swelling around the affected joint/joints, with rapidly progressive disorganisation of the joint. Cartilage is destroyed, the bone ends become grossly distorted, osteophytes appear and fractures around the joint may occur. Clinically the joint appears very warm to the touch, swollen and eventually deformed. Charcot joints are commonly associated with diabetes mellitus.

# IDENTIFICATION OF FACTORS THAT MAY AFFECT PROGNOSIS

It is important as part of the assessment process not only to identify the 'at risk' foot and the presence of complications but also to come to an opinion about the prognosis. This part of the assessment primarily deals with those factors that affect the healing of ulcers. If ulcers fail to heal, there is a greater risk of infection, necrosis and gangrene with the need for subsequent amputation.

The following should be taken into account when assessing the extent of ulceration:

- Site
- Size
- Depth
- Appearance of the edges and base
- Discharge
- Presence of slough
- Presence of infection
- Presence of granulation tissue
- Appearance of surrounding tissues.

Grading systems can be used to assess the extent of ulceration (see Table 9.6). These assessments should be made at every visit. The practitioner should look out for signs and symptoms of infection or incipient gangrene. Table 17.5 summarises the features of a healing, stable and deteriorating ulcer.

**Table 17.5**   Features of deteriorating, stable and healing ulcers

| Deteriorating | Stable | Healing |
|---|---|---|
| Extending | Static | Getting smaller |
| Base very sloughy | Base slough with granulation tissue | Base healthy granulation with epithelial 'islands' |
| Walls steep/undermined | Walls steep/slope inwards | Walls shallow, inward slope |
| Discharge plentiful/purulent/pungent | Discharge scant/serous/slight odour | No discharge, granulation tissue bleeds readily with minor trauma |
| Well defined, wide inflammatory margins | Congested peripheral tissues | Healthy tissues, no congestion, minimal inflammation |
| Likely to get worse, spread | Base may become fibrous and adhere to deeper tissues | May leave a scar once healing is complete |

**Table 17.6**   Factors which may prolong or depress healing

| Factors which prolong or depress healing | |
| --- | --- |
| Internal | Peripheral vascular disease resulting in ischaemia<br>Diabetes mellitus<br>Steroid therapy<br>Penicillamine and other NSAIDs<br>Cytotoxic and immunosuppressant drugs<br>Liver failure<br>Kidney failure<br>Cardiac problems<br>Malnutrition, e.g. lack of vitamins<br>Infection |
| External | Smoking<br>Repeated or sudden trauma<br>Poor hygiene<br>Poor wound care, e.g. adherent dressings<br>Inappropriate use of topical antiseptics and antibiotics<br>Too much activity<br>Cold environment |

Healing will take place if further tissue damage is avoided and infection controlled, in the presence of an adequate blood supply. 'At risk' patients often have a poor healing response and some ulcers may take months or even years to heal. Many factors can delay wound healing (Table 17.6). In some 'at risk' patients the therapeutic regimes that are used to control the disease further increase the likelihood of tissue breakdown, e.g. steroid therapy used to treat rheumatoid arthritis. Information from the primary patient assessment can help the practitioner to detect the presence and extent of these factors.

## CONDITIONS ASSOCIATED WITH AN 'AT RISK' FOOT

There are many conditions which may lead to the development of an 'at risk' foot or leg. The remainder of this chapter examines some of the more common of these conditions.

### Diabetes mellitus

Diabetes mellitus is characterised by chronic hyperglycaemia. It is the most common cause of an 'at risk' foot and is the underlying reason for the majority of non-traumatic lower limb amputations. It affects 2% of the population of the UK,

**Table 17.7**   Complications of diabetes mellitus in the rest of the body

| System/organ | Effect |
| --- | --- |
| Cardiovascular | Coronary artery disease (myocardial infarction)<br>Cerebral artery stenosis and occlusion (CVA, stroke)<br>Postural hypotension |
| Eyes | Background retinopathy<br>Proliferative retinopathy<br>Diabetic maculopathy<br>Cataracts |
| Kidneys | Glomerulosclerosis<br>Urinary tract infections |
| Nerves | Carpal tunnel syndrome<br>Ocular palsies<br>Impotence<br>Gustatory sweating (rare) |

with an incidence that increases with age. Sufferers are prone to develop a range of complications (Table 17.7), a number of which specifically affect the lower limb (Table 17.8). The risk of complications increases with the duration of the disease so no person with diabetes can feel they have escaped the long-term problems.

Diabetes mellitus is due to either a defect in insulin production by the beta islet cells of the pancreas or to factors that oppose the metabolic

**Table 17.8**   Complications of diabetes mellitus in the lower limb

- Neuropathy:   sensory<br>motor<br>autonomic
- Neuropathic ulceration
- Ischaemic ulceration
- Neuroischaemic ulceration
- Charcot's joints (neuroarthropathies), particularly in the tarsal area
- Peripheral arterial disease
- Median arterial calcification
- Microangiopathy (capillary basement membrane thickening and reduced tissue perfusion)
- Glycosylation of protein
- Staphylococcal and candidal skin infections
- Necrobiosis lipoidica and skin bullae
- Granuloma annulare

**Table 17.9** Comparison of insulin-dependent and non-insulin-dependent diabetes mellitus

| IDDM (Type I) | NIDDM (Type II) |
|---|---|
| Younger age of onset | Older age of onset |
| Normal body build or thin at the time of onset | Obese/tendency to overweight |
| European ethnicity | All racial groups, especially the affluent Increased risk in Indians |
| Seasonal onset | |
| HLA-DR3 or HLA-DR4 in 95% of cases | No HLA links |
| 30–50% incidence in identical twins | 90%+ incidence in identical twins |
| Autoimmune | No signs of autoimmunity |
| Insulin deficiency | Insulin resistance (especially if obese) Some insulin deficiency |
| Poor control leads to ketoacidosis | No ketoacidosis |
| Always requires insulin | Diet control Diet control + oral hypoglycaemics Diet control + insulin (in some cases) |

effects of insulin in tissues, or both. There is no clear cause, but it is thought to have a multifactorial aetiology, with both genetic and environmental factors implicated. Untreated, the subject undergoes disturbances of body carbohydrate, fat and protein metabolism. With treatment, using diet on its own or in combination with tablets or insulin, the patient can lead a reasonably normal life provided he/she remains free of complications.

Diabetes commonly occurs in two forms; insulin-dependent (IDDM)/type I diabetes, and non-insulin-dependent (NIDDM)/type II diabetes (Table 17.9). The same long-term complications are seen in both types. IDDM can develop in childhood and there is a familial link with other autoimmune diseases such as thyroid disease. Subjects with IDDM produce none, or only very little, of the insulin that they require for normal metabolism and thus have to rely on an external source of insulin, by injection. Patients who become diabetic as children are at risk of developing secondary foot, eye and kidney complications approximately 10 years after the initial diagnosis.

NIDDM is relatively common among populations that enjoy a relatively affluent lifestyle. It may be present in a subclinical form for years

before it is diagnosed. Therefore, patients who develop NIDDM may already have secondary complications at the time of diagnosis. Subjects retain up to 50% viable beta islet cells, but show a delayed and exaggerated secretion of insulin, with peripheral insulin resistance. Therapy involves stimulating pancreatic secretion and reduction of peripheral resistance to insulin by drug regimes and diet.

The keystone of treatment for diabetes is control of blood sugar levels through dietary intake, with injected insulin in IDDM and oral hypoglycaemic agents such as sulphonylureas and biguanides in some NIDDM. Glycaemic control is monitored by urine and blood tests (Ch. 13). Tight control of blood glucose renders the subject more likely to suffer hypoglycaemic attacks but reduces the likelihood and severity of the late-stage complications (Amiel 1993). Hypoglycaemic attacks occur when blood insulin levels are too high. Hyperglycaemia results from taking too little insulin, poor dietary control, or as the presenting symptom in an undiagnosed diabetic.

The diabetic limb and foot classically shows one of four presenting types. The prime clinical features are presented in Table 17.10; below, specific points are outlined.

**Table 17.10** The four types of diabetic foot

| | |
|---|---|
| Normal | No noticeable changes but at risk from developing fungal, bacterial or viral infections |
| Neuropathic | Warm, with bounding pulses. It can be characterised by Charcot's joints and deep trophic ulceration, with associated infection. The skin may be dry due to reduced sweating as the result of autonomic neuropathy. The neuropathy involves all sensory modalities, as well as motor and autonomic systems. The foot classically assumes a cavoid shape, with inversion of the calcaneus and clawing and triggering of the toes. Prominent joints and areas of callosity are prone to ulceration and possible infection |
| Ischaemic | Cold with thin, dry, atrophic skin. Nail and hair growth is compromised. Pulses are reduced or absent. Muscle bulk is lost in the limb. Intermittent claudication and/or rest pain may be a presenting feature. There may be a history of patchy dry gangrene and painful ulceration, particularly at the tips of digits, or over prominent joints that are subject to pressure |
| Neuro-ischaemic | Similar presentation to the ischaemic foot and limb, in terms of temperature, paucity of blood supply and ulceration. The foot will be relatively pain-free and thus very severely at risk from unconscious damage and infection |

### Normal

Patients with diabetes mellitus are especially prone to develop infections. 20% of diabetics are first diagnosed because they have persistent skin infection (Delbridge et al 1988). The reasons for the increased susceptibility to infection is unclear, but it has been demonstrated that the normal responses to early infection—polymorphonuclear leucocyte function, local cellular response, chemotaxis and phagocytosis—are all depressed in high blood glucose concentrations. When the host response to incidental infection is compromised, opportunistic microorganisms will colonise sugar-rich tissues (Knighton et al 1986). Fungal infections, especially *Candida*, can cause pruritus and intertrigo of the genital areas and interdigital fissures on the feet. Dry fissures around the heels occur in conjunction with dermatophytic infection, anhidrosis and/or autonomic neuropathy.

### Ischaemic

In long-term diabetes arteries are compromised by arteriosclerosis, aggravated by age and hypertension, atheroma and median calcification (Mönckeberg's sclerosis). The ankle/brachial (AB) index is the ratio of the systolic arterial pressure measured at the antecubital fossa and the ankle, a value of 1 being normal. When the arterial supply is reduced by atheroma or stenosis (narrowing of the lumen), the ratio will be less than 1 (e.g. 95/140 = AB 0.68). In cases where there is median arterial calcification, the arteries require a far higher pressure from the inflated cuff to compress them, and the ratio will be greater than 1 (e.g. 220/140 = AB 1.57).

Distal tissues, especially over sites subjected to excess pressure, will not be fully perfused, rendering them susceptible to pain, tissue breakdown and ischaemic ulceration, complicated by secondary infection. Where plantar calluses form they are thin, glass-like and difficult to debride. Isolated, very painful, heloma milliare (seed corns) occur within the dry, inelastic skin. Hyperkeratotic skin lesions and thickened nails may be underlain by tissue breakdown. Tissues subjected to relatively minor trauma from shoe wear or pressure and shear stress from biomechanical anomalies are prone to ulceration. These areas typically include the tips of the digits, areas of tissue over bony prominences such as the lateral aspect of the styloid process at the base of the fifth metatarsal, interdigitally and dorsally over interphalangeal joints. Radiographs of the ischaemic diabetic foot may show calcification of, particularly, the intermetatarsal arteries. This may be due to neuropathy (Edmonds et al 1982).

## Neuropathic

In contrast, the diabetic patient with complications related to neuropathy has easily palpable pulses, which are often bounding and exuberant. The tissues are warm, or even hot, due to the effects of autonomic neuropathy on vasomotor control. It is not unusual to find that the autonomic and sensory neuropathy is worse in one limb, and that foot and leg will be hotter and redder. Blood may be shunted from the arteries to the veins, bypassing arterioles and showing as engorged veins around the ankle and on the dorsum of the foot (Boulton et al 1982).

Doppler sounds in the neuropathic foot can be normal. However, since diabetes renders its sufferers far more prone to arteriosclerosis and atheroma, Doppler sounds are likely to be weakly biphasic or monophasic. The ankle/brachial index is often within the normal range of 0.9–1.1 (Amiel 1993), but the systolic and diastolic blood pressures are usually raised due to the hypertension associated with diabetes.

As well as demonstrating vascular effects, autonomic neuropathy depresses sweat gland activity, causing the skin of the foot to be dry and prone to fissures. Skin infections are common, particularly interdigital *Candida* and dermatophyte infections. Any break in the skin is readily colonised by opportunistic bacteria because of the high levels of glucose likely to be present in tissue fluid, leading to abscesses and pus pockets.

In the neuropathic foot, callosity forms readily at areas of pressure (Sibbaud & Schacter 1984), probably as the result of a neurogenic inflammatory process (Edmonds et al 1986). Plantar pressures are excessively high in the typical diabetic cavoid foot, especially where the plantar fat pad has undergone atrophy, and compromised tissues become subject to further devitalisation. Bullae form at areas of shear stress. Areas of extensive tissue breakdown which rapidly progress to become deep, perforating neuropathic ulcers with undermined walls, and copious exudate may occur as the build-up of exudate remains in situ because of the presence of overlying callosity. Neuropathic ulcers can become very extensive and involve underlying structures such as the deep fascia, joints and bone. They are sometimes complicated by severe spreading cellulitis infection and osteomyelitis. The patient may be quite unaware of the problem, due to the loss of pain sensation (anaesthesia).

Radiographs will show gross abnormality of joints, especially in the tarsal area, where Charcot joints develop as the result of microfractures caused by neurogenic inflammation. Metatarsals undergo resorption to assume a 'licked candy-stick' appearance, and the normal integrity of the metatarsophalangeal joints is lost. These bone changes lead to grossly abnormal foot function and alteration of weightbearing, with deep ulceration of the soft tissues overlying the abnormal joint. It has been observed that reduced subtalar joint motion correlates with neuropathic ulceration (Delbridge et at 1988). Therefore, any reduction in subtalar joint motion in a patient with a potential or actual neuropathy should be continuously monitored, as it can be regarded as a predictor of ulceration.

Neuropathic patients may not necessarily notice that pain sensation has been lost and may damage their feet (Case history 17.1). Neuro-

---

Case history 17.1

**Female, Caucasian aged 62**
I take insulin for my diabetes. I have two injections a day: one of 20 units and one of 16. My husband does them for me. When I lost my sight last year I seemed to lose my confidence. They said at first my sight might come back, but I'm beginning to think now that it won't. I can't feel my feet. Well, that's not quite true. Normally, I wouldn't know I had a foot, but when I got osteomyelitis, I knew all about that. They tried for weeks to get rid of the infection with antibiotics, but in the end they had to take off the big toe and the metatarsal, I think they said. That all started with a bit of plastic. One of my grandchildren had left a little plastic toy on the floor, and of course I didn't see it. In no time I had an ulcer that just wouldn't heal up. I try to keep to my diet, but I've always had a bit of a sweet tooth, so I admit I cheat a bit.

**Table 17.11** Features of neuropathy in diabetes mellitus

| | | |
|---|---|---|
| *Sensory* | | |
| | Symptoms | Non-painful and asymptomatic<br>*or* causes paraesthesia of feet, and occasionally fingers<br>*or* causes shooting pains, and burning sensation especially of the feet at night |
| | Signs | Loss of vibration sense in feet |
| | | Loss of pain sensation |
| | | Reduced or absent limb tendon reflexes |
| | Outcome | Mild to moderate reduction in sensation |
| | | Muscle weakness, and denervation of intrinsic foot muscles → cavoid foot |
| | | Severe impairment of all modalities of sensation (after 20+ years)<br>— glove and stocking anaesthesia<br>— impaired joint position sense, with Charcot's joints, mainly in the feet<br>— sensory ataxia, impaired gait and positive Romberg's sign<br>— deep trophic ulceration<br>— bladder atony and impotence |
| *Autonomic* | | May be asymptomatic or severe |
| | | May accompany sensory polyneuropathy, or manifest as a pure autonomic effect |
| | Signs | *Cardiovascular*<br>— postural hypotension<br>— vagal denervation of the heart, with high resting heart/pulse rates<br>— greater blood flow through superficial tissues = hot, red limb/foot<br><br>*Gastrointestinal tract*<br>— diarrhoea, severe enough to cause faecal incontinence at night<br>— delayed gastric emptying<br><br>*Sudomotor*<br>— facial and upper body sweating at meal times (gustatory sweating)<br>— loss of sweating of feet<br><br>*Endocrine effect*<br>— impaired or upset renin, glucagon or catecholamine release<br>— failure of metabolic response to hypoglycaemia<br><br>*Impotence*<br>— may present as earliest feature of autonomic neuropathy<br>— permanent |
| *Motor* | | |
| | Signs | *Cranial nerve lesions*<br>— those that supply the muscles of the eye (double vision)<br>— facial nerve palsy<br><br>*Isolated peripheral lesions*<br>— lateral cutaneous nerve of the thigh<br>— femoral, sciatic, peroneal nerves affected<br><br>*Diabetic amyotrophy*<br>— proximal, painful, weakness and wasting of legs and digital muscles<br>— anterior compartment syndrome<br>— loss of reflexes, but not loss of sensation<br>— extensor plantar responses<br>— decreased nerve conduction times = radiculopathy |

pathic anaesthesia tends to follow a 'glove and stocking' pattern and affects all modalities of sensation, though not all necessarily to the same extent (Ch. 7). Early signs of impending total loss of sensation are feelings of vague numbness, paraesthesia, shooting pains, hyperaesthesia or atypical sensations such as burning pains. The exacerbation of peculiarities of sensation may be reduced, or halted, by strict attention to the control of the diabetes (Amiel 1993). The features of neuropathy are outlined in Table 17.11. Acute neuropathy presenting early may improve with tight control but chronic, long-standing changes are irreversible.

### Neuro-ischaemic

Some patients with diabetes mellitus develop a combination of neuropathy and ischaemia. The foot is at a greatly increased risk as the normal warning sign of compromised circulation, pain, is absent. The foot and limb will show the typical signs of both chronic ischaemia and neuropathy, resulting in mixed ulcers. Supervening soft-tissue and deep infections complicate the clinical picture. These cases require the most careful management, but even then partial amputation may be unavoidable.

### Secondary infection

This is commonly due to the immuno-compromised state of the diabetic patient. Bacterial infections are an important cause of amputation, coma and death. Any break in the skin may be secondarily infected by bacteria; staphylococcal and streptococcal infections are more common in diabetic than non-diabetic patients. Ulcerated areas can be surprisingly resistant to flagrant infection, even though swabs of their discharge demonstrate high numbers of pathogens, including staphylococci, beta-haemolytic streptococci, faecal streptococci, *Klebsiella* and *Proteus* (Edmonds 1984, Wheat et al 1986). However, once infection is established, it will spread rapidly along deep tissue planes to involve bone, giving rise to deep infections such as osteomyelitis, severe cellulitis and deep plantar abscesses. Infection can lead to obliteration of the blood vessels, resulting in necrosis often seen as dark patches within an area of cellulitis.

Osteomyelitis in its later stages will show on X-ray as darker areas within the bone and loss of cortical integrity (Ch. 11). Early diagnosis of osteomyelitis can be difficult. It is possible to observe early changes using magnetic resonance imaging (MRI) but, as this is a very expensive investigation, the presenting clinical signs of infection, including cellulitis and oedema, raised temperature and lymphadenitis, may be used to diagnose the condition.

Due to profound neuropathy, the patient may be unaware of the severity of the presenting clinical emergency. Thus, any patient with ulcers or neuropathy should be monitored frequently and inspected for signs of possible infection and deep pockets of pus, such as web space infections. Because of autonomic neuropathy or early Charcot joint changes, the neuropathic foot and lower limb may be several degrees warmer and redder that the non-neuropathic foot, without the presence of any infection (Jones et al 1985).

## Rheumatoid arthritis

There are a number of autoimmune disorders which can affect the lower limb (Table 17.12) Of these rheumatoid arthritis is the most common. Rheumatoid arthritis (RA) is a common, chronic,

**Table 17.12**  Autoimmune diseases which may affect the lower limb

- Graves disease
- Atrophic hypothyroidism
- Hashimoto's thyroiditis
- Addison's disease
- Diabetes mellitus Type I (IDDM)
- Vitamin $B_{12}$ deficiency
- Vitiligo
- Hypoparathyroidism
- Myasthenia gravis
- Systemic lupus erythematosus
- Rheumatoid arthritis
- Dermatomyositis
- Polymyositis
- Systemic sclerosis
- Scleroderma
- Vasculitis
- Mixed connective tissue diseases
- Idiopathic thrombocytopenic purpura

Autoantibodies are implicated in the arthritides that arise with other diseases, such as Crohn's disease, and in the development of the vasculitis that characterises many autoimmune diseases

**Table 17.13** Non-articular effects of rheumatoid arthritis

| | |
|---|---|
| Anaemia | Occurs in most cases of RA, and is proportional to the activity of the inflammatory process<br>— normochromic normocytic anaemia of chronic disease—iron deficiency anaemia due to gastric bleeding from NSAID ingestion<br>— haemolytic anaemia<br>— hypersplenism |
| Lungs | Involvement manifests as pulmonary effusions (in 10% of male cases) and obliterative bronchiolitis even in non-smokers |
| Nodules | Can form in the lungs, with pericardial rub being heard in 30% of cases |
| Amyloidosis | The deposition of abnormal protein as a direct result of inflammation may affect the kidneys, and lead to renal failure |
| Vasculitis | Affects kidneys, leading to focal tissue necrosis and loss of function; affects skin particularly around nail folds, causing pinpoint tissue necrosis and a proneness to ulceration |
| Sjögren's syndrome | Keratoconjunctivitis sicca (dry eyes) and xerostomia (dry mouth) |
| Felty's syndrome | Lymphadenopathy proximal to affected joints, splenic involvement, repeated infections and weight loss |

systemic disease of connective tissues, characterised by an inflammatory polyarthritis with progressive joint damage and deformity, depressed healing and skin ulceration. It also affects non-articular joint tissue such as joint capsules and tendons and causes neurological, eye, kidney, lung and heart complications (Table 17.13). Since many of its sufferers have been placed on anti-inflammatory drug regimes such as systemic steroids, side-effects of these should be considered as part of the pathology of the disease (Case history 17.2). It has a high morbidity and causes severe disability. It affects about 2% of the world's population and is evenly distributed between hot and cold climates. The female:male ratio is 3:1, and there is a 5–10% familial incidence. It affects both children and adults, but the greatest incidence is in adults aged 30–40 years.

It is presumed that an unknown antigen is implicated. The formation of antigen–antibody complexes leads to inflammation, particularly in joints. 15% of cases will show an acute presentation, but the majority have an insidious onset with systemic symptoms such as fatigue and fever. Pain is worse on waking, with stiffness taking until mid-morning or later to wear off. Pain increases in the evening, sleep is disturbed

Case history 17.2

**Female, West Indian aged 68**
I was first diagnosed as having rheumatoid arthritis when I was 38. It all started with my foot. I thought I had gout. The outside joint near my little toe came up so swollen and red—I couldn't get my shoe on. I didn't think it could be arthritis as I felt so ill. I'd never had anything like that before. But you know, I had to give up work. They took blood tests and X-rays and told me I had this arthritis. I got a stomach ulcer. They said I took too many pain killers, but I said to them, 'What else do you expect me to do? I got a family to look after!' It's bad enough that I can't get going in the mornings. If I'd have known I was going to end up like this. Look at my hands. My husband says my fingers look like loose bananas. I had to have foot operations, so that now my ankles don't move. At least that takes care of some of the pain, but they had to give me surgical shoes because the steroids made me get ulcers under my feet. I have to have an operation for that next. And now they tell me that I've got diabetes.

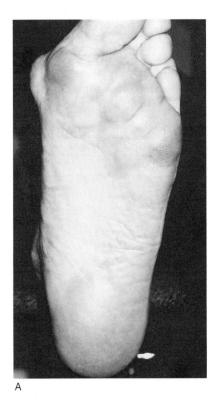

A

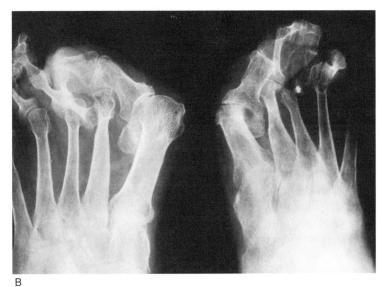

B

**Figure 17.1   A.** Typical appearance of a rheumatoid foot showing hallux valgus and digital deformity   **B.** Radiograph of a rheumatoid foot.

and analgesic and anti-inflammatory drugs are necessary. The synovial linings of affected joints proliferate (pannus formation) and joint surfaces and supporting structures are eroded by a process of enzymic autolysis.

A wide range of body tissues are affected by this disease, rendering the patient prone to pain, ulceration, deformity and reduced tissue viability. Drug regimes that are taken to control the inflammatory process, e.g. steroids, gold salts, non-steroidal anti-inflammatory drugs, exacerbate the tendency to skin ulceration. Because of the inherent disability, the simple day-to-day tasks of self-care, such as combing the hair or cutting toenails, can become impossible.

The small joints of the hands and feet are bilaterally affected, classically the MTPJs/MCPJs and PIPJs. RA may first present as a monoarthritis, such as the knee. In the foot, the fifth MTPJ is likely to be first affected. If a young/middle-aged female presents in clinic with pain and soft-tissue swelling of the fifth MTPJ without an obvious cause, a blood test for

RA is indicated (Renton 1993). Other joints typically affected are wrists and ankles, knees and elbows, shoulders and cervical spine and, later in the disease, the hip joints. New joints are recruited to the pathological process over the first few months of the disease. Involved joints become warm, swollen and very tender, especially on movement, as a result of inflammatory effusions, and the number of swollen joints reflects the activity of the illness.

The fingers and toes show a characteristic lateral deviation at the MCPJs/MTPJs, and the hands and feet show lateral deviation at the wrists and rear foot. Thus the patient can develop gross hallux valgus and a severe valgus deformity at the subtalar joint (Fig. 17.1). Digital joint capsules become weakened and tendons rupture, leading to boutonnière and swan-neck deformity of digits and subluxations. Toes develop hammer deformity and are subject to skin ulceration over prominent joints. Similar processes within the knee, together with wasting of the quadriceps muscle, cause instability of the joint, with profound valgus or varus deviation. The rate of joint deterioration is variable, as the disease follows a pattern of exacerbation and remission. 50% of cases develop significant disability and 10% become seriously disabled, so that all movements are difficult due to loss of strength and joint deformity (Van der Heijde et al 1992).

The knee joint capsule may herniate and rupture posteriorly into the popliteal space—a Baker's cyst—causing severe pain and swelling which can mimic a deep vein thrombosis. Large painful rheumatoid bursae, which are prone to ulceration and sinus formation, form over the plantar aspects of the MTPJs. The normal thickness of the plantar fibro-fatty pad is lost. Tenosynovitis affects the flexor tendons of the hands and feet, causing triggering of digits. Muscles become atrophied through lack of use and the generalised disease process. The intrinsic musculature of the hands wastes, causing 'guttering' of the backs of the hands which is further exacerbated by disuse atrophy. Rheumatoid nodules develop in 20% of cases. These can arise anywhere, but develop particularly over the ulnar surface just distal to the elbow, and anterior tibial surface, just distal to the knee.

Atlanto-axial subluxation in the cervical spine can cause gross neurological problems such as cervical cord compression. It is fortunately rare. More common are carpal and tarsal tunnel syndromes, with a positive Tinel's sign (cutaneous tingling or paraesthesia occurring over the distribution of the nerve if the nerve path is tapped lightly). This occurs as a result of subluxation of the wrist and ankle joints and inflammation (tenosynovitis) of local tendons. A glove and stocking sensory, and sometimes motor, polyneuropathy may occur. Mononeuritis multiplex may arise as a result of vasculitis affecting several nerves at once.

Radiographs give characteristic findings:

- 'Mouse bite' (or mouse ear) erosion on the surface of affected bones
- Early increase in joint space (due to effusions) then later loss of joint space, with thinning of the cortex and loss of cartilage

- Porosis and cystic degeneration of periarticular bone
- Destruction of bone ends, with later joint ankylosis. Thus joints initially affected by rheumatoid arthritis may later develop osteoarthritic changes.

Blood analysis shows anaemia, and a raised erythrocyte sedimentation rate (ESR). Tests for rheumatoid factor are positive in 80% of cases.

## Arterial disease

The term 'arterial disease' includes pathologies that affect large and small arteries:

- Arteriosclerosis
- Median arterial sclerosis
- Atheroma
- Thrombosis
- Embolism
- Vasculitis.

Any of these can affect the arterial supply to the foot and limb and cause the signs and symptoms of chronic ischaemia, to a greater or lesser extent (Plate 35). The blood supply may be completely obstructed or partially obstructed (Case history 17.3). Patients showing signs of limb ischaemia are likely to have similar problems affecting the arteries supplying heart muscle, the central nervous system and kidneys. In these cases foot and limb ischaemia presents as part of a generalised ischaemia, and is thus a manifestation of severe, life-threatening disease (Nelson 1992).

An arterial embolus can cause complete obstruction (acute ischaemia) of the legs. The embolus may have originated from within the heart, as may occur in atrial fibrillation, or by detachment of fragments from a clot or atheroma proximal to the site of occlusion. The leg initially appears deathly pale and stone cold. The patient is in extreme, acute and persistent pain and cannot move the limb. Pulses are absent below the obstruction. Surgery to remove the clot or bypass the obstruction is vital and urgent, but amputation may become necessary as the tissues that have been deprived of an arterial blood supply may necrose.

---

Case history 17.3

**Female, Caucasian aged 94**

I thought that I must be getting rheumatism because my legs were hurting me so much. I did my exercises every morning and it seemed to help for a bit. But the pain didn't ever really go. I used to sleep in my arm chair, as the bedclothes seemed to make the pain worse. My neighbour said I ought to get the doctor in, but I've never seen this new one and didn't fancy the idea. Well in the end I had to give in. When he saw how red my foot was he said, 'My goodness me, what have you been doing to yourself?' A doctor from the hospital came to see me the very next day. He said he was a consultant. He looked at my foot and took my blood pressure in my arm and leg, and listened with a little microphone to the blood. Well to cut a long story short, they put me in hospital straight away. They said they had to do a lot of tests and X-rays, and that the pain wasn't arthritis but circulation. After the tests they said they were pleased with me and I wouldn't have to have my leg off. That was a shock— no one had suggested I should. They said there was a blockage behind my knee and they were going to get rid of it with a little balloon. As soon as I came round from the anaesthetic I knew it had been successful. My leg felt lovely. That was 3 weeks ago. That awful stinging pain started again last week, but this time it's in both legs, and higher up. The consultant was very nice, but he thought that another balloon would not work. He has given me some tablets. I expect they are special leg tablets. I hope they do the trick. I wouldn't want to have both legs off.

---

Chronic ischaemia results from a reduction in the flow of blood to tissues which is either continuous or spasmodic (Raynaud's phenomenon). Arteriosclerosis is the generalised age-related change that occurs in large and small arteries and arterioles. In arteries >1 mm diameter, the changes cause an early compensatory muscular hypertrophy of the vessel's tunica media, which is followed by fibrosis and resultant dilatation of the lumen. The vessel becomes stiff, tortuous and inelastic. Doppler sounds become monophasic. In arteries <1 mm diameter, especially those of the kidney, in addition to median hypertrophy, there is marked thickening of the tunica intima, with resultant narrowing of the lumen. The affected kidney becomes progressively ischaemic, the outcome of which is to increase hypertension and exacerbate the whole problem.

Median artery calcification (Mönckeberg's sclerosis) is a disease of unknown cause, where the tunica media of arteries supplying the lower limb and foot undergo dystrophic calcification. This is seen especially in the elderly, and in patients with diabetes. It is also noted in patients that have previously undergone lumbar sympathectomy, and is therefore considered by some to be a manifestation of autonomic neuropathy.

Atheroma is characterised by the development of fatty, fibrous plaques within the arterial wall. Where atheroma complicates the clinical picture of arteriosclerosis, which is very likely, the condition is referred to as atherosclerosis. Doppler sounds will reflect turbulence in the arterial flow. Atherosclerosis primarily affects medium-sized vessels, rarely being found in vessels of less than 2 mm diameter. As it is a common finding at post-mortem examination of male adults and almost universally in the elderly of both sexes it is considered to be a normal variant of the ageing process. Factors other than age and gender which predispose to its development are familial type, hyper-lipidaemia, cigarette smoking, hypertension and diabetes mellitus. There is a link with the use of the contraceptive pill, heavy alcohol consumption, lack of exercise and obesity. Arterial plaques become colonised by small clots, parts of which may detach, causing distal infarction in cerebral, coronary, renal, optic and digital vessels. Removal or modification of the risk factors that predispose to atheroma does not necessarily reduce the development of atheroma.

Atheromatous disease involving the aorta, iliac and peripheral vessels causes chronic ischaemia of the legs, especially in male smokers of more than 50 years of age. Thromboangiitis obliterans (Buerger's disease) was previously described as a separate disease state. It is now considered to have the same aetiology as atheromatous disease, although it occurs almost exclusively in young men who smoke. Both limbs are usually affected, but it is usually more pronounced in one limb. In very severe cases, arms as well as legs will be involved. X-ray investigation may show calcification of the arteries.

Raynaud's phenomenon affects 5% of the population, the majority of them being young women. The digital arteries show an abnormal vasospastic response to cold stimulus, causing the digits to blanch and stay white or cyanotic for several hours. This episode is followed by reactive hyperaemia, probably under the influence of neuropeptides, during which time the tissues are numb, or burn and are very painful. Problems occur bilaterally, and fingers are more affected than toes. Raynaud's can arise as an idiopathic, isolated problem (primary Raynaud's) or as part of the overall picture of a connective tissue disease, e.g. systemic sclerosis.

## Chronic venous insufficiency

Chronic venous insufficiency presents with a spectrum of characteristic symptoms and signs—telangiectasia (Plate 4), petechiae, haemosiderosis (Plate 6), dependent oedema, varicose eczema, atrophie blanche (Plate 5), varicose veins and stasis (venous) ulceration (Plate 7). Some patients may exhibit all signs while others may only ever be troubled by one. The problems arising from chronic venous insufficiency vary with the degree and extent of the pathology.

Venous insufficiency usually occurs secondary to a previous deep venous thrombosis, although the patient may be unaware of any previous exciting clinical episode (Ch. 6). Vein valves become inefficient, leading to incompetency of the deep and superficial veins, ambulatory venous hypertension and loss of normal capillary fluid exchange. In the early stages the oedema is soft and pitting, but over the years chronic induration and fibrotic changes occur to cause a very firm 'woody' oedema, with the typical signs of chronic venous insufficiency. The medial malleolar areas are first affected, and superficial veins may subsequently become varicosed. Haemosiderosis causes a brownish discoloration of skin that varies from light beige through to black in severe cases. It commonly affects the anterior skin of the lower third of the leg. The discoloration is caused by the deposition of iron-containing pigments within the dermis. The combination of oedema and haemosiderosis can cause irritation and chronic inflammation, dryness of skin and varicose eczema. The skin becomes weakened by scratching and local trauma can easily cause varicose ulceration that can take months or even years to heal. Recurrent ulceration and healing of venous ulcers can lead to the appearance of a 'champagne' leg (Plate 36).

The saphenous veins and their tributaries, when varicosed, can lead to superficial venous thrombosis (thrombophlebitis) and inflammation of the vein wall. Secondary thrombosis can cause the affected portion of the vein to appear red, swollen and distended.

**Varicose veins** are very common as they tend to be associated with the physiological problems imposed by bipedal locomotion. Both the long and short saphenous veins, their tributaries and occasionally the superficial veins of the dorsum of the foot, can be affected. This shows as distention and tortuousness of the superficial veins. The practitioner should be alert to the possible risk of thrombophlebitis and deep venous thrombosis.

### Deep venous thrombosis (DVT)

This can occur in any vein, but it most commonly affects the veins of the pelvis and leg, including the deep veins of the calf. DVT can arise spontaneously or as a complication of prolonged postoperative bed rest and immobility (Case history 17.4). It is found in 60% of hospitalised cases at post-mortem. Other predisposing factors include local damage and inflammation of the vein (such as may arise from repeated injections, cannulation of the vein or thrombophlebitis), varicose veins, local inflammation, a previous history of thrombosis, advanced age or increased blood viscosity, such as occurs with polycythemia, sickle cell anaemia and myeloma. It is a common problem following cerebrovascular accident (CVA) or myocardial infarction. It used to be a severe complication of childbirth, in the days when mothers were expected to 'lie in' for a full month's total best rest following the birth of the baby.

Patients who develop DVT usually present with painful swelling of the calf, with redness or cyanosis and engorgement of the superficial veins. But the extensive, soft, pitting oedema involving much of the lower limb may be the only presenting sign. The condition develops rapidly to a maximum by 48–72 hours. Homan's sign (pain in the calf on dorsiflexion of the foot) may be positive but does not give an absolute diagnosis, as other local problems (such as a ruptured Baker's cyst in patients with rheumatoid arthritis) may cause this phenomenon. When the deep iliofemoral veins are thrombosed, the principal sign is very severe oedema of the leg, causing occlusion of distal veins, so that the limb becomes grossly swollen and cyanotic. A particularly severe, but rare, form manifests as phlegmasia caerulea dolens, where oedema is so severe as to impede arterial flow, causing gangrene of the white, pulseless limb.

The diagnosis of DVT is based on the presenting signs and case history. This is confirmed by venography, where a vein in the dorsum of the foot is injected with contrast medium and the venous system imaged by X-ray. Doppler techniques and plethysmography can also be used. In 50% of cases, a DVT leads to a chronically-swollen limb, with venous eczema, haemosiderosis and a likelihood of ulceration.

Postoperative patients are advised to exercise the leg muscles for a few minutes every hour or so as soon as they can following surgery to reduce the likelihood of a thrombosis developing. If an intravenous clot forms, part of it could detach and pass from the venous side of the circulation and through the heart to lodge in the pulmonary artery, with fatal consequences.

## The oedematous foot and limb

Oedema causes distention of affected tissues (Nelson 1992). It will compromise the efficiency of the microvasculature, the reaction of tissues to trauma, the integrity and texture of overlying skin and the potential for healing of affected tissues.

Oedema occurs as a result of a disruption to the normal mechanism of tissue fluid exchange. It may result due to a systemic or a localised problem and may be uni- or bilateral. Systemic causes result in bilateral oedema and may be due to congestive heart failure or low serum albumen levels associated with kidney or liver failure. Localised oedema may occur due to a variety of causes (Table 17.14) and lead to uni- or bilateral oedema (Young 1991). Chronic venous insufficiency is the most likely cause of unilateral oedema although both legs may be equally affected.

Lymphatic oedema may be either soft and pitting or firm and woody. This form of oedema is due to the pathological accumulation of fluid that fails to be drained from the tissues by a normal lymphatic system. The first signs show as puffiness of the dorsum of the foot, which disappears overnight. Gradually the swelling persists and increases, extending up the calf and in severe cases as far as the thigh. In the later stages it no longer pits nor disappears with bed rest. When oedema develops during the teenage/young adult years, especially in women, it can be due to a congenital deficiency or absence of lymph vessels. Alternatively, it may arise secondary to a proximal obstruction to lymph flow, or removal of a lymph gland, a procedure often undertaken in the treatment of malignant neoplasms. Carcinoma is the most common cause of

**Table 17.14** Causes of localised oedema

| Cause | Onset | Pain | Colour and temperature | Foot involvement |
|---|---|---|---|---|
| Thrombophlebitis | Rapid | Acute | Red/cyanotic<br>Prominent veins<br>Hot, very swollen | Ankle and proximally |
| Chronic venous insufficiency | Slow | Dull discomfort | Brown, haemosiderosis | Distended dorsum veins ankle and proximally |
| Lymphoedema | Slow | Uncomfortable | Normal<br>Slightly cyanotic | Whole foot, including toes |
| Cellulitis | Rapid | Acute | Red, patchy erythema | Depends on site of lymphangitis; hot |
| Ischaemia | Rapid | Acute | White and cold<br>Red and cold<br>Patchy gangrene | Depends on site |
| Muscle rupture or compartment syndrome | Rapid | Acute | Ecchymosis at ankle<br>Hot at injury site | Foot drop if anterior compartment involved<br>No dorsiflexion if calf muscles involved |

secondary lymphoedema arising in patients over 35 years of age.

Cellulitis may result in localised oedema. The onset is sudden, and pain is acute in the non-neuropathic patient. These patients require immediate antibiosis. Residual swelling may persist even after all signs of acute inflammation and infection have cleared (Case history 17.5). The most common portal of entry is an inter-digital fissure associated with dermatomycosis. Cellulitis also presents in patients with diabetes who have severe soft-tissue infections, or osteomyelitis where infection from an ulcer spreads to involve underlying bone.

---

**Case history 17.5**

**Female, Caucasian aged 52**
All the women in my family have big legs. Mine are like tree trunks. They've gradually got like that over the years. They aren't at all soft. In the hot weather they are very uncomfortable. Some years ago I got an infection, cellulitis. The skin over my shins and lower legs just broke open and was oozing clear fluid. Even with bandaging it would not clear, so I ended up in hospital for a couple of weeks until the antibiotics got a hold. Fortunately I haven't had anything quite as bad as that since then. I always wear the elastic stockings, but the swelling never really goes away now. It used to go down a bit at night, but not any more.

---

Severe ischaemia with rest pain induces the patient to keep the legs dependent, even at night, predisposing to oedema. Restoration of blood supply to an ischaemic limb by arterial bypass graft or angioplasty is commonly followed by transient oedema lasting several weeks.

Some medication regimes have the unwanted effect of causing fluid retention, which causes bilateral, soft, pitting oedema in the lower limb. These include non-steroidal anti-inflammatory drugs; antihypertensive drugs (e.g. methyldopa, nifedipine, guanethidine and minoxidil), hormones (e.g. testosterone, progesterone, oestrogen) corticosteroids and monoamine oxidase inhibitors. Ongoing medication with any of these drugs becomes apparent during history taking.

In hyperthyroid patients pretibial myxoedema affects the pretibial region and dorsum of the foot. Garters and tight stockings can cause or aggravate limb oedema, as can prolonged sitting for long periods, such as when driving long distances or travelling by air. Stress fractures will produce swelling of the dorsum of the midfoot, but it is normal for the history to indicate the cause at a very early stage of the consultation. However, a fracture may go unremarked in an osteoporotic patient or where there is a profound sensory neuropathy.

In all of the above cases, the patient history is the clue to the cause of the oedema. The speed of onset may be diagnostic. A rapid onset over the course of a few hours indicates an acute cause, such as thrombophlebitis or cellulitis. A slow progression over several weeks or months suggests chronic venous insufficiency or lymphoedema. A history that links recurrent oedematous episodes with bouts of fever and chills is a strong indication of cellulitis and lymphadenitis. Pain too can be diagnostic. The presence of painful swelling indicates thrombophlebitis, cellulitis, compartment syndrome, severe ischaemia with oedema, or muscle rupture. The swelling of lymphoedema and that due to systemic causes will cause discomfort rather than pain. Examination of the limb can reveal clues as to the likely cause. A diffuse reddish cyanosis with prominent superficial veins suggests deep venous thrombosis. Patchy, reticular or spotty erythema indicates cellulitis. Tender red streaks leading away from an area of inflammation suggest lymphangitis. Ecchymosis around the ankle is a clue to muscle or tendon rupture. Dorsal swelling on the foot, involving the toes and spreading towards the leg, suggests lymphoedema.

## ACQUIRED IMMUNODEFICIENCY SYNDROME (AIDS)

*Pneumocystis carinii* pneumonia tends only to affect subjects who are immunocompromised by malignancy or its treatment. Kaposi's sarcoma is usually only seen in elderly Jewish people or those of Mediterranean or African extraction. In 1981 there was an extraordinary outbreak of these diseases in previously fit young men in Los Angeles and New York. 72% of the cases were practising homosexuals and 17% were intravenous drug abusers. These outbreaks were the first reported episodes of infection with human immunodeficiency virus (HIV).

The human immunodeficiency virus was first isolated in 1983. However, back testing of serum samples has shown that HIV could have originated in central Africa as early as the 1950s. The epidemic appears to have spread from Africa to Haiti, to the USA, then worldwide. In Africa the disease affects both sexes equally, whereas in the Western world the vast majority of the early cases were among homosexual men or intravenous drug abusers. It is rapidly becoming pandemic among both sexes. In 1992, 24% of all new cases in the UK were in heterosexuals. A HIV-positive woman has a 50% chance of infecting her fetus. It is estimated that in some parts of Africa and Asia at least 10% of the population are HIV-positive. Clear evidence is emerging that there are several forms of the causative virus and a preventive vaccine is proving extremely difficult to engineer.

Most patients infected with HIV are shown to have circulating antibodies to HIV viral proteins, but there are those who are seronegative for antibodies. The seropositive HIV patient remains infected and infectious for life. HIV antibodies appear in blood samples (i.e. seroconversion occurs) 5–12 weeks following the initial infection. The HIV antigen test is useful for detecting the presence of early infection, prior to seroconversion. The HIV antibody test is only as reliable as any screening test and therefore requires further tests on fresh samples by another test method before confirmation is made. Since some patients do not raise an antibody response to HIV, a negative HIV antibody test is not absolute reassurance of lack of infection.

Infection with HIV (i.e. seroconversion) can be symptomless or give rise to flu-like symptoms for about a week, and can thus pass unnoticed. The incidence of HIV in a community precedes the development of AIDS by about 5 years. This 'silent period' allows considerable spread among the population before the infection becomes apparent as outward symptoms.

AIDS is defined as the occurrence of a disease indicative of loss of cell-mediated immunity in a person with no known cause for immunodeficiency other than the presence of HIV. In the early stages the patient may develop systemic symptoms, e.g. oral thrush, hairy leucoplakia and repeated episodes of shingles, but does not have a major opportunistic infection or show other features associated with AIDS.

In the early years of the infection the subject remains well. Only 1% of cases die in the early stages of the disease. An early manifestation of HIV is often a skin eruption, such as seborrhoeic dermatitis, especially of the nasolabial folds, or severely pruritic 'itchy folliculitis' of the neck, face, arms or thighs; in Africa 30% of HIV cases show this presentation. The disease progresses, punctuated by intervals of good health. Oral thrush and hairy leucoplakia are important pointers, as 60–80% of patients develop AIDS within 2 years. Shingles (herpes zoster) arising in more than one dermatome simultaneously is often the first manifestation of immuno-suppression in HIV disease. Facial molluscum contagiosum can be considered to be diagnostic of HIV disease and lesions are most widespread in the more severely immunocompromised cases. Common skin infections, such as genital and labial herpes simplex, warts, verrucae, impetigo and dermatophytic eruptions, are more common in HIV-positive individuals, and more difficult to cure (Case history 17.6). Subjects are prone to bouts of chronic diarrhoea due to infection with *Cryptosporidium*, Cytomegalovirus, mycobacteria, *Giardia*, *Salmonella* and *Campylobacter*, leading to severe weight loss.

---

Case history 17.6

**Male, Caucasian aged 41**
I've never had anything wrong with my feet actually. Well, nothing apart from this verruca. It's been a real nuisance. It really hurts at times, and no matter what they do to it, back it comes. They said it was a mosaic wart. That was 4 years ago. They've burnt it, frozen it, put on every sort of acid and padding, but it never really goes, and in fact in the last 6 months it's really started to spread. I seroconverted, became HIV-positive that is, two and a half years ago. I haven't had any serious illnesses, and I haven't got any Kaposi's. My partner got *Pneumocystis carinii* pneumonia. He died. It's odd that, how someone so well can get so ill and die so quickly. He had a really bad attack of shingles on one side of his chest and up his neck last Christmas.

---

Full AIDS is frequently heralded by the development of *Pneumocystis carinii* pneumonia (PCP) or other rare chest infections. 60% of cases of AIDS present with PCP. Some AIDS and HIV-positive patients have contracted a form of tuberculosis that is resistant to the normal range of antitubercular drugs. Kaposi's sarcoma, normally a rare, benign, endothelial cell tumour, was noted in 35% of the first described cases of AIDS in 1981. It is common in homosexuals and heterosexuals with AIDS, but rare in other HIV risk groups. It is thought to be caused by an as yet unidentified opportunistic sarcoma virus that is spread by sexual contact. It is very aggressive in AIDS, affecting all areas of the skin, respiratory and gastrointestinal tracts. About two in three AIDS-related Kaposi's sarcomas present on the lower legs.

Once full AIDS has developed, the subject encounters more and more bouts of overwhelming infection, with serious weight loss and progressive HIV encephalopathy. Two-thirds of AIDS patients are said to suffer from HIV encephalopathy (AIDS dementia complex) with ataxia, paraplegia, paralysis and incontinence if the spinal cord is involved. Peripheral nerve lesions can cause foot drop or slurred speech. Cytomegalovirus eye infections lead to blindness. The total duration of the illness may be from as little as 2 years from seroconversion to 10–20 years—the upper limit is not yet known. It is not clear whether all those who are HIV-positive go on to develop AIDS.

Subjects who are aware of their HIV status are advised to tell as few people as possible; there is no need to make a special point of informing the GP while they are quite well. They are advised to inform the dentist, tattooist, acupuncturist or ear piercer, or any practitioner who is going to perform a surgical procedure.

## OSTEOPOROSIS

Osteoporosis is described as reduced bone mass per unit bone volume. The affected bone shows reduced strength and an increased tendency to fracture in response to episodes of minor trauma. As the problem is one of loss of bone mass, rather than demineralisation, plasma calcium phosphate levels are normal and alkaline phosphatase levels will only be increased if there has been a recent fracture.

**Table 17.15** Features of osteoporosis

| Feature | Description |
|---------|-------------|
| Presentation | Bone pain from fractures—Colles (wrist), femoral neck and vertebrae<br>Nerve pain from nerve root entrapment |
| Epidemiology | Elderly women commonly (lack of oestrogens leads to loss of bone mass) |
| Predispositions | Endocrine diseases (Cushing's disease, diabetes mellitus, thyrotoxicosis)<br>Rheumatoid arthritis<br>Lack of exercise and bed rest<br>Chronic renal failure<br>Sympathetic reflex dystrophy, Sudeck's atrophy<br>Dietary, e.g. anorexia nervosa<br>Smoking<br>Pregnancy |
| Drug-induced | Glucocorticoids, long-term diuretics, heparin |

---

Case history 17.7

**Female, Caucasian aged 89**
They thought I was going to die when I was 8. I had rheumatic fever. Born to hang I was. Mind you, my heart is bad. I get so breathless at the slightest thing. It's not as if I'm a smoker. Look at my legs. Sometimes they are so swollen that they look like I've got wellingtons on. I just have to take my slippers off because even they make my feet sore. I've got this leg ulcer at the moment, where I tripped up and took a layer of skin off my shin. The District Nurse only has to come in twice a week now, but she says I must expect it to take at least 6 months to clear up, so only two more to go. Still, they didn't have to do the skin graft they threatened me with. I wish I weren't so round-shouldered. Do you know, I used to be five foot four. I reckon I'm nearer four foot five now. They said it's all due to my bones crumbling. I get such neuralgia in my shoulder and arm. Sometimes I don't know where to put myself. I asked the doctor at the hospital if I could have HRT, but he only said, 'What, at your age?' You wouldn't think you could break your wrist undoing a jar of jam.

---

Osteoporosis can occur as the result of physiological processes, as well as arising in pathological states (Table 17.15). Physiological osteoporosis occurs as a loss of bone density due to lack of use, such as in prolonged immobility when a plaster cast is worn. It is reversible, and normal bone density is regained once mobility is resumed. Pathological osteoporosis occurs as part of a disease process, or in response to reduced hormone levels or hormonal imbalance. Oestrogens and calcitonin inhibit bone resorption. Excess levels of circulating glucocorticoids lead to excessive bone resorption and osteoporosis, but do not cause demineralisation. By contrast, bone demineralisation occurs in osteomalacia and rickets as the result of vitamin D deficiency, malabsorption or renal disease.

Once established, pathological osteoporosis may result in spontaneous fractures, loss of skeletal alignment, vertebral compression and loss of height, nerve entrapment syndromes, such as sciatica, and severe pain (Case history 17.7). Pathological osteoporosis may remain unnoticed in its early stages, until a fracture occurs. It is very common for elderly ladies to break a hip following a fall.

Older women are particularly prone to osteoporosis. The normal rate of age-related bone mass loss is greatly increased by the absence of circulating oestrogens following the menopause. In addition, exercise, which normally helps to maintain bone density, tends to decline with increasing age. The average intake of calcium in the elderly, at 500–700 mg daily, is roughly 50% of that which is required for an elderly person to maintain bone mass. Non-ambulant patients with neurological deficit, such as those with spina bifida, may show osteoporosis. It also complicates the long-term administration of parenteral, and high doses of topical, steroid drugs.

Osteoporosis should be considered in the diagnosis of the older female who presents with a suspected metatarsal or stress fracture following a period of increased exercise. In the early stages, neither the fracture nor the underlying osteoporosis may be noted on X-ray, as normal radiographic techniques will not demonstrate reduction in bone mass until it has reached an extreme degree (approximately 50%) of loss of density. Alternative means of imaging, e.g. computerised tomography, can confirm osteoporosis at its earliest stages, before the patient develops the clinical signs (Ch. 11).

# SPINA BIFIDA

Dysraphism is a group of congenital conditions that reflect failure of the normal developmental fusion of the foetal neural tube. The most severe form shows as anencephaly, where the brain and cranial vault are absent, or meningoencephalocele, where the brain and meningeal tissue extrude through a fault in the skull. In spina bifida there is exposure of the distal part of the neural tube in the lumbosacral region. In spina bifida occulta, there is failure of fusion of the vertebral arch overlying the spinal cord, without exposure of neural tissues (Fig. 17.2). In spina bifida, a myelocele (where elements of the cord and lumbosacral roots contained within a meningeal sac herniate through a vertebral fault) or a meningocele (where only meningeal tissue protrudes) cause profound neurological complications. Spina bifida is estimated to occur in 3% of the population. Clinically it may only be apparent as a patch of hair (Fig. 17.3) or a dimple near the base of the spine with minor neurological manifestations of the lower limb, as in spina bifida occulta.

The flagrant forms of the condition feature paralysis of the lower limbs and sphincters and profound generalised neuropathy below the level of the neural tube fault. Cases of spina bifida vary in presentation, depending on the extent and position of the developmental fault, but sensory, motor and autonomic neuropathy and talipes equinovarus are present to a lesser or greater extent. If the patient is ambulant,

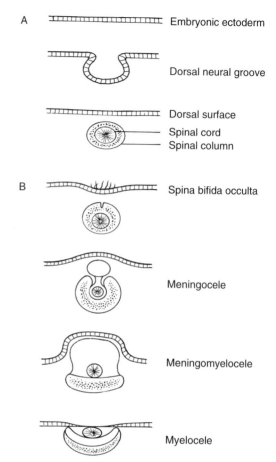

**Figure 17.2 A.** Normal development of the neural tube and spine **B.** Classification of spinal dysraphism.

he/she may have a history of painless trophic ulceration, with or without infection. Fractures

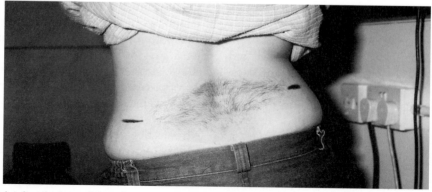

**Figure 17.3** Hair tuft at the base of the spine seen with spina bifida occulta.

of limb bones of which the patient is unaware may occur, due to the combined effects of neuropathy and osteoporosis (Case history 17.8). Non-ambulant patients can suffer severe pressure sores. Spina bifida occulta can present with severe pes cavus or talipes equinovarus with varying amounts of sensory or motor dysfunction. Plantar ulceration may complicate the overall picture.

Case history 17.8

**Male, Caucasian aged 22**
Because I was born with spina bifida, my legs are pretty useless. I have to wear these callipers. I can walk with my crutches, so long as its not too far. I'm learning to drive and as soon as I pass my test Motability are going to get me a car. I've broken my legs loads and loads of times. My mum can always spot a fracture. As soon as she sees a swelling she knows what it is, and carts me off to the hospital. One time when I fell over, I looked down and my foot was pointing behind me. It didn't hurt a bit. I had this really wicked ulcer on my heel. It was after one of my many fractures, and I got this huge pressure sore on my heel. In the end they had to do a skin graft to close it up. My mum has to check my feet and legs every day, because she worries that I'll get gangrene or something.

# HANSEN'S DISEASE (LEPROSY)

Hansen's disease is essentially a disease of tropical climes that can cause profound neuropathy, painless ulceration, blindness, destruction of bone and soft tissues and disfigurement of its victims. It is particularly prevalent in the parts of Africa and Asia that lie between the Tropics of Cancer and Capricorn. Of the 15 million estimated cases world wide, 10 million occur in Asia. Cases that occur in the United Kingdom have usually been contracted abroad. It is a contagious disease and thought to be transmitted via droplet infection.

The infecting organism is *Mycobacterium leprae*. Mycobacteria are acid-fast bacilli which grow extremely slowly within cells, causing a granulomatous reaction in the host. They can multiply within phagocytic cells, resisting intracellular enzymic breakdown, and thus largely resist normal cellular defence mechanisms. *M. leprae* cannot be cultured in vitro.

Following infection, the progress of the disease depends on the gender of the host (males in India are twice as susceptible as females), a genetic susceptibility to the infection and the immunological response of the individual to the mycobacterium. Some subjects show only mild symptoms such as one or more patches of skin hypopigmentation, with erythema but without loss of sensation. Others are severely disabled and disfigured by the disease process. The infecting organism seems to thrive best, and thereby demonstrate the pathology, in the cooler areas of the body, the face and limbs. The greatest effects of the disease process manifest at the extremities—the feet, hands and nose.

In tuberculoid leprosy, in the individual with a good immune response, the disease is localised primarily to the skin. The characteristic lesion is a hypopigmented, anaesthetic (unless on the face) patch of skin, which shows thickened, clearly demarcated edges and central atrophy. The skin of the face, gluteal areas, feet and hands are most commonly affected. The nerve that subserves the area of affected skin can become thickened, palpable and tender. If the nerve has a motor component, subserved muscles will show marked atrophy. Sometimes the skin and nerve lesions may heal spontaneously.

Lepromatous leprosy shows a body-wide distribution. This form of Hansen's disease affects individuals with impaired cell-mediated immunity, such as the malnourished, immunosuppressed, diabetics and AIDS victims. Any organ can be involved in the disease process, but the most obvious effects occur in skin, peripheral superficial tissues and nerves (although nerve involvement may be less pronounced than in the tuberculoid form). At the very early stage patients develop peripheral oedema and rhinitis. Later, skin lesions (macules, papules, nodules or plaques) appear, mainly on the face, gluteal region and limbs. Thickening of the ear lobes and facial skin with thinning of the lateral margins of the eyebrows is noted, described as 'leonine facies'. Generalised infiltration and oedema of the mucous membranes cause exacer-

**Table 17.16** Comparison of the two types of leprosy

| Tuberculoid | Lepromatous |
|---|---|
| Localised | Generalised |
| Good immune responses | Poor immune responses |
| Hypopigmented patches of thickened skin with clear edges (lupus vulgaris) | Peripheral oedema |
| Areas of anaesthesia (but not on face) | Glove and stocking anaesthesia and nerve palsies |
| Nerves to affected areas are thickened and palpable | Inflammation and collapse of nasal septum |
| Severe motor loss | Macules, papules and nodules found anywhere but especially the face |
| Trophic ulceration | Trophic ulceration |
| | Bones of the foot undergo osteoporosis, atrophy and destruction |

bation of rhinitis, leading to laryngitis and hoarseness. The nasal septum may perforate, with collapse and ultimate erosion of the soft tissues of the nose. 'Glove and stocking' anaesthesia, nerve palsies, gynaecomastia and testicular atrophy develop late in the disease. Bones in the fingers and toes undergo neurotrophic atrophy and resorption, leading to characteristic shortening and distortion of the digits (Table 17.16).

The most common presentation of Hansen's disease is a hybrid of tuberculoid and lepromatous forms. Lesions characteristic of this dimorphic presentation of the disease are neither as localised as in tuberculoid nor as widespread as in lepromatous leprosy.

The incubation period of the disease lasts from 2–6 years, but it may be much more or much less. The onset is generally insidious, although an acute presentation may occur in some cases. A tentative diagnosis of Hansen's disease should be made in an individual who presents with hypopigmented skin patches associated with loss of touch and/or temperature sensation and signs of nerve involvement, such as nerve thickening or tenderness, and in whom

acid-fast bacilli have been identified from skin smears. The diagnosis of the disease is made essentially from the clinical presentation and patient history. It is confirmed by growing the organisms in the foot pads of mice. Host resistance can be measured by the lepromin test.

Hansen's disease is still seen in the UK. Quite devastating disfigurement can occur, particularly from the lepromatous form of the disease, where hands, feet or facial features can be eroded (Case history 17.9). A profound sensory neuropathy, analogous to that seen in diabetes mellitus, causes the sufferer to develop trophic ulceration and bone infection, as well as gross distortion of the foot.

---

Case history 17.9

**Male, Asian aged 48**
I've had Hansen's for several years now. It started as a little patch of pale skin on my wrist. I was living in this country at the time. Some of the poor lepers you see at home are really in a bad way with it. I'm lucky. I notice that my feet are going a bit numb. My fingernails and toenails are very thick and look shorter than they used to. My hands are rather clumsy, It's hard to do up buttons and tie bows. The problem is the name of the disease. 'Leper' has such a stigma to it. And some of the cases you see at the hospital clinic are so badly affected. Some of them seem to have hardly any feet or hands. One chap was telling me he was a professional tap dancer, and his feet were size nines. I'd guess his feet are only about six inches long now. He had to spend months in the hospital as they were trying to get his foot ulcers to heel.

---

# AGE

An increasingly elderly population is a feature of the Western world in the 20th century, and will continue to be so into the next millennium, as the 'baby boomers' of the 1940s reach retirement age. Currently, almost one in five of the population is aged over 65 years and one in 17 is over 75 years. The elderly are heavy users of medical, support and care resources. Care of the elderly accounts for almost two-thirds of the health and social services budgets, one in four of hospital admissions and half of hospital bed occupancies.

The elderly form a large part of the client base for Health Service foot care. They form a group that statistically is in greater need of support services, as the typical elderly person is an old lady living alone in poor quality housing, with very little social and family contact, in poor general health and unable to get out and about (Case history 17.10).

---

**Case history 17.10**

**Female, Caucasian aged 87**
My only daughter is in New Zealand. She phones me every Christmas Day. I haven't met her hubby, as they got married after she went out there. She's a grandmother herself now. My neighbours aren't what you could call friendly. We moved in here in 1930 when we first got married. Of course he's passed on now, my husband. Things were not so bad when I could get about a bit, but since I had the stroke, I'm more or less stuck in this chair. The council sends in people to get me up and put me back to bed, and someone else to do my dinner—only out of the freezer though. The problem is, you're always waiting for someone to do things for you. There's not much I can do for myself. Heaven knows what the upstairs of the house is like, it must be 10 years or more since anyone's slept up there. The District Nurse comes in every week to do my leg ulcer. These pads they give you are a godsend. I'm on extra water pills now.

---

Specific health problems of the elderly, which include hypothermia, accidents, urinary incontinence, malnutrition and mental disorders, can result in problems in the foot and lower limb (Table 17.17). Other diseases, such as CVA, transient ischaemic attacks (TIAs), MI, arteriosclerosis, atheroma and diabetes mellitus show an increased incidence with ageing and thus are more often encountered within the elderly population, increasing the number of 'at risk' subjects in this client group.

The process of ageing is intimately associated with senescence. Senescence is the decline in physical and mental functions which, together with the impairment of social adaptation, so typically characterise old age. There are anatomical changes in organs and physiological alterations that lead to reduction in nerve conduction velocity, reduced cardiac output, decreased renal perfusion, poor oxygen uptake and poor breathing capacity. Collagen becomes more rigid and less elastic, with resultant stiffening of joints, exacerbation of deformity and reduction in movement potential. The special senses deteriorate, leading to poor vision and loss of hearing. Neurotransmission in the brain is compromised, leading to Parkinsonism and Alzheimer's disease. Intellectual performance tails off, memory fails, confusion reigns and the subject can finally no longer cope with the tasks of normal living. In contrast, senility refers to the specific disabilities that arise in the elderly in response to disease or trauma.

The older an organism is, the greater the risk of impairment, disease and death. Being elderly means that the patient will not be able to overcome disease easily. The constitutional deterioration renders the elderly person prone to develop pneumonia, particularly if he/she has been bed-bound or has concomitant decreased cardiac or pulmonary function, or chest infection. Pneumonia becomes a common, and fatal, complication following CVA or hip fracture. The elderly become increasingly prone to the effects of generalised arteriosclerosis. As this frequently affects renal, coronary and cerebral vessels, increasingly peripheral and pulmonary oedema will result, exacerbating the tendency to develop pneumonia when other illnesses cause physical deterioration.

The likelihood of tissue breakdown in the foot and lower limb is increased by ischaemia and peripheral oedema. Healing is impaired by poor dietary intake, avitaminosis and poor tissue perfusion. Elderly people are more prone to develop neoplastic disease, as the incidence of neoplasm rises with ageing. The disease state in the elderly is predominantly one of multisystem pathologies, many of which will be chronic degenerative processes that impair healing and general wellbeing.

Typically, the elderly, frail patient presents as suffering from a group of chronic disease states, for which she takes a large number of medications, any or all of which will render her as 'at risk'. Therefore, the assessment of the elderly patient must consider not only the immediate

**Table 17.17**  Problems which may affect the elderly

| Problem | Effects |
|---|---|
| *Hypothermia* | |
| Sign | Patient confused, pale and cold to the touch |
| Causes | Defective thermoregulatory mechanisms and low environmental temperatures |
| Exacerbated by | General infirmity, the effects of stroke, infections and endocrine dysfunction |
| Outcome | Can be fatal, especially in the debilitated patient |
| *Accidents* | |
| Common presentation | Fractured neck of femur and Colles fracture following a fall |
| Predisposing factors | Transient cerebral ischaemia; giddiness due to hypertension, cardiac insufficiency or drug therapy; loss of balance, due to Ménière's disease and other labyrinthine disorders; poor vision, due to cataracts |
| Outcome | 25% mortality following a broken hip; proneness to pneumonia and other opportunistic infections |
| Implications for aftercare | Mobilisation problematic; high demands on domiciliary support services |
| *Urinary incontinence* | |
| Causes | Mechanical obstruction to the neck of the bladder (prostatism), chronic urinary tract infections, mental confusion |
| Exacerbated by | Therapeutic agents such as diuretics given for hypertension or to reduce peripheral oedema |
| Outcome | Embarrassment and distress, profound maceration of skin of feet where slippers are constantly wet |
| *Malnutrition* | |
| Common presentation | General debilitation, poor healing |
| Causes | Poor diet, poor appetite, intestinal disease |
| Outcome | Depressed physical and mental condition; proneness and lack of resistance to disease |
| *Mental disorders* | |
| Common presentation | Memory deterioration, abnormal behaviours, intellectual impairment |
| Classified as | Intrinsic dementia, of vascular/atherosclerotic or non-vascular/senile aetiology *or* extrinsic confusional state, due to endocrine, metabolic, infectious, cardiac failure, respiratory disease or drug-based aetiology |
| Outcome | Need for support and daily cares, inability to maintain regular drug-based therapy programme |

presenting foot or limb problem, but also the overall health status of the patient and its effect on the foot and limb.

Any substance that is used for its therapeutic effects may also produce unwanted toxic or adverse effects. These unwanted effects may occur in up to 20% of an elderly population. Types of unwanted drug reaction include exaggerated but otherwise normal pharmacological actions or aberrant effects. The mechanisms that underlie many drug reactions, such as hepatotoxicity or analgesic neuropathy, are not clear.

**Table 17.18**   Parenteral medications that indicate risk

| Drug | Effects |
|---|---|
| *Steroids* | Given for the treatment of a wide variety of diseases, including RA, polymyalgica rheumatica, autoimmune and hypersensitivity diseases and asthma. Examples include prednisolone. Long-term therapy can cause side-effects that mimic Cushing's syndrome. The dose of steroids should be increased (doubled), in times of serious current illness (such as fever), stress, accident or surgery |
| Side-effects | The current dose should never be stopped suddenly as the adrenal cortex will not be able to respond to the increased demands made on it, and the patient could become seriously ill, suffering in effect an Addisonian crisis (with nausea, vomiting, dangerously low blood pressures, reduced blood glucose and sodium levels, and raised potassium levels) |
| *Anticoagulants* | Given to prevent recurrence of thrombosis. Examples include warfarin and aspirin (though these should never be given together) |
| Side-effects | Blood clotting is reduced, so patients bleed excessively if the skin is cut or injured |
| *Non-steroidal anti-inflammatory drugs (NSAIDs)* | Given to reduce inflammation, such as in prolonged pain states and arthritis. Examples include aspirin and ibuprofen |
| Side-effects | Patients tend to develop gastric irritation and ulceration, leading to chronic anaemia. Fluid retention |
| *Beta-blockers* | Given to regulate the heart. Examples include propranolol |
| Side-effects | Can cause bronchoconstriction, breathlessness and Raynaud's phenomenon |
| *Painkillers* | Given to control chronic pain states. Examples include aspirin, ibuprofen, paracetamol and phenacetin |
| Side-effects | Paracetamol can cause liver damage when dose exceeds $8 \times 500$ mg in 24 hours. Thus, subjects who have taken high doses of paracetamol long term may not be suitable for local analgesia. Phenacetin and other NSAIDs can cause kidney damage, resulting in peripheral oedema that is non-responsive to diuretics |

# MEDICATION

Certain parenteral therapeutic regimes indicate that the patient is actually or potentially 'at risk'. These include steroid therapy, anti-cancer drugs, methotrexate, anticoagulants, aspirin and beta-blockers (Table 17.18). The effects of the prolonged use of steroids are outlined in Table 17.19.

# SUMMARY

This chapter has described a range of conditions which cause a patient to be classified as 'at risk'. Local problems such as corns, callus and loss of depth and resilience of the fibro-fatty padding will accelerate the effects of these conditions. Infections that are normally innocuous, such as tinea and verruca pedis, can become severe in the debilitated or immunocompromised. Normal foot and limb biomechanics can become severely compromised in subjects with connective tissue diseases or neurological deficit, so that the patient is more liable to suffer tissue breakdown. Compromised blood flow or limb drainage will

**Table 17.19** The effects of prolonged steroid use

- Increase in blood pressure
- Peptic ulceration
- Fluid retention leading to oedema
- Urination pattern upset (polyuria and nocturia)
- Insomnia and euphoria or depression
- Weight gain
- Exacerbation of diabetes; symptoms of diabetes
- Menorrhoea
- Osteoporosis and fractures
- Muscle wasting and weakness
- Thinning of skin and ulceration
- Skin striae and easy bruising
- Cataracts
- Proneness to infection—septicaemia, TB, fungal infections
- Inflammatory response dampened

interrupt normal healing processes and render the subject likely to develop ulcers and/or persistent oedema.

The net outcome of these pathological processes is to create tissues in the foot and limb which are not functional or viable. Therefore, patients who present with any of these problems must receive all the care and support that is available, in order to maintain the best possible level of foot and limb health.

## REFERENCES

Amiel S A 1993 Editorial: diabetic control and complications. British Medical Journal 307: 881

Boulton A, Scarpello J H, Weard J D 1982 Venous oxygenation in the diabetic neuropathic foot: evidence of arterio-venous shunting. Diabetologica 22: 6

Delbridge L, Appleberg M, Reeves T 1983 Factors associated with the development of foot lesions in the diabetic. Surgery 93: 71

Delbridge L, Ctercteko G, Fowler C et al 1985 The aetiology of diabetic neuropathic foot ulceration. British Journal of Surgery 72: 1

Delbridge L, Perry P et al 1988 Limited mobility in the diabetic foot: relationship to neuropathic ulceration. Diabetic Medicine 5: 333–337

Edmonds M E 1984 Infection in the diabetic foot. Practical Diabetes 1: 2

Edmonds M E et al 1982 Diabetes and neuropathy. British Medical Journal 284: 928

Edmonds M E, Blundell M P et al 1986 Improved survival of the diabetic foot. Quarterly Journal of Medicine: 60–232; 763–772

Jones E W, Edwards R, Finch R, Jeffcoate W 1985 A microbiological study of diabetic foot lesions. Diabetic

Medicine 2: 213–215

Knighton D R, Fiegel V D et al 1986 Classification and treatment of non-healing wounds. 106th meeting of the American Surgical Association

Mueller M J, Minor S D, Diamond J E, Blair V P 1990 The relationship of forefoot deformity to ulcer location. Physical Therapy 70: 6

Nelson J 1992 The vascular history and physical examination. Clinics in Podiatric Medicine and Surgery 9(1): 1–17

Renton P 1993 Personal communication

Sibbaud R G, Schacter R K 1984 The skin and diabetes mellitus. International Journal of Dermatology 23: 567

Van der Heijde et al 1992 Validity of single variables and composite indices for measuring disease activity in rheumatoid arthritis. Annals of Rheumatic Disease 51(2): 177–181

Wheat J L, Allen S D, Henry M et al 1986 Diabetic foot infections: bacteriologic analysis. Archives of Internal Medicine 146: 1935

Young J 1991 The swollen leg: clinical signs and differential diagnosis. Cardiology Clinics 9: 30

## FURTHER READING

Davies D (ed) 1986 Textbook of adverse drug reactions. Oxford University Press, Oxford

Donaldson R J, Donaldson L J 1988 Elderly people in Essential Community Medicine. MTP Press, Lancaster

Farthing C F, Brown S E, Staughton R C 1988 A colour atlas of AIDS and HIV disease. Wolfe Medical Publications, London

Frykberg R (ed) 1991 The high risk foot in diabetes mellitus. Churchill Livingstone, Edinburgh

Klenerman L 1991 The foot and its disorders. Blackwell, Oxford

Manson-Bahr P E, Bell D 1987 Manson's tropical diseases, 19th edn. Baillière Tindall, London

Melzack R 1988 The challenge of pain. Penguin Books, Harmondsworth

Rook A, Wilkinson D, Ebling F J 1986 Textbook of dermatology, 3rd edn. Blackwell, Oxford

# Index